# Manipal Manual of
# Anatomy

## For Allied Health Science Courses

**Third Edition**

# Manipal Manual of
# Anatomy

## For Allied Health Science Courses

**Third Edition**

### Sampath Madhyastha

Director, Postgraduate Studies (Anatomy)
Faculty of Medicine
Kuwait University, Kuwait

*Former* Additional Professor
Department of Anatomy
Kasturba Medical College, Mangalore
Manipal University
India

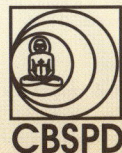

CBSPD

# CBS Publishers & Distributors Pvt Ltd

New Delhi • Bengaluru • Chennai • Kochi • Kolkata • Lucknow • Mumbai
Hyderabad • Jharkhand • Nagpur • Patna • Pune • Uttarakhand

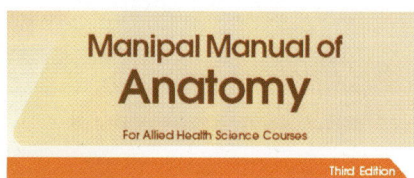

Manipal Manual of
**Anatomy**
For Allied Health Science Courses
Third Edition

ISBN: 978-81-239-2968-2

Copyright © Author and Publisher

**Third Edition: 2016**
  **Reprint: 2017, 2018, 2019, 2020, 2021, 2022, 2023, 2025**
First Edition: 2005
Second Edition: 2007
  Reprint: 2007, 2009, 2010, 2011, 2012, 2014

Published by Satish Kumar Jain and produced by Varun Jain for

**CBS Publishers & Distributors** Pvt Ltd
4819/XI Prahlad Street, 24 Ansari Road, Daryaganj, New Delhi 110 002, India
Ph: 011-23289259, 23266838                    Website: www.cbspd.com
                                              e-mail: delhi@cbspd.com
*Corporate Office:* 204 FIE, Industrial Area, Patparganj, Delhi 110 092
Ph: 011-4934 4934        Fax: 011-4934 4935      e-mail: publishing@cbspd.com; publicity@cbspd.com

**Branches**

• **Bengaluru:** Seema House 2975, 17th Cross, K.R. Road, Banasankari 2nd Stage, Bengaluru 560 070, Karnataka, India
  Ph: +91-80-26771678/79          Fax: +91-80-26771680      e-mail: bangalore@cbspd.com
• **Chennai:** 18/8B, Subbarayan Street, Shenoy Nagar, Chennai 600 030, Tamil Nadu, India
  Ph: +91-44-42032115, 26681266                    e-mail: chennai@cbspd.com
• **Kochi:** 42/1325, 1326, Power House Road, Opp KSEB, Power House, Ernakulam 682 018, Kerala, India
  Ph: +91-484-4059061-65          Fax: +91-484-4059065      e-mail: kochi@cbspd.com
• **Kolkata:** 147, Hind Ceramics Compound, 1st Floor, Nilgunj Road, Belghoria, Kolkata-700056
  West Bengal, India
  Ph: 033-25633055, 033-25633056                   e-mail: kolkata@cbspd.com
• **Lucknow:** Basement, Khushnuma Complex, 7-Meerabai Marg (Behind Jawahar Bhawan), Lucknow 226001, India
  Ph: 0522-4000032                                 e-mail: tiwari.lucknow@cbspd.com
• **Mumbai:** PWD Shed. Gala no. 25/26, Ramchandra Bhatt Marg, Next to JJ Hospital Gate no. 2, Opp. Union Bank of India Noorbaug, Mumbai-400009, Maharashtra, India
  Ph: 022-66661880/89                              e-mail: mumbai@cbspd.com

*Representatives*

• **Hyderabad** 0-9885175004  • **Jharkhand** 0-9811541605  • **Nagpur**      0-8692091830
• **Patna**     0-9334159340  • **Pune**      0-9664372571  • **Uttarakhand** 0-9716462459

*Printed at* Goyal Offset Works Pvt. Ltd., Kundli, Haryana, India

# Preface to the Third Edition

The 2nd edition of Manipal Manual of Anatomy was well accepted by students as well as faculties involved in teaching anatomy to paramedical courses across India. It has been 8 long years since the 2nd edition was released and this is high time for me to look at this manual with new dimension and approach. The first and foremost task was to compile all the guidance and suggestion received from faculties across India. The biggest challenge in writing an anatomy manual for allied health science course (paramedical course) still remains the same as learning objectives for each course is different and more importantly the examination pattern was also different among various health universities. One of the common suggestions I received from the faculties is about the content/information. Many felt that the course content for BSc nursing was too adequate but others felt otherwise. Similar suggestions were brought into notice for the course content of Bachelors of Physiotherapy. Keeping all these suggestions in mind and also carefully evaluating the theory examination papers of various health universities, it decided to make a few changes in the 3rd edition. Information should be sufficient to fulfill the requirements of all paramedical courses offered by all the health universities. The illustration quality has been enhanced with 2 types of illustration. Two-dimensional illustration for understanding the gross anatomy and simple line diagrams which can be reproduced in the exams. At the end an additional chapter named 'Anatomy of certain clinical procedures', which is very much required for all the paramedical students is included. In addition to that a series of sample question papers from various universities were compiled at the end, which would enable the students to prepare for the exams. Clinical emphasis on most relevant areas of human body is included and this would be the highlight of the 3rd edition. The manual has been specially prepared for the students of:

- Physiotherapy
- Occupational therapy
- Nursing
- Speech, language, pathology
- Biotechnology
- Medical laboratory technology
- Bio-medical engineering
- Respiratory therapy technology
- Pharmacy
- Imaging technology
- Nuclear medicine
- Optometry
- Health information science
- Medical transcript

In preparing this manual, it was essential to consider the need of both the students and teachers. With this in mind, the following objectives were formulated

- To provide an accurate and up-to-date text that is visually appealing, interesting, applicable, examination-oriented and readable
- To develop in you a sufficient anatomical vocabulary so that you are conversant with medical terminology
- To identify and clearly state the basic concepts and learning objectives common for all branches of allied health courses
- To provide a correlated and balanced presentation of anatomy at both gross and clinical levels
- To create a book that functions as a solid foundation and information base for students, enabling them to apply the knowledge of anatomy in clinical practice
- To develop an innovative format that encourages the use of the manual not only in the classrooms but also in laboratory as well.

## Text Organization

There are 38 chapters of which 37 chapters are grouped in four sections.

**Section I:** General anatomy
**Section II:** Musculoskeletal system
**Section III:** Organ system
**Section IV:** Nervous system, endocrines and special senses

Sections I and III are common for all the paramedical courses, however sections II and IV are specially designed for BPT and BOT students. Hence the objectives for the remaining paramedical courses were clearly identified before sections II and IV, this would help the students to focus on the required area.

At the end of each section, an exercise section has been formulated which enables students to evaluate themselves by answering objective questions. The model question papers provided at the end will also help the students in preparing for their examinations.

This is another attempt to provide a simple, precise anatomy manual for the students of paramedical courses in one volume. Your suggestions are always welcome.

**Sampath Madhyastha**
madhyast@yahoo.com

# Acknowledgments

My thanks and gratitude to our Chancellor of Manipal University, Dr Ramdas M Pai, who has been conductive for all of my academic accomplishments.

I would like to acknowledge Dr Vinodh Bhat, Vice Chancellor, Manipal University and Dr K Ramnarayan, Vice President, Manipal University for their encouragement.

I wish to acknowledge my teachers, Mr Seetharam Bhat, Dr SN Somayaji and Dr K Ramachandra Bhat for their constant encouragement and support.

I would like to thank my colleague Dr Prameela MD, Associate Professor for her meticulous work in revising the manual.

My sincere gratitude to Mr Satish Kumar Jain, CMD, CBS Publishers & Distributors, New Delhi, Mr YN Arjuna, Sr Vice President—Publishing, Editorial and Publicity, CBSPD, New Delhi and Mr Deepak Rao, Vice President, CBSPD, Bengaluru.

I pay my sincere thanks to my mother Mrs Kamalakshi, wife Prashanthi Madhyastha, my in laws, Professor BS Ramananda and Mrs Rajani Ramananda. Without their support this would not have been possible. Last but not least thanks to my son Pradhan who is my strength and gives all the energy to take up new assignments and tasks every time. This book is dedicated to him.

**Sampath Madhyastha**

# Contents

## Section II  MUSCULOSKELETAL SYSTEM

## Section III  ORGAN SYSTEM

## Section IV   NERVOUS SYSTEM ENDOCRINES AND SPECIAL SENSES

# Section

## I

# General Anatomy

# Introduction to Anatomy

**1**

Human anatomy is the science concerned with the structure of the human body. The term 'anatomy' is derived from the Greek word meaning "to cut up". The dissection of cadavers (dead bodies) has served as the basis for understanding the structure and function of the human body. Most of the terms that form the language of anatomy are of Greek or Latin derivations. In the past, human anatomy was an academic, descriptive science primarily concerned with identifying and naming body structures. Although dissection and description form the basis of anatomy, the importance of human anatomy is in its functional approach and clinical applications. **Human anatomy is a practical, applied science that provides the foundation for understanding physical performance and body health.**

## SUBDIVISION OF HUMAN ANATOMY

1. *Gross anatomy:* It is the study of the structures of a cadaver that can be observed with naked eye. Stringent courses in gross anatomy in professional schools provide the foundation for the students of entire medical or paramedical teaching.

2. *Surface anatomy:* It deals with surface features of the body that can be observed or palpated (felt firmly).

3. *Microscopic anatomy:* It deals with the study of structures with the help of a microscope. The **cytology** (study of cells) and **histology** (study of tissues) are specialities of anatomy that have provided additional understanding of the structure and function of the human body. Certain cells/tissues can be stained by certain dyes (vital stains) which colour selectively the elements in the cell.

4. *Radiological anatomy:* It involves the study of anatomical structures as they are visualised by X-rays,

ultrasound scans or other specialised procedures (CT/MRI scans) performed on living body. In contrast X-ray radio-opaque substances can be ingested or injected for visualizing internal organs. Angiography involves making a radiograph after injecting a dye into the bloodstream. Since radiographs compress the body image with an overlap of organs and tissues, diagnosis is often difficult.

The computerised axial tomography technique (CT or CAT scans) has greatly enhanced the versatility of X-rays, using a computer to display a cross-sectional image similar to that which could only be obtained in an actual section through the body. Magnetic resonance imaging (MRI) and positron emission tomography (PET) are the other techniques used to observe the organ structures of the body.

5. *Surgical anatomy:* It studies anatomical landmarks important for surgical procedures.

6. *Developmental anatomy (embryology):* It examines the changes in form that occur during the period between conception and physical maturity. It is important in medicine because many structural abnormalities can result from errors in development.

## ANATOMICAL TERMS

Though we are familiar with the common terms of many parts and regions of our body, it is essential that we use internationally accepted anatomical names/terms.

## BODY POSITIONS

The following are the positions/postures of the human body during clinical examination/cadaver dissection/anatomical description.

*Anatomical position:* All descriptions of the human body are based on the assumption that the person is:
* Standing erect
* Eyes look straight to the front
* Upper limbs are by the sides of the body, palms facing forward
* Lower limbs are together and digits (toes) pointing forward

*Supine position:* Lying down on back with the face directed upwards.

*Prone position:* Lying down facing the ground.

*Lithotomy position:* Lying down on your back with fully flexed (knees pointing to the roof) and abducted (widely spread) thighs.

## ANATOMICAL PLANES (Fig. 1.1)

These are imaginary planes (lines) that cut through the body when it is in anatomical position. They help in identifying and studying the relative position of a structure/organs in relation to one another. They further help us in making precise surgical incisions.

* *Median plane:* Imaginary vertical plane passing longitudinally through the middle of the body from front to back, dividing it into two equal halves.
* *Sagittal planes:* Imaginary vertical planes passing through the body parallel to the median plane.
* *Coronal planes:* These are imaginary planes passing through the body at right angle to the median plane,

dividing it into anterior (front) and posterior (back) portions.

* *Horizontal planes:* These are imaginary planes passing through the body at right angles to both the median and coronal planes. This plane is parallel to the ground. This plane divides the body into superior (upper) and inferior (lower) parts.
* *Oblique planes:* Any plane other than those mentioned above, they slant or deviate from the other planes.

## TERMS OF RELATIONSHIP (Fig.1.2)

| | | |
|---|---|---|
| Superior (cranial) | – | Nearer to the head |
| Inferior (caudal) | – | Nearer to the feet |
| Anterior (ventral) | – | Nearer to the front |
| Posterior (dorsal) | – | Nearer to the back |
| Medial | – | Nearer to the median plane |
| Lateral | – | Farther from the median plane |

## TERMS OF COMPARISON

Compare the relative positions of two structures with each other.

| | | |
|---|---|---|
| Proximal | – | Nearer to the trunk/point of origin |
| Distal | – | Away from the trunk/point of origin |
| Superficial | – | Nearer to/on the surface |
| Deep | – | Farther from the surface |
| External | – | Towards/on the exterior |
| Internal | – | Towards/in the interior |
| Central | – | Nearer to/towards the center |

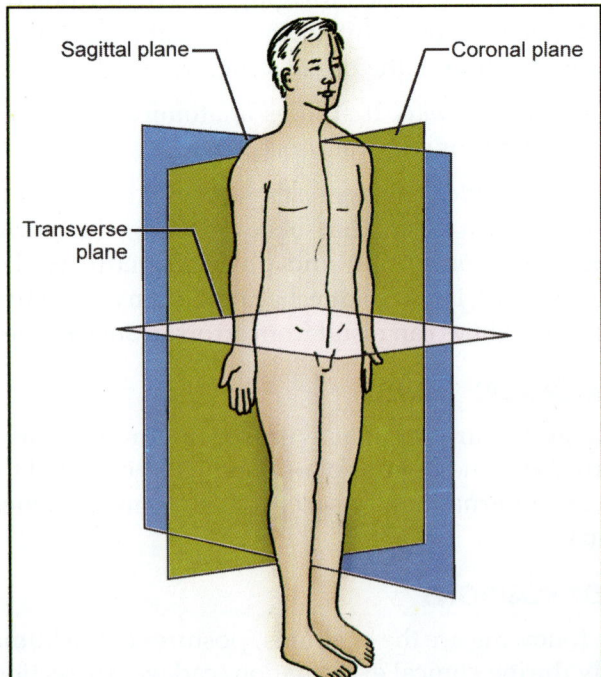

**Fig. 1.1:** Anatomical planes

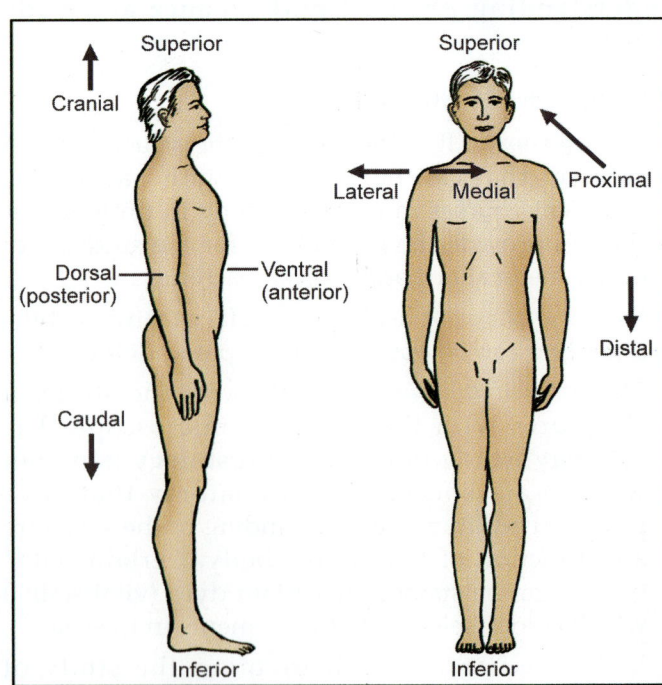

**Fig. 1.2:** Anatomical directions

1

| Peripheral | – | Away from the center |
|---|---|---|
| Parietal | – | External wall of a body cavity |
| Visceral | – | Pertaining to covering of an organ |
| Ipsilateral | – | On the same side of the body |
| Contralateral | – | On the opposite side of the body |
| Evagination | – | Outward bulging of the wall of a cavity |
| Invagination | – | Inward bulging of the wall of a cavity |

## TERMS DESCRIBING MOVEMENTS AT JOINTS

- *Flexion*: Bending/making a decreasing angle between the bones or parts of the body. In this movement there is an approximation of flexor surfaces.
- *Extension*: Straightening of a bent part or making an increasing the angle between bones of the body. In this movement there is an approximation of extensor surfaces.
- *Abduction*: Moving away from the median plane.
- *Adduction*: Moving toward the median plane.
- *Rotation*: Moving around the long axis.
- *Medial rotation*: Inward rotation.
- *Lateral rotation*: Outward rotation.
- *Circumduction*: Circular movement combining flexion, abduction, extension and adduction.
- *Eversion*: Raising the lateral border of the foot.
- *Inversion*: Raising the medial border of the sole of the foot.
- *Pronation*: Rotation of the forearm so that the palm is turned backwards.
- *Supination*: Rotation of the forearm so that the palm is turned forwards.
- *Protrusion*: Moving anteriorly (forward).
- *Retraction*: Moving posteriorly (backward).

## TERMS RELATED TO MUSCLE

- *Origin* is the end of the muscle, which is fixed and shows relatively less movement during contraction.
- *Insertion* is the end of the muscle, which shows relatively more movement during contraction. The origin of the muscle is considered as proximal attachment and insertion as distal attachment.
- *Belly*: The fleshy and contractile part of a muscle.
- *Tendon*: The fibrous, non-contractile part of the muscle.
- *Aponeurosis*: The flattened, sheet of dense connective tissue, which attaches the muscles to the bone/skin.
- *Raphe*: A fibrous band made up of interdigitating aponeurotic fibers of the muscles.

## TERMS RELATED TO VESSELS

- *Arteries*: Carry oxygenated blood away from the heart.
- *Veins*: Carry deoxygenated blood towards the heart.
- *Arterioles*: These are the smallest branches of the arteries within the tissue (with diameter 100 mm or less).
- *Venules*: These are the minute vessels in the tissue, which join to form vein.
- *Capillaries*: Microscopic vessels connecting arterioles to venules.

The umbilical artery and pulmonary artery are exceptions, which carry the deoxygenated blood. The pulmonary vein and umbilical vein carry oxygenated blood.

## BODY ORGANIZATION

Study of the human body will begin with an overview of microscopic anatomy and then proceed to the gross and macroscopic anatomy of each organ system. When considering events from the microscopic to macroscopic scales we are examining several interdependent levels of organization.

To begin with chemical or molecular level of organization. The human body consists of over a dozen different elements, but four of them (hydrogen, oxygen, carbon and nitrogen) account for more than 99% of the total number of atoms.

At the chemical level, atoms interact to form compounds with distinctive properties.

1. *Cellular level*: The cell is the basic structural and functional component of life. It is at the cellular level that such vital functions of life as metabolism, growth, irritability and adaptability, repair and reproduction are carried out.

   Cells are composed of minute particles called atoms, which are bound together to form larger particles called molecules. Certain molecules are arranged into small functional sources called organelles. Each organelle carries out a specific function within the cell. The nucleus, mitochondria and endoplasmic reticulum are organelles.

   The human body contains many distinct kinds of cells; each specialised to perform specific function, e.g. muscle cells, bone cells, fat cells, blood cells and nerve cells.

2. *Tissue level*: Tissues are groups of similar cells that perform specific functions. An example of a

tissue is the muscle within the heart, which functions to contract and pump the blood through the body.

3. *Organ level*: An organ is an aggregate of two or more tissues, integrated to perform a particular function. Each organ usually has one or more primary tissues and several secondary tissues. In the stomach, for example, the inside lining epithelium is considered as primary tissue because it performs the basic functions like secretion and absorption. Secondary tissue of the stomach is the supporting connective tissue with vascular, nervous and muscular tissues.

4. *System level*: The system of the body constitutes the next level of structural organization. A body system consists of various organs that have similar or related functions. Examples of systems are the circulatory system, endocrine system, etc. Certain organs may serve several systems. All the systems of the body are interrelated and function together, constituting the total organism.

## BODY REGIONS (Fig. 1.3)

The human body is divided into several regions that can be identified on the surface of the body. Learning the terminology used with reference to these regions now will make it easier to learn the names of underlying structures later. The major body regions are the head, neck, trunk, upper extremity and lower extremity. The trunk is frequently divided into the thorax and abdomen.

### Head

The head is divided into a facial region (which includes the eyes, nose and mouth) and a cranial region (which covers and supports the brain).

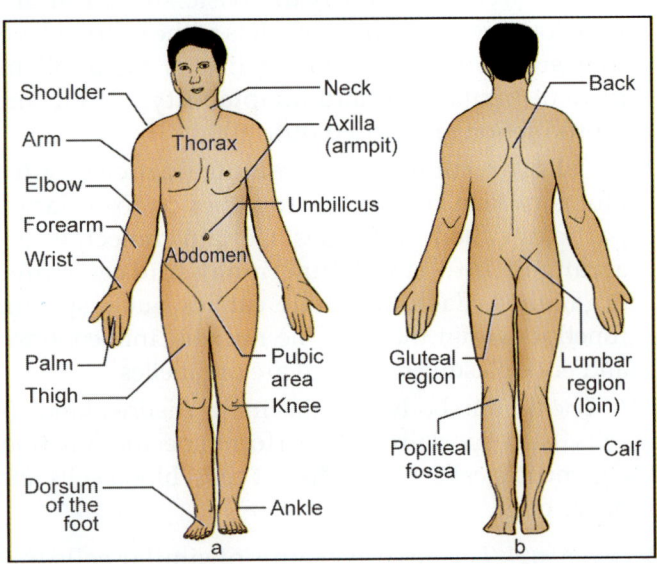

**Fig. 1.3:** Body regions: (a) Anterior view; (b) Posterior view

### Neck

The neck referred to as the cervix or cervical region, supports the head and permits it to move.

### Trunk

#### Thorax

The thoracic region is commonly referred as chest. The mammary region of the thorax surrounds the nipple and in sexually mature females is enlarged as the breast. Between the mammary regions is the sternal region. The armpit is called axilla. The vertebral region, following the vertebral column extends the length of the back.

#### Abdomen

The abdomen is located below the thorax. The umbilicus is a landmark on the front and center of the abdomen. The abdomen has been divided into nine regions in order to describe the location of internal organs.

The pelvic region forms the lower portion of the abdomen. The perineum is the region containing the external sex organs and the anal opening. The center of the backside of the abdomen is called lumbar region. The sacral region is located further down at the point where the vertebral column terminates. The large hip muscles form the buttock or gluteal region.

### Upper Extremity (Upper Limb)

The upper limb is anatomically divided into the shoulder, brachium (arm), antebrachium (forearm) and hand. The front of the hand is referred to as the palm and back of the hand is called dorsum. The fingers are referred as digits.

### Lower Extremity (Lower Limb)

The lower limb consists of thigh, knee, leg and foot. The sole of the foot is referred to as the plantar surface. The dorsum of the foot is the top surface.

### BODY CAVITIES (Fig. 1.4)

Body cavities are confined spaces within the body. During development, the cavity within the trunk is called coelom, which is lined with a membrane that secretes a lubricating fluid. The coelom is portioned by the muscular diaphragm into an upper thoracic cavity, or chest cavity, and a lower abdominopelvic cavity. Organs within the coelom are collectively called viscera. The thoracic cavity is further divided into two pleural cavities by invagination of lungs on either side and a pericardial cavity in the middle by the heart. Similarly

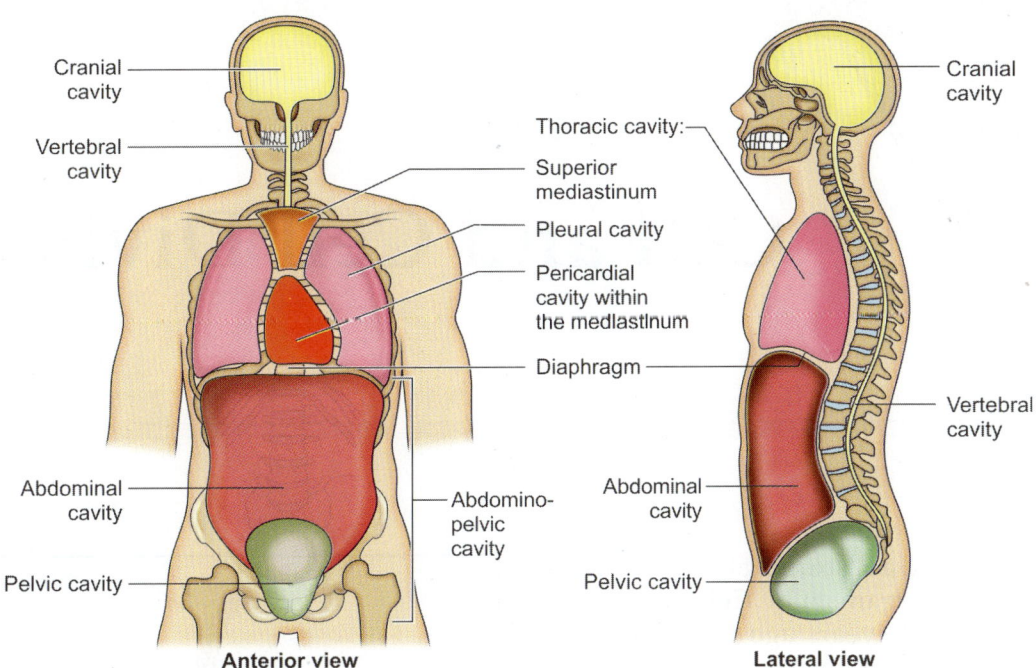

Cranial cavity

Vertebral cavity

Thoracic cavity:

Superior mediastinum

Pleural cavity

Pericardial cavity within the medlastlnum

Diaphragm

Abdominal cavity

Abdomino-pelvic cavity

Pelvic cavity

Cranial cavity

Vertebral cavity

Abdominal cavity

Pelvic cavity

**Anterior view**          **Lateral view**

**Fig. 1.4:** Body cavity

with invagination of some abdominal organs, the abdominal cavity is referred as peritoneal cavity. In addition to these large cavities, there are several small cavities like oral or buccal cavity, middle ear cavities and nasal cavities. The cranial cavity contains brain and its coverings.

# Cell and Cell Division

## 2

The cell can be defined as "structural and functional unit of all living organisms". Cells were first observed more than 300 years ago by the English Scientist Robert Hooke. With the advancement of microscope, a lot of information were obtained. The cell theory was unified in 1838 and 1839 by two German biologists, Matthias Scleiden and Theodor Schwann. Their work laid the foundation for a new science called cytology, which is concerned with the structure and function of cells.

Knowledge of the cellular level of organization is important for understanding the basic body processes of cellular respiration, protein synthesis, mitosis, and meiosis. An understanding of cellular structure gives meaning to the concept of tissue, organs, and system levels of functional body organization. Furthermore, many body dysfunctions and diseases originate in the cells. Although cellular structure and function have been investigated for many years, we still have much to learn about cells. The etiologies, or causes, of a number of complex diseases are yet unknown. Scientists are seeking why and how the body ages. The answer will come only through a better understanding of cellular structure and function.

Some of the cells and their specific functions are listed below:
1. Movement—muscle cell
2. Conductivity—nerve cell
3. Synthesis of enzymes—pancreatic acinar cells
4. Secretion of mucous—mucous gland cells
5. Secretion of steroids—cells of adrenals, testes, ovaries
6. Ion transport—cells of kidney, ducts of salivary glands
7. Intracellular digestion—macrophages
8. Transformation of physical and chemical stimuli into nervous impulses—receptors

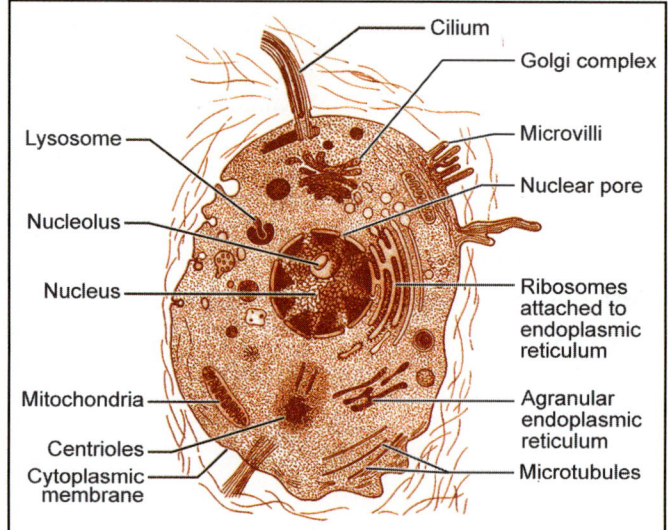

**Fig. 2.1:** Cell and its constituents

9. Metabolic absorption—cells of intestine.

Each cell has a cell membrane enclosing cytoplasm with nucleus (Fig. 2.1).

## CELL MEMBRANE/PLASMA MEMBRANE/PLASMALEMMA

The outermost part of the cell is covered by a membrane called the cell membrane/plasma membrane/plasmalemma. It separates the cell from the "extracellular substance" (the material which lies between the cells). It is extremely thin and delicate membrane and its thickness ranges from 6 to 10 nm.

## STRUCTURE OF CELL MEMBRANE

Under the electron microscope the membrane appears as a trilaminar structure, with outer and inner dark layer and a light layer in between them. Chemically they are made up of phospholipid and protein molecules, externally covered by a coat of glycocalyx (sugar + protein). Each phospholipid molecule has a 'head' and a 'tail'. The head contains phosphate and is water soluble (hydrophilic). The tail consists of two fatty acids and is water insoluble (hydrophobic). Phospholipid molecules line in two rows with their heads lying on the surface and tails pointing at each other (Fig. 2.2).

The permeability of a membrane is a property that determines its effectiveness as a barrier. When substances cannot cross a membrane, it is described as impermeable. When substances can cross the membrane without difficulty, the membrane is freely permeable. Most of the cell membranes fall in-between and are thus said to be selectively permeable. Passage across the membrane may be passive or active. In a passive process ions or molecules move across the cell membrane without any energy expenditure by the cell, e.g. diffusion, osmosis and filtration. The active transport across the cell membrane requires energy in the form of ATP, e.g. pinocytosis, phagocytosis.

In many places, the cell membrane becomes modified to form microvilli and cilia for special functions.

- The *microvilli* increase the surface area for absorption, e.g. cells lining the intestine.
- The *cilia* propel the fluid/particles in one direction. They are motile and larger than microvilli, e.g. cells lining the nasal cavity.
- *Flagellum* is a single hair-like projection from the cell surface. It is present in sperms and is commonly called sperm tail.

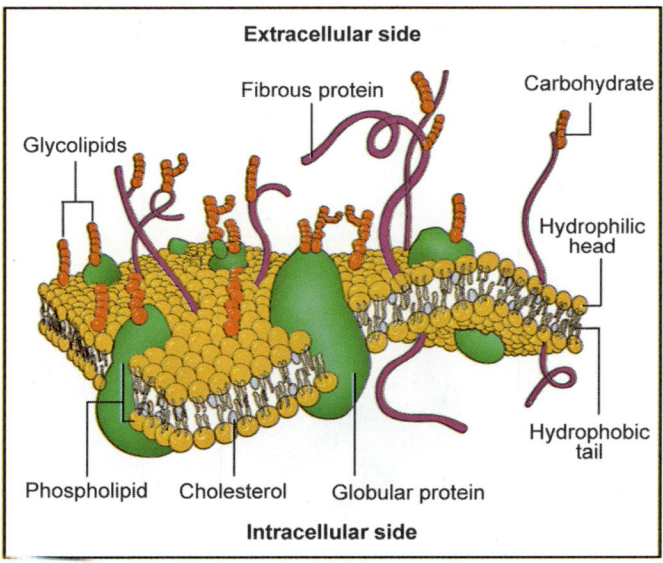

**Fig. 2.2:** Structure of plasma membrane

## CELL JUNCTIONS OR CONTACTS

In tissues like epithelium where cells are closely packed, the following types of cell contacts can occur:
  i. Zonula occludens
 ii. Zonula adherens
iii. Desmosome
iv. Gap junction

### Functions of cell membrane are:

- Maintaining the integrity of the cell
- The semipermeable membrane is involved in endocytosis (phagocytosis) and exocytosis
- Cell membrane bears receptors for specific hormones, enzymes and neurotransmitters
- They serve as identification tags.

## CYTOPLASM

The *cytoplasm* contains the structures concerned with the metabolic processes and products of metabolism. The cytoplasmic bodies are mainly of two types:
1. Organelles (living structural component)
2. Inclusions (non-living accumulations of cell products)

The *cytoplasmic organelles* are ribosomes, endoplasmic reticulum, Golgi apparatus, centrosomes, mitochondria, lysosomes, microbodies (peroxisomes), microtubules and microfilaments. The chemical composition of the cytoplasm is water (75%), proteins (10–20%), lipids (2–3%), carbohydrates (1%), sodium, potassium, magnesium, phosphates, bicarbonates and vitamins.

The cytoplasmic inclusions are classified into organic and inorganic compounds. Organic compounds contain carbon and are formed by living organisms. Proteins, carbohydrates (glycogen granules) and lipids are organic compounds. Inorganic compounds generally lack carbon and are not formed by living organisms. Water and electrolytes (acids, bases and salts) are examples of inorganic compounds.

## ENDOPLASMIC RETICULUM (ER)

Endoplasmic reticulum is a network of intracellular membranes. It can be present in the form of hollow tubes, flattened sheets or round chambers. It synthesises proteins, carbohydrates and lipids. It is also involved in its storage and transport. There are two types of endoplasmic reticulum (Fig. 2.3).

### Rough Endoplasmic Reticulum (Granular)

The membranes of these endoplasmic reticulum are associated with minute particles of RNA called ribosomes. The presence of ribosomes gives the membrane a rough appearance. They synthesize proteins.

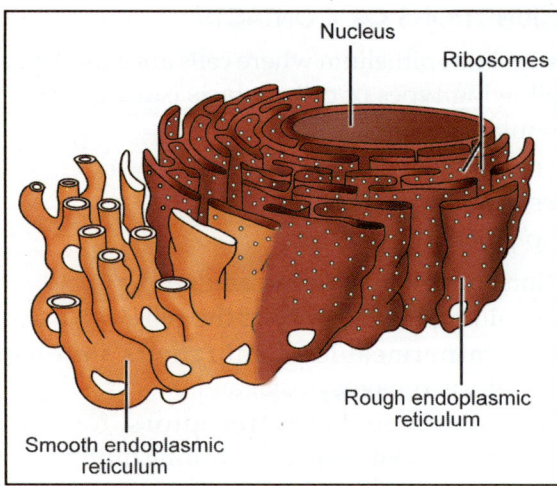

**Fig. 2.3:** Endoplasmic reticulum

## Smooth Endoplasmic Reticulum (Agranular)

The membranes are devoid of ribosomes. These endoplasmic reticulum are involved in lipid cholesterol and carbohydrate metabolism. They are also concerned with steroid hormone synthesis in testes and adrenals.

## GOLGI APPARATUS

- It consists of flattened membrane discs called saccules. A typical Golgi apparatus consists of five to six saccules (Fig. 2.4).
- They lie near the nucleus of the cell.
- They show microvesicles (secretory granules) on their surface.
- They are involved in the process of receiving, concentrating and storing of secretory products (proteins).
- They also secrete polysaccharides.

## RIBOSOMES

- They are small dense granules roughly 25 nm in diameter (10–20 nm).
- Each ribosome consists of roughly 60% RNA and 40% proteins.
- They manufacture proteins using information provided by the DNA of the nucleus.
- There are two types of ribosomes—free and fixed. Free ribosomes are scattered throughout the cytoplasm while fixed ribosomes are attached to the endoplasmic reticulum (Fig. 2.5).

## LYSOSOMES

- They are membrane bound bodies, contain various hydrolytic enzymes (e.g. acid phosphatase).
- They are responsible for intracellular digestive processes and in the breakdown of materials ingested by them.
- They are found in large numbers in macrophages and cells of the reticuloendothelial system. They are often termed as "suicide bags".

## MITOCHONDRIA (Power House of Cells)

- They are found in cells with higher metabolic rates.
- They are sausage-shaped structures, enclosed by two membranes. The inner membrane is thrown into folds called "cristae", which divides the interior into compartments.
- Mitochondria are the sites of production of high-energy compounds (ATP, GTP).
- The dehydrogenase enzyme present in them is responsible for Krebs citric acid cycle, protein and lipid synthesis (Fig. 2.6).

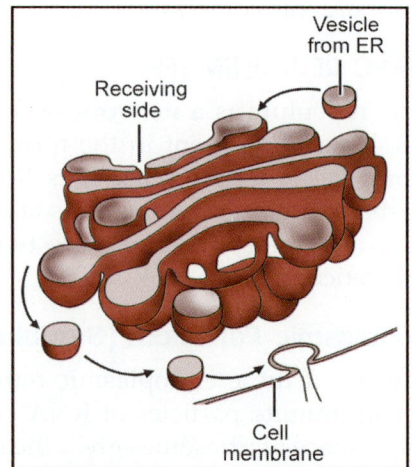

**Fig. 2.4:** Cut section of a Golgi apparatus

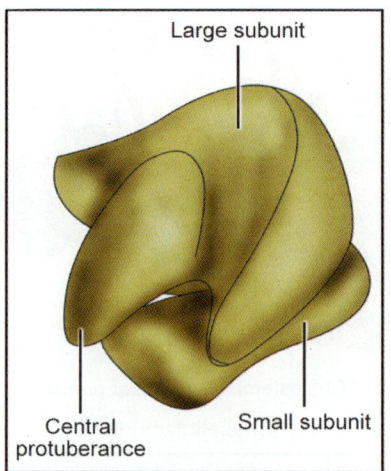

**Fig. 2.5:** Ribosomes

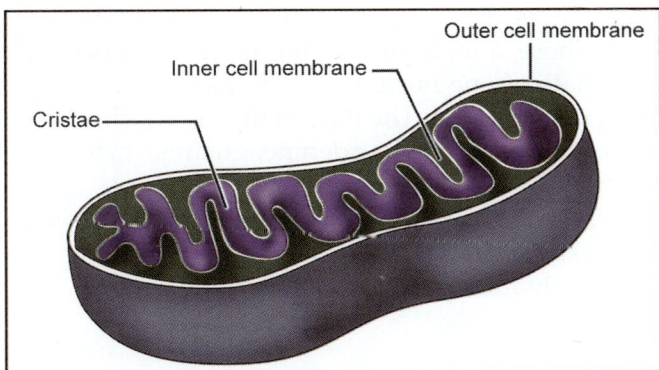

**Fig. 2.6:** Mitochondria

# CENTROSOME

- All cells capable of division contain a pair of structures called "centrioles".
- Centriole is a cylindrical structure composed of short microtubules. There are nine groups of microtubules, with three in each group.
- Centrosome is the cytoplasm surrounding this pair.
- Mature red blood cells and skeletal muscle cells lack centrioles.
- Centrioles direct the movement of chromosomes during cell division. They are said to be absent in nerve cells.

# MICROTUBULES

- They are tubular structures made up of proteins.
- They act as cytoskeleton to maintain cell shape.
- In mitosis, they form the spindle along which the chromosomes move.

# NUCLEUS

- Nucleus is found in all cells except mature erythrocytes (RBCs) and platelets of the blood.
- The shape is normally rounded and placed centrally.
- Nucleus contains the genetic material and influences the metabolic activities of the cells.
- Normally each cell has single nucleus. But some cells have two or more nuclei, e.g. osteoclasts, skeletal muscle.

## Structure of the Nucleus

In a resting cell the nucleus is surrounded by a nuclear membrane. The outer part of the nuclear membrane is continuous with endoplasmic reticulum while its inner surface provides attachment to the ends of the chromatids. The membrane has many gaps called nuclear pores, through which substances can pass from the nucleus to the cytoplasm and vice-versa.

**The cytoplasm of the nucleus (nucleoplasm) contains:**
a. Chromatin material (carriers of genes)
b. Nucleolus—they are rich in RNA and concerned with protein synthesis

*Chromatin:* It is made up of a substance called deoxyribonucleic acid (DNA) and proteins.

*Heterochromatin:* Chromatin fibers are tightly coiled on themselves forming solid mass (inactive).

*Euchromatin:* Coiling of chromatin is not so marked (active). During cell division, the chromatin within the condensed nucleus becomes tightly coiled to form structures called *chromosomes*.

# CHROMOSOMES

Chromosomes are made up of DNA and proteins. The number of chromosomes in each somatic cell is fixed for a given species and in human it is 46. This is referred as the diploid number (diploid = double). However, spermatozoa and ova have 23 chromosomes. This is called haploid number (haploid = half)

Among the 46 chromosomes in a cell 44 are autosomes and two are sex chromosomes. In males the sex chromosomes are X and Y whereas in females it is X and X.

## Structure of the Chromosome

- Each chromosome consists of two parallel rod-like structures called 'chromatids'.
- The two chromatids are joined to each other at a narrow area, which is called 'centromere' (or kinetochore). The chromosomes appear to be constricted in this region and is called 'primary constriction' (Fig. 2.7).

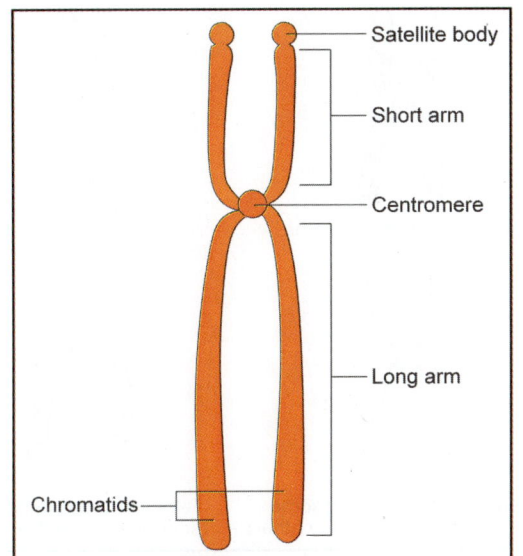

**Fig. 2.7:** A typical submetacentric chromosome

2

- Each chromatid has a long arm (q-arm) and a short arm (p-arm) (centromere is not exactly in the middle of the length of the chromosome).

On the basis of the location of centromere, the chromosomes (Fig. 2.8) are classified into:

*Metacentric chromosome*: The two arms of the chromatid are of equal length.

*Submetacentric chromosome*: One arm of the chromatid is somewhat shorter than the other.

*Acrocentric chromosome*: One arm is much shorter than the other.

*Telocentric chromosome*: Each chromatid has only one arm. The centromere is at one end of the chromosome (Fig. 2.8).

The chromatids of some chromosome show secondary constrictions. Such constrictions are found nearer to one end of the chromatid. The part of the chromatid 'distal' to the constriction is called 'satellite body'. Secondary constrictions are concerned with the formation of nucleoli and are therefore called nucleolar organising regions (NORs).

Each chromosome bears on itself a very large number of functional segments that are called genes.

Chromosomes are made up of nucleic acids called deoxyribonucleic acid (DNA) and ribonucleic acid (RNA).

DNA in a chromosome is in the form of very fine fibers. Each fiber consists of two parallel strands that are together twisted spirally to form 'double helix'. The two strands are linked to each other at regular intervals. Each strand of the DNA fiber consists of a chain of nucleotides. Each nucleotide consists of a sugar-deoxyribose, a molecule of phosphate and a base. The phosphate of one nucleotide is linked to the sugar of the next nucleotide. The base, which is attached to the sugar molecule, may be adenine, guanine, cytosine or thymine.

RNA resembles close to one strand of DNA except for the sugar ribose instead of deoxyribose. Instead of the base thymine RNA contains uracil.

## GENES

Genes are the units of heredity. They are arranged in linear series within the chromosomes. The genes cannot be seen under microscope. A typical gene is composed of a strand of DNA that includes a transcription unit and regulatory sequence (promoter region). Genes are responsible for the synthesis of proteins through transcription from DNA to RNA and translation from RNA to proteins. It is estimated that the human DNA consists about 23000 genes.

Genetic diseases occur due to abnormal genes. Abnormal genes are due to mutation. A change of a base pair of the DNA molecule is known as the gene mutation.

## CHROMOSOMAL ABNORMALITIES

Some of the diseases observed in the humans have genetic and environmental factors as causative agents. The environmental factors can be physical (X-rays and UV rays), chemical (toxic affronts released by factories), or gaseous (harmful gases discharged from refineries). Most of the genetic diseases appear at birth and are called congenital (or birth associated). Genetic disorders can be either due to structural or numerical changes in the chromosome(s) or gene(s) of autosomes or sex chromosomes.

### 1. Numerical Abnormalities

Numerical abnormalities involve the gain or loss of one or more chromosomes known as aneuploidy or the addition of one or more complete haploid complements called euploid.

*Ploidy*: Cells containing multiples of 23 chromosomes are called ploidy. Some cancer cells contain triploid (69 chromosome) and tetraploidy (92 chromosome). Most ploidy conceptions are spontaneously aborted or have short-term survival.

*Trisomy*: The presence of an extra chromosome is called the trisomy 21, 13, 16, 18, X, etc. Down syndrome (trisomy 21) is the most common trisomy in live borns.

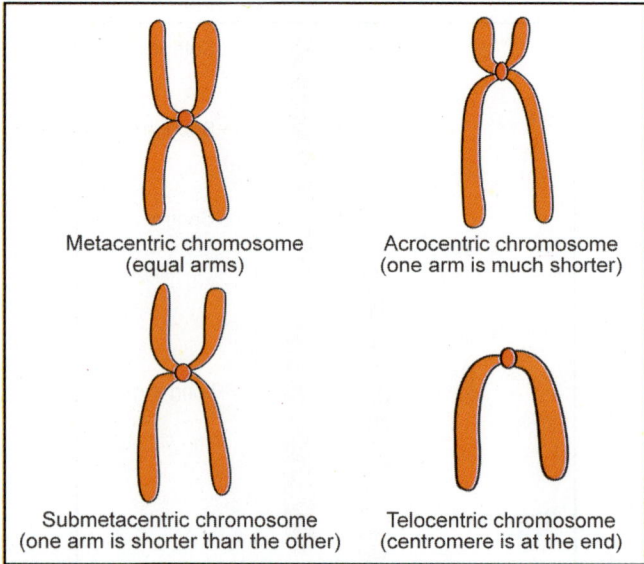

Metacentric chromosome
(equal arms)

Acrocentric chromosome
(one arm is much shorter)

Submetacentric chromosome
(one arm is shorter than the other)

Telocentric chromosome
(centromere is at the end)

**Fig. 2.8:** Different types of chromosomes

*Monosomy*: The absence of a single chromosome is monosomy. Monosomy X (Turner's syndrome) is the most common one.

*Mosaicism*: It is a postzygotic event and occurs after fertilization at an early cell division in the embryos. It results in an individual with two (rarely more) cell lines having different chromosomes constitutions. These numerical abnormalities are usually the result of non-dysjunction, which is the failure of a pair of chromosome to separate normally during either the first or the second meiotic division.

## 2. Structural Abnormalities

*Deletions*: Deletion is caused due to a chromosome break and subsequently loss of genetic material.

*Translocation*: Interchange of genetic material between non-homologous chromosomes. The individual with balanced translocation can be phenotypically normal, but can produce offspring's with unbalanced translocation.

Robertsonian translocation occurs when the long arm of the two acrocentric chromosomes fuses to form one chromosome. Robertsonian translocation occurs only in chromosomes 13, 14, 15, 21 and 22.

*Inversions*: Inversions are common structural anomalies and may be either pericentric (involving centromere) or paracentric (not involving centromere). Individuals with inversion are usually normal in phenotype but can produce offspring's with deletion or duplications.

*Isochromosomes*: This is caused due to an error in cell division when the chromosome divides along the axis perpendicular to its axis of division. The resultant chromosome will be either both 'p' or 'q' arm of the chromosome.

## Genetic disorder involving autosomes

1. *Cri-du-chat syndrome* (genotype: 46, XY, 5p)
   The cause is partial deletion of short arm of chromosome number 5. This incidence occur 1 in 50,000 live births. It is characterized with hypertelorism (eyes are set widely apart) and cry like young kitten. Small mouth, small and receding chin, squint eye and mental retardation are other characters of this syndrome. It is a hereditary congenital syndrome.

2. *Down syndrome* (genotype: 47, XY, +21)
   In gametogenesis two 21 chromosomes are carried due to non-disjunction. Hence it is referred as trisomy 21. This incidence occurs 1.45 per 1000 live births. Maternal age has an effect on incidences of Down syndrome. It is common in children born to elderly women. Mean

pregnancy duration in females carrying a Down syndrome fetus is 270 days instead of 282 days. The Down syndrome is characterized by

- Generalized muscular hypertonia
- Rounded head, flat occiput (back of the skull), large fontanels (unossified areas between the skull bones), hypertelorism and epicanthic folds (skin folds at the medial angle of the eye)
- Short nose with flat bridge, upturned nostrils, small mouth with protruding tongue
- Short and stocky feet
- In 45 percent of the patients there is a unilateral or bilateral palmar crease/simian crease ( a line which joins two opposite ends of the palm horizontally)
- Most individuals with Down syndrome has intellectual disabilities and the severity varies
- In adults secondary sexual characters are weakly manifested, but females with Down can conceive
- Down syndrome often associated with congenital heart disease, umbilical hernia, congenital megacolon, intestinal stenosis
- There are many blood markers to predict the risk of Down syndrome during the first or second trimester which includes alpha fetoprotein, unconjugated estriol and, total hCG (human chorionic gonadotrophin)
- Accurate prenatal diagnosis can be made through amniocentesis or chorionic villus sampling.

## Genetic disorder involving sex chromosomes

1. *Turner syndrome* (genotype: 45,X)
   The individual is female. It is due to the monosomy of the X chromosome (45, XO). The incidence occurs 1 in every 2500–3500 newborns. Turner's syndrome is characterized by:
   - Growth retardation
   - Mostly sterile with underdeveloped ovary
   - Underdeveloped secondary sexual characteristics like pubic hair, breasts and external genitalia are underdeveloped
   - Cubital valgus (patients forearm deviated out), webbed neck, abnormal teeth, squint eyes and auditory defects
   - The patients have normal intelligence, but their behavior is childish.
   - There is no barr body in individuals affected with Turner syndrome

2. *Klinefelter syndrome* (genotype: 47, XXY)
   The individual is male. It is due to the presence of one extra X chromosome (47, XXY).
   The individual is characterized by
   - Gynecomastia (abnormally enlarged breasts) and hypogonadism (underdevelopment of gonads)

• Weak facial hair growth and coarse voice
• Normal intelligence or mild mental retardation
• Low plasma testosterone, high gonadotrophins
• 2–5 cm taller than normal males
• Men with klinefelter syndrome have a single Barr body

## BARR BODIES (SEX CHROMATIN)

• It is observed beneath the nuclear membrane during interphase stage in normal female.
• It is one of the X chromosomes of females, which is highly coiled. It helps in nuclear sexing of the tissues.
• Female with two X chromosomes will have only one Barr body. However, in triple X- syndrome, there are two Barr bodies.

## KARYOTYPING

• It is an orderly arrangement of chromosomes based on their overall size and position of centromere and banding pattern.
• A small quantity of venous blood is collected and suspended in a suitable culture medium in which lymphocytes can multiply.
• The cell division is arrested at metaphase stage by adding colchicin or colcemide to the medium. The cells are then treated with hypotonic saline for proper spreading out of chromosomes.
• A suspension containing cells is spread out on a slide and stained with Giemsa in which the chromosomes are well spread out. A metaphase chromosome plate is then photographed.
• The individual chromosomes are cut from the photographs and are arranged in a proper sequence.
• From this sequential arrangement of chromosomes (karyotype) any abnormalities in their number or form can be identified.

## CELL DIVISION

All nucleated cells can undergo division except highly differentiated cells, e.g. nerve cells.

Cell multiplication is an essential feature of embryonic development, which is necessary after birth for growth and replacement of dead cells. Common type of cell division is mitosis (indirect cell division), in which a parent cell will divide into two daughter cells. The daughter cells will have same number of chromosomes and genetic content as that of the parent cell.

A special type of cell division called meiosis occurs during the formation of gametes (sex cells). In this division, the daughter cell will have half the number of chromosomes. Hence mature sex cells (both male and female) will have haploid (half) number of chromosomes, so that when they fuse (fertilization) the diploid number of chromosomes is restored.

## MITOSIS

For descriptive purpose, this is divided into four phases. The resting phase during which the cell does not divide is described as interphase. During interphase there is synthesis of proteins (Fig. 2.9).

### 1. Prophase

• Chromosomes are long, thin and show spiralization. It produces primary and secondary coils, convert the chromosome into a helical structure.
• Increase in the chromosome diameter and decrease in the chromosome length is observed. Chromosome is double stranded (chromatids) and held together by centromeres.
• Nucleolus is prominent in early prophase but later disappears.
• Nuclear membrane breaks down releasing chromosome.
• Centrioles separate and move towards opposite poles of the cells. Centrioles give rise to microtubules. Central microtubules form 'spindle' and others radiate to form 'astral rays'.

### 2. Metaphase

• Relatively of short duration.
• Chromosomes are sharply defined.
• Chromosome moves towards equator.
• Centromeres of chromosome are attached to the spindle fiber.

### 3. Anaphase

• Active and shortest stages of mitotic division.
• Centromere of each chromosome, containing pair of chromatids splits longitudinally. Original chromosome now splits into two new chromosomes.
• Separated chromosomes move towards each pole of the cell.
• Anaphase chromosome shows different shape, based on position of centromeres, e.g. metacentric, submetacentric, acrocentric and telocentric.

### 4. Telophase

• Stage of reconstruction giving rise to two daughter cells.

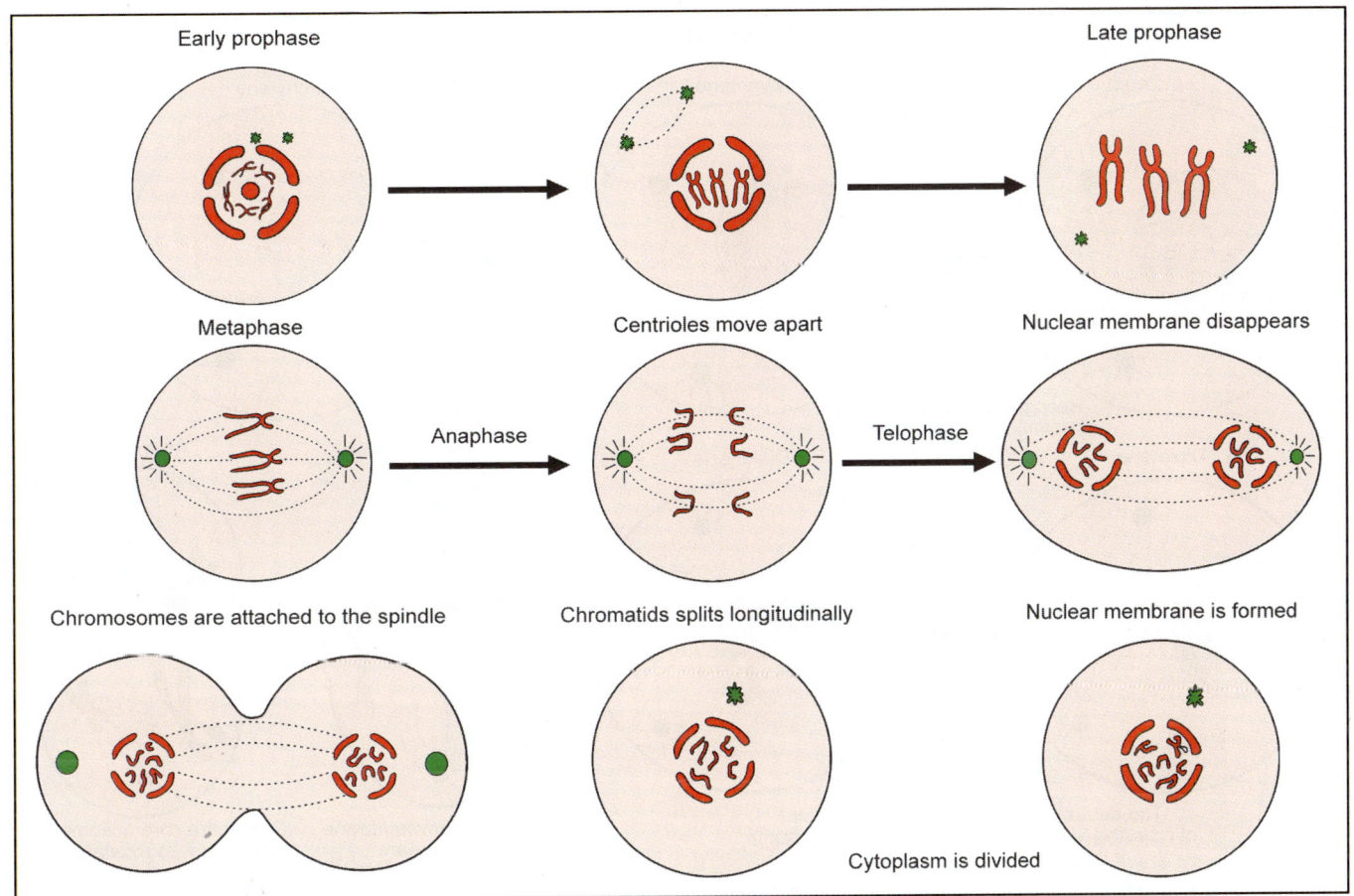

Early prophase

Late prophase

Metaphase

Centrioles move apart

Nuclear membrane disappears

Anaphase

Telophase

Chromosomes are attached to the spindle

Chromatids splits longitudinally

Nuclear membrane is formed

Cytoplasm is divided

**Fig. 2.9:** Mitotic cell division

- Chromosomes become grouped at each pole of the cell, both groups now having diploid number (46).
- Nuclear membrane and nucleoli reappear.
- Spindle and aster disappear.
- Cytoplasm becomes divided into 'two' either by constriction or by new cell membrane formation.
- Each daughter cell receives its compliment of cytoplasmic organelles.

## MEIOSIS

Meiosis consists of two cell divisions—meiotic division first and meiotic division second (Fig. 2.10).

### First Meiotic Division

This is also called the reduction division (chromosome numbers are reduced to half).

*Prophase*: This division is prolonged and divided into a number of stages as follows:

**A. Leptotene**
- Chromosomes are long, slender and thread-like. Each appears-like a string of beads (as in mitosis).

- Chromosomes are double stranded (not visible).
- Individual threads are attached to the nuclear envelope by one end.
- Nucleolus is large and X chromosome is clear.

**B. Zygotene**
- There is a recognition and alignment of homologous chromosomes. So that they become paired. Pairing begins from nuclear envelope. This process is called 'synapsis' (conjugation).
- Each pair of chromosomes is called 'bivalent'.
- Nucleolus and X chromosomes are clearly visible.

**C. Pachytene**
- Chromosomes are shorter and still thicker.
- Each chromosome is formed of two chromatids joined at the centromere. Each 'bivalent pair' consists of four chromatids (tetrads).
- Each chromosome, becomes partially coiled around each other.
- *Crossing over (exchange of DNA)*: A segment of the one of the chromatids (of one chromosome) and a segment of another chromatid (of other chromosome)

2

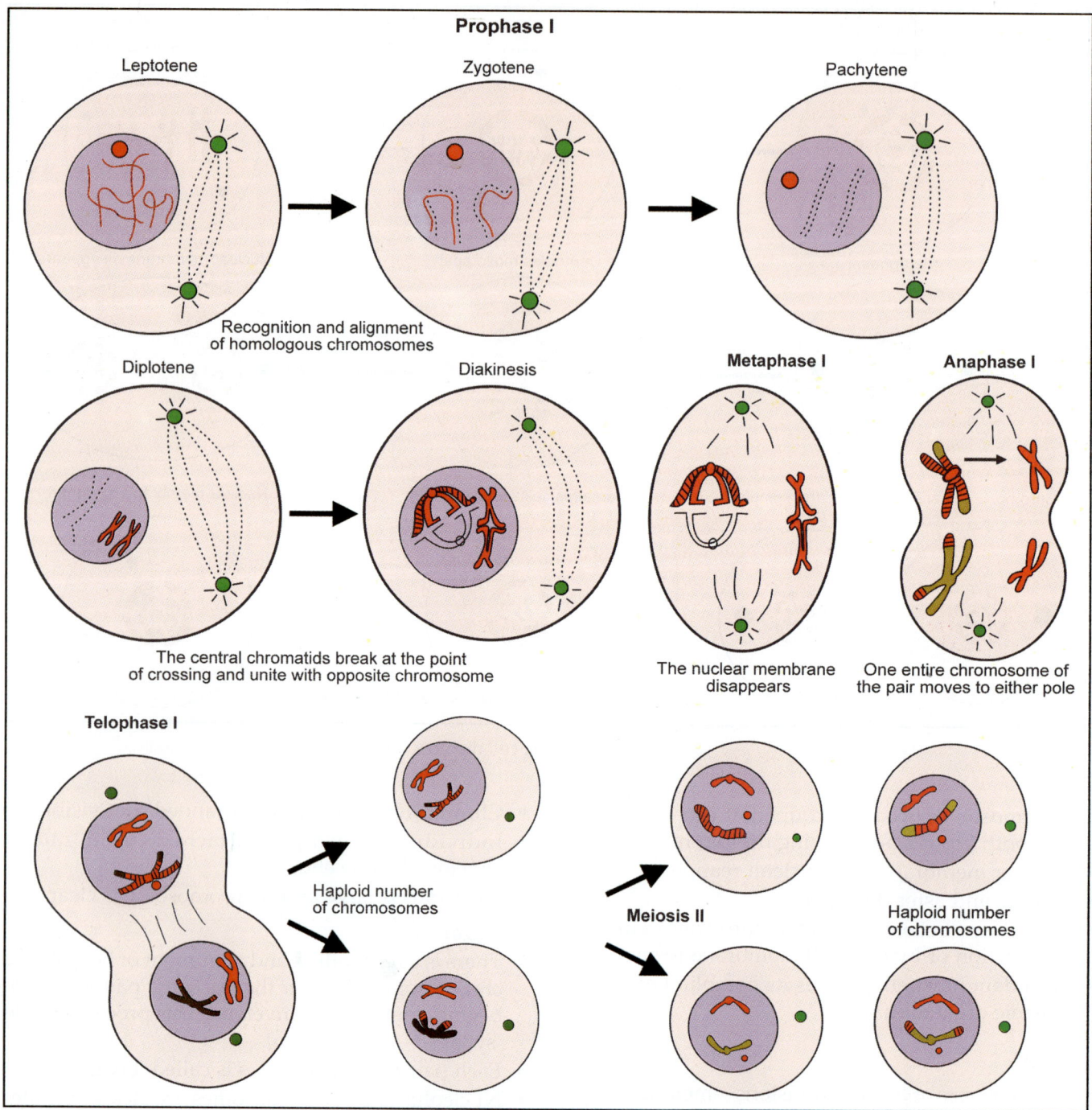

**Fig. 2.10:** Meiotic cell division

exchange their places. Since each segment of chromatid carries specific genes, some of the genes are transferred from one chromosome to other.

**D. Diplotene**

- Cross-shaped configuration is prominent at the point of crossing-over. They are called 'chiasmata'.
- Chromosome surface is still freezy.

**E. Diakinesis**

- Freezy appearance of diplotene is lost.
- Bivalent pairs move away from each other and spreadout against the nuclear membrane.
- Dissolution of nuclear envelope and movement of the bivalent chromosomes towards equator mark the end of the prophase.

*Metaphase I*
- Chromosomes are attached on equator (arms of the chromosomes are on equator and centromeres face the poles).
- Spindle is fully formed and spindle fibers establish connections with centromeres.

*Anaphase I*
- Chromosomes migrate with centromere (they do not split like in meiosis). Hence double stranded chromosomes move towards the pole.
- All chiasmata are lost.

*Telophase I*
- Double stranded chromosomes reach poles.
- Their identity is lost and they appear like mass.
- When the first meiotic division is complete, each daughter cell contains haploid number of chromosomes (23).

## Second Meiotic Division
- This division is same as mitosis.
- The 23 double structured chromosomes divide at the centromere.
- Each daughter cell receives 23 chromosomes.

## RECENT ADVANCES

Advancements in microscopic technology have had a tremendous impact on the science of cytology. In a new process called microtomography, the capabilities of electron microscopy are combined with those of CT scanning to produce high magnification, three dimensional, micrographic images of living cells. With this technology, living cells can be observed as they move, grow and divide. The clinical applications are immense, as scientists can observe living, diseased (including cancerous) cells and their response to various drug treatment.

## Applied Anatomy

1. *Aging*: Although, there are obvious external indicators of aging (graying and loss of hair, wrinkling of skin, loss of teeth and decreased muscle mass) changes due to aging within the cells are not as apparent and not well understood. The mitochondria may change in structure and number and Golgi apparatus may fragment. Also, lipid vacuoles tend to accumulate in the cytoplasm. Extracellular substances also change with age. Collagen and elastic fibers change in quality and numbers. Elastic fibers deterioration in the wall of the blood vessels cause arteriosclerosis in aged persons.

2. *Cancer*: Mitotic rates are usually well controlled and in normal tissue the rate of cell division balances cell loss or destruction. When that balance breaks down, the tissue begins to enlarge. A tumor or neoplasm is a mass or swelling produced by abnormal cell growth and mitosis. In a benign tumor the cells remain within the connective tissue capsule. Such tumor seldom threatens an individual life. Surgery can usually remove the tumor if its size or position disturbs tissue function.

Cells in a malignant tumor are no longer responding to normal control mechanisms. These cells divide rapidly, spreading into the surrounding tissues and they may also spread to other tissues and organs. This spread is called metastasis. The term cancer refers to an illness characterised by malignant cells. Cancer cells gradually lose their resemblance to normal cells. They change size and shape. Organ function begins to deteriorate as the number of cancer cells increases. Cancer cells compete for space and nutrients with normal cells.

# Tissue of the Body

# 3

A group of cells having similar origin, structure and function is called a tissue.

*Types*: There are four types of basic tissues in the body:
1. Epithelial tissue
2. Connective tissue
3. Muscular tissue
4. Nervous tissue

Cartilage and bone are specialized connective tissues.

## EPITHELIAL TISSUE

It is a layer of cells, which covers the external surface (skin) or lines the internal surface of gastrointestinal, respiratory, and urogenital tracts.

## Functions

- *Protection*: It protects the body surface from drying or bacterial invasion.
- *Transport*: Mucous and particulate matters are carried to epithelial surface. Fluid may pass through the cell.
- *Secretion*: The cells secrete the product synthesized, either to the lumen or blood.
- *Excretion*: May excrete metabolic waste products.
- *Absorption*: It absorbs essential substances from the lumen of the GIT and kidney tubules (where it is called reabsorption).
- *Lubrication*: Peritoneum, pleura and pericardial epitheliam serve this function.
- *Sensory*: In the skin (touch sensation), nasal mucosa (smell sensation) and tongue (taste sensation), it serves as sensory organ.

## Types of Epithelium

Epithelium is classified into simple, pseudostratified and stratified varieties.

### Simple Epithelium

Single layer of cells resting on a basement membrane (Fig. 3.1).

1. *Simple squamous*: Irregular flat cells with height less than width.

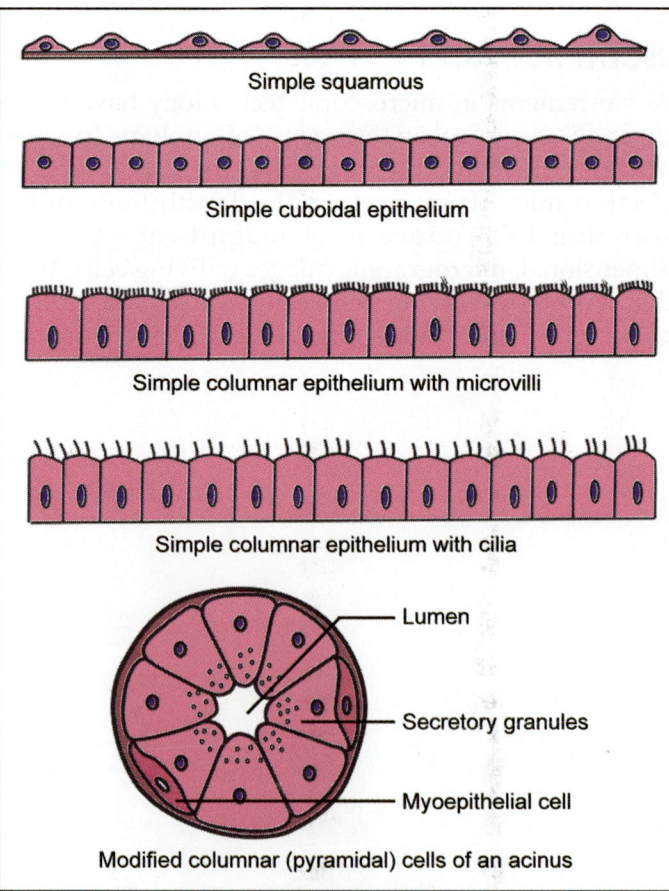

Simple squamous

Simple cuboidal epithelium

Simple columnar epithelium with microvilli

Simple columnar epithelium with cilia

Lumen

Secretory granules

Myoepithelial cell

Modified columnar (pyramidal) cells of an acinus

**Fig. 3.1:** Simple epithelial tissue

- *Distribution*: Alveoli of the lungs.
- Bowman's capsule and loop of Henle of kidney.
- Mesothelium lining the peritoneum, pleura and pericardial cavities.
- Endothelial cells lining blood vessels.

2. *Simple cuboidal*: Height and width are nearly equal and nuclei are central in position.
- *Distribution*: Thyroid follicles
- Ducts of many glands
- Surface of the ovary (germinal epithelium).

3. *Simple columnar*: Height of the cells is greater than width. Nuclei are elongated and placed towards the base.
- *Distribution*: Small bronchi and bronchioles, uterine tube.
- Ependyma lining the cavities of the brain. Efferent ductules of the testes.

**Non-ciliated simple columnar**

*Distribution*: Lining of gastrointestinal tract from stomach to rectum.
  Gallbladder (with brush border).

## Pseudostratified Columnar Epithelium

Single layer of epithelial cells resting on a basement membrane.

- Some cells are shorter and do not reach the lumen, while tall cells reach the lumen.
- The nuclei of the cells therefore lie at different levels. This gives the impression of stratification (false stratification).

**A. Pseudostratified non-ciliated**
- *Distribution*: Male urethra (membranous and penile parts)
- Auditory tube
- Vas deferens

**B. Pseudostratified ciliated**
- *Distribution*: Upper part of the respiratory tract (trachea and larger bronchi).

## Stratified Epithelium

Epithelium is made up of many layers of cells. They are found in areas, which are subjected to friction.

**A. Stratified squamous non-keratinised**

Epithelium is made up of many layers of cells. Basal cells resting on the basement membrane are columnar or low cuboidal.

- Superficial cells are squamous and flat, hence called stratified squamous epithelium (Fig. 3.2).

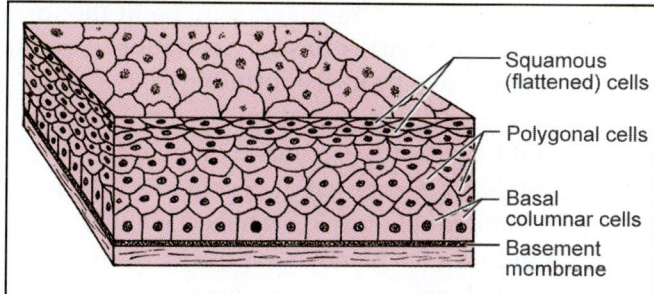

**Fig. 3.2:** Stratified squamous epithelium

- *Distribution*: Epithelium lining mouth, pharynx and esophagus, anal canal, vagina and cornea.

**B. Stratified squamous keratinised epithelium**

The superficial layer consists of non-living cells with keratin in their cytoplasm. They are tough and water-resistant.
  *Distribution*: Epidermis of the skin.

**C. Stratified cuboidal epithelium**

It consists of few layers of cuboidal cells.
  *Distribution*: Ducts of sweat glands.

**D. Stratified columnar epithelium**

It consists of two or more layers of cells.
  Basal cells are polyhedral, while superficial cells are columnar.
  *Distribution*: Male urethra (membranous part).

## Transitional Epithelium (Urothelium)

This is a stratified epithelium with three to four layers of cells. The deepest cells are columnar or cuboidal.
  The middle layers are made up of polyhedral or pear-shaped cells. The cells of the surface are large and are shaped like an umbrella.
  *Distribution*: Renal pelvis, ureter, urinary bladder and proximal part of the urethra.
Transitional epithelium can be stretched considerably without being damaged. When stretched the cells become flattened. Presence of a glycoprotein membrane on the surface cells is believed to protect the underlying tissue from toxic substances present in the urine.

## Glandular Epithelium

The epithelial cells are specialized to perform secretary function. Such epithelial cell in-groups constitute glands (single epithelial cell can also be a gland-unicellular).
  There are *two* main types of glands:
  1. *Exocrine glands*: When the secretion from the gland is poured through duct system, they are called exocrine glands, e.g. salivary gland.

The secretary part of the gland may be in the form of rounded sac (or acini) or flask shaped tube (alveoli). Exocrine glands may be in the form of:

- Unicellular gland, e.g. goblet cells.
- Simple tubular gland, e.g. intestinal glands.
- Simple alveolar gland, e.g. it represents a stage in the development of simple branched glands.
- Compound tubular gland, e.g. mucous glands.
- Compound alveolar gland, e.g. mammary gland.
- Compound tubuloalveolar gland, e.g. salivary gland.

Depending upon the nature of secretion, the exocrine glands may be classified into mucous glands and serous glands. The mucous glands secrete 'mucopolysaccharide' and secretions of serous glands are watery in nature rich with proteins.

**Glands are also classified into:**

*Apocrine gland:* The luminal part of the cell disintegrates as a part of secretion. The basal part will regenerate, e.g. mammary gland.

*Holocrine gland:* The cell itself will be disintegrated as a part of secretion, e.g. sebaceous gland.

*Merocrine gland (epicrine gland):* The secretion is discharged without disintegrating the cell. Most of the glands belong to this type.

2. *Endocrine glands:* These glands are 'ductless' and pour their secretion directly into the bloodstream. Their secretion is called 'hormone'. The cells of the endocrine glands are usually arranged in cords or in clumps with rich network of blood capillaries around them.

## CONNECTIVE TISSUE

- Connective tissue has formed elements (fibers and cells) and amorphous substance (ground substance).
- This tissue binds various other tissues of the body.

**Components of the connective tissue:** Connective tissue has two components—cells and matrix, which has fibers and ground substance.

- *Cells:* Seven types of cells are found in the connective tissue.
- *Fibers:* The connective tissue fibers are of three types, collagen, elastic and reticular fibers (Fig. 3.3).

## Collagen Fibers

- In fresh state, they appear white and therefore are also called white fibers.
- It contains a protein called 'collagen', which is derived from tropocollagen.
- Collagen fibers run in straight or wavy bundles. The individual fibers do not branch but bundles themselves can branch.

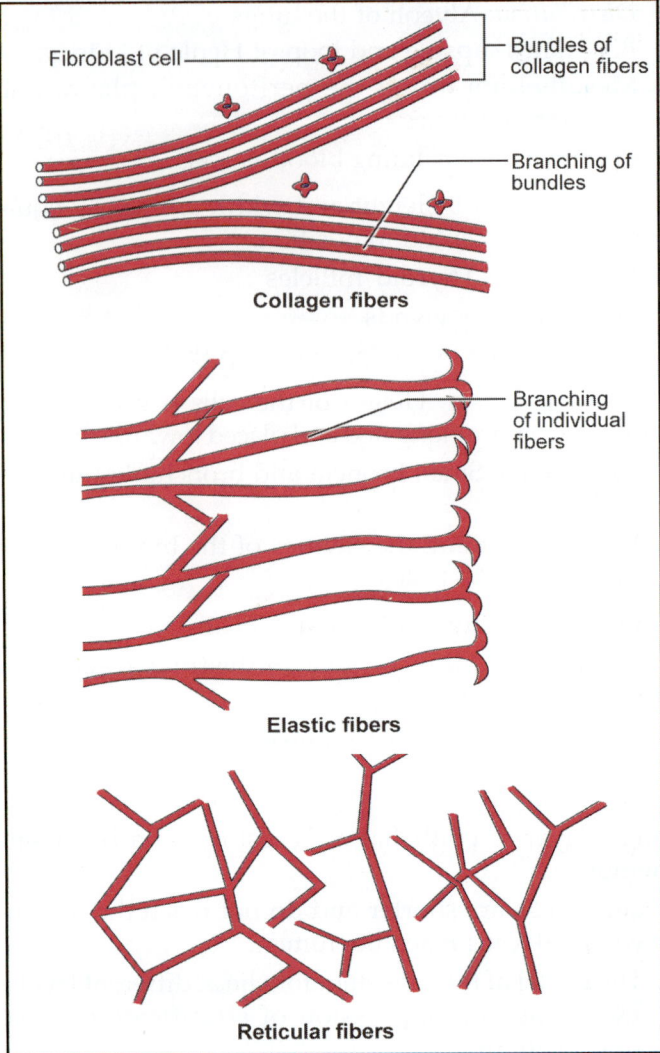

**Fig. 3.3:** Connective tissue fibers

- The fibers are soft but strong and flexible but they are not elastic.
- Collagen fibers are formed and maintained by 'fibroblasts'.
- They are found in all types of connective tissue.
- The individual collagen fibers are 1–12 µm in diameter.
- Depending upon their diameter, they are classified into four types:

### Types and distribution

- *Type I:* (Diameter of about 250 nm). They are found in tendons, ligaments, aponeurosis, bone and meninges.
- *Type II:* (Diameter of about 20 to 100 nm). This variety is found in cartilages.
- *Type III:* They are also called 'reticular fibres', which is discussed in next page.

- *Type IV*: They form the basement membrane of the epithelium.

## Reticular Fibers

- These are similar to collagen fibers (type-III) in chemical structure.
- They are thin fibers showing branching and hence form a network or a reticulum.
- They do not run in bundles.
- These fibers form the skeletal framework of the lymphatic organs.

### Distribution

- Basement membrane of the epithelial tissue
- Walls of the blood vessels
- Lymphatic organs.

## Elastic Fibers

- Elastic fibers are thin and highly elastic.
- These fibers branch and anostomose with each other but do not form bundles.
- In bulk they appear yellow, hence also called yellow elastic fibers.
- Elastic fibers can be stretched (like a rubber band) and return to their original length when tension is released. The cut ends of the fibers show spiralling and kinking.
- Elastic fibers are made up of proteins called 'elastin'. They are digested by the enzyme elastase. Elastin contains amino acid valine and also rich in 'glycine' and 'proline'.

### Distribution

- Loose connective tissue
- Walls of the blood vessels
- Ligamentum flava
- Capsules of the glands

## Ground Substance (Intercellular substance)

The ground substance consists of water, carbohydrates, lipids and proteins. They together constitute matrix. The carbohydrates are in the form of mucopoly-saccharides, which may be either sulfated or non-sulfated, in combination with hyaluronic acid.

- Chondroitin 4—sulphate in cartilage matrix
- Chondroitin 6—sulphate in cartilage matrix
- Chondroitin sulphate B in skin and cornea
- Hyaluronic acid in synovial fluid, soft connective tissue, vitreous humor.

## Cell Types

1. *Fibroblasts*: Each cell is flattened or fusiform in shape with centrally placed nucleus. The cell shows numerous processes. They are responsible for the formation of collagen, reticular and elastic fibers. They help in healing of wounds (Fig. 3.4a).

2. *Macrophages (histiocytes or clasmatocytes)*: These cells are less numerous than the fibroblasts. Their cytoplasm has hydrolytic enzymes. These cells are phagocytic in function. They phagocytose bacteria and other foreign bodies. Macrophages are classified into fixed and wandering varieties. The fixed type is attached to the reticular fibers of the connective tissue. They are irregular in shape. The wandering type is free and become ovoid (Fig. 3.4b).

3. *Plasma cells*: These cells are numerous in mucous and submucous coats of the gut. The cells are rounded in shape with eccentrically placed nucleus. These cells produce antibodies to counteract the actions of antigens in defense mechanism of the body. The antibodies may be stored within the cell itself in the form of Russell's body.

4. *Mast cells*: Each cell is rounded in shape with a centrally placed nucleus. They are present in the

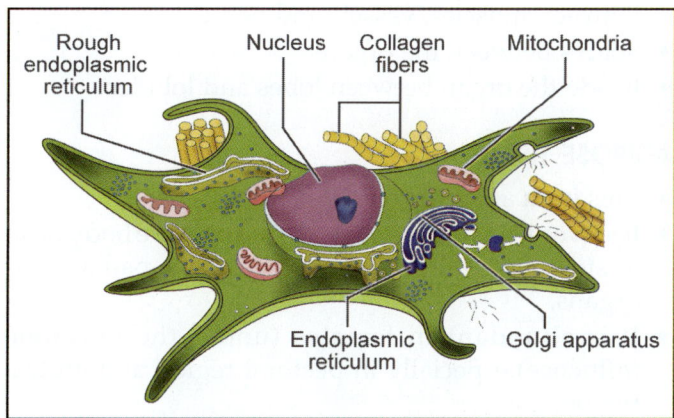

**Fig. 3.4a:** Fibroblast cell

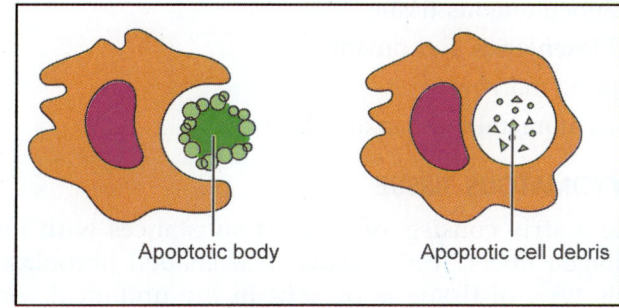

**Fig. 3.4b:** Macrophage cell (histocyte)

3

fibrous capsule of the liver, along the blood vessels, beneath the mucosa of alimentary and respiratory tracts. They secrete heparin, which is an anti-coagulant. They also produce histamine, which causes allergic reactions.

5. *Pigment cells*: They are present in the iris and choroid of the eye.

6. *Reticular cells*: These are present in the reticular connective tissue. They produce reticular fibers. They are also phagocytic in function.

7. *Fat cells (adipocytes)*: These cells are polygonal in shape with eccentrically placed nucleus. The cyto-plasm contains large amount of fat. They are numerous in adipose tissue.

### AREOLAR TISSUE

It is the most common connective tissue where collagen and elastic fibers are loosely arranged. The ground substance is semifluid in nature. They have plenty of fibroblasts and macrophages. They are traversed by nerves and vessels.

#### Distribution

- Subcutaneous tissue
- Submucous coat in the gastrointestinal tract
- Between muscles, vessels and nerves
- Spaces between the organs
- Inside the organ between lobes and lobules

### ADIPOSE TISSUE

- This is an aggregation of fat cells.
- It serves as insulating material to conserve body heat, as storage depot for food, as protective pad around organs.
- It is abundant in females (under the hormone influence) especially in pectoral region and gluteal region.

#### Distribution

- Subcutaneous tissue
- Mesenteries and omenta
- Bone marrow
- Ischiorectal fossa, axilla, bony orbit.

### MYXOMATOUS TISSUE

The matrix consists of mucoid substances with few collagen fibers. It also shows star shaped fibroblasts. This type of tissue is present in the umbilical cord (Wharton's jelly) and vitreous body of the eye.

### RETICULAR TISSUE

- It consists of network of reticular fibers.
- These fibers are associated with specialized fibroblasts called 'reticulocytes'.
- This type of tissue is present in lymphatic organs and bone marrow.
- Connective tissues form the internal framework of the body. It is the main constituent of fascia.

### SKIN (INTEGUMENT)

Skin covers the entire external surface of the body including external auditory meatus and lateral aspect of tympanic membrane.

Structurally skin is complex and highly specialized lamina having an area between 1.2 and 2.2 $m^2$. The thickness ranges from about 1.5 to 4.0 mm.

Skin protects against micro-organisms, toxic substances, dehydration, ultraviolet radiation and friction. It acts as a sensory receptor and has role in excretion, vitamin D metabolism, and the regulation of blood pressure and body temperature.

The outer surface of the skin presents various markings which are referred as 'skin lines'. They include:

1. *Flexure lines:* Externally visible grooves of the epidermis near or opposite the joints.

2. Tension lines over the surface of hairy skin.

3. Papillary ridges forming parallel lines on thick hairless skin of the hands and feet.

4. Striae gravidarum bands appear after rapid local expansion of underlying structure (after pregnancy/linea albicantes)

5. Voight lines are boundary lines between darker and lighter areas on the upper limbs.

6. *Mongolian spots:* Blue-grey patches on trunk.

7. *Naevi (moles):* Accumulation of pigment cells in the epidermis.

#### Lines of Cleavage (Langer's line)

Skin is normally under tension. In the dermis of the skin there are collagen fibers arranged in parallel rows. This direction of rows of collagen is known as Langer's line.

These Langer's lines tend to run longitudinally in limbs, horizontally in the neck and trunk.

A surgical incision along the rows of collagen fibers causes minimum disruption of collagen and leaves minimum amount of scar.

## Types of Skin

The fundamental structure of skin of the entire body is similar, but there are local variations like degree of keratinization, size and number of hairs, pigmentation, vascularity, innervation and others. On this basis skin is classified into 2 types.

1. **Thin hairy skin (Hirsute)** constitutes great majority of body's covering
2. **Thick hairless skin (Glabrous)** forming the surfaces of palms of hand, soles of feet and flexor surfaces of digits.

## Microscopic Structure of the Skin

Skin is made up of two distinct layers (Fig. 3.5)

1. *Epidermis:* It is the outer layer of the skin made of stratified squamous keratinized epithelium. Developmentally it is from surface ectoderm and is avascular. It receives its nutrition by diffusion from dermis.

2. *Dermis:* It is deeper connective tissue layer. Developmentally it is mesodermal in origin and is vascular.

*Epidermis:* In this layer, there is a continuous replacement of cells. The cells are arranged in many layers. The living cells from the basal layer are transferred to the surface as dead cells with accumulation of 'Keratin' in their cytoplasm. These cells are called **"Keratinocytes"**. But there are other cell types in epidermis which are not engaged in this replacement. These include pigment forming melanocytes, phagocytic Langerhans' cells and neurally associated cells like Markel cells (Meissner's corpuscles, Pacinian corpuscles in dermis). The cell layers from deep to superficial are as follows—stratum basale, stratum spinosum, sratum granulosum, stratum lucidum and stratum corneum. The width of these layers differs in thick and thin skin.

The junction between the epidermis and the dermis presents zigzagging interdigitations between upward projection of dermis (dermal papillae) and downward projections of the epidermis (epidermal ridges).

Epidermis is mainly consists of keratinocytes. The different layers of the epidermis represent process of keratinization (a living cell from stratum basale getting transformed to a dead cell). The process involves 4 overlapping stages: cell renewal (mitosis), cell differentiation (keratinization), cell death (apoptosis), and the sloughing of dead cells from the surface (exfoliation). The entire process takes 15 to 30 days.

1. *Stratum basale:* A single layer of columnar (mostly) and cuboidal cells attached to basement membrane (basal lamina). These cells give rise to the keratinocytes in all other superficial layers.

2. *Stratum spinosum (prickle cell layer):* It contains more mature keratinocytes with several layers. The polygonal cells are placed closely and it gives spiny appearance and is called prickle cell layer.

3. *Stratum granulosum:* In this layer, drastic changes in keratinocyte structure occur. The cells become flattened and accumulate basophilic granules called keratohyalin. Their pycnotic nuclei begin to disintergrate and other cellular organelles degenerate.

4. *Stratum lucidum:* The layer is found only in thick skin. It stains strongly than stratum corneum with acidic stain. It appears as translucent band of flattened keratinocytes whose nuclei and intercellular borders are not visible.

5. *Stratum corneum:* It consists of closely packed layers of flattened dead cells with keratin filaments in their cytoplasm. Dead cells are continuously exfoliated from the surface and replaced by cells from the deeper layers.

## Other Cell Types in Epidermis

1. *Langerhans' cells:* These cells are derived from bone marrow cells. The 'star' shaped cell bodies of Langerhans' cells are situated in stratum spinosum and their branched dendrites are insinuated between the surrounding cells.

The function of Langrhans' cell is cellular defense. They are particular in detecting, binding and presenting antigens to local lymphocytes. It is a part of immune mechanism of skin. This is important in cell mediated immunity to epidermal viral infection, in elimination of epidermal cancers, etc.

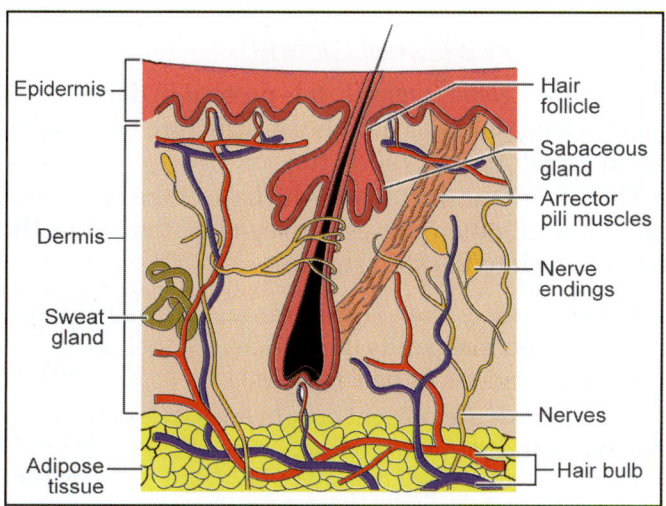

Epidermis —

Dermis —

Sweat gland —

Adipose tissue —

Hair follicle

Sabaceous gland

Arrector pili muscles

Nerve endings

Nerves

Hair bulb

**Fig. 3.5:** Skin-schematic

2. *Epidermal melanocytes:* These cells lie in stratum basale in contact with basal lamina. They are derived from the neural crest cells. They provide a pigment shield against ultraviolate light from sun. Melanocytes are more in face, mucosal orifices, external genitalia nipple and areola.

   In amphibia, these cells are abundant and are responsible for quick changes in the colour of the skin.

3. *Merkels cells:* These cells are present is the stratum spinosum. It acts as a mechanoreceptors and nerve fibers terminate in them.

*Dermis:* Mechanically dermis provides strength to skin by its collagen fibers and elastin content. The dermis can be divided into 2 zones, a narrow superficial papillary layer and deeper reticular layer.

Papillary layer lies immediately deep to epidermis consists of extensive network of capillaries. It provides mechanical anchorage, metabolic support and trophic maintenance to the overlying tissue. The superficial surface of this layer is marked by numerous papillae which interdigitate with recess in the base of epidermis. The papillae are few and small in thin skin whereas larger and closely aggregated in thick skin. The reticular layer consists of many arterio-venous anastomoses that help to regulate the blood pressure and body temperature.

*Meissner's corpuscular nerve endings:* They are present in papillary layer of the dermis. These corpuscles are believed to be responsible for touch.

Reticular layer is rich in strong collagen fibers and also elastic fibers. The layer also contains adipose tissues and capillaries.

## Appendages of the Skin

### Hair

- Hairs are filamentous (Fig. 3.5), keratinized structures which assist thermoregulation, provide some protection and have sensory function.
- The distribution of hair differs in different parts of the body and also differs in two sexes.
- The length varies from less than a millimeter to a meter.
- The structures that form hairs and maintain their growth are called hair follicle. The hair follicle consists of shaft and root. The visible part on the surface is called shaft and embedded part is called root.

*Hair shaft:* It is made of keratin filaments. It shows 3 concentric zones, the cuticle, cortex and medulla.

*Hair root:* It is covered by several layers which includes: Outermost connective tissue sheath, external root sheath and internal root sheath composed of Henle's layer and Huxley's layers.

## Arrector Pili Muscles (Fig. 3.5)

These are non-striated (smooth) muscles which link between hair follicles and papillary layer of the dermis. Contraction of these muscles tends to pull the hair more vertically and skin in the region of its attachments gets elevated while neighboring region which gives attachment to this muscle is depressed to give rise to 'goose skin'. The muscle is supplied by sympathetic nerves. The Arrector pili contract and hairs stand erect in response to cold, fear and anger.

### Sebaceous Glands (Fig. 3.5)

- Sebaceous glands are present in dermis of almost whole body except palms and sole.
- The gland secretes an oily substance called sebum to skin surface and hairs.
- The gland consists of clusters of acini. The duct of the gland opens at the apical portion of hair follicle.
- Wherever hair follicle is absent, the duct opens directly into skin surface (e.g. lips, corners of mouth, nipple).
- Sebaceous glands are numerous over face, which cause 'acne' in adult with retention of secretion.
- The sebaceous gland assists in water proofing of epidermis, discourages blood sucking ecto-parasites and contributes to the characteristic body odor.

### Sudorific Glands (Sweat Glands)

*Eccrine sweat gland (typical):* It is present in dermis. The gland is long unbranched tubular structure with highly coiled secretory part called fundus.

The wall of the duct fuses with base of the epidermal papillae and lumen passes between keratinocytes. The duct opens into the skin surface.

*Apocrine sweat gland:* These are large sweat glands unlike, endocrine glands they discharge their secretion into apical regions of hair follicles.

These glands are present only in few parts of the body like axilla and perineal region.

## Applied Anatomy

*Cyanosis:* When hemoglobin is poorly oxygenated, both the blood and the skin appear blue, a condition called cyanosis. Skin often becomes cyanotic during heart failure or severe respiratory disorders. In black people, the skin is too dark to reveal the color of the underlying vessels, but cyanosis is apparent in the mucous membranes and nail beds.

*Erythema:* Infection, inflammation or allergic reaction of the skin cause superficial capillary engorgement. This makes skin abnormally red. This sign is called erythema. In jaundice yellowish pigment called bilirubin builds up in the blood, giving yellowish appearance to the skin and white of the eye.

*Albinism:* It is a genetic disorder causing specific trait. The enzyme responsible for conversion of tyrosine to melanin (DOPA pathway) is deficient. These groups of individuals are more prone for dermal cancers.

*Lacerations:* It refers to skin cuts or tears. It can be superficial or deep. Superficial cuts do not interrupt the continuity of the dermis. Deep cuts penetrate the deep layers of the dermis and require approximation of the cut edges of the dermis by suturing or stitches.

*Wound healing:* Lacerations (cuts), abrasions, and burns cause structural damage to the skin. In the process of healing the fibroblasts initially proliferate to secrete mainly type III collagen fibers. Subsequently most of these fibers are replaced by type I collagen. Small, shallow wounds are typically recovered by keratinocytes arising from the stratum basale. In wounds that remove the epidermis from a larger area, keratinocytes in the external root sheath of hair follicles divide and migrate to replace the epidermal tissue. Eventually normal epidermal and dermal architecture may be restored. Larger and deeper wounds, in which the hair follicles are lost are destroyed, may never be completely recovered by normal epidermis, thus may leave a scar at the site.

## Fasciae

It is a connective tissue layer presents deep to the skin. It is further divided into superficial fascia and deep fascia. The superficial fascia is mainly composed of adipose tissue, which provides insulation and padding and lets the skin or underlying structure move independently.

The deep fascia is mainly made up of connective tissue fibers. They also surround the muscle groups, blood vessels, nerves binding some structure together or allowing the structures to glide smoothly over each other. In the limbs the deep fascia forms compartments between flexor and extensor group of muscles. Deep fascia forms retinacula around the joint to hold the tendons of the muscle. The deep fascia also provide thick protective coat for arteries like carotid sheath, axillary sheath and femoral sheath. In few places the deep fascia gives attachment to the underlying muscles. Understanding of the arrangement of the fascial planes, their extent and attachments are important for surgeons.

# Cartilage and Bone

## 4

Cartilage is a specialised dense connective tissue. It is hard but not rigid like bone. It can be bent and also brought back into its original form when bending force is withdrawn. This cartilage forms the 'skeletal' basis of some parts of the body (auricle of the ear, external nose).

At the time of birth, many parts of the skeletal framework of the newborn are made up of cartilage. Later this cartilage will be converted into bones by a process called 'ossification'. However, depending on the functional need, some of them remain as cartilages even in adults (Fig. 4.1).

### General Features

- They are rigid structures, hence provide protection and support the organs. They can withstand the effects of pressure, pull or torsion.
- They are present in the body where elasticity and rigidity is required.

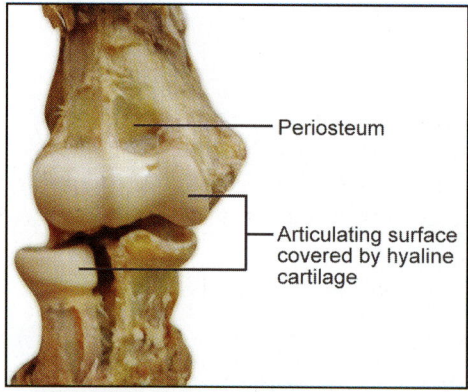

**Fig. 4.1:** Articular cartilage

- They are avascular structures, nourished by diffusion from adjacent tissues.
- Repair of cartilage is slow and takes time due to its avascularity.
- There are three types of cartilages—hyaline, elastic and fibrocartilage.

**Cartilage consists of:**
1. Cells called chondrocytes
2. Fibers
3. Ground substance

Based on the type of fibers present in the matrix, the cartilages are classified into three types—hyaline, elastic and white fibrocartilage.

### 1. HYALINE CARTILAGE (Fig. 4.2a)

- It appears transparent glass like in fresh condition.
- It is covered by a vascular fibrous membrane called 'perichondrium'. This perichondrium has an outer fibrous layer and inner cellular layer. The cellular layer consists of chondroblasts (immature chondrocytes).
- It has a homogeneous matrix, which is glassy and transparent in appearance.
- The matrix contains collagen fibers (type II) which run in parallel bundles.
- The chondrocytes are placed in 'lacunae' of the matrix.
- They are arranged in-groups of two, four and six (isogenous group). This arrangement is called the '*cell nest condition*'.
- The ground substance is made up of carbohydrates and proteins. The carbohydrates are glycosaminoglycans. It includes chondroitin 4-sulphate and hyaluronic acid.
- The fibers cannot be seen under light microscope because the refractive index of the fibers and ground substance is same and hence it is homogeneous.

## Distribution

1. Costal cartilages of the ribs.
2. Cartilage covering the articulating surfaces of the bones.
3. Cartilages of the larynx—thyroid and cricoid cartilage.
4. The tracheal rings.

## 2. ELASTIC CARTILAGE (Fig. 4.2b)

Structurally the elastic cartilage is mainly made up of elastic fibers and the chondrocytes. The surface of the elastic cartilage is covered by 'perichondrium'.

Elastic cartilage is more flexible than hyaline cartilage.

## Distribution

- Pinna of the external ear
- Epiglottis, corniculate and cuneiform cartilages of the larynx.
- Medial part of the auditory tube

## 3. FIBROCARTILAGE (WHITE FIBROCARTILAGE) (Fig. 4.2c)

- Structurally the white fibrocartilage contains mainly thick bundles of collagen fibers (type I) and a few chondrocytes.
- It has no perichondrium.
- It is very tough and strong but resilient.
- It has great tensile strength and considerable elasticity.

## Distribution

- Articular disc of the temporomandibular joint and sternoclavicular joint.
- Intervertebral discs present between the bodies of vertebrae.
- Glenoidal labrum of shoulder joint.
- Acetabular labrum of hip joint.
- Menisci of the knee joint.

## Growth of the Cartilages

**Cartilages grow by two mechanisms**

In **appositional** growth, cells of the perichondrium (chondroblasts) undergo repeated division. These cells produce cartilaginous matrix and are transformed into chondrocytes. This differentiation gradually increases the size of the cartilage. Chondrocytes within the cartilage matrix also undergo division, and the daughter cells produce additional matrix. This cycle enlarges the cartilage rather as a balloon is inflated; the process is called **interstitial growth**. Neither interstitial nor apositional growth occurs in adult cartilages and they cannot repair themselves after a severe injury.

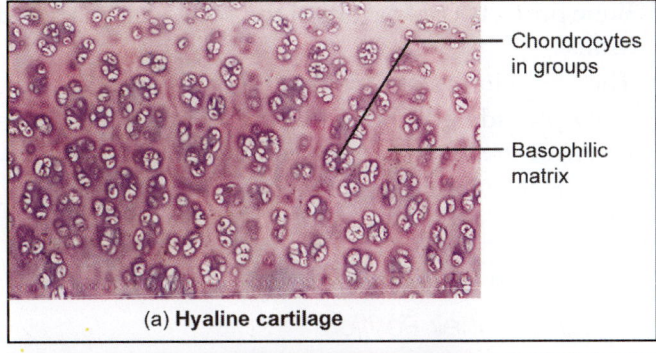

**(a) Hyaline cartilage**

— Chondrocytes in groups

— Basophilic matrix

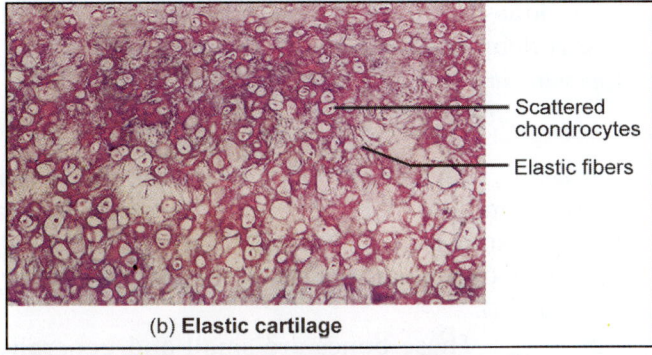

**(b) Elastic cartilage**

— Scattered chondrocytes

— Elastic fibers

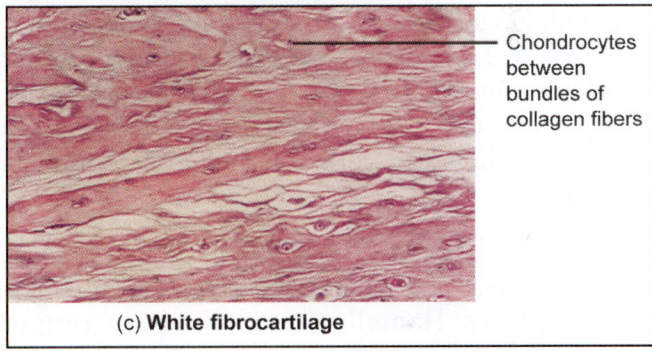

**(c) White fibrocartilage**

— Chondrocytes between bundles of collagen fibers

**Fig. 4.2a to c:** Types of cartilage (H & E stained)

The cartilage tissue grows rapidly during youth, but has little capacity for regeneration and healing in adults. Adult cartilage regenerates poorly because chondrocytes have lost capacity for division. The little healing that occurs within adult cartilage is due to the ability of the surviving chondrocytes to secrete more extracellular matrix.

### BONE

Bone is a highly vascular living connective tissue in which the matrix is calcified by the deposition of calcium phosphate.

The human skeleton consists of **206** bones.

## FUNCTIONS OF THE BONE

- Bone provides supporting framework and shape for the body.

4

- Bone protects vital organs of the body (e.g. heart and brain).
- They help in transmission of the body weight.
- They provide attachment to the muscles and act as levers of the joints helping in locomotion.
- Bone is the storehouse of calcium salts.
- Involved in erythropoiesis.

### Classification of the Bone

#### According to their Position

1. *Axial*: Bones forming the axis of the body, e.g. skull, ribs, vertebrae.
2. *Appendicular*: Bones of the limbs.

#### According to the Shape

1. *Long bones*: They have three parts: Upper end, lower end and a middle shaft. The ends of these bones take part in forming the joint (articulates with other bone), e.g. bones of limbs (humerus, ulna, radius, femur, tibia, fibula).
2. *Short bones*: These bones are small and generally cuboidal in shape, e.g. carpal and tarsal bones.
3. *Flat bones*: These bones are expanded and are flat, e.g. sternum, scapula, ribs, and parietal bone.
4. *Irregular bone*: The shape is irregular without any proper outline, e.g. vertebrae, sphenoid, temporal bones, etc.

#### According to Gross Structure

1. *Compact (lamellar bone)*: Structurally it is made up of bony plates (lamellae) which are arranged compactly, e.g. outer cortical part of the long bone.
2. *Spongy bone (cancellous)*: Structurally it is made up of bony plates, which are arranged irregularly leaving spaces in between them. It gives a spongy appearance, and e.g. flat bones, irregular bones and ends of the long bone.
3. *Diploic bone*: It consists of inner and outer tables of compact bone with an interval, which is occupied by bone marrow and diploic veins, e.g. most of the cranial bones (parietal, frontal, occipital).

#### According to the Development

All the bones are developed from the mesoderm.

1. *Membranous bones*: The mesenchymal tissue (mesoderm) is directly transformed into a bone, e.g. clavicle, bones of the face and cranial vault.
2. *Cartilaginous bones*: The mesenchymal tissue is first transformed into a 'cartilage'. Later cartilage undergoes ossification to form bones, e.g. majority of the limb bones and bones at the base of the skull.

### SPECIAL TYPES OF BONES

1. *Pneumatic bones*: These are flat or irregular bones with hollow spaces in their body. These spaces contain air, e.g. ethmoid, maxilla, and mastoid part of temporal bone.
2. *Sesamoid bones (sesamoid = seed-like)*: These bones develop within the tendon of some muscles.
   - They do not possess periosteum and Haversian system.
   - They ossify after birth.
   - They minimise the friction and also change the direction of the pull of a muscle.

For example, pisiform bone (in the tendon of flexor carpi ulnaris muscle), patella (in the tendon of quadriceps femoris muscle), fabella (in the tendon of lateral head of gastrocnemius muscle).

### MACROSCOPIC STRUCTURE OF A BONE (Fig. 4.3)

- The long bone consists of two ends (epiphysis) and a shaft (diaphysis).
- The shaft consists of a cylindrical cavity inside called **'medullary cavity'**, which is filled with bone marrow. The outer (cortical) part of the shaft is made up of compact bone.
- The two ends of the long bone are filled with tiny plates of bone containing numerous spaces. This is referred as 'spongy bone' to which the medullary cavity does not extend.
- The outer surface of the bone is covered by a highly vascular connective tissue membrane called 'periosteum' except at the articular surfaces. This articular surface is covered by articular cartilage, usually hyaline type.

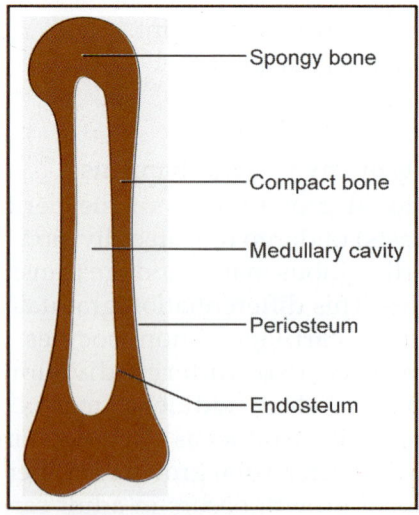

**Fig. 4.3:** Adult long bone

- The medullary cavity is lined by another connective tissue membrane called 'endosteum'.

## BONE MARROW

It is the vascular connective tissue present in the cavity (medullary cavity) of the bone. The bone marrow differs in composition in different bones and at different ages. It occurs in two forms, yellow marrow and red marrow. The red marrow is actively engaged in the production of blood cells. The yellow marrow derives its colour from the large quantity of fat cells it contains. At birth the red marrow is present throughout the skeleton. After about fifth year of postnatal life, the red marrow is gradually replaced in the long bones by yellow marrow.

### Microscopic Structure

An adult long bone consists of following components:
- Bone cells
- Matrix

### COMPACT BONE (Fig. 4.4a and b)

- The compact bone is made up of 'lamellae'.
- Lamellae are thin plates of bone consisting of collagen fibers embedded in ground substance.

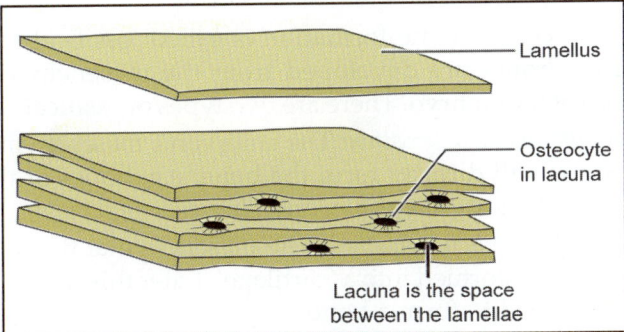

**Fig. 4.4a:** Lamellar bone

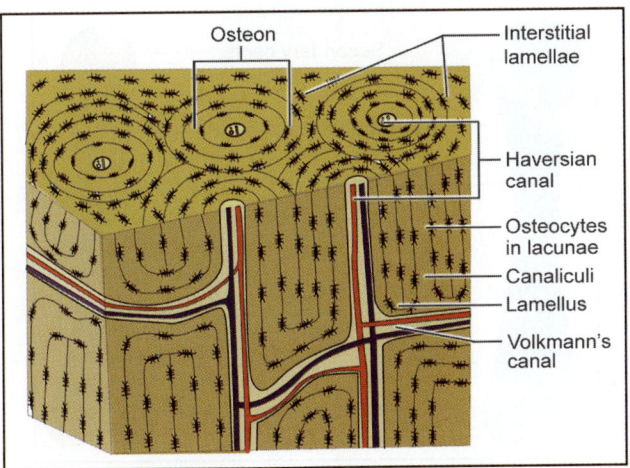

**Fig. 4.4b:** Haversian system of bone

- Lamellae are placed one over another.
- The spaces between the lamellae are called 'lacunae'.
- Lacunae are occupied by osteocytes.
- The adjacent lacunae are connected through canaliculi, which are occupied by cytoplasmic processes of osteocytes.
- Most of the lamellae are arranged in the form of concentric rings that surround a 'Haversian canal', which is present at the center of each ring.
- Haversian canals are placed parallel to medullary cavity and they are occupied by blood vessels and nerve fibers.
- Adjacent Haversian canals are connected by Volkman's canal.
- One Haversian canal and lamellae around it constitute a Haversian system or an Osteon (Fig. 4.4b).

### Matrix (Ground Substance)

The matrix of the bone consists of both organic and inorganic constituents.

**a. Organic constituent (25% of the matrix)**
- It is mainly made up of collagen fibers.
- These collagen fibers are embedded in proteins, carbohydrates and water.
- The collagen fibers are responsible for toughness and resilience of bone. These fibers are synthesized by osteoblasts.
- Chondroitin sulphate is another important organic constituent of the bone.

**b. Inorganic constituent (75% of the matrix)**
- Following mineral salts are present:
  Calcium phosphate (85%)
  Calcium carbonate (10%)
  Small amount of calcium fluoride and magnesium phosphate.
- Most of the calcium, phosphate and hydroxyl ions are in the form of needle-shaped crystals called 'hydroxyapatite crystals'.
- These crystals lie parallel to collagen fibers.

### BONE CELLS

### Osteoblasts

- These are bone forming cells.
- They are more numerous in periosteum.
- The cells are ovoid, triangular or cuboidal in shape with oval nucleus.

4

- These cells are responsible for laying down the organic matrix of bone including the collagen fibers.
- They are responsible for calcification of the matrix.

## Osteocytes

- These are mature bone cells.
- They are derived from osteoblasts after they have laid down the matrix.
- They are present in the 'lacunae' of the bone between the lamellae.
- Osteocytes show many cytoplasmic processes, which establish connections with other osteocytes.
- Osteocytes maintain the integrity of the lacunae and thus keep open the channels for diffusion of nutrients.

## Osteoclasts

- These are bone removing cells and found in relation to the surfaces of the bone.
- Osteoclasts are multinucleated large cells (diameter varies from 20 to 100 µm).
- The lysosomes present in their cytoplasm contain 'acid phosphatase'.
- Osteoclasts are involved in demineralization and removal of bone matrix.
- Osteoclasts are stimulated by parathyroid hormone.

## Periosteum

The external surface of the bone is covered by a connective tissue membrane called 'periosteum' except the articular surface.

The periosteum consists of outer fibrous layer and inner cellular layer consisting of osteoblasts.

## Parts of the Developing Long Bones (Figs 4.5 and 4.6)

1. *Epiphysis* is the part of the bone, which develops from the secondary center of ossification, e.g. ends of the long bones.

**Types of epiphyses**

a. *Pressure epiphyses:* They ossify from centers exposed to pressure at the joints, e.g. epiphysis of the head of the femur.

b. *Traction epiphyses:* They ossify from centers subjected to tension by the pull of the muscle, e.g. greater and lesser trochanters of the femur.

c. *Atavistic epiphyses:* These epiphysis are formed by centers of ossification which are believed to represent the skeletal elements which were separate in some lower vertebrates, e.g. coracoid process of scapula.

2. *Diaphysis* is the part of the bone, which develops from the primary center of ossification, e.g. shaft of the long bones.

3. *Metaphysis* is the zone of the bone where active growth is seen. It is present at the junction of the epiphysis and diaphysis of the long bones.

## Ossification

The process of bone formation is called 'ossification'. All the bones are developed from the mesenchymal tissue of the embryo. There are two types of ossification:

1. *Membranous ossification:* The embryonic mesenchymal tissue will directly form the bone, e.g. bones of the cranial vault, mandible, and clavicle.

2. *Cartilaginous ossification:* The mesenchymal tissue is first transformed into a 'cartilage'. Later this cartilage is ossified to form a bone.

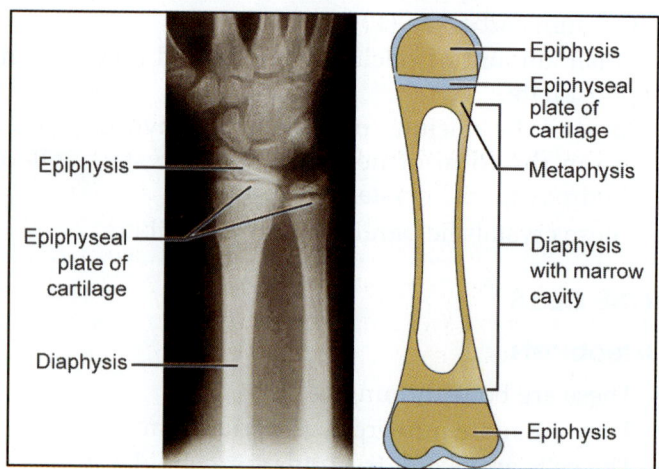

**Fig. 4.5:** Typical growing long bone

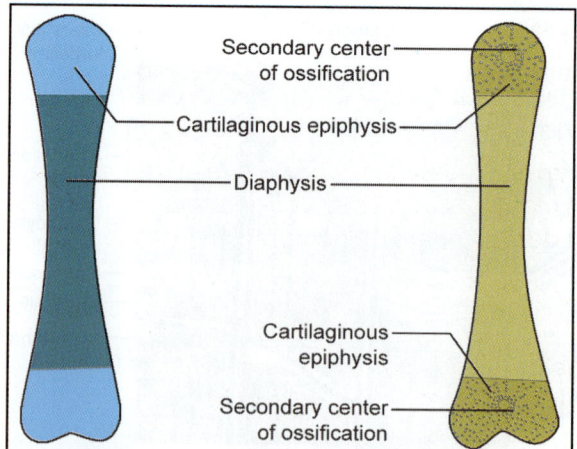

**Fig. 4.6:** Formation of a typical long bone

## Ossification of a Long Bone

The ossification begins in one or more areas of future bone model. These areas are called centers of ossification.

### Primary Center of Ossification

The ossification starts in the central part of the cartilaginous model (i.e. at the center of the future shaft). The portion of the long bone developed from this primary center of ossification is called 'diaphysis'. The primary center of ossification normally appears before birth.

### Secondary Center of Ossification

These centers appear at the two ends of the long bone usually after birth. The portion of the long bone developed from secondary center of ossification is called 'epiphysis'.

The two ends of the diaphysis, which are actively involved in growth, are called 'metaphyses'.

In a long bone between epiphysis and diaphysis is a part of the cartilage remains unossified until epiphysis fuses with diaphysis and it is called 'epiphyseal plate'. They also undergo ossification at puberty.

### Laws of Ossification

1. The epiphysis which ossifies first (or appears first) unites (fuses) with the diaphysis last and the epiphysis which ossifies last fuses first. Exception: lower end of the fibula.
2. The end of a long bone where epiphysis appears first and fuses last is called the 'growing end' of the bone.
3. The direction of nutrient artery is always away from the growing end.
4. In the long bones, growing ends fuse with the shaft at about 20 years and the opposite ends at about 18 years.

### Intramembranous Ossification (Dermal Ossification)

This type of ossification normally occurs in the deeper layers of the dermis, and the bones that result are often called dermal bones, e.g. clavicle. It involves following steps:

#### Step 1

Osteoblasts first cluster together and start to secrete the organic components of the matrix.

The matrix consists of collagen fibers then mineralised through crystalization of calcium salts.

The location in a bone where ossification first occurs is called primary ossification center. As ossification proceeds, it traps some osteoblasts inside bony pockets; these cells differentiate into osteocytes.

#### Step 2

The developing bone grows outward from the ossification center in small struts, called spicules. Although, osteoblasts are still being traped in the expanding bone, mesenchymal cell division continues to produce additional osteoblasts.

Bone growth is an active process and osteoblasts require oxygen and a supply of nutrients. Blood vessels that branch between the spicules meet these demands.

#### Step 3

Over the time, the bone assumes the strucure of spongy bone. Although, initially the intramembranous bone resembles spongy bone, subsequent remodelling around the trapped blood vessels can produce compact bone.

### Cartilaginous Ossification (Endochondral Ossification)

It begins with the formation of a hyaline cartilaginous model. It involves the following steps:

#### Step 1

As the cartilage enlarges, chondrocytes near the center of the shaft increase greatly in size and surrounding matrix begins to calcify. Deprived of nutrients these chondrocytes die and disintegrate.

#### Step 2

Cells of the perichondrium surrounding this region of the cartilage develop into osteoblasts. The perichondrium has now been converted into a periosteum and the inner organic layer soon produces a thin layer of bone around the shaft of the cartilage.

#### Step 3

While these changes are under way, the blood supply to the periosteum increases. Capillaries and osteoblasts migrate into the cartilage invading the space left by the disintegrating chondrocytes. The calcified cartilaginous matrix breaks down and osteoblasts replace it with spongy bone. Bone development proceeds from this primary center of ossification located in the shaft towards the ends of the cartilaginous model.

#### Step 4

While the diameter is small, the entire diaphysis is filled with spongy bone but as it enlarges osteoblasts erode

4

the central portion and create a bone marrow cavity. Further growth involves two distinct processes, an enlargement in diameter and an increase in the size.

## Bone Development and Growth

The growth of the skeleton determines the size and proportions of our body. The bony skeleton begins to form about six weeks after fertilization.

Bone growth continues through adolescence.

## Factors Regulating the Bone Growth

- Normal bone growth requires constant dietary source of calcium and phosphate salts.
- Vitamin A and C are essential for normal bone growth and remodelling. These vitamins are obtained from the diet.
- Vitamin D plays an important role in normal calcium metabolism by stimulating the absorption and transport of calcium and phosphate ions into the blood.
- The thyroid gland secretes the hormone calcitonin, which stimulates osteoblasts to produce new matrix.
- The secretion of parathyroid stimulates osteoclast activity.
- Growth hormone produced by the pituitary and thyroxin from the thyroid gland stimulate the bone growth.

## Blood Supply to a Long Bone (Fig. 4.7)

1. *Nutrient artery*: It enters the shaft through a nutrient foramen with one or two veins. On reaching the bone marrow cavity they divide into ascending and descending branches.
2. *Epiphyseal arteries*: They are several in numbers and enter the bone near the ends.
3. *Metaphyseal arteries*: They enter the bone along the line of attachment of capsular ligament (near the articular end).
4. *Periosteal arteries*: They are numerous and enter the bone along the muscular attachment.

Branches of all these arteries form a rich sinusoidal plexus in bone marrow. Many branches from the plexus enter Haversian canal.

These vessels provide blood to the superficial osteons of the shaft. During endochondral ossification, these vessels also enter the epiphyses providing blood to the secondary ossification centers. Following the closure of epiphyses all these sets of vessels becomes extensively interconnected.

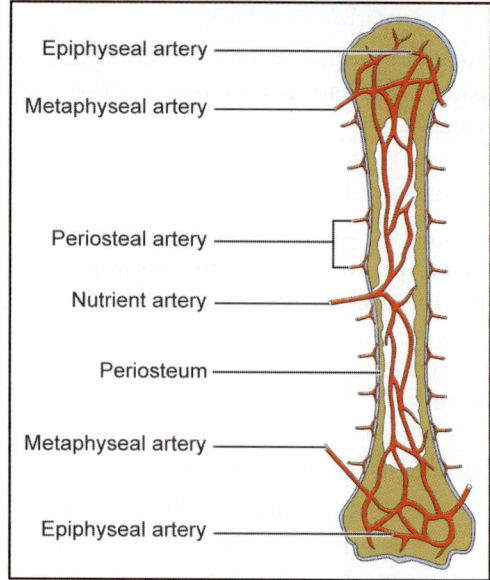

**Fig. 4.7:** Blood supply to a long bone

## Nerve Supply to the Bone

Bones are innervated by sensory nerves and injuries to the bone can be very painful.

## Applied Anatomy

A long bone that is taken from a fresh cadaver and soaked in a solution of weak acid for several weeks will maintain its original form but will look leathery and can be easily tied into a knot. The acid dissolves away the bone's mineral, leaving only the organic component (mainly collagen). The fact that a demineralised bone can be knotted demonstrates the great flexibility provided by collagen fibers within the bone. This fact also confirms that without its mineral content, bone bends too easily to support weight.

**Bone remodeling:** Bone remodeling may involve a change in the shape or internal architecture of a bone or a change in the total amount of minerals deposited in the skeleton. Osteoblasts and osteoclasts remain active even after the epiphyseal plates have closed. As one osteon forms through the activity of osteoblasts, another is destroyed by osteoclasts. The turnover rate for the bone is quite high. Each year almost one fifth of the adult skeleton is demolished and is rebuilt or replaced.

**Injury and repair:** Despite its mineral strength, bone may crack or even break if subjected to extreme loads or stresses from unusual directions. The damage produced constitutes a fracture. Healing of a fracture usually occurs even after severe damage, provided the blood supply and the cellular components of the endosteum and periosteum survive.

A fracture is the cracking or breaking of a bone. Radiographs (X-rays) are often used to diagnose the position and extent of fracture. Most fractures are caused by injuries and few results from diseases that weaken the bones. The following are the descriptions of several kinds of traumatic fracture:

1. Simple or closed: The fracture bone does not break through the skin.
2. Compound or open: The fractured bone is exposed to the outside through an opening in the skin.
3. Partial (fissured): The bone is completely broken
4. Complete: The fracture has separated the bone into two pieces
5. Capillary: A hair like crack occurs within the bone
6. Commumuted: The bone is splintered into small fragments
7. Spiral: The fracture line is twisted as it is broken
8. Avulsion: A portion of the bone is torn off.
9. Greenstick: In this incomplete break, one side of the bone is broken and the other side is bowed

When a bone fractures, medical treatment involves realigning the broken ends and then immobilizing them, until new bone tissue is formed and the fracture is healed. The methods of immobilization include tape, splints, casts, straps, wires and steel pins.

When bone is fractured the surrounding periosteum is usually torn and blood vessels in both tissues are ruptured. A blood clot called a fracture hematoma, soon forms throughout the damaged area. During healing of fracture a cartilaginous mass called a 'bony callus' fills the gap within the fragmented bone.

**Assessment of bone age:**

The knowledge of ossification of each bone is important in forensic science and anthropology. The sites where ossification appears, the rate at which they grow and time of fusion epiphyses with diaphysis for every bone is important even in clinical medicine. This knowledge is also important because the epiphyseal plates (cartilaginous structures) appear radiolucent (dark) could be mistaken for a fracture. The age of a young person can be determined from X-ray by assessing the ossification centers.

Loss of arterial supply to an epiphysis or other parts of a bone results in vascular necrosis of bone tissue. In children the disorders of epiphysis due to avascular necrosis is referred as 'osteochondroses'.

**Osteoporosis:** A reduction in organic and inorganic components of bone to a degree that compromises normal function. The bone becomes brittle, lose their elasticity, and fracture easily. Bone scanning will reveal the reduction of bone mass.

**Osteomalacia:** A softening of bone due to a decrease in the mineral content.

**Achondroplasia:** A condition resulting from abnormal epiphyseal activity. The epiphyseal plate grows unusually slow and the individual develops short, stocky limbs. The trunk is normal in size and sexual and mental development remains unaffected.

**Rickets:** A disorder that reduces the amount of calcium salts in the skeleton. It is characterised by a 'bowlegged' appearance.

# Muscles

**5**

Muscle is a contractile tissue, which brings movement of the body.

*Types*: There are three types—skeletal, cardiac and smooth muscles.

## SMOOTH MUSCLES (NON-STRIATED/INVOLUNTARY)
(Fig. 5.1a)

1. Each muscle fiber is an elongated spindle shaped cell with a single nucleus placed centrally.
2. The length of the smooth muscle is highly variable (15–500 μm).
3. They often aggregate to form bundles and fascicles.
4. They are found in the walls of gastrointestinal tract, respiratory tract, urogenital tract, blood vessels and a few muscles of the eye. They are arranged circularly inside and longitudinally outside in the walls of the gastrointestinal tract, urogenital tract, etc.
5. They do not exhibit cross striations and are smooth in form, supplied by autonomic nerves, hence involuntary.
6. They are made up of actin and myosin filaments.
7. These muscles respond slowly to stimuli, being capable of sustained contractions, therefore do not fatigue easily.

8. There are two types of smooth muscles—multi-unit and unitary.
   a. *Multi-unit smooth muscles*: Nerve fibers establish direct contact with several myocytes. Muscles contract under nervous stimulus, e.g. smooth muscles of iris and large arteries.
   b. *Unitary smooth muscles*: They have their own rhythmic contractility that is independent of nerve supply. Contraction of muscle is stimulated by stretch. However, the nerve supplying them can alter the rate of contraction, e.g. smooth muscles of the stomach, intestine, uterus and ureter.

## CARDIAC MUSCLE (STRIATED/INVOLUNTARY)

1. It forms the myocardium of the heart, shows striations but is involuntary. It is meant for automatic and rhythmic contractions.
2. Each muscle fiber has a single rounded nucleus placed centrally.
3. Each muscle fiber branches and anastomoses with the neighbouring fibers at intercalated discs.
4. Myocytes are about 80 μm long and 15 μm broad.

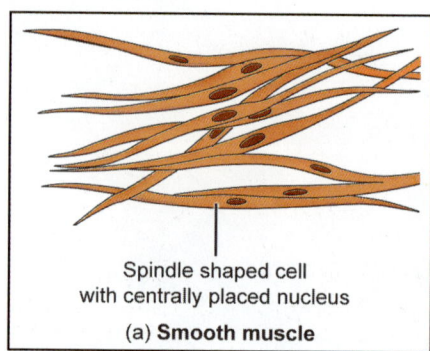

Spindle shaped cell
with centrally placed nucleus

**(a) Smooth muscle**

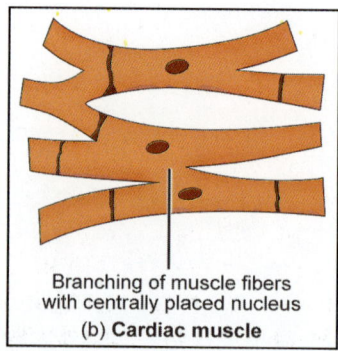

Branching of muscle fibers
with centrally placed nucleus

**(b) Cardiac muscle**

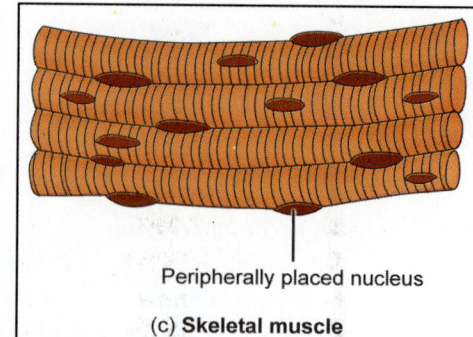

Peripherally placed nucleus

**(c) Skeletal muscle**

**Figs 5.1a to c:** Types of muscle fibers

5. The sarcoplasm contains more number of mitochondria and less number of myofibrils and sarcoplasmic reticulum when compared to skeletal muscle (Fig. 5.1b).

## SKELETAL MUSCLES (STRIATED/VOLUNTARY) (Fig. 5.1c)

1. These are most abundant, found attached to the skeletal system.
2. They exhibit cross striations under the microscope.
3. They are supplied by somatic (cerebrospinal) nerves, hence under voluntary control.
4. Each muscle fiber is a multinucleated cylindrical cell containing a group of muscle fibrils, e.g. muscles of the limb and body wall.

### Arrangement of the Muscle Fibers (Fig. 5.2)

The arrangement of muscle fibers varies according to the direction, force and range of movement at a particular joint. The force of contraction is directly proportional to the number and size of muscle fibers, and the range of movement is proportional to the length of the fiber.

The fascicles of the muscle can be parallel or oblique. When fascicles are obliquely set to the line of pull, the power of contraction is more, but range of movement is less.

Unipennate, e.g. palmar interossei of hand

Bipennate, e.g. rectus femoris

Multipennate, e.g. middle fibers of deltoid

### Lubricating Mechanisms for the Muscles

*Synovial bursa*: Bursa is a lubricating device to minimise the friction. Structurally, it is a closed sac of synovial membrane with synovial fluid. Bursa is often present around the joint but it can be subcutaneous. Bursa can communicate with joint cavity.

*Synovial sheaths*: The tendinous part of the muscle while passing deep to fibrous bands is surrounded by synovial sheath.

### Blood Supply

The blood vessels and nerves enter the muscle at a point called neurovascular hilum. The arteries branch repeatedly to form arteriole and capillaries in the muscle.

### Connective Tissue Support to the Muscle (Fig. 5.3)

A connective tissue membrane called endomysium surrounds each muscle fiber. Similar membrane covering each bundle of muscle fibers (fascicles) is called perimysium. Epimysium surrounds the entire muscle.

### Microscopic Structure of the Skeletal Muscle (Figs 5.4 and 5.5)

Each muscle is made up of a number of muscle fibers.

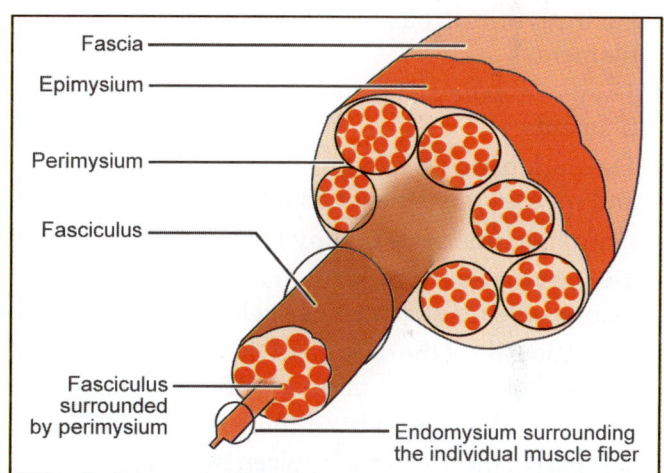

**Fig. 5.3:** Connective tissue framework of a skeletal muscle (transverse section)

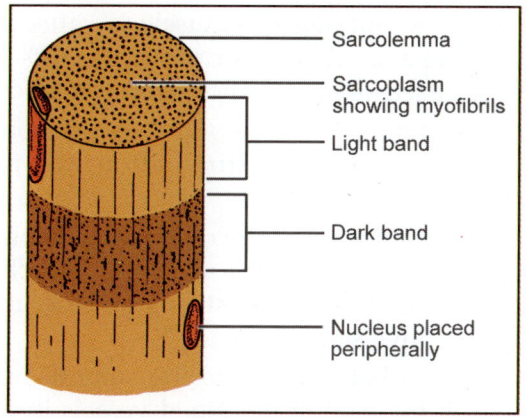

**Fig. 5.4:** An individual muscle fiber

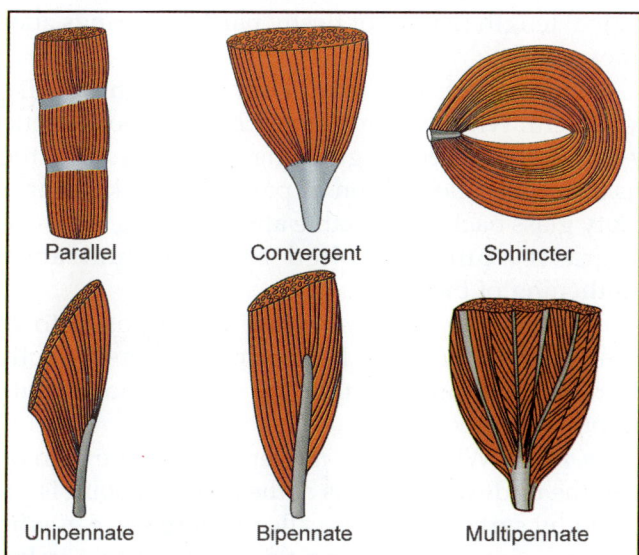

**Fig. 5.2:** Arrangement of fasciculi of skeletal muscle

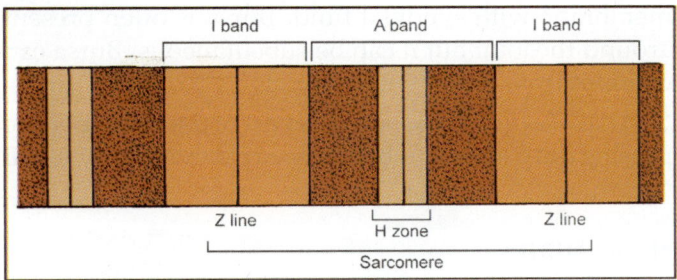

**Fig. 5.5:** A myofibril showing transverse bands

- Each muscle fiber is multinucleated and shows striations. They are also called myocytes and their length varies from 1–300 mm.
- The outer membrane of the muscle fiber is called sarcolemma and its cytoplasm is called sarcoplasm.
- The sarcoplasm shows many peripherally placed nuclei and large number of myofibrils.
- Each myofibril shows alternate dark and light bands.
- Dark bands are known as A bands (anisotropic) and the light bands as I bands (isotropic).
- Each myofibril has two protein filaments (myo-filaments).
- They are called actin (thin) and myosin (thick) filaments.
- The dark band (A band) is the area where the actin and myosin filaments overlap each other.
- Only actin filaments occupy the light band (I band).
- This arrangement of actin and myosin filament is responsible for striations of skeletal muscle.
- In the middle of the dark band there is a light H band where there are no actin filaments.
- In the middle of the I band there is a dark Z line.
- The part of the myofibril between two Z lines is called sarcomere.

## NERVE SUPPLY

- The nerve supplying the muscle is called motor nerve. However, this motor nerve has 60% motor fibers, 40% sensory fibers and also autonomic fibers.
- The motor fibers are axons of the ventral horn cells of the spinal cord. On stimulation, the muscle contracts.
- The sensory fibers arise from muscle spindles (stretch receptors present in the muscle) which give information about the status of the muscle (proprioceptive sensation).
- Autonomic fibers innervate the smooth muscles present in the wall of the blood vessels inside the skeletal muscles.

## NEUROMUSCULAR JUNCTION

A nerve supplying a muscle is composed of both motor and sensory components. As the motor portion of the nerve penetrates a muscle, it plays into a number of branching neuron processes called axons. The terminal ends of axons contact the sarcolemma of muscle fibers by means of motor end plates. Each axon may split into enough branches to serve dozens of muscle fibers. The area consisting of the motor end plate and the sarcolemma of the muscle fiber is known as the neuromuscular junction. Acetylcholine is a neurotransmitter chemical stored in synaptic vesicles at the terminal end of the axons. A nerve impulse reaching the terminal end of an axon causes the release of acetylcholine into the neuromuscular cleft of the neuromusclular junction. As this chemical mediator contacts the sarcolemma, it initiates physiological activity within the muscle fiber, resulting in contraction.

## MOTOR UNIT

A motor unit consist of a single motor neuron and the aggregation of muscle fibers innervated by the motor neuron. When a nerve impulse travels through a motor unit, all of the fibers served by it contract simultaneously to their maximum. Most muscles have an innervation ratio of one motor neuron per 100–150 muscle fiber. Muscle capable of precise movements, such as an eye muscle, may have an innervation ratio of 1:10. Massive musles that are responsible for gross body movements, such as those of the thigh may have an innervation ratio exceeding 1:500.

## ACTION OF MUSCLE

When a muscle contracts, it shortens by 30% of its original length (length of fleshy part) and brings about a movement.

*Agonists (prime movers):* They bring the desired movement. When a prime mover helps opposite action by active controlled lengthening against gravity, then this action is called action of paradox, e.g. keeping an empty glass back on the table after drinking is assisted by gravity but controlled by a gradual active lengthening of biceps brachii.

*Antagonists (opponents):* They are opposite to the prime movers, but they help prime movers by active controlled relaxation so that the desired movement is smooth and precise.

*Synergists:* When prime movers cross more than one joint, the undesired actions at the proximal joint is prevented by certain muscles called synergists, e.g. when making a tight fist by long flexors, the wrist is kept fixed in extension by the synergists (extensors of wrist).

## Applied Anatomy

**Muscle pull:** Skeletal muscles are limited in their ability to lengthen. Muscle cannot elongate beyond 1/3rd of its resting length with its bony attachments, beyond which the muscle sustain damage, which is often referred as muscle pull.

**Rigor mortis:** When death occurs, circulation ceases and the skeletal muscles are deprived of nutrients and oxygen. The calcium ions accumulate inside the sarcoplasm, which results in locking of the muscles in contracted position. All the skeletal muscles of the body are involved. This condition is called rigor mortis.

**Muscle hypertrophy:** Excessive increase in the activity of muscle results increase in number of myofibrils. This causes enlargement of the muscles / hypertrophy. Hypertrophy occurs in muscles that have been repeatedly stimulated. A champion weight lifter or body builder is an excellent example of hypertrophied muscular development.

**Muscle atrophy:** When a skeletal muscle is not stimulated by a motor neuron on a regular basis, it losses muscle tone and mass. The muscle becomes flaccid and the muscle fiber becomes smaller and weaker. This reduction in muscle size, tone and power is called atrophy.

**Paralysis:** The loss of power of contraction is called paralysis. It may be due to the injury to the nerve supplying it or the disease of the muscle itself. It is characterized by sudden and involuntary tightening of muscle fibers.

**Polio:** Progressive paralysis of muscles due to destruction of CNS motor neurons (ventral horn cells of the spinal cord) by the poliovirus.

**Fibrosis:** A process in which excess amounts of connective tissue develops, making muscles less flexible.

# Joints

**6**

The articulation between two or more bones is called joint.

Joints are classified into two types on the basis of presence or absence of joint cavity. They are:

1. *Synarthroses (without joint cavity):* Which is further divided into fibrous and cartilaginous variety.
2. *Diarthroses (synovial joints):* Which are mobile with synovial joint cavity.

## FIBROUS JOINTS

In this type of joint, the articulating surfaces of the bones are connected by fibrous tissue, and thus very little movement is possible. Following are the types of fibrous joints:

1. *Sutures:* Sutural ligament (fibrous connective tissue) connect the bones without allowing movement, e.g. many skull bones are held together by sutures (Fig. 6.1).
2. *Syndesmosis:* The articulating parts of the bones are connected by interosseus ligament, e.g. inferior tibiofibular joint.
3. *Gomphosis (peg and socket):* For example, tooth in its bony socket.

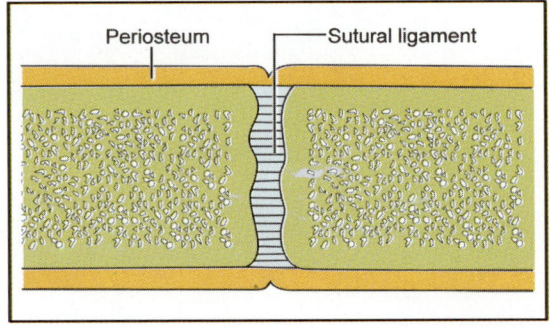

**Fig. 6.1:** Sutural variety of fibrous joint

## CARTILAGINOUS JOINTS

In these joints articulating surfaces are connected by a cartilage. There are two types of cartilaginous joints:

1. *Primary cartilaginous joint (synchondrosis):* The articulating ends of the bones are connected by a plate of hyaline cartilage. These joints are temporary because after certain age the cartilaginous plate is replaced by bone (it will ossify into a bone). These joints are immovable (Fig. 6.2a), e.g. (i) joint between the epiphysis and diaphysis of a growing long bone, (ii) joint between the body of the sphenoid and basilar part of the occipital bone.

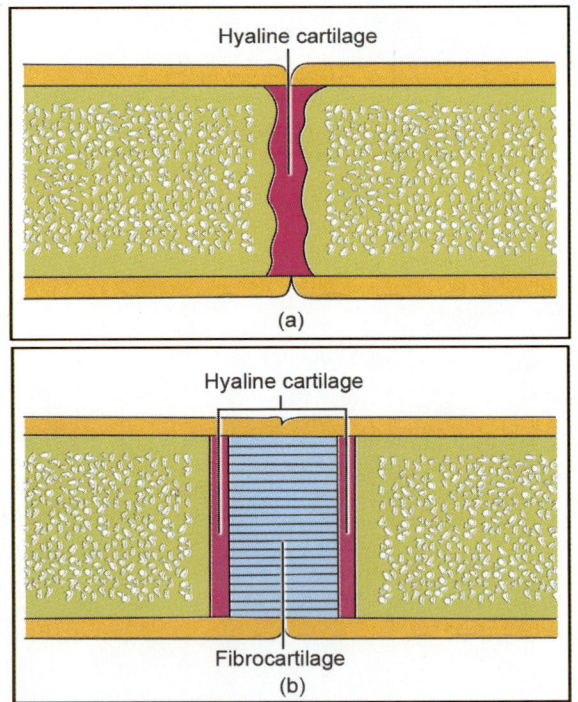

**Fig. 6.2a and b:** (a) Primary cartilaginous joint; (b) Secondary cartilaginous joint

2. *Secondary cartilaginous joint (symphysis)*: The articulating surface is covered by hyaline cartilage. However, an articular disc is present between the articulating surfaces. This articular disc is a white fibrocartilage. These joints are permanent (except symphysis menti). These joints allow a limited movement (Fig. 6.2b), e.g. pubic symphysis, manubriosternal joint, intervertebral joints between the bodies of vertebrae.

## SYNOVIAL JOINT

In a synovial joint the articular surfaces of the bones are separated by a joint cavity filled with synovial fluid. Synovial joints are highly mobile.

### Structure of a Typical Synovial Joint (Fig. 6.3)

1. *Articular surface*: The articulating surface is smooth and is covered by hyaline cartilage (in some cases by white fibrocartilage, e.g. temporomandibular joint). This articular cartilage is avascular, non-nervous and nourished by synovial fluid. These articular cartilages provide slippery surface for the free movement.

2. *Joint cavity*: The space between the articulating surfaces is called joint cavity, which is filled with synovial fluid. In some joints, the cavity is divided into two compartments by the presence of an articular disc or meniscus (complex joint). A fibrous capsule externally closes the joint cavity.

3. *Fibrous capsule*: Structurally, it is made up of collagen and elastic fibers, which provide strength and elasticity respectively. Functionally, it holds the two bones and prevents their dislocation. It is attached to the margins of the articulating surfaces. It has stretch receptors, which are innervated by nerve fibers. They carry the information from the joint (proprioceptive information) and also execute reflexes to protect the joint from any sprain. Fibrous capsule has rich vascular plexus.

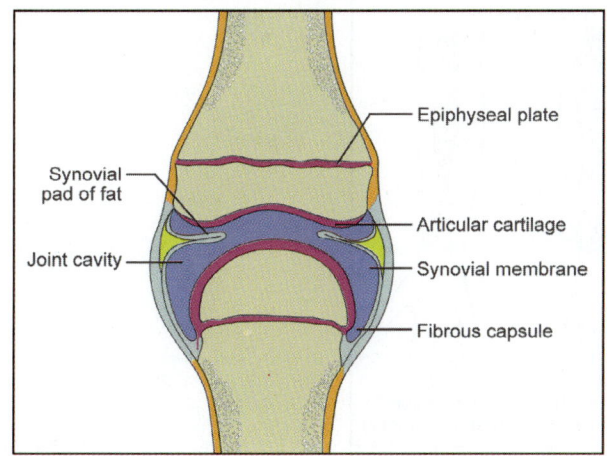

Synovial pad of fat

Joint cavity

Epiphyseal plate

Articular cartilage

Synovial membrane

Fibrous capsule

**Fig. 6.3:** Typical synovial joint

4. *Synovial membrane*: The fibrous capsule is lined by synovial membrane on its inner aspect. It is a highly vascular and cellular connective tissue membrane. They secrete synovial fluid and also hyaluronic acid, which maintains viscosity of the fluid.

5. *Synovial fluid*: It is a viscous fluid present in the joint cavity. It contains hyaluronic acid, monocytes, lymphocytes, macrophages and traces of protein. It provides nutrition to the articular cartilage and also lubrication to the joint.

6. *Ligaments*: The synovial joint is stabilized by ligaments outside or inside the fibrous capsule. They may be thickened portions of the fibrous capsule or separate structures. These ligaments permit desirable movements and prevent undesirable ones. Their main function is to maintain stability of the joint. The tone of the muscles around the joint is an important factor in maintaining the stability.

### Types of Synovial Joints

Synovial joints are classified into many subtypes according to the shape of the articular surfaces and types of movement occurring in them.

1. *Plane joints*: In these joints, the articular surfaces are flat permitting only sliding movement, e.g. acromioclavicular joint and joints between the articular processes of the vertebrae.

2. *Hinge joints*: These joints resemble the hinge on a door. Only flexion and extension movements are possible, e.g. elbow joint, knee joint (modified hinge), and ankle joint.

3. *Pivot joints*: In these joints, there is a central pivot or an axis surrounded by a bony or ligamentous ring. In this joint either the pivot or the ring rotates. Rotation is the only movement possible, e.g. atlantoaxial joint, superior radioulnar joint.

4. *Condylar joints*: A condylar articulation is structured so that an oval, convex articular surface of one bone fits into an elliptical, concave depression on another bone. This permits angular movement in two directions as in an up-and-down and side-to-side motion, e.g. temporomandibular joint, knee joint.

5. *Ellipsoid joints*: In these joints, there is an elliptical convex articular surface that fits into an elliptical concave articular surface. The movements are flexion, extension, abduction and adduction, but rotation is not possible, e.g. wrist joint.

6. *Saddle joints*: In these joints, the articular surfaces are reciprocally concavoconvex and resemble a saddle on a horse's back. This joint permits flexion, extension, abduction and rotation, e.g. carpometacarpal joint of the thumb.

6

7. *Ball and socket joints:* In these joints, a ball-shaped head of one bone fits into a socket-like concavity of another. This arrangement permits very free movements, including flexion extension, abduction, adduction, medial and lateral rotation and circumduction, e.g. shoulder joint and hip joint.

### Blood Supply to a Synovial Joint

The epiphysial branches of the artery supplying the bone form a periarticular plexus close to the attachment of fibrous capsule. Numerous minute vessels arising from this plexus pierce the fibrous capsule and form a rich vascular plexus on the outer surface of the synovial membrane. The blood vessels of the synovial membrane supply capsule, synovial membrane and the epiphysis. Before the fusion of epiphysis with metaphysis these vessels do not anastamose with metaphyseal arteries. However, after fusion, the communications between epiphyseal and metaphyseal arteries are established.

### Nerve Supply to a Synovial Joint

The nerve supplying the joint contain sensory and autonomic fibers. The sensory fibers are *proprioceptive*

in function. They provide the information regarding position and movement of the joint. They are concerned with reflex control of posture and locomotion. They also convey pain sensation from the joint. The autonomic fibers provide motor fibers to the blood vessels. The capsule and ligaments possess a rich nerve supply and specialized receptors (Golgi tendon end organs).

### Hilton's Law

It claims that, a motor nerve supplying a muscle which acts on a joint also supplies skin covering that particular joint.

### Movements at Synovial Joints

Movements at synovial joints are produced by the contraction of skeletal muscles that span the joints and attached to the bones articulating. In these actions, the bones act as levers, the muscles provide the force, and the joints are the fulcra or pivots (Figs 6.4 and 6.5).

The range of movement at a synovial joint is determined by the structure of the individual joint and the arrangement of the associated muscle and the bone. The movement at hinge joint, e.g. occurs in only one plane, whereas the structure of a ball and socket joint

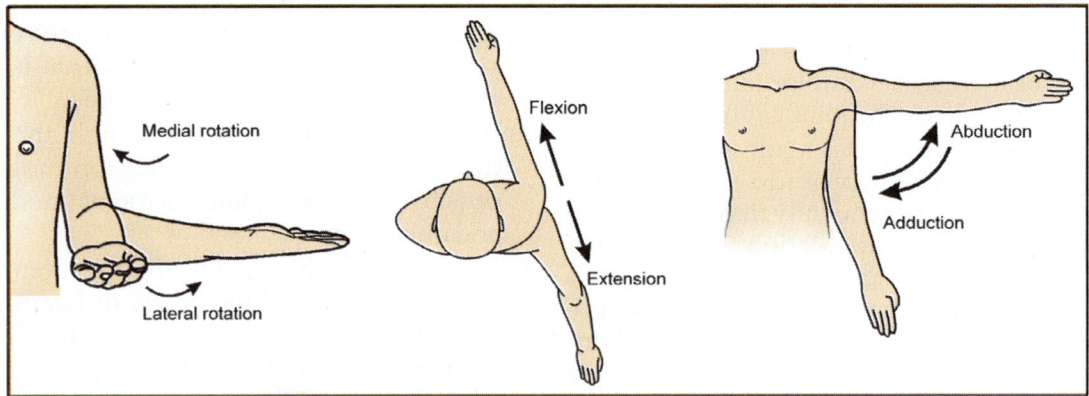

**Fig. 6.4a:** Movements at the shoulder joint

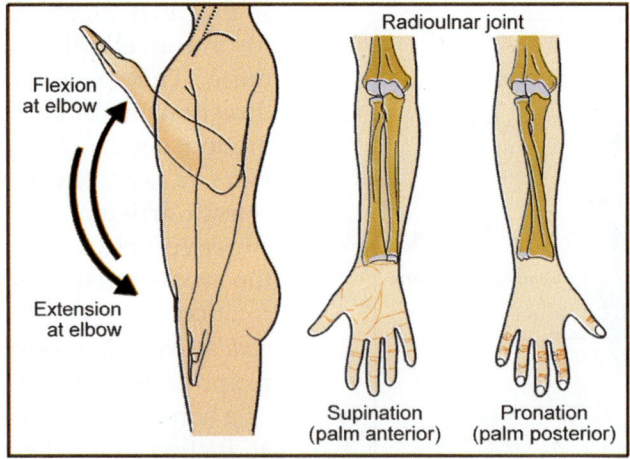

**Fig. 6.4b:** Movements of the upper limb

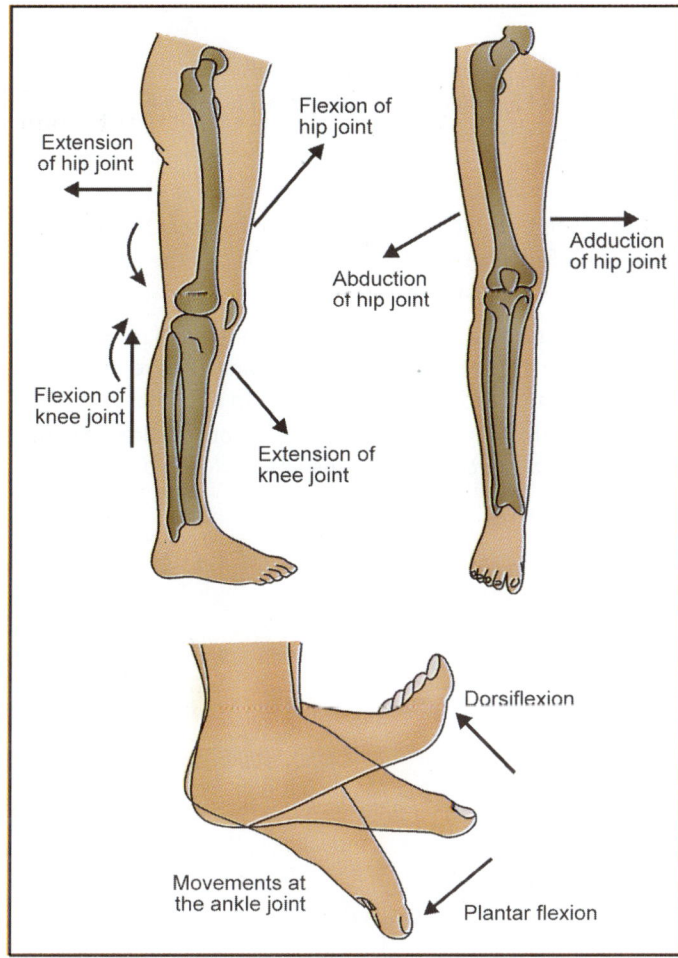

**Fig. 6.5:** Movements at the lower limb

180°. The exception to this is the ankle joint, in which there is a 90° angle between the foot and leg in the anatomical position. Examples of extension are the straightening of the elbow or knee joints from flexion positions. Hyperextension occurs when a part of the body is extended beyond the anatomical position so that the joint angle is greater than 180°. An example of hyperextension is tipping the head backwards.

3. *Abduction:* Abduction is the movement of a body part away from the main axis of the body or away from the midsagittal plane, in a lateral direction. Examples of abductions are moving the arms sideward and away from the body or spreading the fingers apart.

4. *Adduction:* The opposite of abduction is the movement of a body part towards the main axis of the body. In the anatomical position the arms and legs have been adducted towards the midplane of the body.

## Circular Movements

Joints that permit circular movement are composed of a bone with a rounded or oval surface that articulates with a corresponding cup or depression on another bone. The two basic types of circular movements are rotation and circumduction.

1. *Rotation:* Rotation is the movement of the body part around its own axis. There is no lateral displacement during this movement. Examples are turning the head from side to side in a 'no' motion.

   Supination (rotation of the forearm in which the palm of the hand being turned anteriorly) and pronation (rotation of the forearm in which the palm being turned posteriorly) are the specialised rotations of forearm.

2. *Circumduction:* Circumduction is the circular, conelike movement of a body segment. The distal extrimity forms the circular movement and proximal attachment forms the pivot. The example for circumduction is the bowling action (in cricket) at shoulder joint.

   Eversion (elevating lateral border of the foot), inversion (elevating the medial border of the foot), protraction, retraction, elevation and depressions are the special movements described in certain joints (Fig. 6.6).

permits movements around many axes. Joint movements are broadly classified as angular and circular.

## Angular Movements

Angular movements increase or decrease the joint angle produced by the articulating bones. Following are the types of angular movements:

1. *Flexion:* Flexion is a movement that decreases the joint angle on an anteroposterior plane. Examples of flexion are the bending of the elbow or knee. Flexion of the elbow joint is a forward movement, whereas flexion of the knee is a backward movement. Flexion in most joints is simple to understand, such as flexion of the neck as the head is bowed. In the ankle joint the flexion occurs as the dorsum of the foot is elevated. This movement is frequently called dorsiflexion. Pressing the foot forward is plantar flexion.

2. *Extension:* In extension, which is the reverse of flexion, the joint angle is increased. Extension returns the body to the anatomical position. In an extended joint the joint angle between the articulating bone is

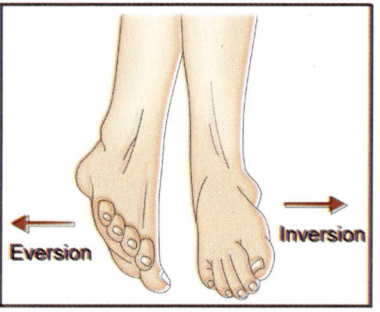

**Fig. 6.6:** Inversion and eversion

## Applied Anatomy

**Dislocation (luxation):** The articulating surfaces of the bones are forced out of position. This displacement can damage the articular cartilages, tear ligaments or distort the joint capsule. The capsule and ligaments are innervated by nerves and hence dislocation is very painful. The damage accompanying a partial dislocation or subluxation is less severe.

**Sprain:** The ligamentous tear is called sprain which causes severe pain in the joint.

Age related structural changes in the articular cartilages are main cause of joint problems in elderly people often affecting the weight bearing joints like knee and hip. The articular cartilage becomes less effective shock absorber as a result the articulation becomes vulnerable to repeated friction that occurs during joint movement. This can cause severe pain.

**Arthritis:** It is the inflammation of the joint(s). It can be caused by a variety of diseases. The joint is swollen and movements are restricted and painful (rheumatic arthritis, rheumatoid arthritis). Osteoarthritis is a degenerative joint disease in elderly people characterized by stiffness, discomfort, and pain. It usually affects the weight bearing joints-like hip and knee.

**Arthroscopy:** It is a procedure by which the joint cavity can be examined through an arthroscope. This procedure not only helps in identifying joint abnormalities (such as torn menisci), but some surgical procedures can also be performed during this procedure.

# Blood Vessels and Lymphatic System

**7**

Blood vessels and lymphatic vessels are tubular channels, which carry nutrients to the tissue and metabolites back from the tissue into circulation (Fig. 7.1).

Heart acts as a pumping organ which pumps oxygenated blood (arterial blood) to all the parts of the body through arteries. The deoxygenated blood (venous blood) is brought back to the heart by veins, which is later carried to the lungs for oxygenation.

## ARTERIES

- They carry blood away from the heart.
- They branch like trees on their way to different parts of the body.

- The tiny branches of arteries are called 'arterioles' with diameter greater than 0.3 mm.
- Arteries are thick walled, being uniformly thicker than the accompanying veins.
- The lumen is smaller than that of the veins accompanying it.
- Arteries do not have any valves.

### Structure of an Artery

The basic structure of the artery and the vein is almost same with few differences. Figure 7.2 shows the different layers of the wall of the blood vessels.

- The wall of the artery is made up of three layers, tunica intima, media and adventitia (from inside to outside).

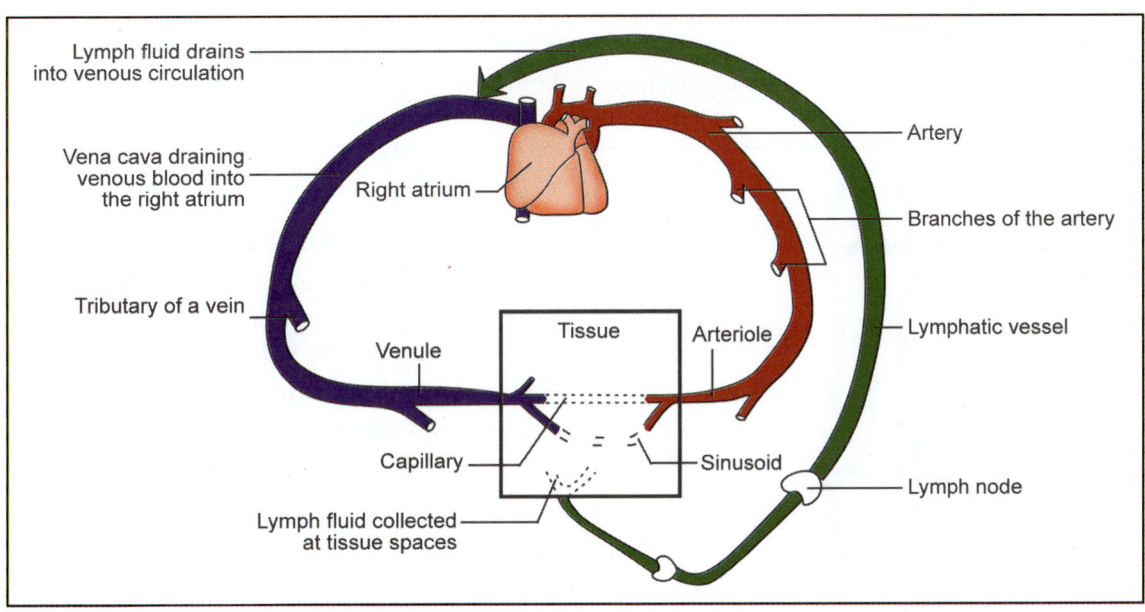

**Fig. 7.1:** Organization of blood vessels

43

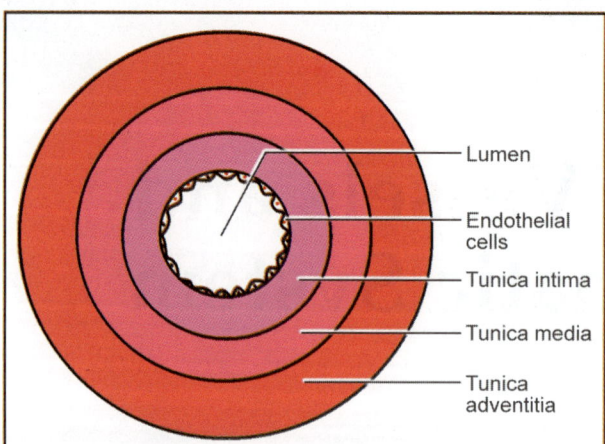

**Fig. 7.2:** Layers of blood vessels

- Endothelium is the lining epithelium and is part of the tunica intima.
- Tunica media is the thickest of all the three coats, which is made up of elastic fibers and smooth muscles.
- The large arteries contain more elastic fibers and medium sized artery has more smooth muscles.
- Small arteries called 'vasa vasorum' nourish the wall of the large artery.
- Internal elastic lamina is a membrane formed by elastic fibers just deep to the endothelium of the tunica intima. It is better defined in medium sized arteries.

## VEINS

- They bring blood from various tissues of the body back into the heart.
- The veins are formed by the union of many tributaries (like a river).
- The small veins are called 'venules', they join to form veins, which further form large veins and finally vena cavae before entering the heart.
- Veins are thin walled, being thinner than the arteries.
- Their lumen is larger.
- Veins have 'valves' which are reduplications of endothelium. They maintain the unidirectional flow of blood even

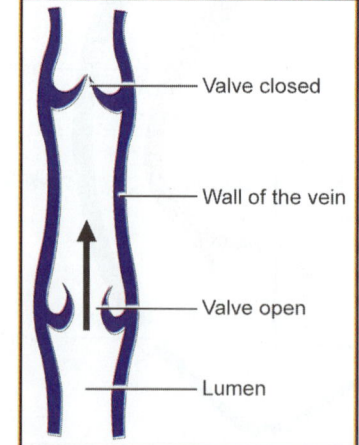

**Fig. 7.3:** Valves inside the veins

against gravity (Fig. 7.3). However, some of the veins do not have valves, e.g. emissary veins and veins of the vertebral column.

## Structure of a Vein

- The wall of the veins is made up of three layers like arteries—tunica intima, media and adventitia (from inside to outside). Endothelium is the lining epithelium and is part of the tunica intima. Tunica media has a mixture of connective tissue and a few smooth muscle fibers.
- Tunica adventitia is the thickest and best developed in large veins. Tunica adventitia has large amount of smooth muscle fibers along with collagen and elastic fibers.
- The muscular and elastic tissue content of the venous wall is much less than that of the arteries.
- The walls of the larger veins are supplied by nutrient vessels called 'vasavasorum', which may penetrate up to the tunica intima.

## Blood Supply to the Wall of the Blood Vessels

The large arteries (of more than 1 mm diameter) and veins are supplied by nutrient vessels called vasavasorum. They form a capillary network in tunica adventitia and outer part of the tunica media. The inner portion of the vessel wall (tunica intima) is nourished directly by diffusion from the luminal blood. However, in the veins, the vessels may penetrate up to the intima, probably because of the low venous pressure. Minute veins accompanying the arteries drain the blood from the outer part of the arterial wall. Lymphatics are also present in the adventitia.

## Nerve Supply to the Blood Vessels

They are supplied by non-myelinated sympathetic fibers, which are vasoconstrictor in function (with exception). Myelinated nerve fibers are believed to be sensory in function.

## Capillaries (Capillus = hair)

These are microscopic blood vessels within the tissue. They have single layer of endothelial cells resting on a basement membrane, without any outer coats (Fig. 7.4a).
- Capillaries have arterial and venous ends.
- The diameter of a capillary is 6–8 microns, however, the capillaries of skin and bone marrow have larger diameter.

## Sinusoids

- Sinusoids replace capillaries in certain organs like liver, spleen, bone marrow and endocrine glands.

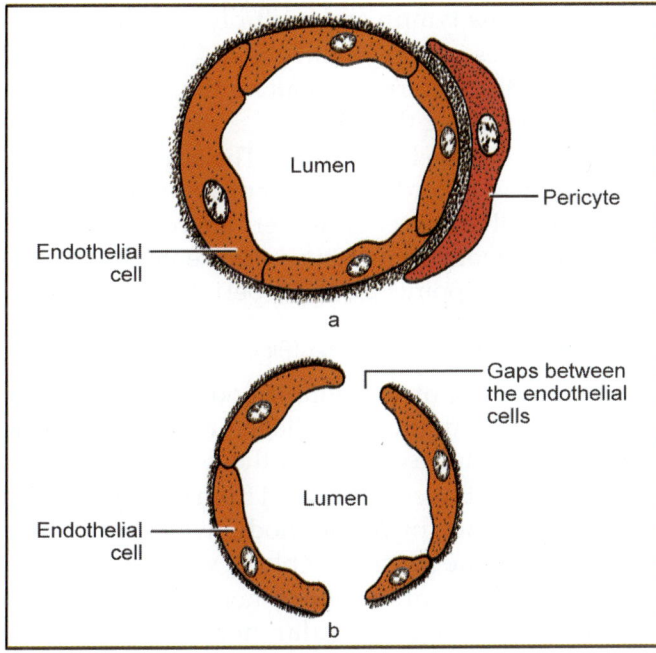

**Fig. 7.4:** Cross-section: (a) Continuous capillary, (b) sinusoid

- The lumen of the sinusoid is large and irregular.
- Their wall is thinner and incomplete with spaces between endothelial cells.
- The basal lamina of endothelial cells is replaced by fine reticular fibers (Fig. 7.4b).

## ANASTOMOSIS

A precapillary or postcapillary communication between the neighbouring vessels is called anastomosis.

## Types

1. *Arterial anastomosis:* The terminal branches of arteries or arterioles join with each other to form anastomosis, e.g. palmar arch, plantar arch, circle of Willis, intestinal arcades. On sudden occlusion of a main artery, the anastomosis may facilitate a collateral circulation.

2. *Venous anastomosis:* It is the communication between the veins or tributaries of the vein, e.g. dorsal venous arch of hand and foot.

3. *Arteriovenous anastomosis:* It is the direct communication between the arteries and veins. There will be a network of capillaries between the arteriole and venule. When the organ is at rest the blood bypasses these capillaries (Fig. 7.5). The arteriovenous anastomosis is observed in skin, nasal cavity, lips, mucous membrane of the alimentary canal, erectile tissue, tongue, thyroid gland, etc.

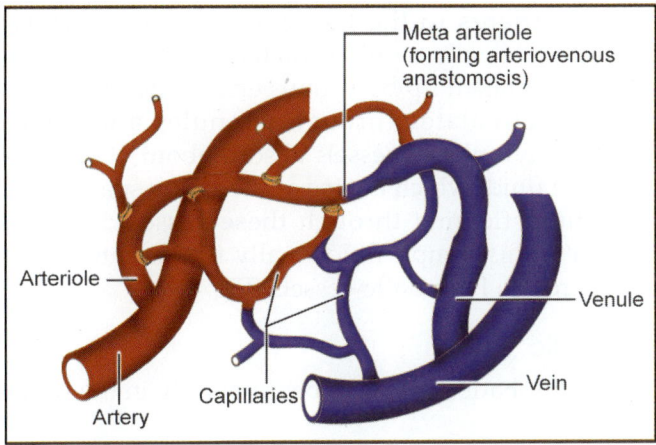

**Fig. 7.5:** Microcirculation at capillary level

## End Arteries

Arteries which do not anastomose with their adjacent arteries are called end arteries. Occlusion of an end artery causes severe ischemia resulting in death of the tissue. Occlusion of central artery of retina results in permanent blindness.

*Examples:* (i) Central artery of retina, (ii) central branches of cerebral arteries and (iii) vasae rectae of the mesenteric arteries.

### Types of Circulation

1. *Systemic circulation:* The arterial blood ejects from left ventricle, then ascending aorta. Then the arterial tree branches repeatedly to form microscopic vessels within the tissue or organ to provide nutrition. The venous blood from these tissue/organs enter venous tree which finally drain into right atrium. The blood flow is from left to the right.

2. *Pulmonary circulation:* The venous blood from the right ventricle goes to lung through pulmonary arteries. In the lung they get oxygenated and returns back to left atrium through pulmonary veins.

3. *Portal circulation:* The two ends of the vessels are capillaries. It begins from capillaries and ends in capillaries. For example, the venous blood from the wall of the stomach, intestine (having absorbed nutrients) begins from capillaries in the wall of stomach or intestine. These portal vessels end in liver again by breaking into capillaries/sinusoids. Portal system is also present in pituitary gland.

## LYMPHATIC SYSTEM

Lymphatic system is a drainage system, which removes larger particles from the tissue fluid.

The lymphatic system consists of:

- Lymph vessels
- Lymphoid organs
- Circulating lymphocytes

7

The nutrients to the tissue are given by artery, arteriole and finally capillaries at tissues. The fluid from the tissue is taken up by venous end of the capillaries and then circulates through vennules and veins. However, lymphatic vessels absorb about 10–20% of the tissue fluid, which begins at the tissue spaces. The tissue fluid flowing through these vessels is called **"lymph"**. This lymph fluid finally drains into larger veins through lymphatic vessels (Fig. 7.1).

## Lymphatic Vessels

- The lymphatic capillaries begin blindly in the tissue spaces.
- Lymphatic vessels are connected to each other forming a network.
- The superficial lymphatic vessels accompany veins while deep lymphatic vessels accompany arteries.
- Larger lymphatic vessels are named, e.g. thoracic duct.
- Lymph nodes are present in relation to the lymphatic vessels.
- The caliber of lymphatic capillary is greater and less regular than blood capillaries.
- Lymph fluid is colorless but in the intestine it is milk-white due to absorption of fat. It is called **chyle**.
- Lymphatic capillaries are absent in brain, spinal cord, bone marrow and other avascular structures.

## Lymphoid Organs

Lymphatic organs are classified into central and peripheral parts.

a. Central lymphatic organs are bone marrow and thymus.
- The lymphoid stem cells are produced by bone marrow except during early fetal life (produced by spleen and liver).
- The stem cell undergoes differentiation in these central lymphatic organs and becomes competent.
- Bone marrow differentiates the B lymphocytes, which are capable of synthesizing antibodies.
- Thymus differentiates immunologically competent but uncommitted T lymphocytes.

b. Peripheral lymphatic organs include lymph nodes, spleen, tonsil and lymphoid tissue present in the wall of the gastrointestinal and respiratory tracts.
- The B and T lymphocytes reach peripheral lymphatic organs where they proliferate and mature into immunocompetent cells.

## Lymph Nodes

- Lymph nodes are oval or bean-shaped structures present in the course of small lymphatic vessels.
- They filter the lymph and multiply lymphocytes.
- Lymph nodes are present in-groups. The superficial lymph nodes are arranged along the veins and the deep nodes along the arteries.
- Each lymph node has a hilum. The artery enters the node and vein and one efferent lymphatic vessel emerge at this place. However, afferent lymphatic vessels are many in number, which enter the lymph node at many points along its periphery.

## Structure of a Lymph Node (Fig. 7.6)

1. Outer covering of the lymph node is made up of connective tissue fibers (collagen and a few elastic fibers) which form capsule of the lymph node.
- Number of trabeculae extend from the capsule into the substance of lymph node, which provide a media for the passage of blood vessels.
- The substance of the lymph node shows reticular fibers forming irregular network on which lymphocytes are placed.

2. The substance of the lymph node is divided into **outer cortex** and **inner medulla**.
- The cortex is absent at the hilum.
- Lymphocytes are arranged in the form of follicles (or nodules) in the cortex. Each lymphatic follicle consists of densely packed lymphocytes outside and large lymphocytes (lymphoblasts) called germinal center in the middle.

3. The medulla shows medullary cords where lymphocytes are arranged in irregular masses with spaces in between them called medullary sinuses. These **medullary sinuses contain lymph fluid.**

4. Apart from the lymphocytes, the lymph node also has macrophages, plasma cells and reticulocytes.

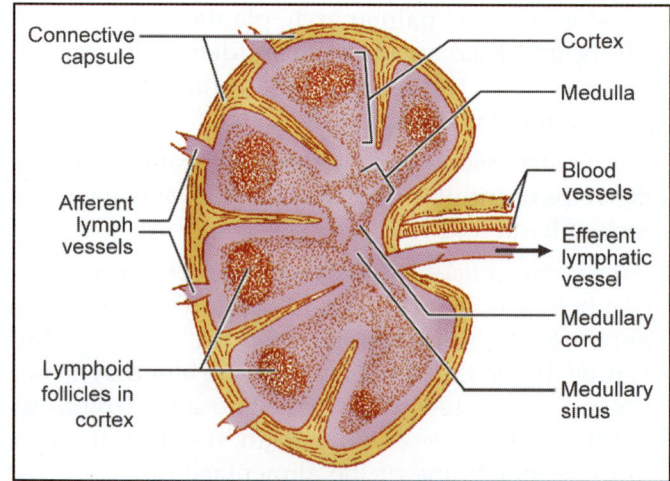

**Fig. 7.6:** Structure of a lymph node

5. The afferent lymphatic vessel entering the lymph node at multiple sites opens into a subcapsular sinus. The subcapsular sinuses are connected with medullary sinuses through radiating cortical sinuses. The lymph collected in the medullary sinuses is drained out from the lymph node by efferent lymphatic vessel (Fig. 7.6).

## Functions of the Lymphoid System

1. Lymphatic vessels drain large protein molecules from the tissue places. Thus cellular debris and foreign particles (dust particles inhaled into the lungs, bacteria and other micro-organisms) are drained by this system.
2. Lymphatic vessels help in transportation of fat from the gut.
3. Lymph node serves the following functions:
   • They filter the lymph and prevent the foreign particles entering into the bloodstream.
   • The foreign particles are phagocytosed by macrophages.
   • They lymphocytes multiply in the lymph nodes.
   • These lymphocytes provide both humoral and cellular immunity against the antigens.

## Applied Anatomy

**Hemorrhage:** (bleeding) It is a flow of blood (bleeding). Arterial hemorrhage causes spurting of bright red blood and venous haemorrhage cause oozing (steady stream) of dark blood

**Arteriosclerosis:** In old age the arteries become stiff. It is a thickening and toughening of arterial wall. The amount of blood flow through these arteries is reduced which can rise the systolic blood pressure.

**Atherosclerosis:** A type of arteriosclerosis characterised by changes in the endothelial lining. A fatty mass of tissue is projected into the lumina of the vessels.

**Ischemia:** It refers to reduction of blood supply to an organ or region as consequences of atherosclerosis or a thrombus formation or occlusion of a vessel by adjacent structure. Arterial occlusion resulting in ischemia is characterized by **5 Ps—pallor (pale), pain, puffiness, pulselesness and paralysis** (involving muscles)

**Infarction:** It refers to death or necrosis of an area of tissue or an organ resulting from reduced blood supply. Such infarction in heart causes heart attack, stroke in brain and gangrene in distal parts of the limbs.

**Arteritis:** An inflammation of an artery is called arteritis. Inflammation of a vein is called 'phlebitis'.

**Thrombosis:** It is the coagulation of blood in the vessels. The clot thus formed is termed as thrombus.

**Embolism:** An obstruction of blood vessel, usually an artery by a thrombus, fat cells, air, etc.

**Aneurysm:** A permanent dilatation of an artery usually with rupture of the internal and middle coats. The thoracic aorta and the innominate artery (brachiocephalic trunk) are usually affected.

**Varicose veins:** This refers to abnormally dilated and twisted superficial veins, which more frequently affects the limbs. The walls of the vein become weak and do not withstand the pressure resulting in its dilation. The valves becomes incompetent, thus the blood flow towards the heart is unbroken causing more pressure to the valves. Varicose vein can also occur due to inflammation of valves.

**Lymphadenopathy:** It refers to chronic or excessive enlargement of lymph node.

**Lymphomas:** A malignant cancers consisting of abnormal lymphocytes or lymphocytic stem cells.

**Autoimmune disorder:** A disorder that develops when the immune response mistakenly targets normal body cells and tissues.

**Lymphangitis:** Inflammation of the lymphatic vessels can occur while draining an infected area. The lymphangitis are marked on the skin as painful red lines and swollen lymph nodes.

**Elephantiasis:** The filarial parasite in the lymphatic vessel may block it and results in edema (elephantiasis) in the peripheral area of the drainage.

*Cancer spread through lymphatic vessels:* Cancer can invade the adjacent tissue by direct contact and spread into distant sites (metastasis) by lymphatic vessels or blood vessels. Lymphatic route is the most common way of metastasis. Hence lymphatic drainage of those organs which are commonly involved in cancer should be studied in greater detail which is helpful in the diagnosis of the primary site of the cancer. From the affected organ the cancer spread in the direction of lymph from that organ, hence it is important to know proximal and distal sets of lymph nodes for each organ. Understanding of lymphatic drainage of an organ helps in:
1. To know what nodes are likely to be affected when a tumor is identified in an organ or a tissue
2. To be able to locate the likely sites of primary cancerous sites, when enlarged node is detected.

7

# Nervous Tissue

The human nervous system is the most complex physical system known to mankind. At present our understanding of this complex system seems to be very rudimentary. This system provides a complex mechanism by which the living organism can react to the ever-changing external and internal environment and thus enabling the survival of human species.

## NERVOUS TISSUE

Nervous tissue consists of two types of cells: Neurons and neuroglial cells.

### Neurons

- Neurons are basic structural and functional units of the nervous system.
- They respond to physical and chemical stimuli.
- They conduct the impulses and release specific chemical regulators.
- Neurons cannot divide mitotically, but some neurons can regenerate.

### Microscopic Structure of a Neuron (Fig. 8.1)

The principal components of the neurons are:
- Cell body
- Dendrites
- Axon

### *Cell Body* (Fig. 8.2)

- The cytoplasm of the cell body is covered by a cell membrane with centrally placed nucleus.
- The cytoplasm presents numerous mitochondria, Golgi complex, ribosomes and lysosomes.
- It has been said that centrioles are absent in neurons, however, recent electron microscopic studies have confirmed the presence of centriole.

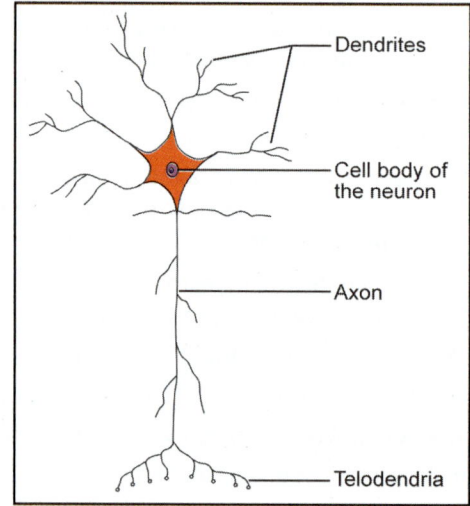

**Fig. 8.1:** Parts of the neuron

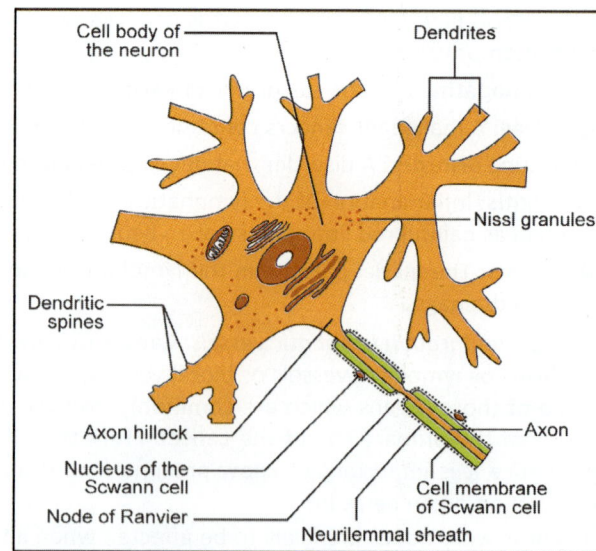

**Fig. 8.2:** Schematic presentation of a neuron

48

- The most characteristic feature of the cytoplasm of the neuron is presence of granular material called 'Nissl substance' (Nissl bodies/granules). This Nissl substance is composed of rough endoplasmic reticulum.
- The cytoplasm of the neuron also shows 'neurofibrils' which consist of microfilaments and microtubules.
- The cytoplasmic processes of neurons are of two types—Dendrites and axons.

### Dendrites

- These are branched processes that extend from the cytoplasm of the cell body.
- Their function is to receive stimuli and conduct impulses to the cell body.
- Some dendrites present minute 'spines' that increase their surface area.
- The dendrites contain 'Nissl substance' which is absent in the axons. The Nissl-free zone extends partly to the cell body and is called axon hillock.

### Axon

- Axon is the long cytoplasmic extension from the cell body.
- The term 'nerve fiber' is commonly used with reference to either an axon or an elongated dendrite.
- Axons conduct impulses away from the cell body.
- Their length varies from few millimeters in the CNS to over meter in the PNS.
- Side branches called collateral branches extend for a short distance from the axons.

### Types of Neurons (Fig. 8.3)

According to the number of cytoplasmic processes they may be classified into:

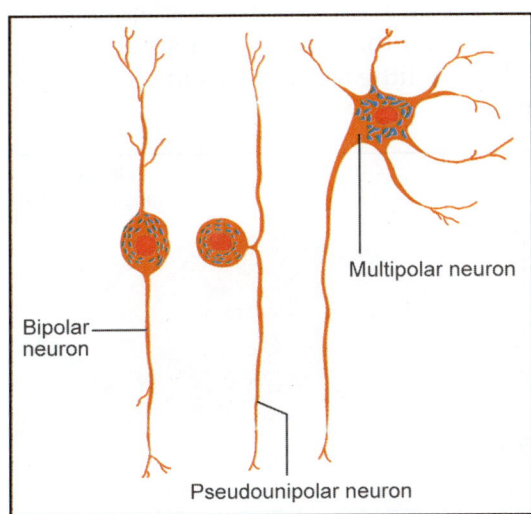

**Fig. 8.3:** Types of neuron

- Unipolar neurons/pseudounipolar neurons, e.g. mesencephalic nucleus and dorsal root ganglia of spinal nerves.
- Bipolar neurons, e.g. spiral and vestibular ganglion of the internal ear.
- Multipolar neuron. Majority of the neurons are multipolar.

According to the length of axon, the neurons are classified into:

Golgi type I—with long axons, e.g. neurons of cerebral cortex.

Golgi type II—with short or no axons, e.g. interneuron's of spinal cord.

### NEUROGLIA (GLIAL CELLS)

- These are non-excitable supporting cells of the nervous tissue.
- They are more numerous than neurons and have limited mitotic capacity.
- There are many varieties of neuroglial cells.

**1. Astrocytes**

- These cells are stellate in appearance.
- They are present at the site of blood–brain barrier.
- They regulate the passage of molecules from the blood to brain.
- Astrocytes are the primary glycogen stores in the central nervous system (CNS).

**2. Oligodendrocytes**

- These cells form myelin sheath around the axons in CNS.

**3. Microglial cells**

- These are small cells with flat cell body and a few short cellular processes.
- They are found along the perivascular coat of blood vessels in CNS.
- They are phagocytic in function and act as macrophage cells of the CNS.

**4. Ependyma**

- These are simple columnar cells with non-motile cilia, lining the cavities of the brain (ventricles) and central canal of the spinal cord.

**5. Schwann cells**

- These cells provide myelin sheath for the PNS.

8

## Synapse

The junction between the neurons is called synapse. Synapses may be of various types depending on the parts of neurons that come in contact.

1. *Axodendritic synapse*: It is the most common type where axon terminals contact with dendrites.
2. *Axosomatic synapse*: Axon terminal synapses with cell body of another neuron.

The impulses are transmitted across a synapse by specific neurotransmitters like acetylcholine, noradrenaline, dopamine, serotonin, histamine, glycine, GABA (gamma amino butyric acid) and certain polypeptides.

## Nerve Fiber

A nerve fiber or a nerve can be defined as 'collection of cytoplasmic processes (mainly axons) of neurons'.

**Myelination**

- Myelination is a process in which a neuroglial cell surrounds a portion of the axons or dendrite to provide support and to facilitate the conduction of impulses
- If the axons are covered with a myelin sheath, then the nerve is myelinated. Myelinated nerve fibers are found in peripheral nerves and in the white matter of the CNS. The grey matter of the brain and spinal cord is mostly composed of non-myelinated fibers. Structure of myelinated peripheral nerve fiber (inside to outside).
- *Axoplasm*: The cytoplasm of the axon, which contains neurofibrils and mitochondria.
- *Axolemma*: It is a semi-permeable membrane covering the axoplasm.
- *Myelin sheath (medullary sheath)*: Myelin sheath is formed by Schwann cells in peripheral nervous system, which are arranged in linear manner along the axon. The Schwann cells undergo spiraling around the axon and deposit concentric layers of lipids and proteins. The sheath is interrupted at intervals by 'node of Ranvier' where adjacent Schwann cells meet.
- *Neurilemmal sheath*: It is the outer cell membrane of the Schwann cells. Neurilemmal sheath is absent in the nerves of central nervous system. Peripheral nerves, if damaged, may regenerate. Nerves within the CNS cannot regenerate after injury due to the absence of neurilemmal sheath and endoneurium.
- *Endoneurium*: It is the outermost connective tissue covering of the nerve fiber. The nerve fibers are grouped in fasciculi and connective tissue covering them is called 'perineurium'. A nerve consists of numerous fasciculi, which are enclosed by connective tissue membrane called 'epineurium'.
- Functionally, nerves resemble like electric wires. Like the electric current flowing though the wires, the impulses (sensory and motor) are conducted through the nerves.
- The myelin sheaths act as an insulator of nerve fiber and reduce the loss of electrical activity into the surrounding tissue by dispersion. The node of Ranvier helps in faster conduction of impulses.

## Spinal Nerves

- These nerves arise directly from the spinal cord.
- There are 31 pairs of spinal nerves.
- It includes 8 cervical, 12 thoracic, 5 lumbar, 5 sacral and 1 coccygeal nerves.

### Formation of a Typical Spinal Nerge (Fig. 8.4)

- Each spinal nerve arises from the spinal cord by two roots.
- Ventral root is motor, which arises from the anterior grey horn of the spinal cord. Dorsal root is sensory which shows a ganglion called 'dorsal root ganglion'.
- The ventral and dorsal roots join to form mixed spinal nerve trunk, which again divides into ventral and dorsal rami.
- At certain places, ventral rami of the spinal nerves join together and branch to form nerve plexus, e.g. cervical plexus, brachial plexus, lumbar plexus and sacral plexus of nerves.

**Dermatome:** A dermatome is an area of the skin supplied by a single spinal segment. The dermatome representation differs in trunk and limbs. In trunk there they are arranged successively one below another and each dermatome extending anterior and posterior midline. There is a considerable overlapping of adjacent dermatomes so that injury to a single spinal nerve results in very little sensory loss in the corresponding dermatome.

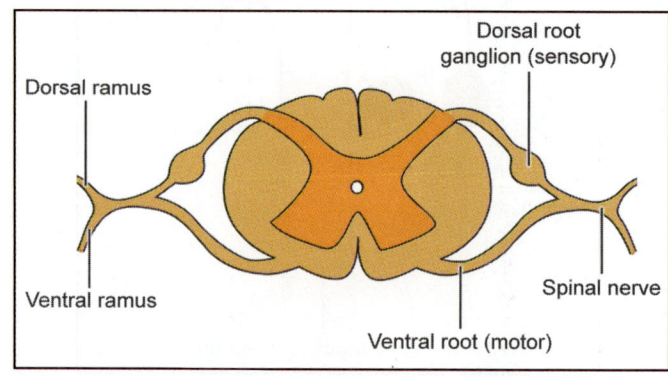

**Fig. 8.4:** A typical spinal nerve formation

## Some of the Important Terminologies used in the Nervous System

1. Nerve is a collection of nerve fibers outside the central nervous system.
2. Sensory nerves carry information from the peripheral part to the CNS, e.g. cutaneous nerve, optic nerve, vestibulocochlear nerve.
3. Motor nerve is the nerve which carries impulses from the CNS to the target structure.
4. Grey matter is the collection of cell bodies of neurons within the central nervous system. Such aggregation, when it is smaller in size is referred as 'nucleus' (not to be confused with nucleus of a cell).
5. White matter is mainly collection of nerve fibers with few supporting glial cells in the central nervous system.
6. Ganglia is collection of cell bodies of neurons outside the central nervous system.
7. *Root value*: The root value of a nerve refers to its segmental origin from the spinal cord. For example, the root value of axillary nerve is $C_5$ and $C_6$. It means the axillary nerve is derived from fifth and sixth cervical segments of the spinal cord.

## Cranial Nerves

There are 12 pairs of cranial nerves, which arise directly from the brain.

Following are the cranial nerves:

1. Olfactory
2. Optic
3. Oculomotor
4. Trochlear
5. Trigeminal
6. Abducent
7. Facial
8. Vestibulocochlear
9. Glossopharyngeal
10. Vagus
11. Accessory
12. Hypoglossal

## Applied Anatomy

**Irritation of a nerve or nerve injury:**

- Irritative lesion (compression) of sensory nerve result in reduced sensation (hypesthesia) or altered sensation (paresthesia)
- Destructive lesion of sensory nerve result in a loss of sensory modality
- Irritative lesion of motor nerve result in weakness of skeletal muscle (paresis)
- Destructive lesion of motor nerve result in paralysis of skeletal muscle

When nerves are stretched, severed or crushed, their axons degenerate distal to the lesion because they depend on the cell bodies for survival. If the axon is damaged with intact cell body, regeneration and restoration of function is possible. In crushing type of injury the connective tissue coverings of the nerve is intact, which guides the cut ends of the axons to grow to their destination. But a cutting nerve injury requires surgical intervention because regeneration of axons requires apposition of the cut ends by suture through epineurium. Compression of blood vessels supplying the nerve can also cause nerve degeneration.

CNS axons with myelin sheath formed by oligodendrocytes do not regenerate if cut. Myelinated axons in the PNS have the capacity to regenerate due to neurolemmal sheath of Schwann cells.

**Demyelination:** The progressive destruction of myelin sheath in the CNS and PNS, leading to a loss of sensation and motor control. Demyelination is associated with heavy metal poisoning, diphtheria and multiple sclerosis.

**Neuralgia:** A severe pain along the distribution of a nerve.

# Self-Assessment Exercise

☞ Select the Single Best Response Questions

☞ Short Note Questions

☞ Brief Essays

☞ Major Questions

## Select the Single Best Response Questions

1. **Which of the following processes requires energy (ATP) for movement across the cell membrane?**
   A. Osmosis
   B. Phagocytosis
   C. Diffusion
   D. None of the above

2. **Which of the following is/are cell contacts?**
   A. Zonula occludens
   B. Desmosome
   C. Zonula adherens
   D. All of the above

3. **Which of the following structures is known to maintain the shape of a cell?**
   A. Nucleus
   B. Mitochondria
   C. Microtubules
   D. Ribosomes

4. **When the two arms of the chromatid are of equal length, the chromosome is called:**
   A. Metacentric chromosome
   B. Acrocentric chromosome
   C. Telocentric chromosome
   D. None of the above

5. **Which of the following syndromes is associated with presence of an extra X chromosome?**
   A. Cri du chat syndrome
   B. Down syndrome
   C. Klinefelter's syndrome
   D. Turner's syndrome

6. **Which of the following stages of mitosis involves splitting of chromosomes?**
   A. Telophase
   B. Anaphase
   C. Metaphase
   D. Prophase

7. **The shortest stage of mitotic cell division is:**
   A. Anaphase
   B. Prophase
   C. Telophase
   D. Metaphase

8. **In karyotyping, chromosomes are identified in:**
   A. Telophase stage
   B. Prophase stage
   C. Anaphase stage
   D. Metaphase stage

9. **In which of the following stages of the meiotic division does "crossing over" of the chromosome occur?**
   A. Leptotene
   B. Zygotene
   C. Pachytene
   D. Diplotene

10. **Alveoli of the lungs are lined by:**
    A. Simple squamous epithelium
    B. Simple cuboidal epithelium
    C. Simple columnar epithelium
    D. Pseudostratified columnar epithelium

11. **Transitional epithelium lines:**
    A. Mucous membrane of the stomach
    B. Epidermis of the skin
    C. Mucous membrane of the trachea
    D. None of the above

12. **The secretory unit of the mammary gland is an example for:**
    A. Compound tubuloalveolar gland
    B. Compound alveolar gland
    C. Compound tubular gland
    D. Simple alveolar gland

13. **The gland in which the entire cells is discharged during secretion is called:**
    A. Merocrine gland
    B. Holocrine gland
    C. Apocrine gland
    D. None of the above

14. **Which of the following cells is responsible for synthesis of collagen fibers?**
    A. Fibroblasts
    B. Lymphocytes
    C. Plasma cells
    D. Macrophages

15. **Which of the following sentences is incorrect regarding the collagen fibers?**
    A. They are formed by fibroblasts
    B. They consist of a protein called 'collagen'
    C. The individual fibers branch and anastamose
    D. Tendon of the muscle is made up of collagen fibers

16. **Which of the following cells is involved in phagocytosis?**
    A. Fibroblast
    B. Mast cells
    C. Histiocytes
    D. Plasma cells

17. **Mast cells are involved in:**
    A. Production of antibodies
    B. Production of histamine
    C. Phagocytosis
    D. Wound healing

18. **Myxomatous tissue is found in:**
    A. Vitreous body of the eye
    B. Lymphatic organs
    C. Bone marrow
    D. Mesenteries

19. **Which of the following structures is made up of elastic cartilage?**
    A. Costal cartilage
    B. Thyroid cartilage
    C. Tracheal rings
    D. Pinna of the external ear

20. Which of the following statements is incorrect regarding hyaline cartilage?
    A. It is highly vascular
    B. It is made up of collagen fibers
    C. It can ossify to form a bone
    D. Its matrix is homogeneous

21. Intervertebral disc is an example for:
    A. Hyaline cartilage    B. Spongy bone
    C. Elastic cartilage    D. Fibrocartilage

22. Following are the examples for fibrocartilage *except*:
    A. Glenoidal labrum
    B. Epiglottis
    C. Menisci of the knee joint
    D. Intervertebral discs

23. Which of the following bones is an example for pneumatic bone?
    A. Parietal bone    B. Mandible
    C. Hyoid bone    D. Maxilla

24. Following are the sesamoid bones *except*:
    A. Malleus    B. Fabella
    C. Pisiform    D. Patella

25. The part of the long bone developed from secondary center of ossification is called:
    A. Epiphysis    B. Diaphysis
    C. Metaphysis    D. None of the above

26. Which of the following statements is incorrect regarding the compact bone?
    A. Lamellae are made up of collagen fibers
    B. Osteocytes are present between the lamellae
    C. Lamellae with Haversian canal constitute an osteon
    D. Volkmann's canals are placed parallel to the medullary cavity

27. Which of the following bones is an example for dermal bone?
    A. Femur    B. Hip bone
    C. Clavicle    D. Humerus

28. Which of the following bones violates the laws of ossification?
    A. Tibia    B. Fibula
    C. Radius    D. Ulna

29. Which of the following statements is incorrect regarding the structure of a skeletal muscle?
    A. The dark band is the area where the actin and myosin filaments overlap each other
    B. Only myosin filaments occupy the light band

C. The H band traverse the middle of the dark band
D. The Z line is in the middle of light band

30. Which of the following muscles is an example for bipennate muscle?
    A. Middle fibers of deltoid
    B. Rectus femoris
    C. Palmar interossei
    D. Flexor carpi ulnaris

31. The inferior tibiofibular joint is an example for:
    A. Primary cartilaginous joint
    B. Syndesmosis
    C. Gomphosis
    D. Secondary cartilaginous joint

32. Which of the following joints is an example for pivot variety of synovial joint?
    A. Atlanto-occipital joint
    B. Elbow joint
    C. Ankle joint
    D. None of the above

33. Which of the following arteries is an example of an end artery?
    A. Superficial palmar arch
    B. Mesenteric artery
    C. Central artery of retina
    D. None of the above

34. Which of the following structures is an example for a lymphatic vessel?
    A. Thoracic duct    B. Bile duct
    C. Cystic duct    D. Parotid duct

35. Following are the lymphatic organs *except*:
    A. Spleen    B. Thymus
    C. Thyroid gland    D. Palatine tonsil

36. The internal elastic lamina is well-defined in:
    A. Medium sized vein
    B. Large vein
    C. Medium sized artery
    D. Large sized artery

37. The wall of the large artery mainly consists of:
    A. Collagen fibers    B. Elastic fibers
    C. Smooth muscles    D. Reticular tissue

38. Unipolar neurons are found in:
    A. Mesencephalic nucleus
    B. Spiral ganglion
    C. Sympathetic ganglion
    D. Vestibular ganglion

**39. Which of the following cells in CNS are phago-cytic in function?**
A. Oligodendrocytes    B. Astrocytes
C. Schwann cells    D. Microglial cells

**40. Collection of cell bodies of the neurons outside the central nervous system is called:**
A. Nucleus    B. Ganglion
C. Grey matter    D. White matter

**41. The neuroglial cells that form myelin sheaths in the peripheral nervous system are:**
A. Astrocytes    B. Schwann cells
C. Microglial cells    D. Oligodendrocytes

**42. Neurotransmitters are stored in synaptic vesicles within the:**
A. Sarcolemma    B. Motor units
C. Axon terminals    D. Myofibrils

**43. Muscles capable of highly dexterous movements contain:**
A. One motor unit per muscle fiber
B. Many muscle fibers per motor unit
C. Few muscle fibers per motor unit
D. Many motor units per muscle fiber

**44. The site at which a nerve impulse is transmitted from the motor nerve ending to the skeletal muscle is the:**
A. Sarcomere
B. Neuromuscular junction
C. Myofilament
D. Z line

**45. An interosseus ligament is characteristic of:**
A. Suture    B. Synchondrosis
C. Symphysis    D. Syndesmosis

**46. Specialised bone cells that reabsorb bone tissue are:**
A. Osteoblasts    B. Osteocytes
C. Osteons    D. Osteoclasts

**47. Cardiac muscle fiber has:**
A. Striations
B. Intercalated discs
C. Rhythmical contractions
D. All of the above

**48. Cartilage is slow in healing following an injury because:**
A. It is non-living
B. It is avascular
C. Its chondrocytes cannot reproduce
D. It has a semisolid matrix

**49. The organelle that combines protein and carbohydrates and stores them for secretion is the**
A. Golgi apparatus
B. Rough endoplasmic reticulum
C. Smooth endoplasmic reticulum
D. Ribosomes

**50. The phase of mitosis in which the chromosomes line up at the equator of the cell is called?**
A. Prophase    B. Metaphase
C. Anaphase    D. Telophase

**51. Which of these organelles contains strong hydro-lytic enzymes?**
A. Lysosome    B. Golgi apparatus
C. Ribosome    D. Mitochondria

**52. Layers or aggregations of similar cells that perform specific functions are called:**
A. Organelles    B. Tissues
C. Organs    D. Glands

**53. Most of the arteries in the body contain oxygen-rich blood with the exception of the:**
A. Aorta    B. Renal arteries
C. Pulmonary arteries    D. Coronary arteries

## Short Note Questions (3 marks)

1. Cell membrane
2. Meiotic cell division
3. Chromosomes
4. Mitochondria
5. Golgi complex
6. Nucleus
7. Ribosomes
8. Collagen fibers
9. Elastic fibers
10. Macrophages
11. Fibroblasts
12. Epiphysis
13. Cardiac muscle
14. Smooth muscles
15. Neuroglial cells
16. Bone marrow
17. Periosteum
18. Capillaries and sinusoids
19. Structure of a nerve fiber
20. Fibrous joint
21. Structure of an artery
22. Structure of a vein
23. Karyotyping

24. Down syndrome
25. Klinefelter's syndrome
26. Turner's syndrome

## Brief Essays (5 or 6 marks)

1. Write briefly on the structure and functions of cell membrane.
2. Give an account of the structure and types of chromosomes.
3. Name the different types of exocrine glands giving examples to each variety.
4. Write briefly about the structure and distribution of collagen fibers.
5. Write briefly about the structure and distribution of hyaline cartilage.
6. Give an account of ossification centres. What are the laws of ossification?
7. Name the different types of epiphysis. Give examples to each type.
8. Give an account of the blood supply to a long bone.
9. Write briefly about the structure and functions of cardiac muscle.
10. Give an account of the structure and distribution of smooth muscles.
11. What are agonists, antagonists and synergists?
12. Draw a neat-labelled diagram of a neuron. Write briefly about its structure.
13. Write briefly on cartilaginous joint.
14. Give an account of the different types of fibrous joints.
15. Enumerate the structural differences between the arteries and veins.
16. Write briefly about different types of vascular anastomosis. What are their significance?
17. Write briefly about the neuroglial cells.
18. With the help of a diagram, show the formation of a typical spinal nerve. What is a spinal segment?

## Major Questions (10 marks)

1. Draw a neat-labeled diagram of normal human cell. Add a note on the structure and functions of cellular organelles and nucleus. *(3+5+2)*
2. Give a brief account of stages of mitotic cell division. Enumerate the differences between mitotic and meiotic cell division. *(7+3)*

3. Write briefly about the steps involved in first meiotic cell division.
4. Discuss the genetic disorders involving autosomes and sex chromosomes. *(5+5)*
5. Classify the epithelial tissue giving examples to each variety. List the functions of the epithelium. *(6+4)*
6. Give an account of the structure, distribution and functions of different types of connective tissue fibers.
7. Give an account of the structure and distribution of different types of cartilage *(7+3)*
8. Classify the bones according to their shape, giving examples. Write briefly about the functions of the bone. *(6+4)*
9. Discuss the structure and functions of different types of bone cells. Add a note on the matrix of the bone. *(6+4)*
10. Give an account of steps involved in endochondral ossification. Name the bones developed by endochondral ossification. *(8+2)*
11. Discuss the macroscopic and microscopic structure of a long compact bone. *(3+7)*
12. Discuss the microscopic structure of a skeletal muscle with the help of a diagram.
13. Classify the joints giving examples to each variety. Discuss the structure of a typical synovial joint. *(3+7)*
14. Discuss the structure of a typical synovial joint. Name the different types of synovial joints giving examples. *(6+4)*
15. Give an account of the structure and functions of a lymph node. *(6+4)*
16. Classify the neurons according to their cytoplasmic processes, giving examples. Discuss the microscopic structure of a neuron. *(3+7)*

## Answers to Single Best Response Questions

| | | | | | |
|---|---|---|---|---|---|
| 1. B | 2. D | 3. C | 4. A | 5. C | 6. B |
| 7. A | 8. D | 9. C | 10. A | 11. D | 12. B |
| 13. B | 14. A | 15. C | 16. C | 17. B | 18. A |
| 19. D | 20. A | 21. D | 22. B | 23. D | 24. A |
| 25. A | 26. D | 27. C | 28. B | 29. B | 30. B |
| 31. B | 32. D | 33. C | 34. A | 35. C | 36. C |
| 37. B | 38. A | 39. D | 40. B | 41. B | 42. C |
| 43. C | 44. B | 45. D | 46. D | 47. D | 48. B |
| 49. A | 50. B | 51. A | 52. B | 53. C | |

# Musculoskeletal System

*Section*

## II

## LEARNING OBJECTIVES FOR BSC NURSING

1. Be able to identify the bones of the upper and lower limbs and to explain their major parts.
2. Be able to explain the specific parts of the bones articulating and forming various joints (for example, capitulum of the lower end of the humerus articulate with head of the radius, trochlea of the lower end of the humerus articulate with trochlear notch of the ulna to form elbow joint).
3. Be able to name the muscles in different regions of the limb and also able to give their nerve supply and actions.
4. Be able to explain the articulations, major ligaments, movements with muscles producing for—shoulder, elbow, wrist, hip, knee and ankle joints.
5. Be able to explain mammary gland with its blood supply and lymphatic drainage.
6. Be able to explain cubital fossa with its clinical relevance.
7. Be able to name the arteries supplying the upper and lower limb mentioning their major branches.
8. Be able to explain the distribution of median, ulnar and radial nerves and their effect of injury.
9. Be able to explain the distribution of femoral, obturator, sciatic, peroneal nerves and their effect of injury.
10. Be able to identify the different parts of the vertebrae and also differences between cervical, thoracic and lumbar vertebrae.
11. Be able to explain the formation of thoracic cage.
12. In a given skull be able to identify the major bones forming it.
13. Be able to identify the major foramina in the base of the skull (also in the cranial cavity) and to list the structures passing through it.
14. Be able to explain the functions, major openings, nerve supply and applied anatomy of the diaphragm.
15. Be able to name the muscles of the thoracic and abdominal wall.
16. Be able to name the muscles of the scalp, face and infratemporal fossa with their nerve supply and actions.
17. Be able to explain the boundaries and contents of the inguinal canal and its applied anatomy.
18. Be able to name the muscles of the neck and to explain the attachment and action of sternocleidomastoid muscle.
19. Be able to name the extraocular muscles of the eye with their nerve supply and actions.

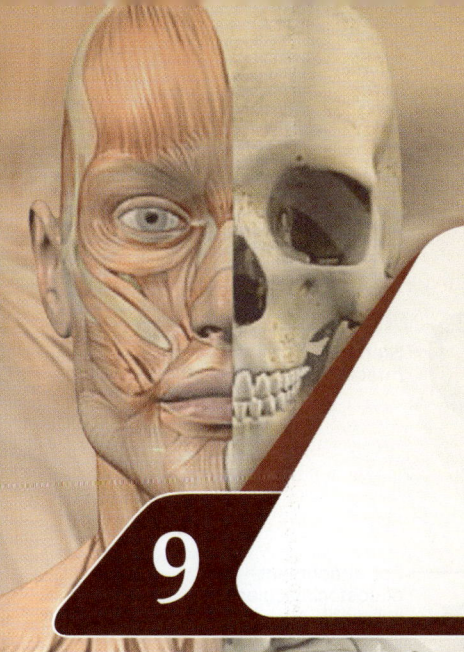

# Bones of the Limbs

**9**

## CLAVICLE (COLLAR BONE)

It is a prominent subcutaneous bone present on either side of the neck connecting the trunk with the upper limb (Fig. 9.1).

Medially, it articulates with the manubrium sterni at the sternoclavicular joint.

Laterally, it articulates with the acromial process of the scapula at the acromioclavicular joint.

The medial 2/3 of the clavicle is convex forwards.

Its superior surface is subcutaneous, medial end is expanded and lateral end is flat.

The inferior surface of the lateral end presents an elevation called conoid tubercle and a ridge called trapezoid ridge (Fig. 9.2).

### Applied Anatomy

Fractured clavicle can compress the subclavian artery or brachial plexus. In case of fracture the medial end is pulled by sternocleidomastoid muscle and lateral end is pulled down by deltoid muscle. The clavicle is commonly fractured at the junction between the two curvatures of the bone, as it is the weakest point of the clavicle (at the junction of medial 2/3 and lateral 1/3).

### Peculiarities of Clavicle

1. It is the only long bone placed horizontally in the body.
2. It is subcutaneous and can be easily palpated.
3. It is the first bone to ossify in the body.
4. It is the only long bone with two primary centers of ossification for shaft.
5. It is the only long bone to ossify in membrane.
6. It has no medullary cavity.

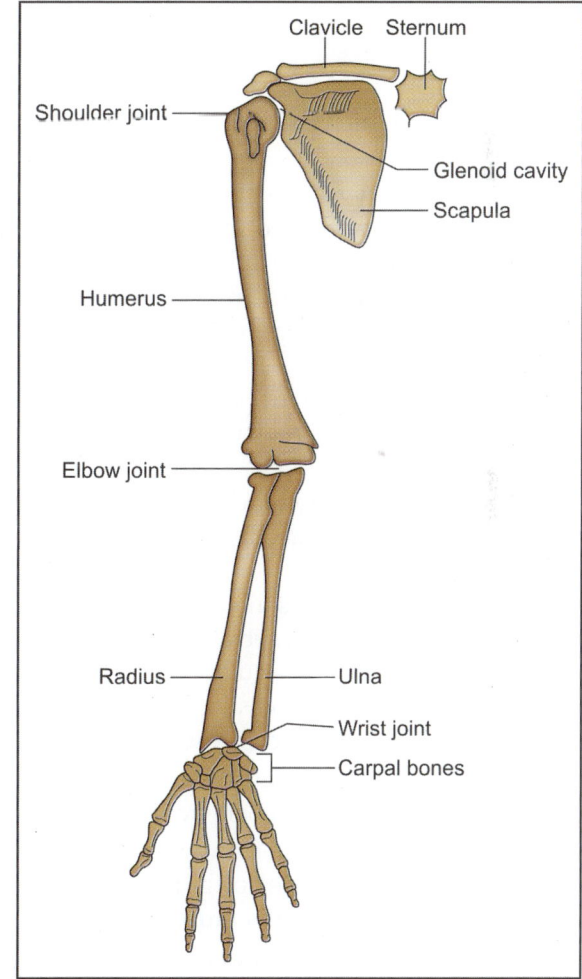

**Fig. 9.1:** Skeleton of the upper limb

## SCAPULA (SHOULDER BLADE)

This bone is placed in the scapular region behind the upper 7 ribs. It gives attachments to many muscles

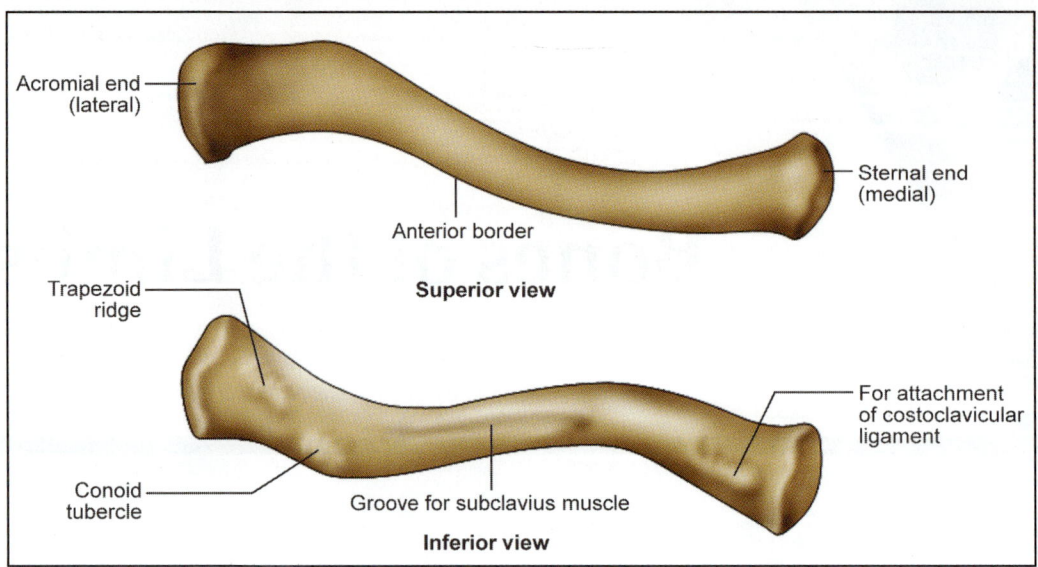

**Fig. 9.2:** Right clavicle—superior view and inferior view

(scapular muscles) which connect the upper limb with trunk.

Scapula presents two surfaces and three borders.

a. Costal surface is also called 'subscapular fossa'. It provides attachment to the subscapularis muscle.

b. Dorsal surface is divided into an upper supraspinous and lower infraspinous fossa by spinous process.

   i. Superior border—It presents 'suprascapular notch' for the transmission of suprascapular nerve and vessels.

  ii. Lateral border—It extends below the glenoid cavity and provides attachment to teres major and minor muscles.

 iii. Medial border—It faces the vertebral column and provides attachment to serratus anterior on costal surface and levator scapulae and rhomboideus muscles on dorsal surface.

Scapula also presents three processes (Figs 9.3 and 9.4)

1. *Acromion process:* It articulates with the lateral end of the clavicle at the acromioclavicular joint.

2. *Coracoid process:* It is a small forward projection from the scapula. Its tip provides origin to short head of biceps and corachobrachialis muscle.

3. *Spinous process:* It can be felt in the living as a ridge on the back. It is present on the dorsal aspect of scapula, continues laterally, as the acromion process.

The glenoid cavity of the scapula articulates with the head of the humerus (bone of the arm), to form the shoulder joint.

### Applied Anatomy

Paralysis of a muscle called serratus anterior causes winging of the scapula. The medial border of the scapula becomes prominent on the back and arm cannot be abducted.

### HUMERUS

Humerus is the bone of the arm. It has an upper end, lower end and a shaft in-between (Figs 9.3 and 9.4).

### Upper End

• *Head:* It is rounded and covered by articular cartilage. It articulates with glenoid cavity of the scapula to form shoulder joint.

• *Greater tubercle:* Greater tubercle is a long elevation behind the lesser tubercle. It has three impressions for the insertions of supraspinatus, infraspinatus and teres minor muscles.

• *Lesser tubercle:* The lesser tubercle is the prominent, sharp projection on the anterior aspect of the upper end. It receives the insertion of subscapularis muscle.

• *Bicipital groove (intertubercular sulcus):* It is an area between the greater and lesser tubercles. The floor of the sulcus provides insertion to latissimus dorsi, medial lip of the groove for teres major and lateral lip for pectoralis major muscle.

   a. *Surgical neck:* It is the junction between the upper end and shaft of the humerus. Axillary nerve and posterior circumflex humeral artery wind around it.

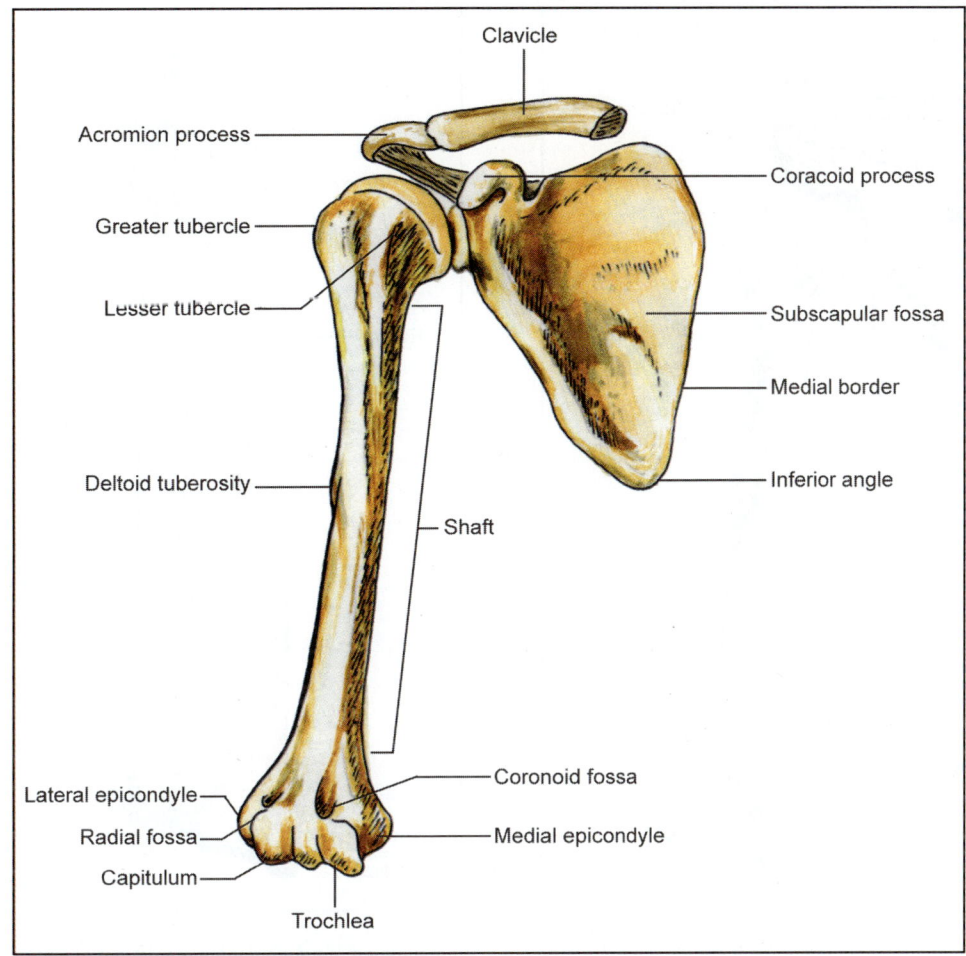

**Fig. 9.3:** Humerus and scapula—anterior view

b. *Anatomical neck:* It is the constricted portion adjoining the head. It provides attachment to the capsule of the shoulder joint.

c. *Morphological neck:* It is the line joining the epiphysis with diaphysis and connects the two tuberosities.

## Shaft

It is cylindrical and connects the upper and lower ends. It has following important features.

### Radial Groove (spiral groove)

The middle 1/3 of the posterior surface is crossed by a groove called the radial groove. It is related to the radial nerve and the profunda brachii artery.

## Lower End

- *Capitulum* is a rounded projection on the lateral side and articulates with the head of the radius (elbow joint).

- *Trochlea* is a pully shaped area, present medially, and articulates with the trochlear notch of ulna (elbow joint).

- *Medial epicondyle:* A subcutaneous prominent bony projection on the medial side of the elbow. It is crossed posteriorly by the ulnar nerve. It gives origin to all the superficial flexor muscles of the forearm (common flexor origin).

- *Lateral epicondyle:* It is on the lateral side but smaller than the medial epicondyle. It provides origin to all the superficial extensor muscles of the forearm (common extensor origin).

- *Coronoid fossa:* Present just above the trochlea to accommodate the coronoid process of the ulna in a flexed elbow.

- *Radial fossa:* Present above the capitulum, to accommodate the head of the radius in a flexed elbow.

- *Olecranon fossa:* It is present posteriorly and accommodates the olecranon process of the ulna in an extended elbow.

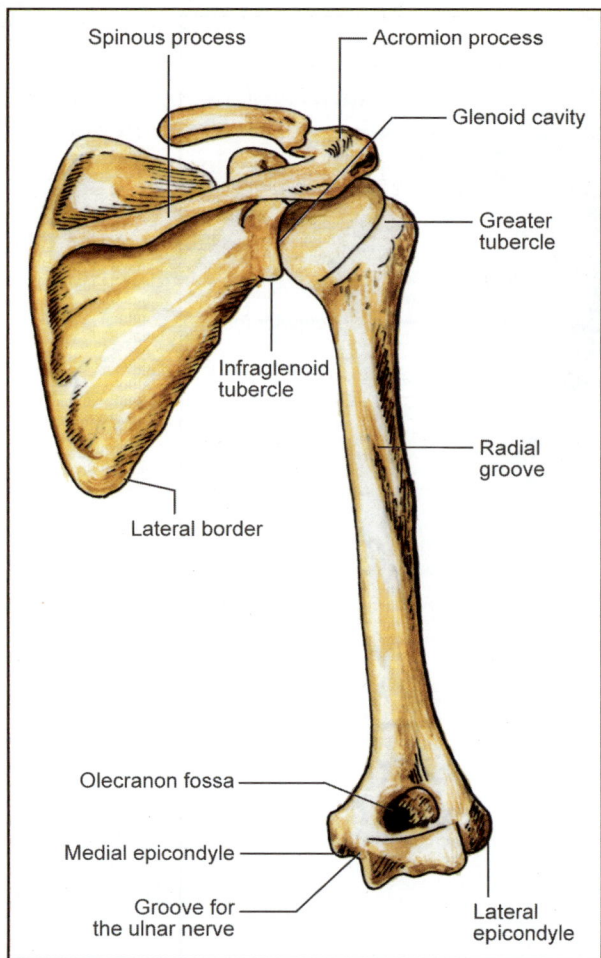

Fig. 9.4: Humerus and scapula—posterior view

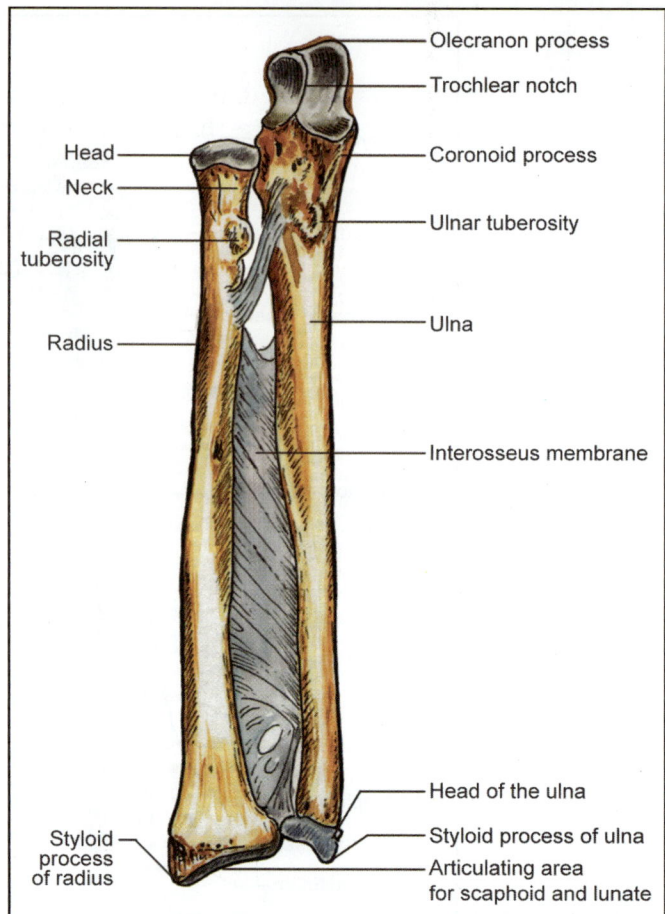

Fig. 9.5: Radius and ulna—anterior view

## Applied Anatomy

- The fracture affecting the surgical neck can damage axillary nerve, which leads to paralysis of deltoid muscle and cause difficulty in abducting the shoulder. The skin sensation over the deltoid is also lost.
- Fracture affecting the shaft can cause damage to radial nerve which may result in 'wrist drop' and sensory loss in the back of the forearm and lateral part of the dorsum of the hand.
- Supracondylar fracture can damage median nerve and brachial artery. Compression of brachial artery deprives blood supply to forearm and hand which eventually cause Volkman's ischemic contracture.
- Fracture affecting the medial epicondyle can damage ulnar nerve which leads to 'clawhand' with sensory loss in the medial side of the palm and medial one and a half finger.

## RADIUS

Radius is the lateral bone of the forearm. It has two ends (upper and lower) and a shaft (Figs 9.5 and 9.6).

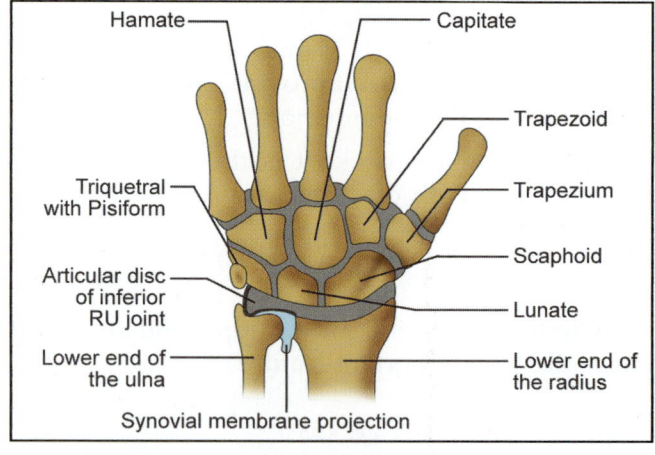

Fig. 9.6: Carpal bone articulations

## Upper End

- *Head:* It is a disc-shaped structure separated from the shaft by neck. Its upper surface articulates with the capitulum of humerus (elbow joint). Medial margin of the head articulates with radial notch of the ulna to form the superior radioulnar joint.

- *Neck:* It is the lower constricted part of the bone below the head.
- *Radial tuberosity:* It is below the medial part of the neck and provides insertion to the biceps brachii muscle.

## Shaft

It is the elongated cylindrical part connecting the two ends. It presents three borders and three surfaces. The interosseus (medial) border provides attachment to interosseus membrane.

## Lower End

- Inferior surface of the lower end articulates with scaphoid laterally and lunate medially (wrist joint).
- Lister's tubercle: The posterior aspect of the lower end presents a tubercle called dorsal tubercle (or Lister's tubercle).
- Styloid process: It is a conical projection from the lower end at the lateral aspect.
- Medial part of the lower end (ulnar notch) articulates with the head of the ulna to form the inferior radioulnar joint. This part also gives attachment to the articular disc of the inferior radioulnar joint.

## Applied Anatomy

*Colles' fracture:* A fall on the outstretched hand results in fracture of distal end of the radius. The distal fractured fragment is displaced upwards and posteriorly by brachio-radialis muscle. This produces 'dinner fork deformity'.

*Smith's fracture:* It is the reverse of Colles' fracture. It is produced by a fall on the back of the hand. The distal fractured element is displaced forwards and upwards.

## ULNA

It is the medial bone of the forearm. It has the following parts—upper end, shaft and lower end (Fig. 9.5 and Fig. 9.6).

## Upper End

The important parts include:

*Olecranon process:* It projects forwards from the upper most part of the ulna. It bends forward, forming a beak like projection. It occupies the olecranon fossa of the humerus, when the elbow is extended. Triceps muscle is inserted into its superior surface.

*Coronoid process:* It is a shelf-like projection from the upper end and anterior part of the shaft below the olecranon process. Its anterior aspect bears a rough

impression, called the ulnar tuberosity which provides insertion to brachialis muscle.

*Radial notch:* Lateral surface of the coronoid process presents a radial notch, to articulate with head of the radius to form the superior radioulnar joint. Its margins provide attachment to annular ligament.

*Trochlear notch:* It is between the olecranon and coronoid process. It articulates with trochlea of the humerus.

## Shaft

It has three borders and three surfaces. The lateral (interosseus) border provides attachment to the interosseus membrane.

## Lower End

- *Head:* Its lateral part articulates with the ulnar notch of the radius (inferior radioulnar joint). Its inferior surface is separated from the carpal bones by an articular disc of the inferior radioulnar joint.
- *Styloid process:* It projects from the posteromedial aspect of the lower end. It is palpable on posteromedial part of the wrist. It lies 1.25 cm above the level of the tip of the styloid process of the radius.

## Applied Anatomy

Fracture of shaft of ulna may be associated with fracture of radius. Fracture of olecranon process occurs if one falls on the point of elbow.

## CARPAL BONES

The skeleton of the hand is made up of carpal, metacarpal and phalangeal bones.

Carpal bones are 8 in number, and are arranged in proximal and distal rows.

*Proximal row consists* (from lateral to medial side)
- Scaphoid
- Lunate
- Triquetral
- Pisiform

*Distal row consists* (from lateral to medial side)
- Trapezium
- Trapezoid
- Capitate
- Hamate

Among these bones, scaphoid and lunate articulate with the lower end of the radius to form the wrist joint. The distal row of carpal bones articulates with the metacarpal bones (Fig. 9.7).

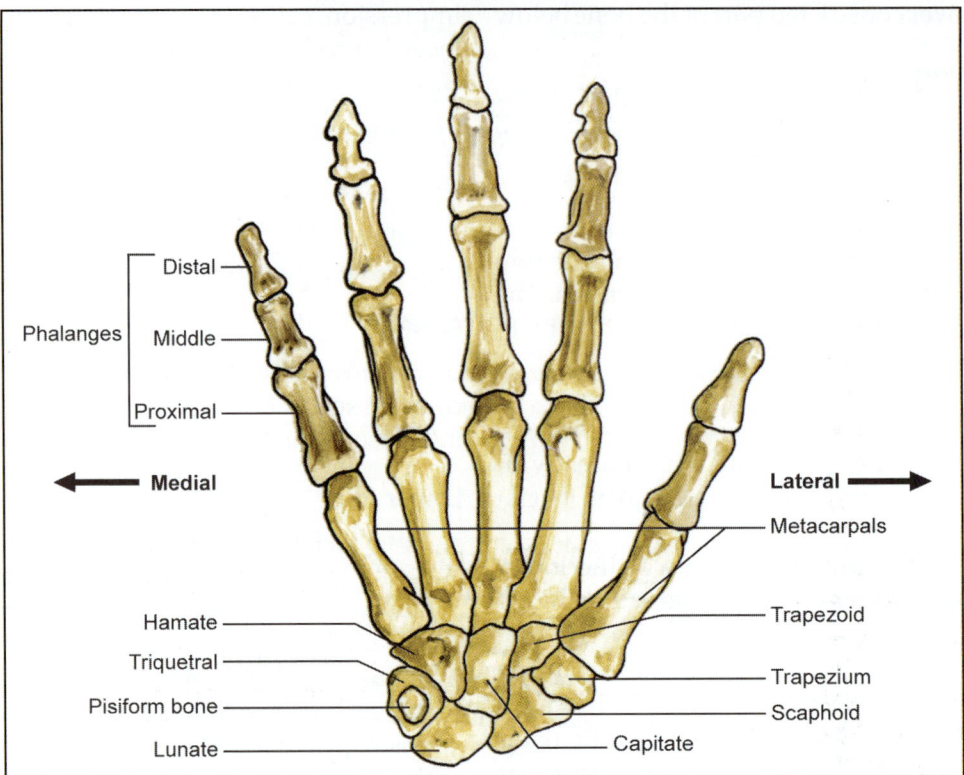

**Fig. 9.7:** Bones of the hand—dorsal view

## Applied Anatomy

*Scaphoid fracture:* Scaphoid is the most common carpal bone to be fractured due to fall on the outstretched hand. In scaphoid fracture there will be tenderness in the anatomical snuff box as well as over the volar aspect of the scaphoid. A fracture affecting the scaphoid between its proximal and distal segments can leads to avascular necrosis of its proximal segment. This is because the artery supplying the scaphoid enters through distal segment and then proceeds to proximal segment.

A fall on outstretched hand can cause fractures of scaphois, radius and clavicle.

*Lunate dislocation:* Though it is uncommon, its forward dislocation can cause carpal tunnel syndrome.

## Metacarpal Bones

There are five metacarpal bones, which are numbered from lateral to medial side. Each metacarpal bone has a head (placed distally), a shaft and a base (at the proximal end).

## Phalanges

There are 14 phalanges in each hand, 3 for each finger and 2 for thumb. Each phalanx has a base, a shaft and a head.

## Applied Anatomy

- *Bennett's fracture:* Fracture involving the base of the 1st metacarpal bone.
- *Mallet finger:* The distal phalanx undergoes extreme flexion due to detachment of extensor tendon from the distal phalanx.

### LOWER LIMB (Fig. 9.8)

### HIP BONE (INNOMINATE BONE)

It is an irregular bone, forming the skeleton of the gluteal region (Figs 9.9 and 9.10). It is made up of three parts:

1. Pubis
2. Ilium
3. Ischium

### Pubis

It forms the anteroinferior part of the hip bone. It has body, superior and inferior ramus.

*Body:* It presents the following features:
- Pubic crest—A ridge along the upper border of the body of the pubis.

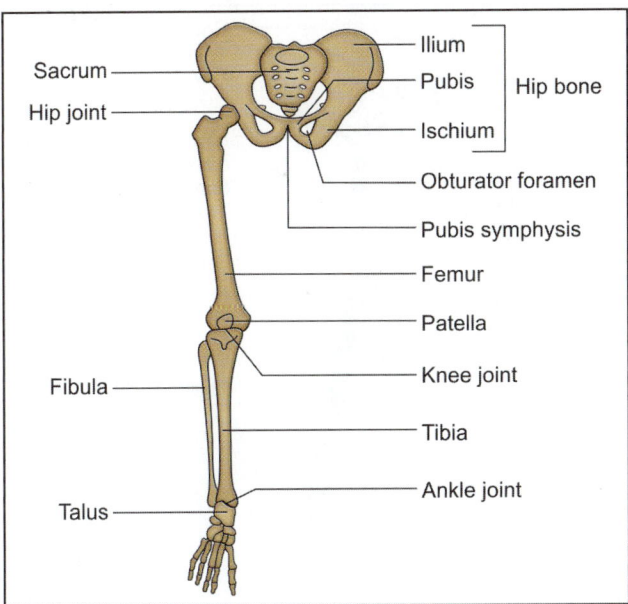

**Fig. 9.8:** Skeleton of the lower limb

- Pubic tubercle—It is the lateral end of the pubic crest. It provides attachment to the medial end of the inguinal ligament.
- Pubic symphysis—The right and left pubic bone meet in a median joint called pubic symphysis (a secondary cartilaginous joint).

*Superior ramus:* It extends from the body to the acetabulum. It presents:

- Pecten pubis—It extends from the pubic tubercle to iliopubic eminence.

- Obturator crest—It extends from the pubic tubercle to acetabular notch.

*Inferior ramus:* It extends from the body to ramus of the ischium. Together with ramus of the ischium it forms 'conjoint ischiopubic ramus'.

### Ilium

It forms the upper expanded bony plate of hip bone. It has the following important features.

- *Iliac crest:* It is the upper border of the ilium. The highest point of the iliac crest is situated at the level of the interval between the spines of L3 and L4 vertebrae where lumbar puncture is done. The anterior end of the iliac crest is called anterior superior iliac spine and the posterior end is called the posterior superior iliac spine. The anterior border of the ilium extends from the anterior superior iliac spine to the acetabulum. Its lowest part presents a prominence called anterior inferior iliac spine. It gives attachment to the straight head of the rectus femoris muscle and iliofemoral ligament of the hip joint.
- *Greater sciatic notch:* It is the curved notch on the posterior border of ilium, just below the posterior inferior iliac spine. This notch is converted into greater sciatic foramen by two ligaments (sacrotuberous and sacrospinous ligaments). This foramen transmits nerves (sciatic nerve) and vessels to the lower limb.
- Ilium presents two surfaces.

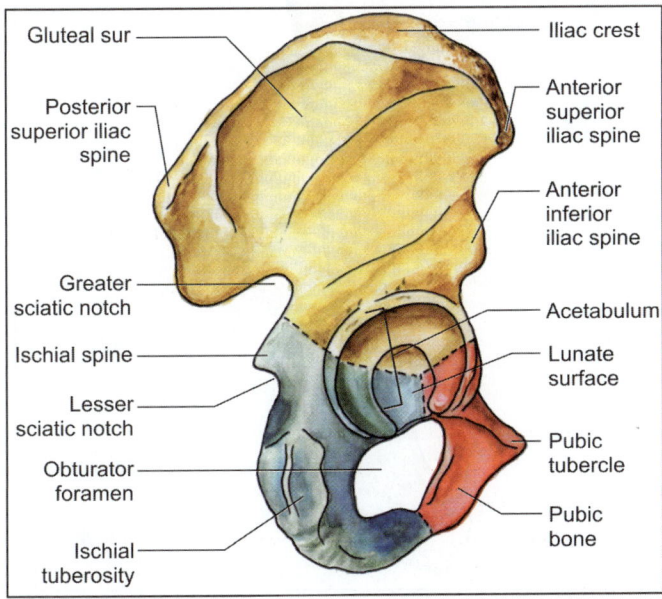

**Fig. 9.9:** Hip bone—external surface

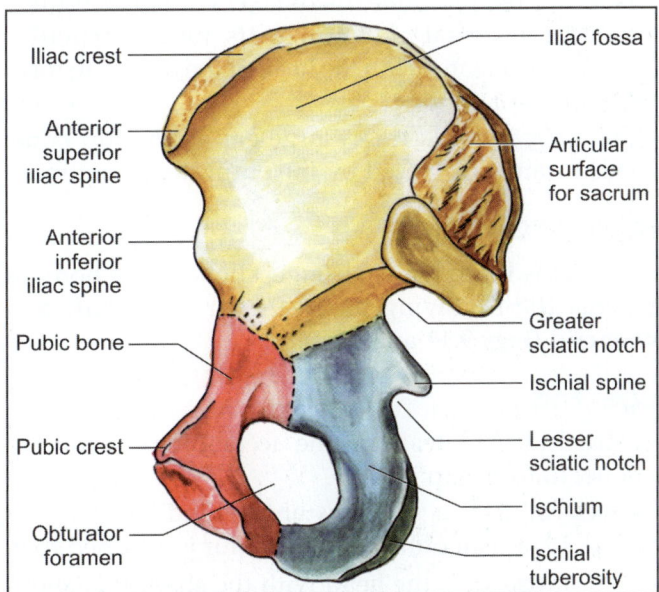

**Fig. 9.10:** Hip bone—internal surface

- Outer gluteal surface provides attachment to gluteus maximus, medius and minimus muscles.
- Inner surface presents iliac fossa in front and sacropelvic surface behind.

  Iliac fossa provides attachment to iliacus muscle. It forms false pelvis. Caecum with appendix is located in the right iliac fossa and sigmoid colon on the left iliac fossa.

  The sacropelvic surface presents 'auricular' (ear-shaped) surface for the side of the sacrum to form sacroiliac joint.

## Ischium

It forms the posteroinferior part of the hip bone. It consists of body and ramus. It presents an ischial spine and an ischial tuberosity.

- *Ischial tuberosity:* The lower end of the body forms 'ischial tuberosity'. The upper part of the ischial tuberosity provides origin to semimembranosus (on lateral side) and semitendinosus with long head of biceps femoris muscle (on medial side). The lower part provides origin to the hamstring part of the adductor magnus muscle.
- *Ischial spine:* The posterior border of the body of ischium presents spine like projection called 'ischial spine'. Above the ischial spine is the greater sciatic notch and below is the lesser sciatic notch. Lesser sciatic notch is also converted into a foramen by sacrotuberous and sacrospinous ligaments.
- *Ramus of the ischium:* It arises from the lower part of the body and joins the inferior ramus of the pubis (conjoint ischiopubic ramus)
- *Acetabulum:* It is a cup shaped cavity on the lateral aspect of the hip bone. Its deficient lower margin is called the acetabular notch. Its lunate articular surface articulates with the head of the femur, to form the hip joint.
- *Obturator foramen:* It is a large gap in the hip bone. This foramen is closed by the obturator membrane.

## FEMUR (THIGH BONE)

Femur is the longest and strongest bone of the body. It presents the following parts: Upper end, shaft and lower end (Figs 9.11 and 9.12).

## Upper End

- *Head:* It articulates with the acetabulum of the hip bone, to form hip joint.

  Fovea capitis is a pit below and behind the center of head. Ligament of head of the femur is attached to it.
- *Neck:* It connects the head with the shaft. It is about 5 cm in length.

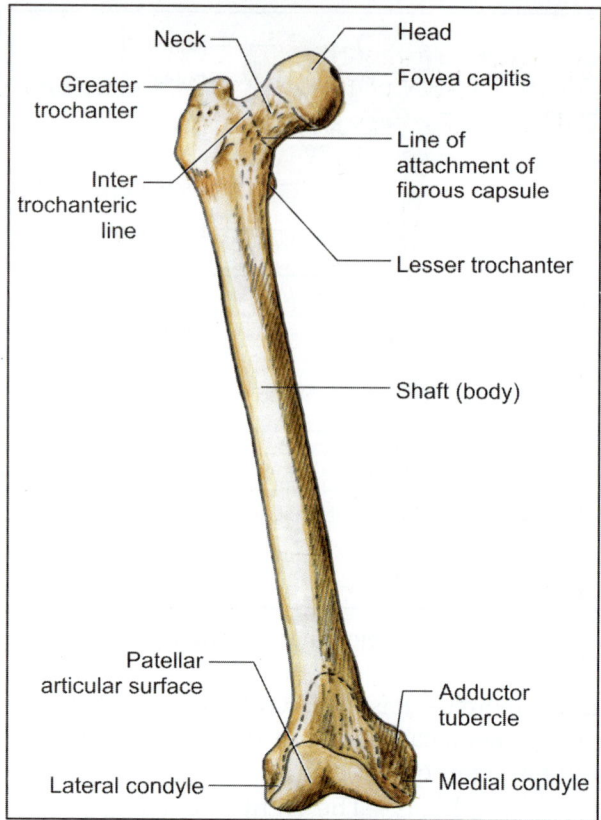

**Fig. 9.11:** Femur—anterior view

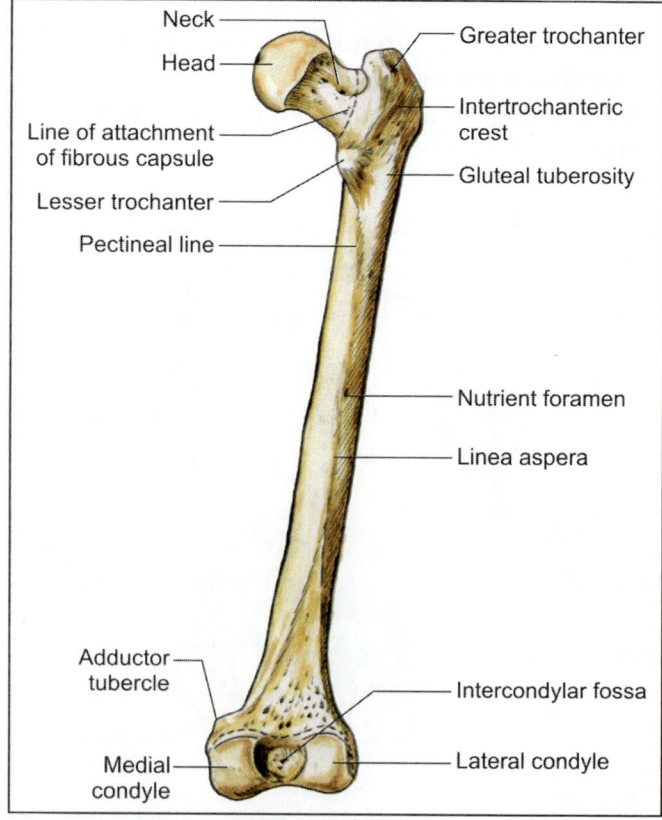

**Fig. 9.12:** Femur—posterior view

## Neck Shaft Angle

It is the angle between the lower border of the neck and medial border of the shaft. It is about 125°. The medial part of the neck is intracapsular.

- *Greater trochanter:* This is a large prominence at the upper part of the junction of the neck with the shaft.
- A ridge on the upper part of medial surface receives insertion of obturator internus, superior and inferior gemelli.
- Trochanteric fossa is a depression in the lower part of medial surface. It receives insertion of obturator externus.
- The anterior surface of the greater trochanter receives the insertion of gluteus minimus muscle.
- The lateral surface of the greater trochanter provides insertion to gluteus medius muscle.
- Apex of greater trochanter receives insertion of piriformis muscle.
- Lesser trochanter is a conical eminence, present on the posteroinferior part of the neck. It receives the insertion of iliopsoas muscle.
- *Intertrochanteric crest:* It connects greater trochanter and lesser trochanter (junction between neck and shaft) posteriorly. Quadrate tubercle is an elevation in this crest and receives insertion of quadratus femoris muscle.
- *Intertrochanteric line:* It connects greater trochanter and lesser trochanter (junction between neck and shaft) anteriorly. The capsule of the hip joint is attached to this line.

## Shaft

The posterior surface of the shaft presents a bony ridge called 'linea aspera' with medial and lateral lips. The medial lip of the linea aspera continues upwards as spiral line and lateral lip as gluteal tuberosity. Below, the medial lip continues as medial supracondylar line and lateral lip as lateral supracondylar line. The linea aspera provides attachment to many muscles.

## Lower End

*Condyles:* The lower end of the femur is widely expanded to form two large condyles (medial and lateral). Posteriorly the two condyles are separated by a gap called intercondylar fossa.

The condyle presents two articular surfaces.

The patellar surface articulates with the patella anteriorly (part of the knee joint).

The tibial surface on the inferior aspect articulates with the condyles of the tibia (the knee joint).

## Applied Anatomy

- The common site of fracture is neck in old age.
- Coxa vara is a condition in which the neck shaft angle is reduced
- The fracture of the neck may damage the blood vessels supplying neck and head (neck is intracapsular). It may lead to necrosis of head.
- Medicolegal importance: The epiphyseal center for the lower end of femur appears just before birth in the ninth month of intrauterine life. Hence, its presence provides a proof for viability of the baby.
- In case of supracondylar fracture the distal segment is pulled backwards by gastrocnemius muscle which may injure the popliteal artery.

## PATELLA (KNEE CAP)

The patella is the largest sesamoid bone in the body developed in the tendon of the quadriceps femoris muscle. It is situated in front of the lower end of femur, about 1 cm above the knee joint.

The patella has an apex, base, medial and lateral borders, anterior and posterior surfaces. The base, medial and lateral borders receive insertion of quadriceps femoris muscle. The apex provides attachment to ligamentum patellae. The anterior surface is separated from skin by a prepatellar bursa. The upper part of the posterior surface articulates with condyles of femur Fig. 9.13).

The upper part of its posterior surface articulates with the femur.

The apex of the patella is directed downwards and provides attachment to ligamentum patellae.

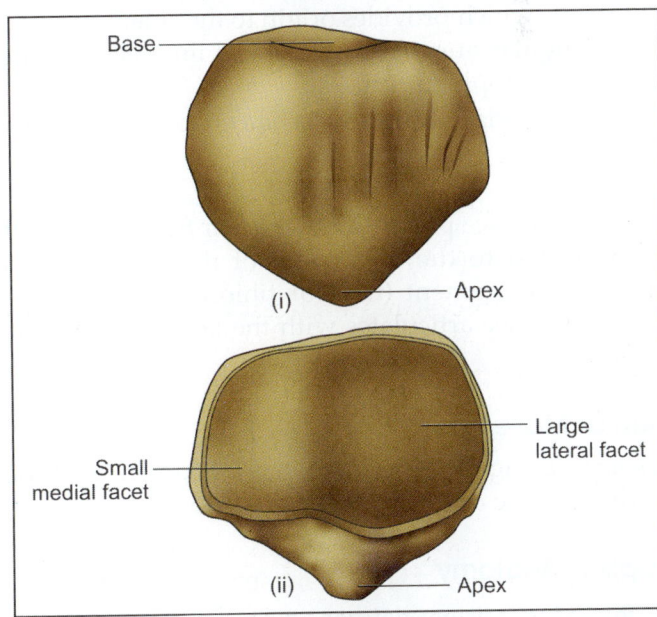

**Fig. 9.13:** Patella: (i) anterior view, (ii) posterior view

## Applied Anatomy

Patella tends to be displaced laterally, however, this tendency is minimised by forward projection of lateral condyle of femur. The patella can be fractured by a direct blow.

## TIBIA

Tibia is the medial and larger bone of the leg. It has the following important parts: upper end, shaft and lower end (Figs 9.14 and 9.15).

Upper end is expanded to form two large condyles.

- *Medial condyle:* Its superior surface articulates with medial condyle of the femur (knee joint). A groove on the posterior aspect of the medial condyle receives the insertion of the semimembranosus muscle.
- *Lateral condyle:* Its superior surface articulates with lateral condyle of the femur (knee joint). Posteroinferiorly it presents a fibular facet for the head of the fibula (superior tibiofibular joint).
- *Intercondylar area:* It is the rough area between the superior articular surfaces of medial and lateral condyles. It provides attachment to cruciate ligaments and ends (horns) of menisci.
- *Tibial tuberosity:* It is a prominent elevation in the upper anterior part of the tibia. It gives attachment to the ligamentum patellae.

## Shaft

The medial surface is subcutaneous. Its upper part receives the insertions of sartorius, gracilis and semitendinosus muscles.

The posterior surface presents an oblique ridge called soleal line, which provides origin to the soleus muscle. The triangular area above the soleal line receives the insertion of popliteus muscle.

Its lateral surface provides attachments to many muscles.

## Lower End

Its lateral surface presents a triangular fibular notch. It is connected to the lower end of the fibula by an interosseus ligament (inferior tibiofibular joint). Its inferior surface articulates with the talus, to form the ankle joint.

## Medial Malleolus

A short, strong process, which projects down from the medial surface of the lower end of tibia.

## Applied Anatomy

- In rickets (calcium deficiency) tibia is often involved leading to bowlegs. The outward curving of the tibia is

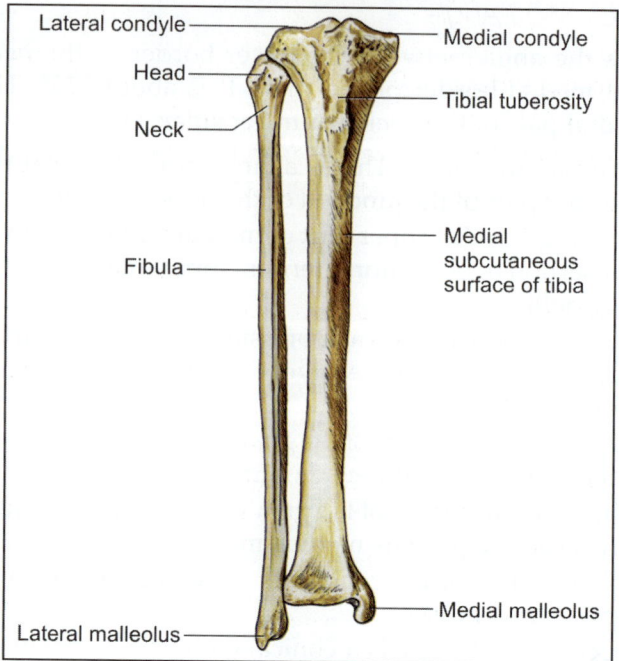

**Fig. 9.14:** Tibia and fibula—anterior view

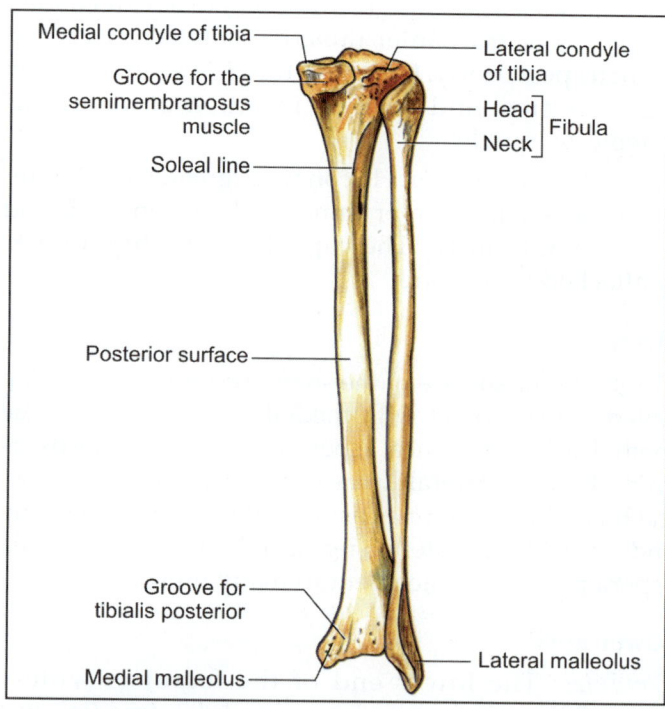

**Fig. 9.15:** Tibia and fibula—posterior view

referred as genu valgum and inward curving is referred as genu varum.
- Upper end of the tibia is one of the commonest sites for acute osteomyelitis.
- Tibia is commonly fractured at the junction of the upper 2/3 and lower 1/3 of shaft.

- Bone grafts are easily obtained from the subcutaneous medial surface of the tibia.
- Invertion at the subtalar joint is associated with external rotation of talus. It can leads to fracture of medial and lateral malleolus. This is called Pott's fracture.

## FIBULA

Fibula is the lateral bone of the leg. It has the following parts: upper end, shaft and lower end (Figs 9.14 and 9.15).

- *Upper end (head):* It is expanded in all directions. The superior surface bears an articular facet, to articulate with the lateral condyle of the tibia (superior tibiofibular joint). The apex of the head is called styloid process. It provides attachment to biceps femoris muscle.
- The constriction below the head is called the neck of the fibula. The common peroneal nerve winds round the neck.
- Shaft is narrow elongated part, which connects the two ends.
- *Lower end (lateral malleolus):* Its medial surface articulates with the talus (ankle joint).

The medial surface also presents a depression called the malleolar fossa.

### Applied Anatomy

- The common peroneal nerve is commonly injured near the neck of the fibula.
- Fibula is the ideal spare bone for a bone graft.
- *Violation of law of ossification:* The epiphyseal center for lower end of fibula appears between one and two years and that of the upper end appear between third and fourth years. The fusion of the lower end (epiphysis) with shaft (diaphysis) takes place earlier (at around sixteenth year) when compared to the upper end (which join the shaft by eighteen years).
- Law of union of ossification: The center (secondary) which appears first fuses last with the diaphysis and vice versa).

## TARSAL BONES

The skeleton of the foot is formed by tarsal bones. There are 7 tarsal bones arranged in two rows (Figs 9.16 and 9.17).

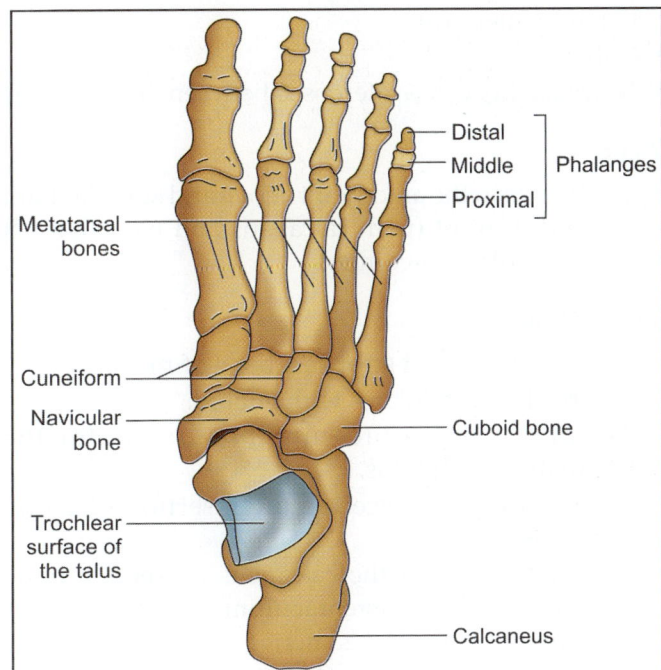

**Fig. 9.16:** Articulated foot—superior view

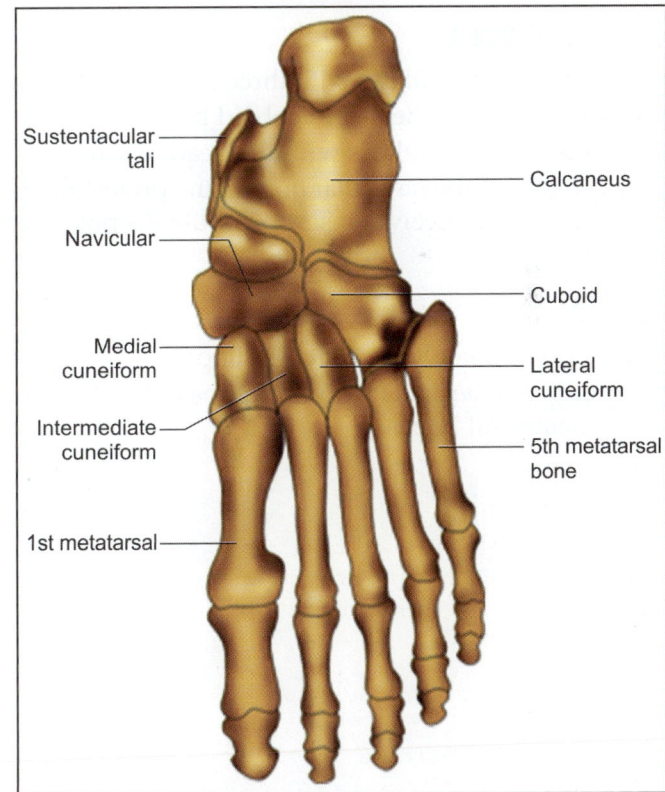

**Fig. 9.17:** Articulated foot—inferior view

### Proximal Row Presents

- Talus (above the calcaneum)
- Calcaneus

### Distal Row

- Medial cuneiform
- Intermediate cuneiform

9

- Lateral cuneiform
- Cuboid
- Navicular bone (it is interposed between the two rows)

## TALUS

It participates in the ankle joint above and subtalar joint below and in front (with calcaneus and navicular). It has no muscular attachment.

## CALCANEUS

- It is the largest and strongest bone of the foot.
- Anteriorly it articulates with cuboid.
- Its upper surface presents three facets for the articulation with talus.
- Its posterior part receives the insertion of tendo calcaneus.
- The medial part of the calcaneus presents a bony projection called 'sustentaculum tali'. It provides attachment to spring ligament.
- The lower most part of the posterior surface is covered by dense fibro-fatty tissue. It supports the body weight in standing position.

## NAVICULAR BONE

- Anteriorly it articulates with three cuneiform bones.
- Laterally, it is connected to cuboid bone.
- Posteriorly it articulates with the head of talus.
- Tuberosity of the navicular bone is the projection on medial side. It receives insertion of tibialis posterior muscle.

## CUBOID

- It is approximately cuboidal in shape.
- Anteriorly it articulates with the bases of 4th and 5th metatarsal bones.

- Posteriorly it articulates with calcaneum.
- Medially it articulates with lateral cuneiform bone and connected with navicular bone.
- The plantar surface of the cuboid presents a groove, which is traversed by the tendon of peroneus longus muscle.

## CUNEIFORM BONES

- These are three wedge shaped bones, named medial, intermediate and lateral cuneiforms.
- The posterior end of each cuneiforms articulates with navicular bone. Their anterior ends articulate with the bases of 1st, 2nd and 3rd metatarsal bones.
- Medial cuneiform bone receives the insertion of tibialis anterior and peroneus longus muscles.

## METATARSALS

There are 5 metatarsal bones, which are numbered from medial to lateral side. Proximally they articulate with the cuneiform and cuboid bones. Distally they articulate with the phalanges.

## PHALANGES

There are 14 phalanges in each foot, 2 for the great toe and 3 for each of the other toes. These phalanges are smaller than the phalanges of the hand.

### Applied Anatomy

- Forceful dorsiflexion may fracture the neck of the talus.
- Fracture of the calcaneus occurs, when a person falls on his heals from the height.
- Removal of navicular bone is an alternative technique in treatment of congenital flat foot.
- Fracture of the base of the 5th metatarsal is common.

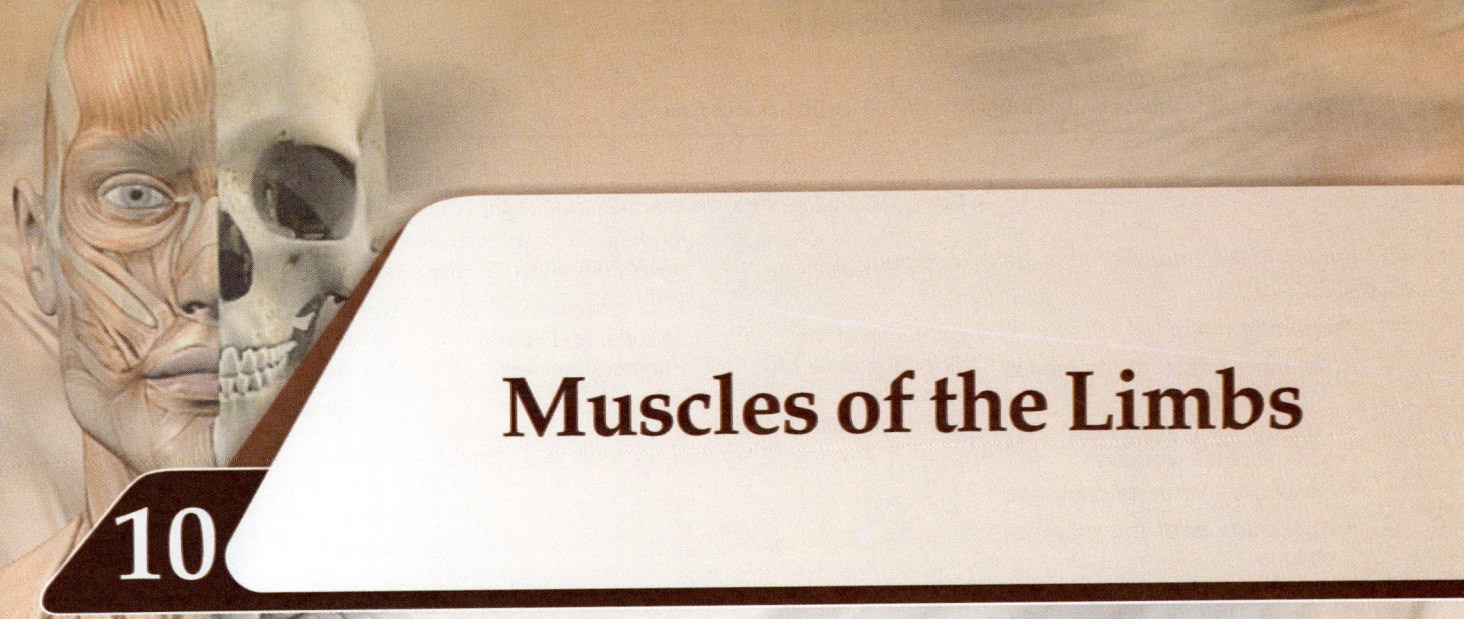

# Muscles of the Limbs

## 10

### PECTORAL REGION

These muscles connect the upper limb with trunk on its anterior aspect. These muscles mainly acts on the shoulder joint (Fig. 10.1). The breast or mammary gland is present in the pectoral region and is discussed below.

The name of the muscles, their attachment, actions and nerve supply is listed in Table 10.1.

Paralysis of serratus anterior muscle results in a condition called 'winging of the scapula'. The medial margin of the scapula becomes prominent on the dorsal side.

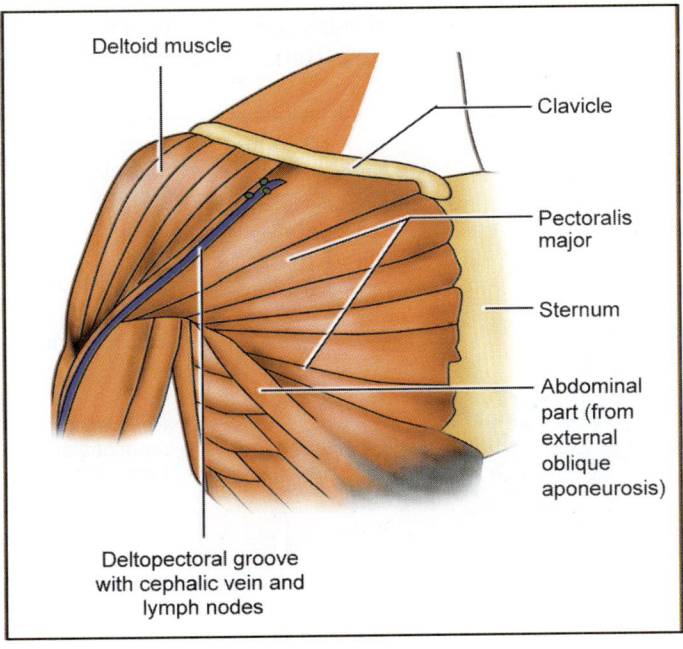

**Fig. 10.1:** Pectoralis major muscle

### MAMMARY GLAND (THE BREAST)

It is rudimentary in males and is well developed in females after puberty. It is an accessory organ of the female reproductive system and provides milk to the newborn (Figs 10.2 and 10.3).

*Situation:* It is situated in the superficial fascia of the pectoral region.

### Structure

*Nipple:* It is a conical projection in the skin covering the mammary gland. The lactiferous ducts draining the milk from the alveoli pierce the nipple.

A pigmented circular area surrounding the nipple is called areola. It has plenty of modified sebaceous glands and they enlarge during pregnancy and lactation.

*Glandular tissue:* Some fibrous tissue extends from the skin to pectoral fascia forming suspensory ligaments. Involvement of these ligaments in carcinoma of the breast, makes it more fixed and retracted. The gland consists of 15–20 lobes. Each lobe consists of many alveoli. The alveoli are lined by columnar epithelium during lactation. The alveoli are drained by lactiferous ducts. The secretion is controlled by the hormone prolactin secreted by the anterior lobe of the pituitary gland.

The bulky constituent of the mammary gland is fat. Some fibrous tissue extends from the skin to pectoral fascia forming suspensory ligaments.

*Arterial supply:* Mammary gland is supplied by branches of the following arteries (Fig. 10.3):

a. Internal thoracic artery.
b. Branches from axillary artery.
c. Branches from the posterior intercostal arteries.

**Table 10.1:** Muscles of the pectoral region

| Name of the muscle and its origin | Insertion | Nerve supply | Actions | |
|---|---|---|---|---|
| 1. **Pectoralis major**<br>• Anterior surface of the medial half of the clavicle<br>• Lateral part of the anterior surface of the sternum<br>• Second to sixth costal cartilages<br>• Aponeurosis of the external oblique | Lateral lip of the bicipital groove of humerus (intertubercular sulcus) | Medial and lateral pectoral nerves | Medial rotation<br>Adduction<br>Flexion | At shoulder joint |
| 2. **Pectoralis minor**<br>Third to fifth ribs | Medial margin and superior surface of the coracoid process of the scapula | Medial and lateral pectoral nerves | Along with serratus anterior protracts the scapula | |
| 3. **Subclavius**<br>Junction of first rib and its costal cartilage | Undersurface of the middle third of the clavicle | Nerve to subclavius from upper trunk of brachial plexus | It steadies the clavicle during shoulder joint movement | |
| 4. **Serratus anterior**<br>By 8 fleshy digitations from outer surfaces of upper 8 ribs | Medial border of the scapula on the costal surface | Nerve to serratus anterior (long thoracic nerve) | Protracts the scapula around the chest wall in pushing and punching movements | |

The venous blood drains into internal thoracic, axillary and posterior intercostals veins.

*Lymphatic drainage:* The lymph from the breast mainly drains into axillary (about 75%) and internal mammary group (about 20%) of lymph nodes and posterior intercostal nodes (5%) (Fig. 10.3). Breast is the frequent site of carcinoma.

### Applied Anatomy

• Breast is the frequent site of carcinoma, which is manifested as painless hard lump in the initial stage. Through lymphatic communications cancer may spread from one breast to the other or into the peritoneal cavity and spread into abdominal organs like liver or ovary.

• The posterior intercostal veins communicate with internal vertebral venous plexus. Hence a carcinoma of the

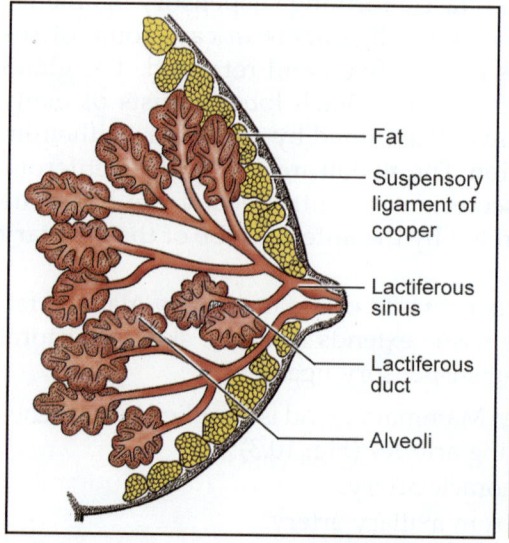

**Fig. 10.2:** Structure of the mammary gland

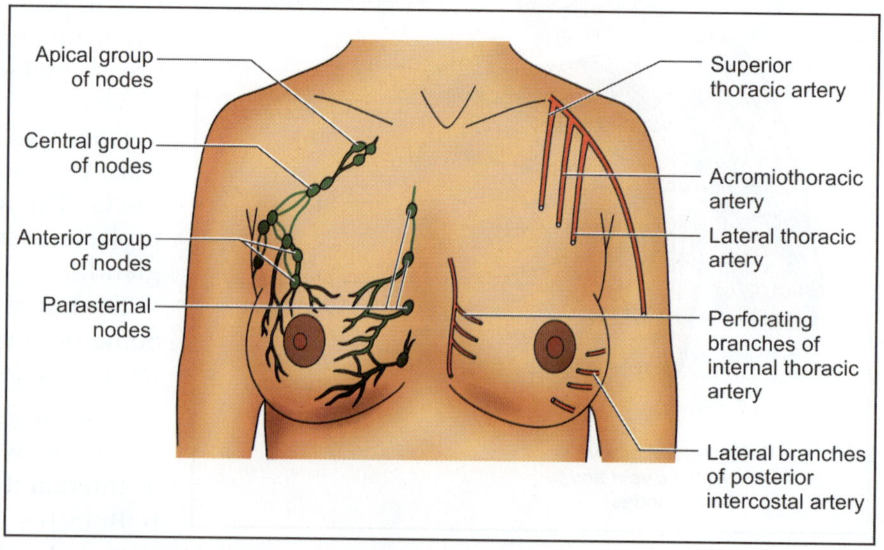

— Fat
— Suspensory ligament of cooper
— Lactiferous sinus
— Lactiferous duct
— Alveoli

Apical group of nodes — 
Central group of nodes — 
Anterior group of nodes — 
Parasternal nodes — 

— Superior thoracic artery
— Acromiothoracic artery
— Lateral thoracic artery
— Perforating branches of internal thoracic artery
— Lateral branches of posterior intercostal artery

**Fig. 10.3:** Blood supply and lymphatic drainage of the mammary gland

mammary gland can spread into vertebral column and skull through these venous communications.

- The blockage of superficial lymphatic vessels in case of carcinoma results in edema of the overlying skin. The edema does not occur at the points where the ducts of the sweat gland open on the skin. This gives resembles of an orange peel (peau d'orange appearance) to the mammary gland.

- In case of carcinoma of the mammary gland the anterior axillary group is first to be involved. For confirmation of diagnosis, biopsies of the axillary lymph nodes are necessary.

- The surgical removal of the mammary gland is called 'mastectomy', which is necessary in case of carcinoma of the gland along with the removal of axillary lymph nodes.

- During removal of axillary lymph nodes, the nerve to serratus anterior, the nerve to latissimus dorsi and intercostobrachial nerves are likely to be injured. Involvement of nerve to serratus anterior can cause difficulty in overhead abduction at the shoulder joint and winging of the scapula. Involvement of intercostobrachial nerve may lead to loss of cutaneous sensation in the arm pit and upper medial part of the arm.

- Mammography is an X-ray of the mammary gland to detect the malignancy.

- Though the mammary gland is rudimentary in males, abnormal enlargement of male mammary gland is referred as gynecomastia. It is a feature of Klinefelter's syndrome (XXY).

- Accessory nipples may be found anywhere along the milk line which extends from axilla to the inguinal region.

## MUSCLES OF THE BACK

These muscles connect the upper limb to the vertebral column. Their names, attachments, nerve supply and actions are listed in Table 10.2 and Figs 10.4 and 10.5.

**Table 10.2:** Muscles of the back

| Name of the muscle and its origin | Insertion | Nerve supply | Actions |
|---|---|---|---|
| **1. Trapezius** (Fig. 10.1)<br>• Medial part of the superior nuchal line of the occipital bone<br>• Ligamentum nuchae (fibrous structure connecting cervical spines)<br><br>• Spinous processes and supraspinous ligaments of all 12 thoracic vertebrae | • Upper fibers inserted to posterior border of the lateral one third of the clavicle<br>• Middle fibers to medial border of the acromion and upper lip of the crest of the spine of scapula<br>• Lower fibers to the triangular area at the medial end of the spine of the scapula | Spinal part of the accessory nerve and ventral rami of $C_3$ and $C_4$ nerves are proprioceptive | • Upper fibers elevate the scapula<br><br>• Middle fibers retract the scapula<br>• Upper and lower fibers acting together with serratus anterior rotates the scapula for overhead abduction at shoulder joint. |
| **2. Latissimus dorsi** (Fig. 10.1)<br>• Lower 6 thoracic spines and their supraspinous ligaments<br>• Spines of all the lumbar and sacral vertebrae through the posterior layer of thoracolumbar fascia<br>• Outer lip of the iliac crest<br>• Lower 4 ribs<br>• Inferior angle of the scapula | The muscle forms a tendon and is inserted to the floor of the bicipital groove | Nerve to latissimus dorsi from posterior cord of the brachial plexus | Extension<br>Medial rotation<br>Adduction ⎫<br>Helps in climbing ⎬ At shoulder (lifting the trunk) ⎭ joint |
| **3. Rhomboideus minor**<br>• Lower part of the ligamentum nuchae<br>• Spinous processes of $C_7$ and $T_1$ vertebrae | Medial border of the scapula on the dorsal aspect | Nerve to rhomboideus ($C_5$) | Retract the scapula |
| **4. Rhomboideus major**<br>Spinous process of $T_2$ to $T_5$ vertebrae and their supraspinous ligaments | Medial border of the scapula on the dorsal aspect (from spine to inferior angle) | Nerve to rhomboideus ($C_5$) | Retract the scapula |

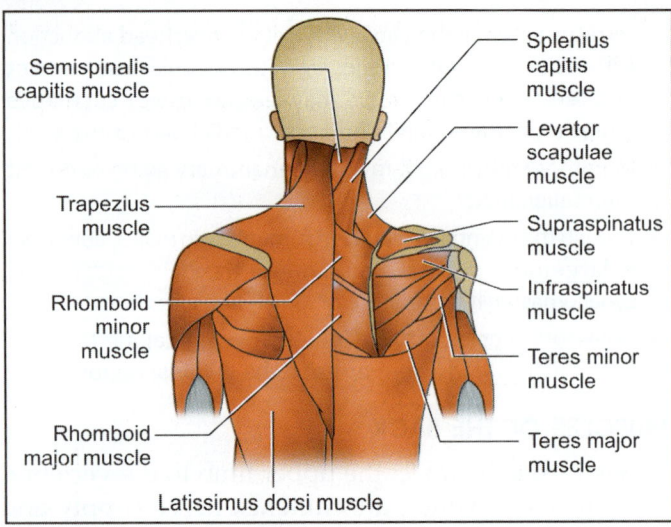

**Fig. 10.4:** Trapezius and latissimus dorsi muscles

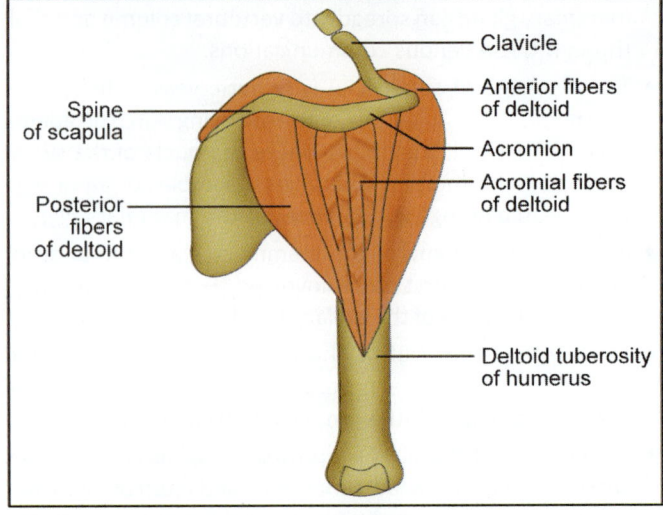

**Fig. 10.5:** Deltoid muscle

## MUSCLES OF THE SCAPULAR REGION

These muscles acts on shoulder joint. Their name, attachments, nerve supply and actions are listed in Table 10.3. The deltoid muscles is explained below.

### 1. Deltoid

Deltoid is a powerful muscle that surrounds the shoulder. Intramuscular injections are often given into the deltoid (Fig. 10.5).

### Origin

The anterior fibers arise from anterior border of the lateral 1/3rd of the clavicle.

The middle fibers are multipennate and arise from lateral margin of the acromion process.

The posterior fibers arise from lower lip of the crest of the spine of the scapula.

### Insertion

Deltoid tuberosity of the humerus.

| Table 10.3: Muscles of the scapular region | | | |
| --- | --- | --- | --- |
| Name of the muscle and its origin (Fig. 10.4) | Insertion | Nerve supply | Actions |
| **2. Supraspinatus** <br> Medial 2/3rd of supraspinous fossa of scapula | Tendon passes beneath the coracoacromial arch and inserted into upper impression of greater tubercle of humerus | Suprascapular nerve ($C_{5, 6}$) | Initiates the abduction at shoulder joint (first 15°) |
| **3. Infraspinatus** <br> Medial 2/3rd of the infraspinous fossa of scapula | Middle impression of the greater tubercle of the humerus | Suprascapular nerve ($C_{5, 6}$) | Lateral rotation at shoulder joint |
| **4. Teres minor** <br> Upper 2/3rd of the lateral border of the scapula | Lowest impression of the greater tubercle of humerus | Axillary nerve ($C_{5, 6}$) | Lateral rotation at the shoulder joint |
| **5. Teres major** <br> Lower 1/3rd of the lateral border of the scapula | Medial lip of the bicipital groove of humerus | Lower subscapular nerve ($C_{5, 6}$) | Medial rotation and adduction at shoulder joint |
| **6. Subscapularis** <br> Medial 2/3rd of the subscapular fossa of the scapula | Lesser tubercle of the humerus | Upper and lower subscapular nerves ($C_{5, 6}$) | Medial rotation and adduction at shoulder joint |

### Nerve Supply

Axillary nerve.

### Actions

Anterior fibers cause flexion and medial rotation at shoulder joint.

Posterior fibers cause extension and lateral rotation of the shoulder joint.

Middle fibers abduct the arm at shoulder joint from 15° to 90°.

### Structures under Cover of the Deltoid

1. Shoulder joint
2. Coracoid process of the scapula, upper end of the humerus
3. Axillary nerve
4. Anterior and posterior circumflex humeral vessels
5. Muscles include—insertion of pectoralis minor, subscapularis, supraspinatus, infraspinatus, origins of short and long heads of biceps, long head of triceps.

## Axilla (arm pit)

It is a space situated between the upper part of the arm and the chest wall. It is pyramidal in shape with its apex directed towards the root of the neck.

It has an anterior, posterior, medial and lateral walls. The apex is blunt and is called cervicoaxillary canal. The brachial plexus and axillary artery enter the axilla through this canal.

The boundaries of the axilla are:

*Anterior wall:* Pectoralis major, pectoralis minor and subclavius muscles.

*Posterior wall:* Subscapularis, latissimus dorsi and teres major.

*Medial wall:* Upper four intercostal spaces (upper thoracic wall).

*Lateral wall:* Shaft of the humerus with coracobrachialis and short head of the biceps brachii muscle.

### Contents

1. Axillary artery and vein
2. Infraclavicular part of the brachial plexus
3. Axillary lymph nodes
4. Axillary pad of fat.

### Applied Anatomy

1. Axilla has abundant axillary hairs. Infections of the hair follicles and sebaceous glands give rise to boils.
2. Examinations of axillary lymph nodes are important in clinical practice.
3. An abscess originating from the cervical vertebrae can track down to the axilla along the neurovascular bundle.

## MUSCLES OF THE FRONT OF THE ARM (FLEXOR COMPARTMENT) (Figs 10.6 to 10.8)

Their names, attachments, nerve supply and actions are listed in Table 10.4. The biceps brachii is discussed below.

### 1. Biceps Brachii

*Origin:* It has two heads of origin. The short head arises from the tip of the coracoid process along with coracobrachialis. The long head arises from the supraglenoid tubercle of the scapula within the shoulder joint cavity (Figs 10.6 to 10.8).

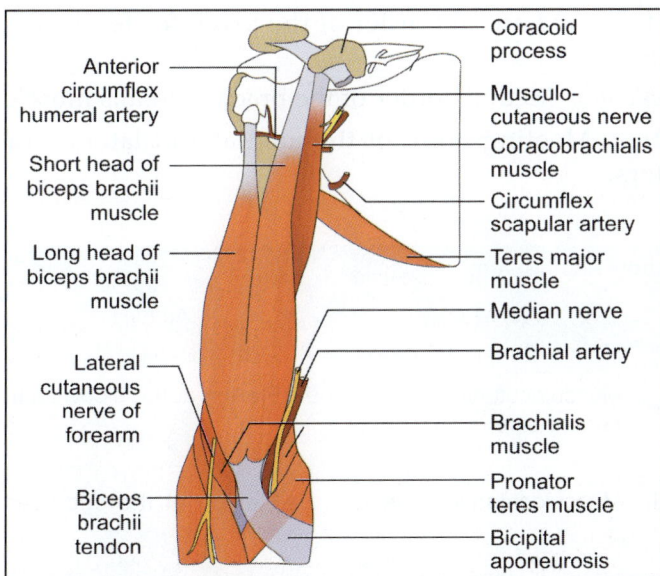

**Fig. 10.6:** Biceps brachii and coracobrachialis muscles

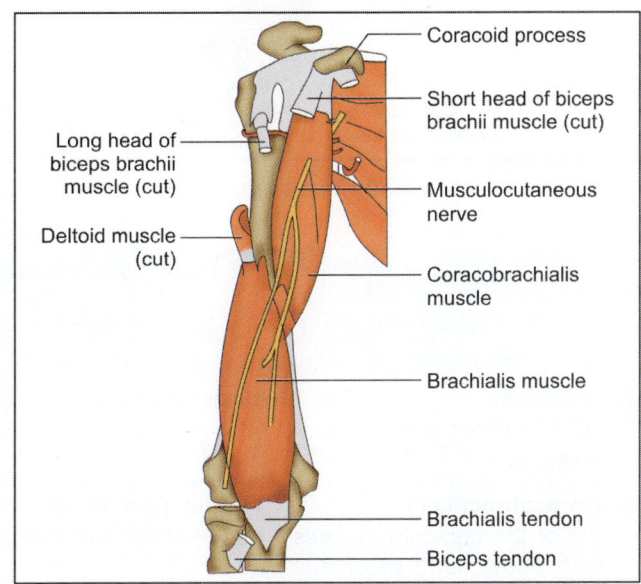

**Fig. 10.7:** Brachialis and coracobrachialis muscles

10

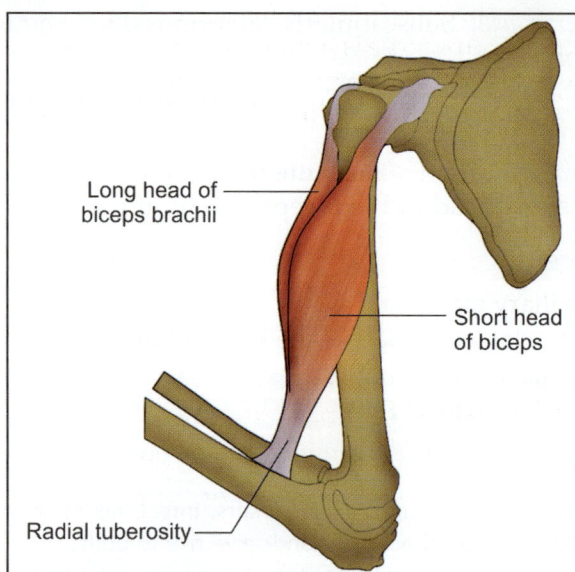

**Fig. 10.8:** Biceps brachii muscle

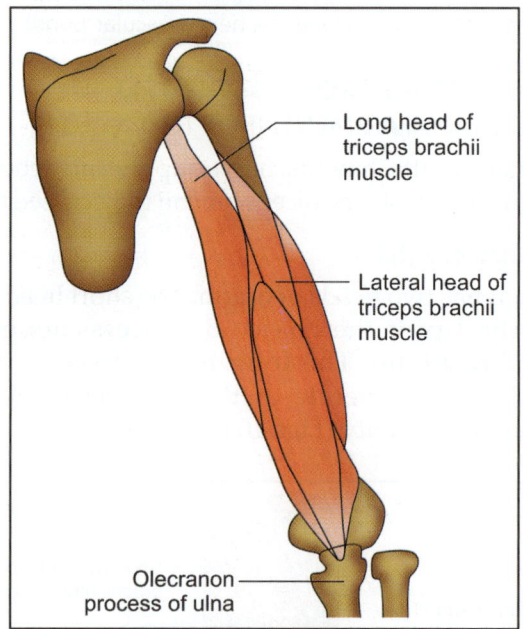

**Fig. 10.9:** Triceps brachii

*Insertion:* The two heads join in the front of the arm. It is inserted by a tendon to the tuberosity of the radius.

*Nerve supply:* Musculocutaneous nerve

*Actions:* It supinates the forearm at radioulnar joint and flexes the elbow joint.

## MUSCLES OF THE BACK OF THE ARM (POSTERIOR OR EXTENSOR COMPARTMENT)

### Triceps

Only one muscle occupies this area, called triceps. It has three heads of origin (Fig. 10.9).

*Origin:* The long head arises from the infraglenoid tubercle of the scapula.

The lateral head arises from a ridge above the radial groove of the humerus.

The medial head arises from the posterior surface of the humerus below the radial groove.

*Insertion:* To the olecranon process of the ulna.

*Nerve supply:* It is supplied by radial nerve.

*Action:* It is a chief extensor of the elbow joint.

### CUBITAL FOSSA

This is a triangular space situated on the front of the elbow (homologous with the popliteal fossa present on the back of the knee) (Fig. 10.10).

### Boundaries

*Base:* An imaginary line connecting the two epicondyles of the humerus.

*Medially:* Lateral border of the pronator teres muscle.

*Laterally:* Medial border of the brachioradialis muscle.

*Apex:* Meeting point of the medial and lateral borders.

| **Table 10.4:** Muscles in front in the arm | | | |
|---|---|---|---|
| Name of the muscle and its origin | Insertion | Nerve supply | Actions |
| 2. **Brachialis**<br>Lower half of the front of the humerus | Ulnar tuberosity | Musculocutaneous nerve and radial nerve | Flexion at the elbow joint |
| 3. **Coracobrachialis**<br>Tip of the coracoid process with short head of biceps brachii | Middle part of the medial border of the humerus | Musculocutaneous nerve | Flexion at the shoulder joint |

10

*Roof:* The roof is formed by skin superficial fascia with median cubital vein, medial cutaneous nerve of the forearm, lateral cutaneous nerve of the forearm, deep fascia with bicipital aponeurosis (Fig. 10.11). The medial cubital vein is connected with deeper veins by perforating veins which perforates bicipital aponeurosis. This makes median cubital vein more fixed and hence often selected for intravenous injections.

*Floor:* The floor is formed by brachialis muscle in the upper part and supinator muscle in the lower part.

## Contents (from medial to lateral side)

1. *Median nerve:* Further down it leaves the fossa by passing between the two heads of the pronator teres muscle.

2. *Brachial artery:* It terminates in the fossa at the level of the neck of the radius by dividing into ulnar and radial arteries. The blood pressure is recorded by auscultating the brachial artery in front of the elbow medial to the tendon of biceps brachii. Among the terminal branches radial artery is superficial and ulnar is deep. The ulnar artery passes deep to the deep head of the pronator teres muscle.

3. *Tendon* of the biceps brachii muscle.

4. *Radial nerve:* It appears on the lateral side between brachialis and brachioradialis muscles. It also terminates by dividing into a superficial branch and deep branch (posterior interosseous nerve). The superficial branch is cutaneous supplies skin of the lateral part of the dorsum and dorsal side of the

lateral three and a half finger. The posterior interosseous nerve is motor and supplies muscles of the back of the forearm which are responsible for extension at the wrist joint.

## MUSCLES OF THE FRONT OF THE FOREARM

It consists of superficial and deep groups. These muscles mainly cause flexion at the elbow and wrist joints. Hence, this compartment is called the flexor compartment.

### Superficial Muscles (Table 10.5 and Fig. 10.12a)

These superficial muscles have a common origin from the medial epicondyle of the humerus (common flexor origin).

1. Pronator teres—pronates the forearm
2. Flexor carpi radialis—flexes the wrist joint
3. Palmaris longus—flexes the wrist joint
4. Flexor carpi ulnaris—flexes the wrist joint
5. Flexor digitorum superficialis (sublimus). This muscle divides into four tendons for medial four fingers. Each tendon extends up to the middle phalanx. They flex the fingers.

All these muscles are supplied by median nerve except flexor carpi ulnaris, which is supplied, by ulnar nerve.

### Deep Muscles (Table 10.6 and Fig. 10.12b)

1. Flexor digitorum profundus—this muscle also divides into four tendons for medial four fingers. Each tendon extends up to distal phalanx of the finger. They also flex the fingers.
2. Flexor pollicis longus—the tendon of this muscle passes into thumb and it flexes the thumb.

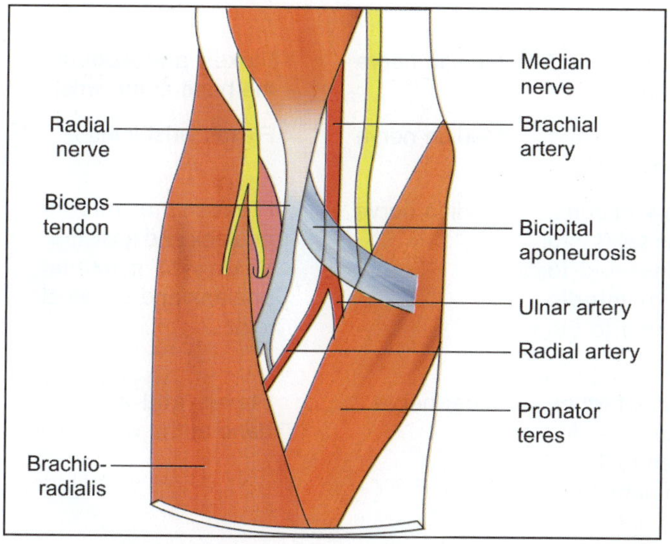

**Fig. 10.10:** Contents of the cubital fossa

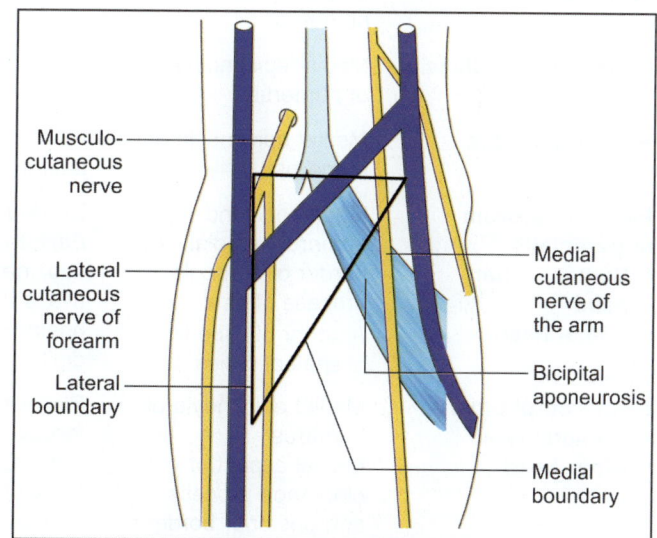

**Fig. 10.11:** Roof of the cubital fossa

10

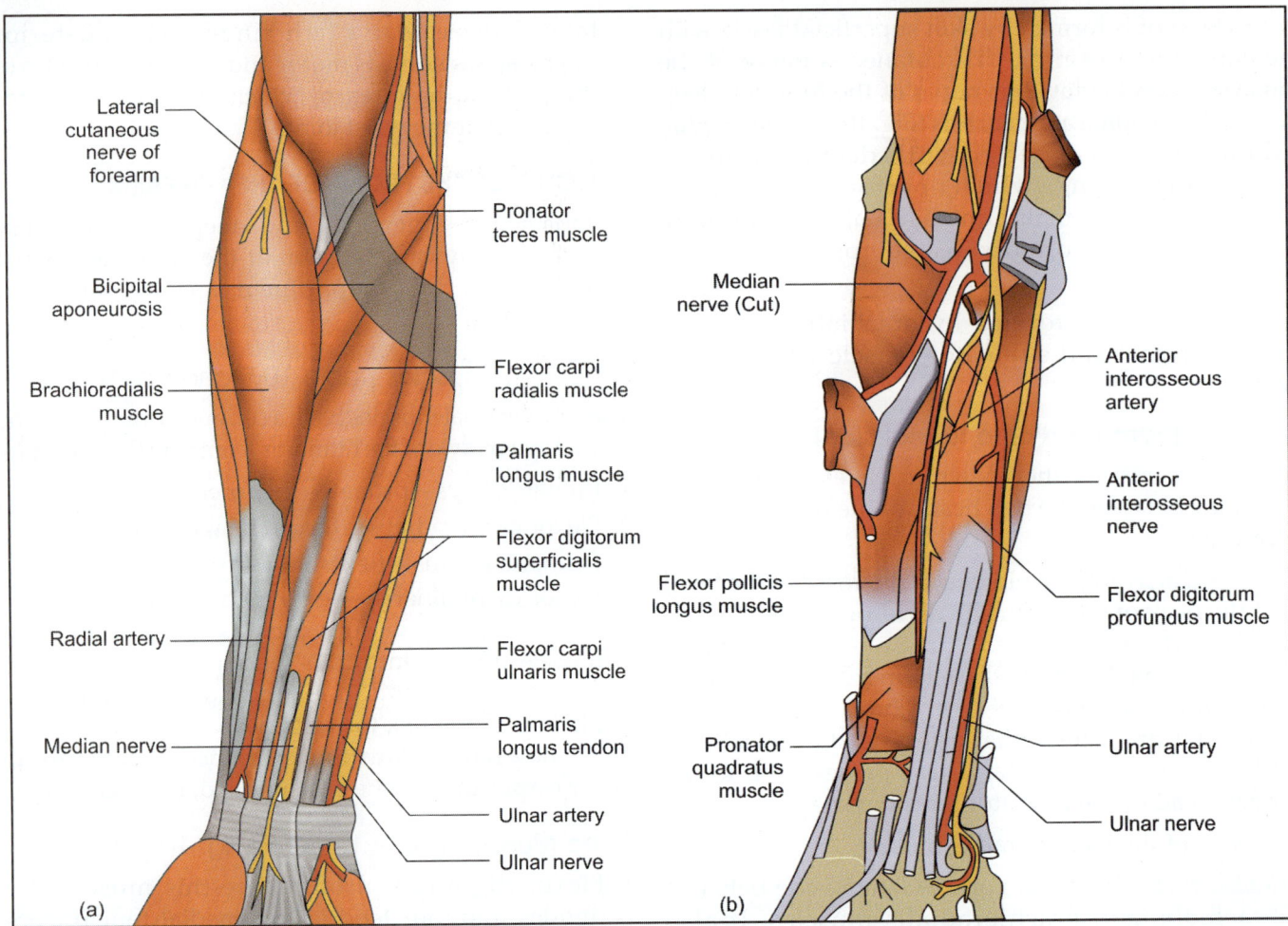

**Fig. 10.12a and b:** (a) Superficial muscles of the front of forearm; (b) deep muscles of the front of the forearm

**Table 10.5:** Superficial flexor muscles of the forearm

| Muscle | Origin | Insertion | Nerve supply | Actions |
|---|---|---|---|---|
| **Pronator teres** | Medial epicondyle of humerus | Middle of lateral aspect of shaft of radius | Median nerve | Pronation of forearm |
| **Flexor carpi radialis** | Medial epicondyle of humerus | Bases of second and third metacarpals | Median nerve | Flexes and abducts the hand at the wrist |
| **Palmaris longus** | Medial epicondyle of humerus | Flexor retinaculum and palmar aponeurosis | Median nerve | Flexes wrist joint |
| **Flexor digitorum superficialis**<br>• **Humero ulnar head**<br>• **Radial head** | Medial epicondyle of humerus; medial border of coronoid process of ulna<br>Anterior oblique line of shaft of radius | Divided into 4 tendons. Each tendon splits into two, gets inserted to the sides of middle phalanx of 2nd to 5th digits | Median nerve | Flexes the middle phalanx and assists in flexing of proximal phalanx and the wrist joint |
| **Flexor carpi ulnaris**<br>• **Humeral head**<br>• **Ulnar head** | Medial epicondyle of humerus<br>Medial aspect of olecranon process and posterior border of ulna | Pisiform bone; further tendon extends and gets inserted to the hook of the hamate and base of fifth metacarpal bone | Ulnar nerve | Flexes and adducts hand at the wrist joint |

3. Pronator quadratus—it is a quadrangular muscle connecting the lower ends of ulna and radius. It causes pronation of forearm at radioulnar joints.

The long tendons of these muscles (flexor digitorum superficialis, flexor digitorum profundus and flexor pollicis longus) while passing through the hand (over the carpal bones) are held in position by a fibrous band called flexor retinaculum (Table 10.6).

## Flexor Retinaculum of the Hand

It is a modified deep fascia with thick transversely running glistening fibers present opposite to the level of carpal bones. Functionally, it holds the long flexor tendons in their position during movements of the wrist joint.

### Attachments

Medially, it is attached to the pisiform bone and the hook of the hamate. However a superficial slip is attached to the pisiform bone making a tunnel (Guyon's canal) for the passage of ulnar vessels and nerves.

Laterally, it is attached to the tubercle of scaphoid and the crest of the trapezium. A deep slip on the lateral side is attached to medial lip of the groove of trapezium forms a tunnel for the passage of flexor carpi radialis tendon.

### Structures Passing Superficial to it

1. Ulnar nerve and vessels
2. Palmaris longus tendon
3. Palmar cutaneous branch of the ulnar nerve
4. Palmar cutaneous branch of the median nerve
5. Superficial palmar branch of the radial artery

### Structures Passing Deep to the Flexor Retinaculum

1. Median nerve
2. Tendons of flexor digitorum superficialis
3. Tendons of flexor digitorum profundus
4. Tendon of flexor pollicis longus

The tendons of superficialis and profundus are enclosed in a common synovial sheath called ulnar bursa, while tendon of flexor pollicis longus has a separate synovial sheath called radial bursa.

*Carpal tunnel:* It is an osseofibrous tunnel between superficially placed flexor retinaculum and palmar surface of the carpal bone on the deeper side. All the structures passing deep to the flexor retinaculum are the contents of the carpal tunnel. Among them, median nerve is clinically significant because in case of inflammation of these tendons in the carpal tunnel the nerve is likely to be compressed. This is

| Table 10.6: Deep muscles of the front of the forearm | | | | |
|---|---|---|---|---|
| *Muscle* | *Origin* | *Insertion* | *Nerve supply* | *Actions* |
| **Flexor digitorum profundus** | Upper 3/4 of anterior and medial surface of shaft of ulna. Upper 3/4 of posterior border and medial surface of olecranon and coronoid processes of ulna. Adjoining anterior surface of interosseous membrane | Forms 4 tendons for medial 4 digits. Passes deep to flexor retinaculum to enter the palm. Perforates the tendon of flexor digitorum superficialis at the level of proximal phalanx. Inserted to palmar surface of base of distal phalanx. | Medial half by ulnar nerve. Lateral half by anterior interosseous nerve. | Flexes the distal phalanx combined with the action of flexor digitorum superficialis. Flexes other joints of digits, fingers and wrist. Acts better when wrist is extended. Flexes the distal phalanx of thumb |
| **Flexor pollicis longus** | Upper 3/4 of anterior surface of shaft of radius; adjoining anterior surface of interosseous membrane | Passes deep to the flexor retinaculum to enter the palm. Inserted into palmar surface of distal phalanx of the thumb | Anterior interosseous nerve | Flexes the proximal joints that is crossed by the tendon |
| **Pronator quadratus** | Oblique ridge on the lower 1/4 of anterior surface of shaft of ulna and adjoining medial area | Superficial fibers—lower 1/4 of anterior surface and anterior border of radius. Deep fibers—triangular area above ulnar notch | Anterior interosseous nerve | Superficial fibers—pronates the forearm. Deep fibers—fixes the lower ends of radius and ulna |

10

referred as 'carpal tunnel syndrome' which will be discussed after explanation of median nerve in the hand.

## MUSCLES OF THE BACK OF THE FOREARM

This compartment (extensor) consists of superficial and deep groups. These muscles mainly cause extension at the wrist joint. These muscles are supplied by radial nerve (or its branch called posterior interosseous nerve). Paralysis of these muscles causes 'wrist drop'.

Before passing into the dorsum of the hand, the tendons of these muscles are held in their proper position by a fibrous band called extensor retinaculum.

### Superficial Muscles (Table 10.7 and Fig. 10.13a))

1. Anconeus—extends the elbow joint
2. Brachioradialis—flexes the elbow joint
3. Extensor carpi radialis longus—extends and abducts the wrist.

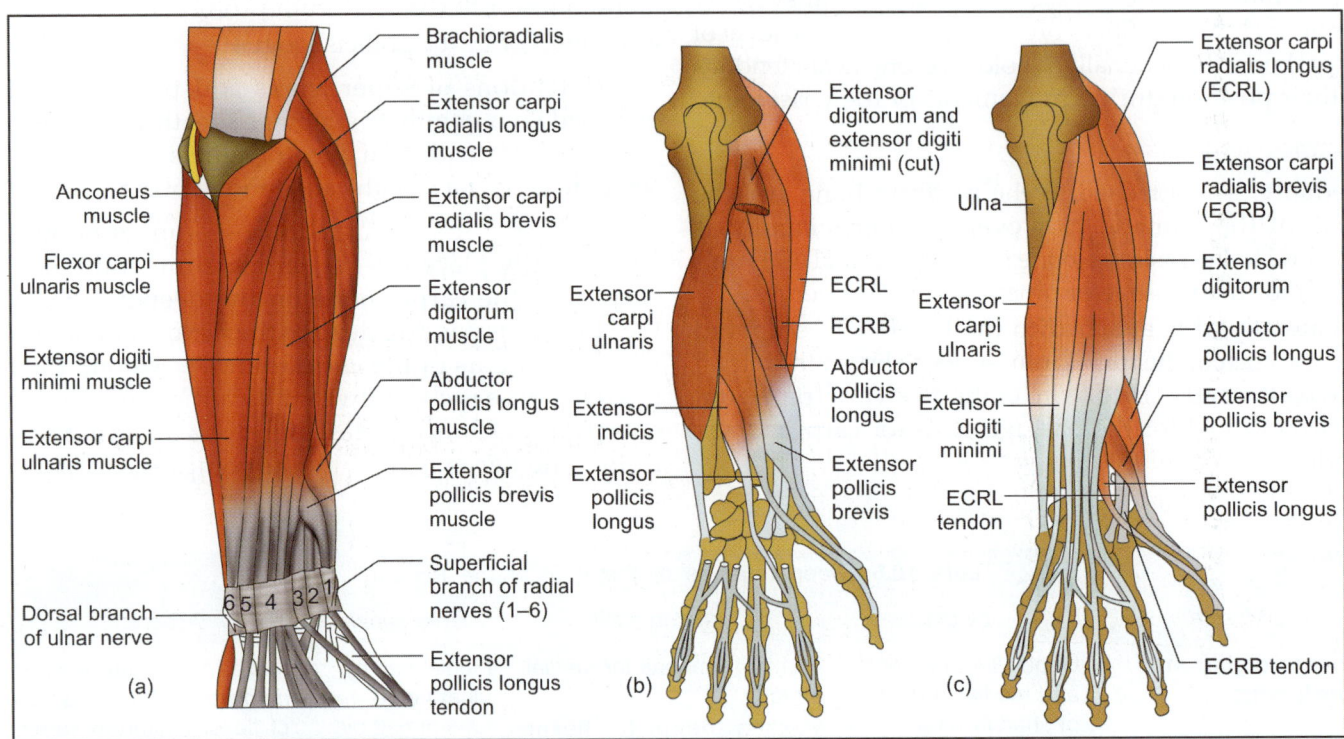

**Fig. 10.13a and b:** (a) Superficial extensors of the forearm; (b) deep extensors of the forearm; (c) deep extensors of the forearm

| Muscle | Origin | Insertion | Nerve supply | Actions |
|---|---|---|---|---|
| Anconeus | Lateral epicondyle of humerus | Lateral surface of olecranon process of ulna | Radial nerve | Extends the elbow joint |
| Brachioradialis | Upper 2/3rd of lateral supracondylar ridge of humerus | Base of styloid process of radius | Radial nerve | Flexes the forearm at elbow joint in mid prone position |
| Extensor carpi radialis longus | Lower 1/3rd of supracondylar ridge of humerus | Posterior surface of base of 2nd metacarpal | Radial nerve | Extends and abducts hand at wrist joint |
| Extensor carpi radialis brevis | Lateral epicondyle of humerus | Posterior surface of base of 3rd metacarpal | Radial nerve (deep branch) | Extends and abducts hand at wrist joint |
| Extensor digitorum | Lateral epicondyle of humerus | Bases of middle phalanx of 2nd–5th digits | Radial nerve (deep branch) | Extends the digits of hand |
| Extensor digiti minimi | Lateral epicondyle of humerus | Dorsal digital expansion of little finger | Radial nerve (deep branch) | Extensor of metacarpophalangeal joint of little finger |
| Extensor carpi ulnaris | Lateral epicondyle of humerus | Bases of 5th metacarpal | Radial nerve (deep branch) | Extends and adducts the hand at wrist joint |

Table 10.7: Superficial muscles of the back of forearm (Fig. 10.13a)

10

4. Extensor carpi radialis brevis—extends and abducts the wrist.
5. Extensor digitorum—it divides into four tendons for medial four fingers.
6. Extensor digiti minimi—extends the little finger.
7. Extensor carpi ulnaris—extends and adducts the wrist joint.

### Deep Muscles (Table 10.8, Fig. 10.13b and c)

1. Supinator
2. Abductor pollicis longus—abducts the thumb
3. Extensor pollicis brevis—extends the thumb
4. Extensor pollicis longus—extends the thumb
5. Extensor indicis—extends the index finger.

### Extensor Retinaculum of the Wrist

It is formed by the modification of the deep fascia present at the back of the wrist. Functionally it holds the long extensor tendons in their respective position during the movements at the wrist joint.

### Attachments

Medially it is attached to the pisiform and triquetral bones. Laterally to the anterior border of the lower end of the radius.

From the under surface of the retinaculum septa passes deep and is attached to the dorsal surface of the distal end of the radius forming 6 osseofascial compartments. Each compartment is traversed by extensor tendons with their synovial sheaths. The compartment and their contents from lateral to medial side are:

1. Abductor pollicis longus
   Extensor pollicis brevis
2. Extensor carpi radialis longus (ECRL)
   Extensor carpi radialis brevis (ECRB)
3. Extensor pollicis longus
4. Four tendons:
   Extensor digitorum
   Extensor indicis
   Posterior interosseous nerve
   Anterior interosseous artery
5. Extensor digiti minimi (between radius and ulna)
6. Extensor carpi ulnaris

### INTRINSIC MUSCLES OF HAND

The elevation, proximal to the thumb (lateral side of hand) is called thenar eminence. The underlying muscles produce this elevation. The muscles are (Fig. 10.14):

1. Abductor pollicis brevis
2. Flexor pollicis brevis
3. Opponens pollicis
4. Adductor pollicis

All these muscles act on the thumb. They are all supplied by the median nerve except adductor pollicis, which is supplied by the ulnar nerve.

The elevation on medial side of the hand is called hypothenar eminence. It is produced by the underlying muscles.

| | | Table 10.8: Deep muscles of back of forearm (Fig. 10.13b and c) | | |
| --- | --- | --- | --- | --- |
| Muscle | Origin | Insertion | Nerve supply | Actions |
| **Supinator** | Lateral epicondyle of humerus, Annular ligament of superior radioulnar joint, supinator crest of ulna and a depression behind it | Neck and complete shaft of upper 1/3rd of radius | Radial nerve (deep branch) | Supination of forearm in extended elbow |
| **Abductor pollicis longus** | Posterior surface of shaft of radius and ulna | Base of first metacarpal on the dorsal surface | Radial nerve (deep branch) | Abducts and extends thumb |
| **Extensor pollicis brevis** | Posterior surface of shaft of radius | Base of proximal phalanx of thumb | Radial nerve (deep branch) | Extends metacarpophalangeal joint of thumb |
| **Extensor pollicis longus** | Posterior surface of shaft of ulna | Base of distal phalanx of thumb | Radial nerve (deep branch) | Extends distal phalanx of thumb |
| **Extensor indicis** | Posterior surface of shaft of ulna | Dorsal digital expansion of index finger | Radial nerve (deep branch) | Extends the metacarpophalangeal joint of index finger |

10

1. Palmaris brevis (lies under the skin)
2. Abductor digiti minimi
3. Flexor digiti minimi
4. Opponens digiti minimi

These muscles (except palmaris brevis) act on the little finger. They are supplied by ulnar nerve.

### LUMBRICAL MUSCLES

These are small worm like muscles, four in number, counted from lateral to medial side. They are attached to the tendon of flexor digitorum profundus. The tendon of each muscle is inserted into dorsal digital expansion (on the dorsal aspect of the metacarpophalangeal joint). The 1st and the 2nd are supplied by the median nerve, the 3rd and 4th are supplied by the ulnar nerve. Functionally they flex the metacarpophalangeal joints and extend the interphalangeal joints (Fig. 10.14).

### INTEROSSEOUS MUSCLES (OR INTEROSSEI)

There are two groups. The superficial group is called palmar interossei and the deep group is called dorsal interossei. There are four palmar interossei, which cause adduction of fingers. There are four dorsal interossei, which cause abduction of the fingers. The ulnar nerve supplies both palmar and dorsal interossei (Figs 10.15 and 10.16).

All the interossei and lumbricals have a common action—flexion at metacarpophalangeal joint and extension at the interphalangeal joints. Hence paralysis of these muscles (injury to the ulnar nerve T1 segment of the spinal cord) results in 'clawhand' (extension at metacarpophalangeal joint and flexion at the interphalangeal joint).

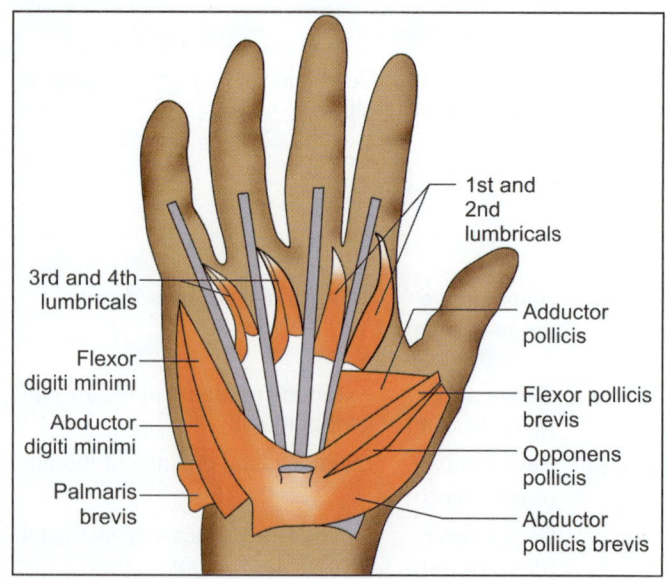

Fig. 10.14: Superficial extensors and deep extensors of the forearm

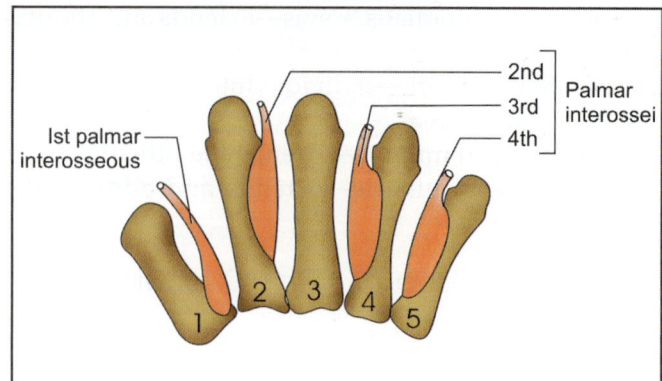

**Fig. 10.15:** Palmar interossei

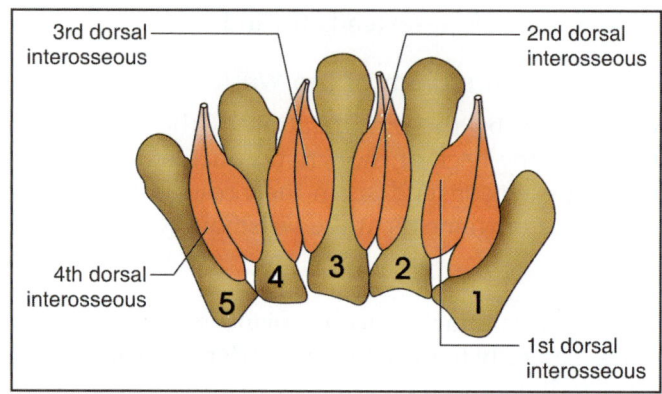

**Fig. 10.16:** Dorsal interossei

### Summary

The muscles of the upper limb are placed in two compartments in arm and forearm. The posterior compartment is extensor compartment and their muscles are supplied by radial nerve. The anterior compartment is flexor compartment. The flexor compartment of the arm is supplied by musculocutaneous nerve. The flexor compartment of forearm is mainly supplied by medial nerve and partly by ulnar nerve. Most of the muscles of the hand are suplied by ulnar nerve and a few by median nerve.

### MUSCLES OF THE LOWER LIMB

### MUSCLES OF THE ANTERIOR (EXTENSOR) COMPARTMENT OF THE THIGH

It includes muscles from the posterior abdominal wall and the iliac region. They are psoas major and iliacus. These muscles are the flexors of the hip joint. The remaining muscles mainly extend the knee joint (hence extensor muscles) (Fig. 10.17).

### Sartorius

*Origin:* Anterior superior iliac spine.

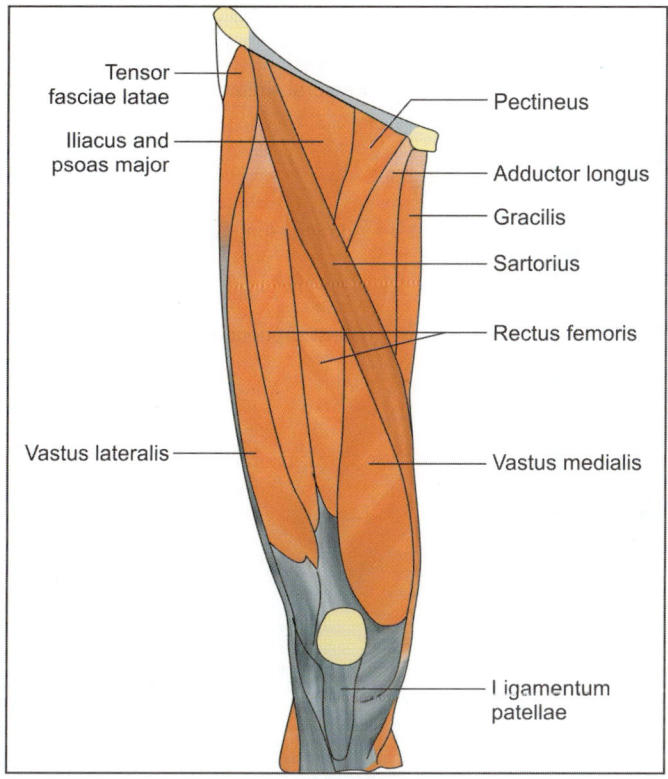

**Fig. 10.17:** Muscles in front and medial side of the thigh

*Insertion:* The muscle descends obliquely downwards and medially inserted into upper part of the medial surface of the tibia

*Nerve supply:* Anterior division of the femoral nerve

*Actions:*

On hip joint: Flexion, abduction and lateral rotation

On knee joint: Flexion and medial rotation.

## Quadriceps Femoris

- It is the bulky muscle in the front of the thigh. It consists of four parts—vastus medialis, vastus lateralis, vastus intermedius and rectus femoris.
- Each muscle has different origin from the femur but rectus femoris arises from the hip bone. Hence, it crosses the hip joint.
- All the four parts of the quadriceps femoris join to form a common tendon, which is inserted into base of the patella.
- *Nerve supply:* Posterior division of the femoral nerve.
- *Actions:* It is a powerful extensor of the knee. Rectus femoris in addition to extending the knee also flexes the hip joint.

## FEMORAL TRIANGLE

It is a triangular depression in the upper part of the thigh. The base of the triangle is directed upwards and apex downwards (Fig. 10.18).

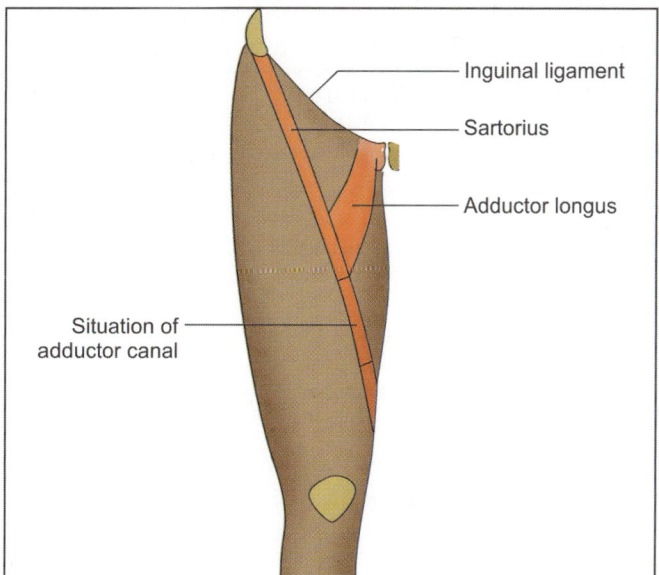

**Fig. 10.18:** Femoral triangle—boundaries

## Boundaries

*Base*—inguinal ligament

*Laterally*—medial border of sartorius

*Medially*—medial border of adductor longus muscle

*Apex:* Meeting point of the medial and lateral borders (apex continues as adductor canal).

*Roof:* Skin, Superficial fascia (with superficial inguinal lymph nodes, terminal part of the great saphenous vein, superficial arteries and cutaneous nerves).

Deep fascia (fascia lata) which shows an opening called 'saphenous opening'.

*Floor (from medial to lateral side):* Adductor longus, Pectineus, Iliopsoas muscles.

*Contents* (Fig. 10.19)

1. Femoral artery and its branches
2. Femoral vein and its tributaries
3. Femoral nerve and its branches
4. Deep inguinal lymph nodes

## Femoral Sheath

It is a fascial sheath enclosing the proximal part of the femoral artery and vein. It has anterior and posterior wall, which are connected by septa. Hence, the sheath is divided into three compartments (Figs 10.20a and b).

a. Lateral arterial compartment encloses femoral artery and femoral branch of genitofemoral nerve.

b. Middle venous compartment encloses femoral vein.

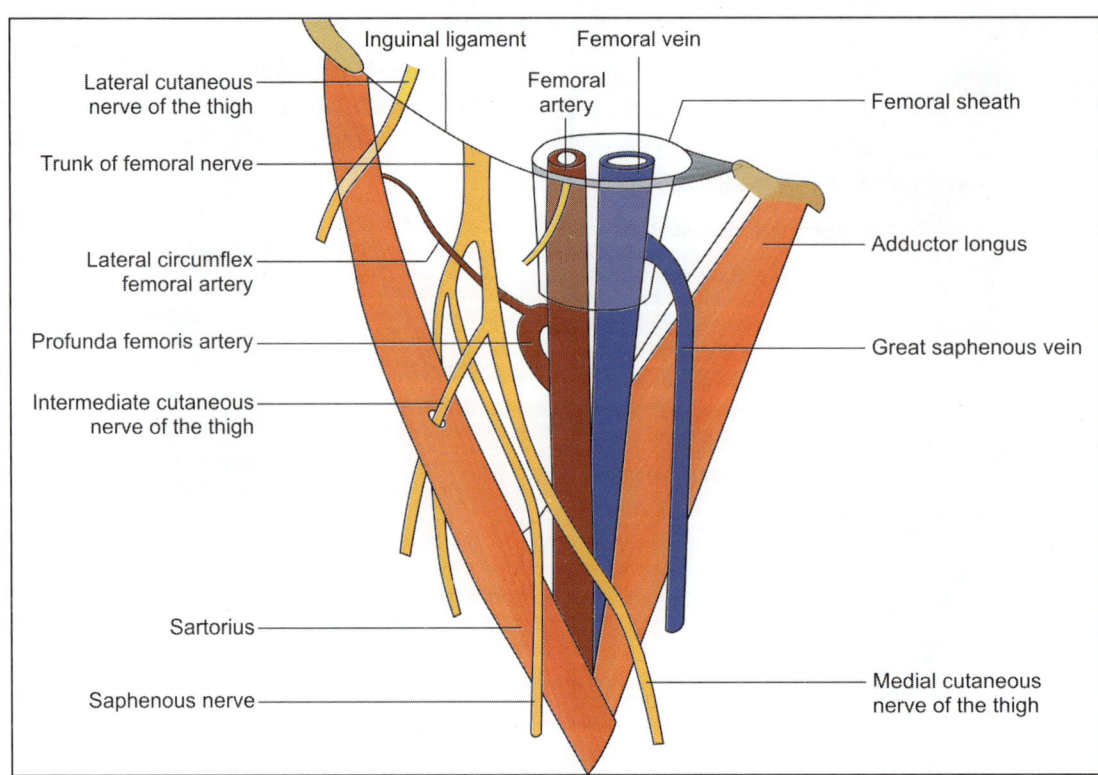

**Fig. 10.19:** Femoral triangle—contents

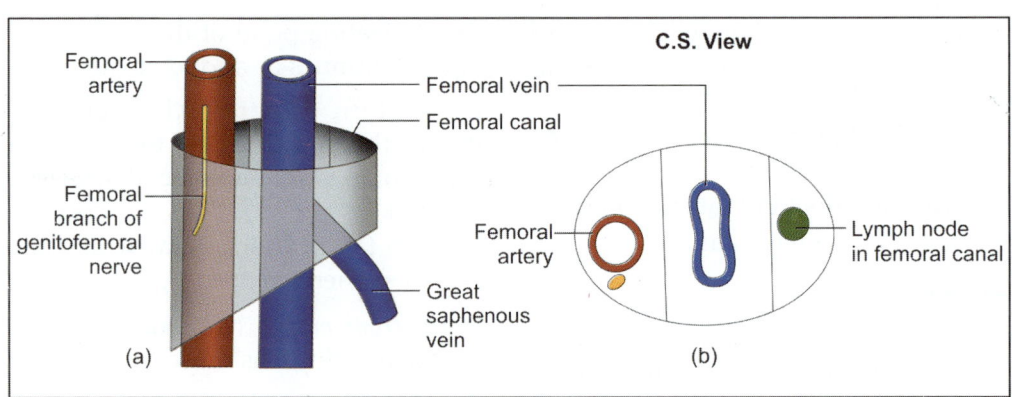

**Fig. 10.20a and b:** Femoral sheath and contents

c. Medial compartment is very short (1.25 cm long) and is called 'femoral canal'. The upper part of the canal opens into abdominal cavity at femoral ring. The canal is occupied by a lymph node.

The femoral hernia can occur through this canal and it is common in females.

**Iliopsoas muscle:** It comprises two muscles, namely psoas major and iliacus. The psoas major takes origin from the lumbar vertebral bodies while iliacus arises from iliac fossa of the ilium bone. The two muscles join together to form iliopsoas passes deep to the inguinal ligament and inserted into the lesser trochanter of the femur. The psoas is tendinous and fleshy fibres of the iliacus joins it. The muscle is chief flexor of the hip joint (Fig.10.21).

**Tensor fasciae latae:** This muscle is located at the junction of the gluteal region and the thigh.

*Origin:* It takes origin from the anterior part of the iliac crest.

*Insertion:* It is inserted into the upper part of the iliotibial tract.

*Nerve supply:* Superior gluteal nerve.

*Action:* It is an abductor and medial rotator of the hip joint. Through the ilio-tibial tract it maintains the extended position of the knee joint.

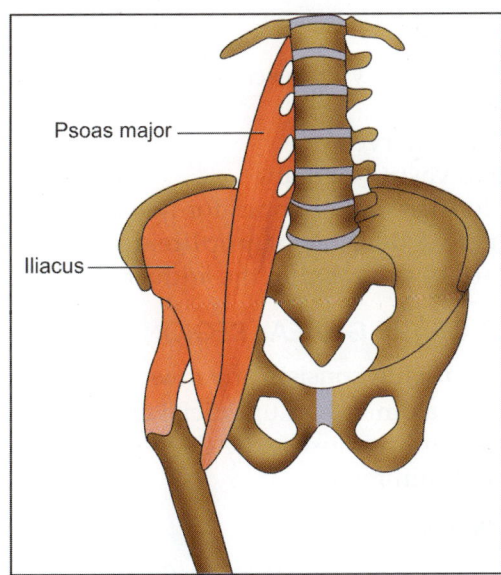

**Fig. 10.21:** Iliopsoas muscle

## MUSCLES OF THE MEDIAL (ADDUCTOR) COMPARTMENT OF THE THIGH

The muscles are pectineus, adductor longus, brevis, magnus, obturator externus and gracilis (Table 10.9).

All these muscles mainly cause adduction at the hip joint. They are all supplied by the obturator nerve.

### Adductor Magnus Muscle

It belongs to both adductor and hamstring (posterior) compartments and is supplied by nerves of the both compartments (Fig. 10.22a).

#### Attachment

a. Inferior ramus of the pubis—fibers from this origin extend almost horizontally to be inserted into shaft of the femur along the medial margin of the gluteal tuberosity.

b. Ramus of the ischium—fibers arising from this origin extend obliquely downwards to be inserted into medial lip of the linea aspera and upper part of the medial supracondylar line of the femur.

c. Ischial tuberosity—fibers from this origin passes almost vertically downwards to be inserted into adductor tubercle (just above the medial epicondyle) of the femur by a tendon. This part constitutes the hamstring component.

#### Nerve Supply

Adductor component is supplied by posterior division of the obturator nerve and hamstring component is supplied by sciatic nerve.

| | | Table 10.9: Muscles of medial compartment of thigh | | |
|---|---|---|---|---|
| Muscle | Origin | Insertion | Nerve supply | Actions |
| **Adductor longus** | Narrow tendon from front of body of pubis | Linea aspera in middle 1/3 between the vastus medialis and adductor brevis and magnus | Anterior division of obturator nerve | Adductors of thigh at hip joint |
| **Adductor brevis** | Anterior surface of body of pubis  Outer surface of inferior ramus of pubis  Outer surface of ramus of ischium | Line extending from lesser trochanter to linea aspera | Anterior or posterior division of obturator nerve | Adduction and flexion of hip joint |
| **Gracilis** | Medial margin of lower half of body of pubis. Inferior ramus of pubis  Adjoining part of ramus of ischium | Upper part of medial surface of tibia behind sartorius and in front of semitendinosus | Anterior division of obturator nerve | Flexor and medial rotator of thigh  Weak adductor |
| **Pectineus** | Pectin pubis  Upper half of pectineal surface of superior ramus of pubis  Fascia covering pectineus | Line between lesser trochanter to linea aspera | Anterior fibers— femoral nerve  Posterior fibers— anterior division of obturator nerve | Flexor and adductor of thigh |

10

## Actions

The adductor components adducts the thigh and hamstring part extends the thigh at hip joint.

The muscle presents five openings for the passage of perforating arteries (upper 4 openings), and the femoral vessels (the 5th opening).

## ADDUCTOR CANAL (SUBSARTORIAL CANAL)

It is an intermuscular space situated in the middle 1/3 of the medial part of the thigh. It connects the apex of the femoral triangle to popliteal fossa, at hiatus magnus (last opening in the adductor magnus muscle) (Fig. 10.22b).

### Boundaries

Anteriorly—vastus medialis
Posteriorly—adductor longus above
              adductor magnus below
Medially (roof)—a fibrous membrane connecting the anterior and posterior walls. Sartorius muscle is placed above this fibrous membrane.

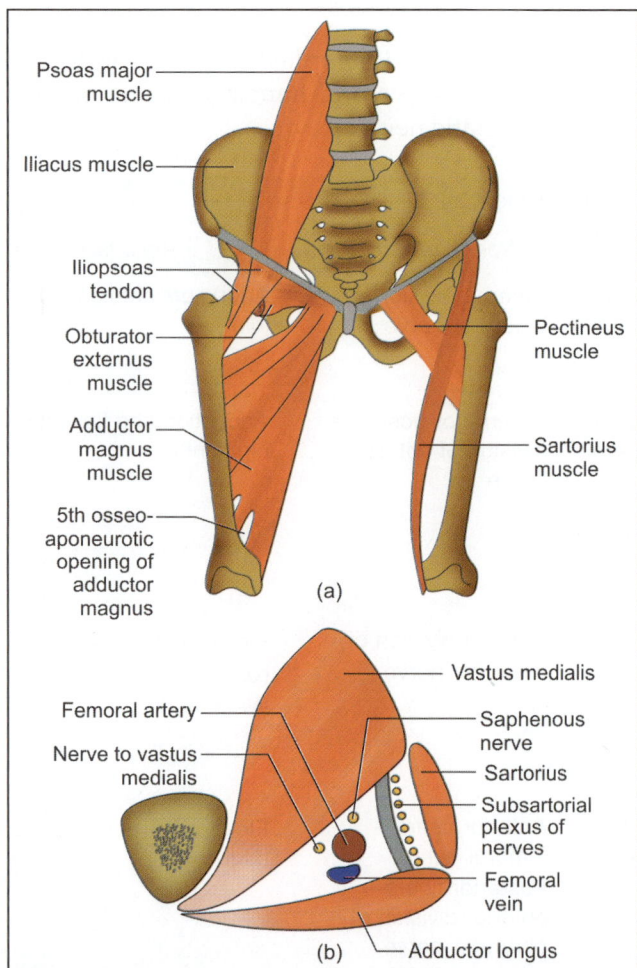

**Fig. 10.22a and b:** (a) Adductor magnus; (b) adductor canal—cross-section

## Contents

1. Femoral artery with descending genicular branch
2. Femoral vein
3. Saphenous nerve
4. Nerve to vastus medialis
5. Posterior division of obturator nerve

In surgical dealing of popliteal aneurysm, the femoral artery is ligated in the adductor canal.

## MUSCLES OF THE GLUTEAL REGION

The gluteal region consists of 9 muscles.

Gluteus maximus is a superficial and bulky muscle. All the remaining muscles lie deep to it (e.g. gluteus medius and minimus).

## Gluteus Maximus

It is the largest and most superficial muscle of the gluteal region (Figs 10.23 and 10.24).

### Origin

- From the gluteal surface of the ilium above and behind the posterior gluteal line.
- From the posterior layer of the thoracolumbar fascia covering the erector spinae muscle.
- From the dorsal surface of the lower part of the sacrum and coccyx.
- From sacrotuberous ligament.

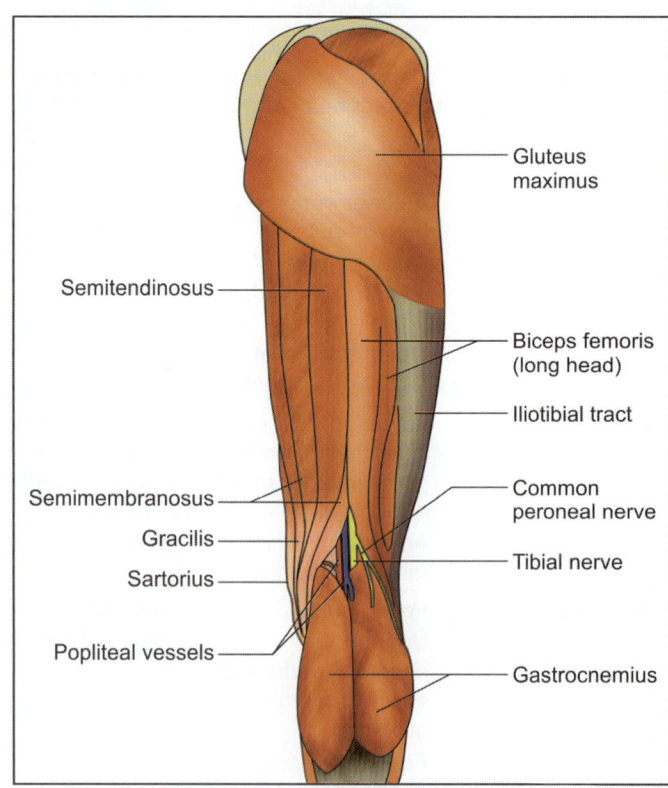

**Fig. 10.23:** Hamstring muscles

**10**

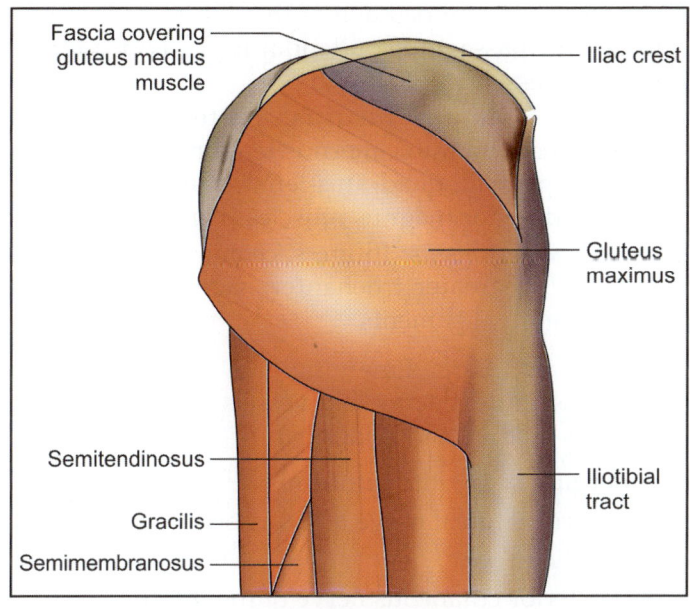

Fascia covering gluteus medius muscle

Iliac crest

Gluteus maximus

Semitendinosus

Gracilis

Semimembranosus

Iliotibial tract

**Fig. 10.24:** Gluteus maximus muscle

*Insertion:* One fourth of the muscle (deep fibers of the lower half) is inserted into gluteal tuberosity of the femur.

The remaining 3/4 of the muscle (deep fibers of the upper half and the whole of superficial fibers) is inserted into upper part of the iliotibial tract. (Iliotibial tract is the thickened part of the deep fascia [fascia lata] on the lateral side of the thigh).

*Nerve supply:* Inferior gluteal nerve

*Actions:* Extension of the hip joint (in running and climbing). In standing position the hip joint is kept in extended position by hamstring muscles. It is also a lateral rotator and abductor of the hip joint.

### Gluteus Medius (Fig. 10.25)

*Origin:* Gluteal surface of the ilium between the posterior and anterior gluteal line of the hip bone. The muscle passes downwards, forwards and laterally.

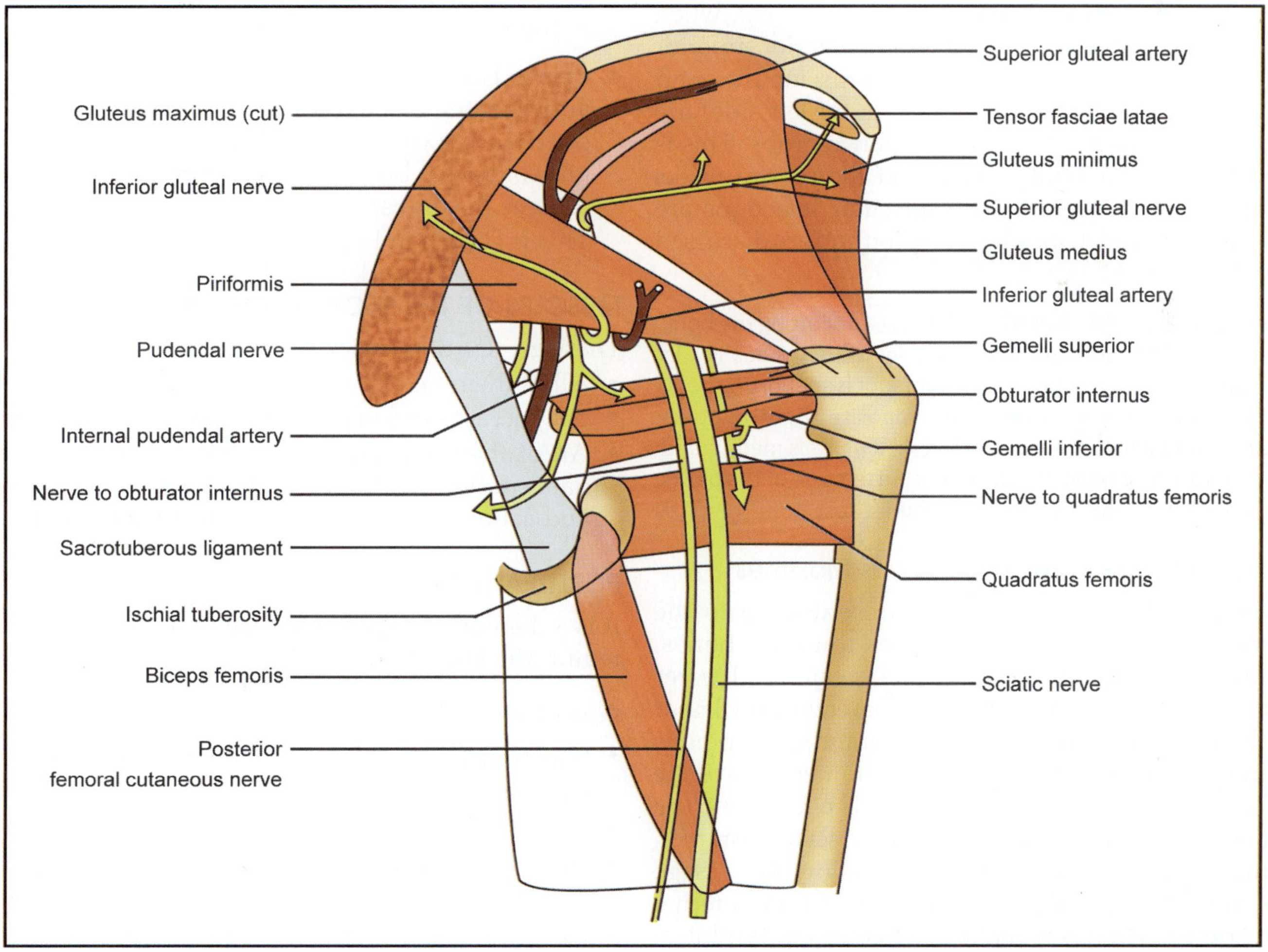

Gluteus maximus (cut)

Inferior gluteal nerve

Piriformis

Pudendal nerve

Internal pudendal artery

Nerve to obturator internus

Sacrotuberous ligament

Ischial tuberosity

Biceps femoris

Posterior femoral cutaneous nerve

Superior gluteal artery

Tensor fasciae latae

Gluteus minimus

Superior gluteal nerve

Gluteus medius

Inferior gluteal artery

Gemelli superior

Obturator internus

Gemelli inferior

Nerve to quadratus femoris

Quadratus femoris

Sciatic nerve

**Fig. 10.25:** Gluteus medius and minimus muscles

10

*Insertion:* It is inserted into the lateral surface of the greater trochanter of the femur.

*Nerve supply:* Superior gluteal nerve.

### Gluteus Minimus

*Origin:* Gluteal surface of the ilium between anterior and inferior gluteal line of the hip bone.

*Insertion:* It is inserted into the anterior surface of the greater trochanter.

*Nerve supply:* Superior gluteal nerve

### Actions of Gluteus Medius and Minimus

1. Abductors of the hip joint.
2. Anterior fibers of both muscles act as medial rotators of the hip joint. These two actions are exerted when its attachment to the greater trochanter is acting as insertion.
3. When its attachment to the hip bone acts as insertion, it tends to pull the hip bone towards the femur, which is required to raise the opposite hip. Hence it prevents the unsupported side of the pelvis from sagging downwards during locomotion, e.g. when right foot is off the ground the right anterior superior iliac spine is raised by left gluteus medius and minimus muscle. If these muscles (of left side) are paralysed the right side of the pelvis drops. This is called Trendelenburg's sign and the person walks with a lurching gait. Intramuscular injections are often preferred in the gluteal region and are discussed in Chapter 38.

> *Trendelenburg's test:* When both feet are supporting the body weight, the anterior superior iliac spine of two sides lies in the same horizontal plane. When right foot is supporting body weight, the left foot is raised by opposite (right) gluteus medius and minimus muscles. If the right gluteus medius and minimus are paralysed, the unsupported left side of the pelvis drops indicating positive Trendelenburg's test.

### Structures under Cover of Gluteus Maximus

There are plenty of structures present deep to the gluteus maximus, which includes muscles, bones, ligaments, nerves and vessels. The greater and lesser sciatic notches are converted into greater and lesser trochanter foramina by sacrotuberous and sacrospinous ligaments. The greater trochanter foramen allows the passage of piriformis muscle, which is a key structure under gluteus maximus. The greater sciatic foramen connects the pelvis and gluteal region allow the passage of nerves from sacral plexus and vessels from internal iliac arteries. The lesser sciatic notch connects the gluteal region with the perineum through pudendal canal. The foramen allows the passage of the obturator internus muscle and passage of pudendal nerve and internal pudendal vessels to perineum.

1. *Muscles:* Gluteus medius, gluteus minimus, piriformis, obturator internus tendon, superior and inferior gemelli, quadratus femoris and upper part of the adductor magnus muscles (Fig. 10.26).
2. *Bones and ligaments:* Ilium, sacrum, coccyx, ischial tuberosity, greater trochanter, sacrotuberous and sacrospinous ligaments.
3. *Nerves and vessels:* Emerging above the piriformis: Superior gluteal nerve and vessels (passes between gluteus medius and minimus)

   Emerging below the piriformis:
   - Inferior gluteal nerve and vessels
   - Sciatic nerve
   - Posterior cutaneous nerve of the thigh
   - Pudendal nerve
   - Nerve to obturator internus
   - Nerve to quadratus femoris muscle
   - Internal pudendal vessels.
4. *Bursae:* Trochanteric bursa (between gluteus maximus and greater trochanter), ischial bursa (between gluteus maximus and ischial tuberosity) and gluteofemoral bursa (between ventral lateralis and gluteus maximus).

This is shown in Fig.10.26.

## MUSCLES OF THE BACK OF THE THIGH

These groups of muscles are called hamstring muscles.
- All of them take origin from ischial tuberosity.
- They act as flexors of knee and extensors of the hip joint.
- All of them are supplied by the sciatic nerve. The name of the muscles, their attachment, nerve supply and actions are listed in Table 10.10 and Fig. 10.26.

## POPLITEAL FOSSA

It is a diamond shaped space, behind the lower 1/3 of femur, the knee joint and the upper part of the tibia.

### Boundaries (Fig. 10.27)
- Superomedially—semimembranosus and semitendinosus muscles.
- Superolaterally—biceps femoris muscle
- Inferomedially—medial head of gastrocnemius muscle
- Inferolaterally—lateral head of gastrocnemius muscle

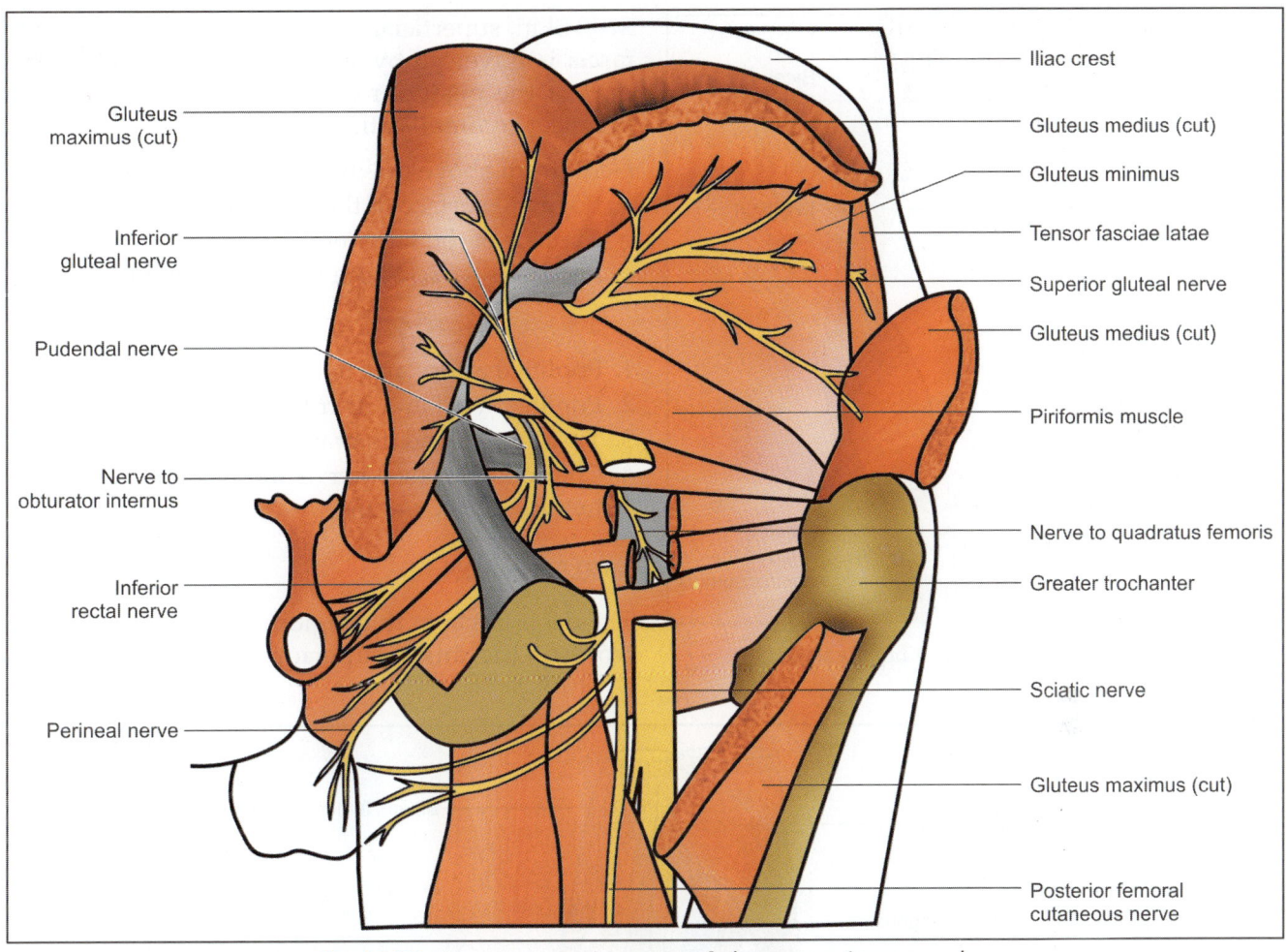

Iliac crest

Gluteus maximus (cut)

Gluteus medius (cut)

Gluteus minimus

Inferior gluteal nerve

Tensor fasciae latae

Superior gluteal nerve

Pudendal nerve

Gluteus medius (cut)

Piriformis muscle

Nerve to obturator internus

Nerve to quadratus femoris

Greater trochanter

Inferior rectal nerve

Sciatic nerve

Perineal nerve

Gluteus maximus (cut)

Posterior femoral cutaneous nerve

**Fig. 10.26:** Structures under cover of gluteus maximus muscle

| Table 10.10: Muscles of the posterior compartment of the thigh | | | |
|---|---|---|---|
| Name of the muscle and its origin | Insertion | Nerve supply | Actions |
| 1. **Semimembranous** Superolateral part of the ischial tuberosity. It is membranous in upper part and becomes fleshy in lower part | Its tendon is inserted into a groove on the posterior surface of the medial condyle of tibia. Oblique popliteal ligament is an expansion from the insertion of this muscle. | Sciatic nerve (tibial component) | Flexion at knee and extension at hip joint |
| 2. **Semitendinosus** Inferomedial part of the ischial tuberosity along with long head of biceps femoris | Upper part of the medial surface of the tibia (behind the insertions of sartorious and gracilis) | Sciatic nerve (tibial component) | Flexion at knee and extension at hip joint |
| 3. **Biceps femoris** It has 2 heads of origin a. Long head: Inferomedial part of the ischial tuberosity along with semitendinosus b. Short head: Lower part of the lateral lip of the linea aspera and upper part of lateral supracondylar line of femur. | Head of the fibula in front of styloid process | Sciatic nerve (long head-tibial component, short head peroneal component of sciatic nerve) | Flexion at knee and extension at hip joint |

10

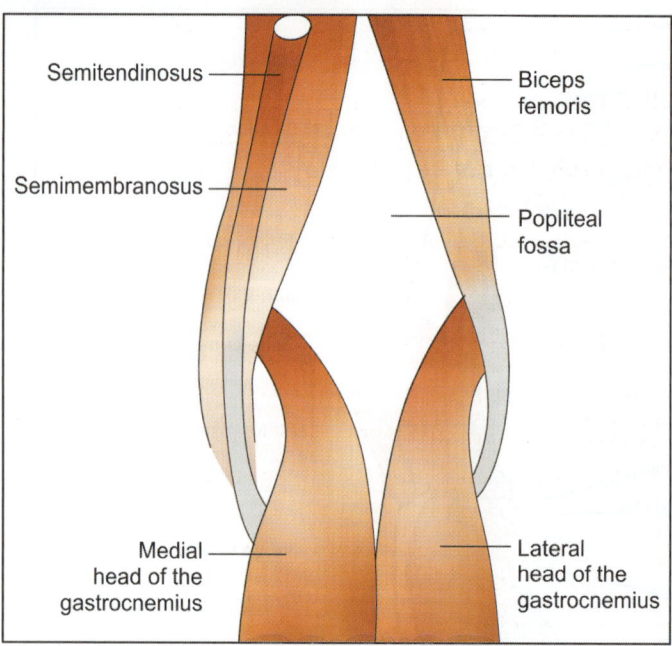

**Fig. 10.27:** Boundaries of the popliteal fossa

*Roof:* Skin, superficial and deep fascia. The superficial fascia is traversed by small saphenous vein, terminal part of the posterior cutaneous nerve of thigh and peroneal communicating nerve.

*Floor* (from above downwards)
a. Popliteal surface of the femur
b. Capusle of the knee joint
c. Popliteus muscle with fascia covering it

*Contents* (Fig. 10.28)
1. Popliteal artery and its branches
2. Popliteal vein and its tributaries
3. Tibial nerve and its branches
4. Common peroneal nerve and its branches
5. Lymph nodes and fat.

## ANKLE REGION

The deep fascia in this region forms two retinacula in front of the ankle-superior and inferior extensor

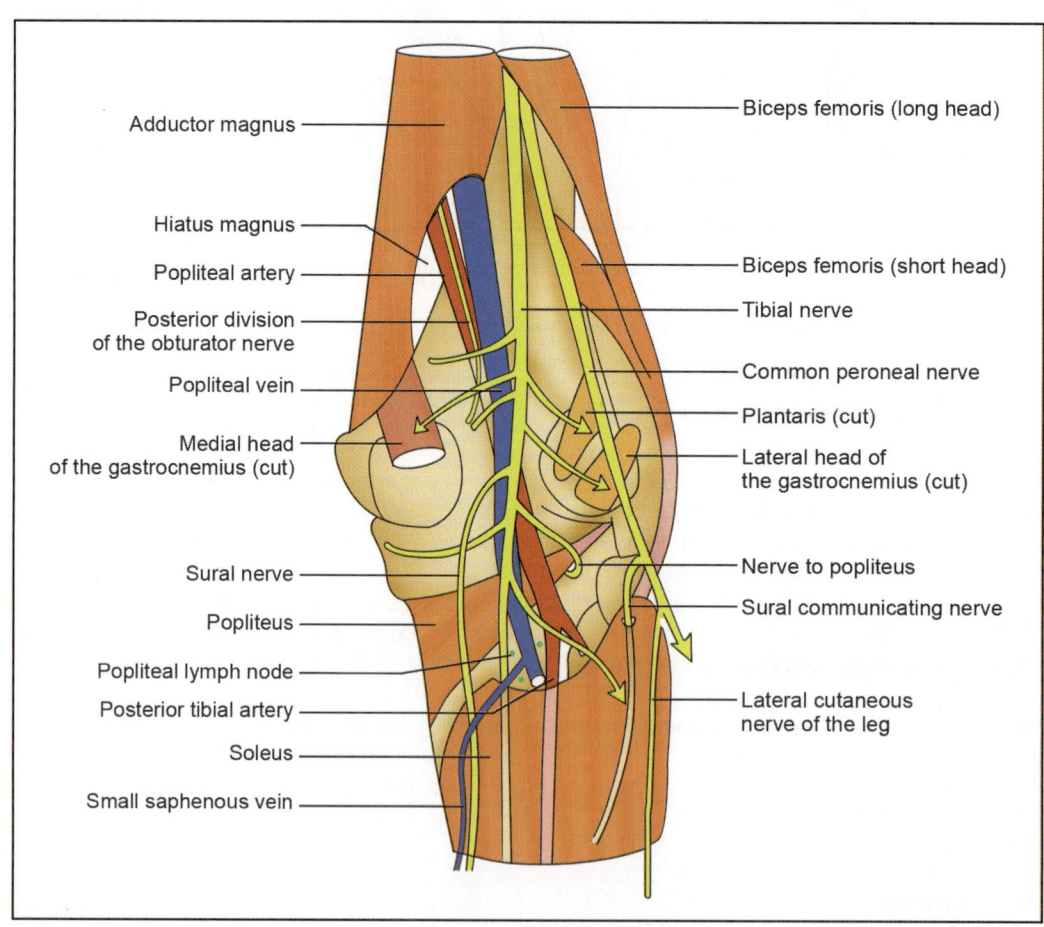

**Fig. 10.28:** Contents of the popliteal fossa

retinacula. The superior retinacula is present in front of the ankle at the lower part of the leg and the inferior on the dorsum of the foot.

## Superior Extensor Retinaculum

It is thick deep fascia present in front of the ankle. It holds the extensor tendons in their position during movement of the joint.

### Attachments

*Medially:* Lower part of the anterior border of the tibia.

*Laterally:* Lower part of the anterior surface of the fibula.

### Structures Passing Superficial to the Retinaculum

1. Great saphenous vein
2. Saphenous nerve
3. Superficial peroneal nerve

### Structures Passing Deep to the Retinaculum

**Following structures passes from medial to lateral side:**

1. Tibialis anterior
2. Extensor hallucis longus
3. Anterior tibial vessels
4. Deep peroneal nerve
5. Extensor digitorum longus
6. Peroneus tertius

The tendons of these muscle has separate synovial sheath which allows frictionless movement.

## Inferior Extensor Retinaculum

It is a thick modified deep fascia present on the dorsum of the foot. It is 'Y' shaped with the stem of the 'Y' present on the lateral side.

### Attachments

The stem is attached to the upper surface of the calcaneus in its anterior part.

Medially, the upper band is attached to the medial malleolus and the lower band passes to the medial margin of the foot and continues with deep fascia of the sole (plantar aponeurosis).

The relations of the retinaculum (structures passing superficial and deep) are similar to the superior extensor retinaculum except for anterior tibial artery, it is dorsalispedis artery (dorsalispedis artery is the continuation of the anterior tibial artery).

## MUSCLES OF THE ANTERIOR COMPARTMENT OF THE LEG

All these muscles pass into the dorsum of the foot. They mainly bring Dorsi flexion at the ankle joint. All these muscles are supplied by deep peroneal nerve (Table 10.11).

The muscles are explained in Table 10.11 and Fig. 10.29:

> *Shin splints:* It is a condition results from injury to the tibialis anterior muscle. It is common in people who are not used to exercise regularly.
>
> *Anterior compartment syndrome:* This also results from excessive usage of leg muscle as in severe exercise or long distance running. It leads to swelling in the muscles of the leg especially in the anterior compartment where muscles are tightly held by deep fascia. The muscular swelling may compress the veins which cause accumulation of the fluid in this compartment. The increased pressure in this compartment can compress deep peroneal nerve and anterior tibial artery. Arterial compression can cause gangrene of the foot. To relieve the pressure the deep fascia of the leg is cut along the whole length of the anterior compartment. Fracture of the tibia with bleeding inside can also cause anterior compartment syndrome.

## Peroneal Retinacula

These are modified deep fascia present lateral to the ankle. It hold the tendons of the lateral compartment muscles during the movement of the ankle joint.

*Superior peroneal retinaculum:* It extends from lateral malleolus to the lateral surface of the calcaneus. The tendon of the peroneus longus and brevis are enclosed in with a common synovial sheath, where tendon of peroneus longus is superficial.

*Inferior peroneal retinaculum:* Above it is attached to the anterior part of the superior surface of the calcaneus where it becomes continues with the stem of the inferior extensor retinaculum and below the lateral surface of the calcaneus. The tendon of the peroneus brevis with its separate synovial sheath occupies the upper compartment beneath the retinaculum, while tendon of the peroneus longus in the lower compartment with its synovial sheath. A peroneal trochlea or tubercle separates the two tendons.

**Table 10.11:** Muscles of anterior compartment of leg

| Muscle | Origin | Insertion | Nerve supply | Actions |
|---|---|---|---|---|
| **Tibialis anterior** | Lateral condyle of tibia. Upper 2/3rd of lateral surface of shaft of tibia Adjoining interosseous membrane | Inferomedial surface of medial cuneiform and adjoining part of base of the first metatarsal | Deep peroneal nerve | Dorsiflexor and invertor of foot Maintains medial longitudinal arch of foot |
| **Extensor hallucis longus** | Posterior part of middle 2/4th of medial surface of shaft of fibula. Upper part of inter-osseous membrane | Dorsal surface of base of distal phalanx of great toe | Deep peroneal nerve | Dorsiflexes the foot and extends the metatarsophalangeal, proximal and distal interphalangeal joints of great toe |
| **Extensor digitorum longus** | Lateral condyle of tibia Upper 1/4 and anterior half of middle 2/4th of medial surface of shaft of fibula Upper part of interosseous membrane | Divides into four tendons for lateral four toes Tendons of 2nd, 3rd, 4th digits are joined by tendon of extensor digitorum brevis laterally which together forms the dorsal digital expansion and gets inserted to bases of middle and distal phalanx | Deep peroneal nerve | Dorsiflexes the foot and extends the metatarsophalangeal, proximal and distal interphalangeal joints of 2nd to 5th toes |
| **Peroneus tertius** | Lower 1/4th of medial surface of shaft of fibula Adjoining interosseous membrane | Medial part of dorsal surface of base of 5th metatarsal | Deep peroneal nerve | Dorsiflexor and evertor of foot |
| **Extensor digitorum brevis** | Anterior part of superior surface of calcaneum | Divided into 4 tendons for medial 4 toes. The first tendon (extensor hallucis brevis) is inserted to dorsal surface of base of proximal phalanx of great toe Lateral three tendons joins the lateral side of tendons of extensor digitorum longus and thereby to dorsal digital expansion of 2nd, 3rd and 4th toes. | Lateral terminal branch of deep peroneal nerve | First tendon extends the great toe at meta-tarsophalangeal joint, while the latter three extends 2nd, 3rd and 4th digits at metatarso-phalangeal joints and interphalangeal joints |

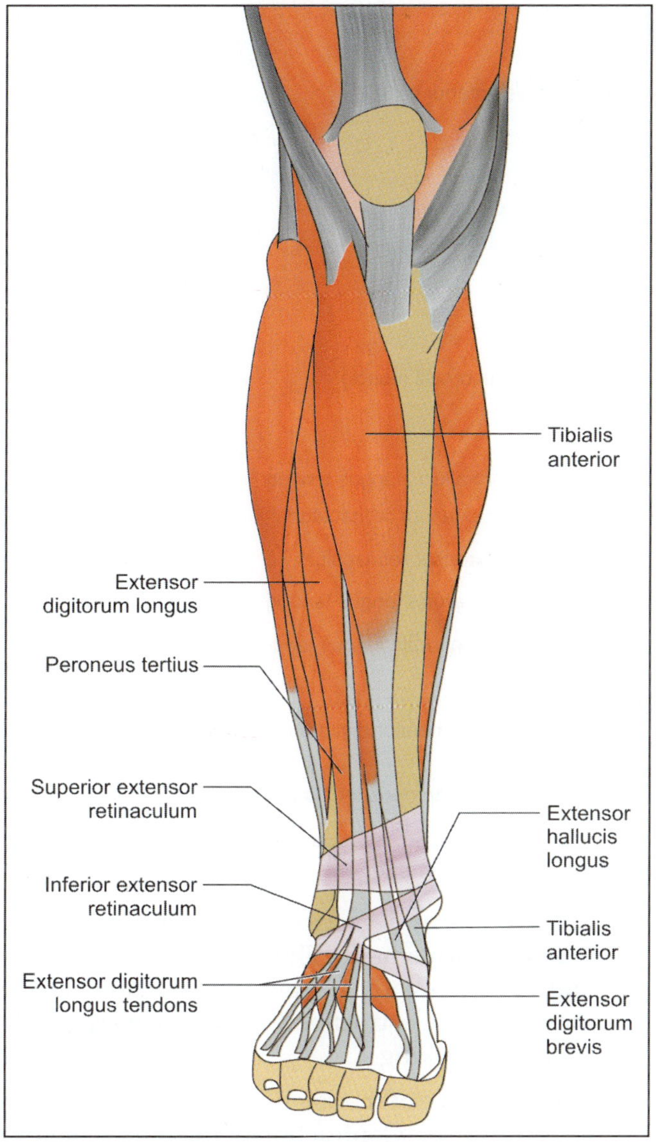
Tibialis anterior
Extensor digitorum longus
Peroneus tertius
Superior extensor retinaculum
Extensor hallucis longus
Inferior extensor retinaculum
Tibialis anterior
Extensor digitorum longus tendons
Extensor digitorum brevis

**Fig. 10.29:** Muscles of the anterior compartment

## MUSCLES OF THE LATERAL COMPARTMENT OF THE LEG

These muscles are supplied by superficial peroneal nerve. Both these muscles cause evertion at subtalar joint and mid tarsal joints (Table 10.12 and Fig. 10.30).

### Flexor Retinaculum of the Ankle

It is a thick modified deep fascia present behind the medial malleolus. It holds the deep muscles of the back of the leg that are entering the sole during movement of the ankle joint (Fig.10.31).

#### *Attachments*

*Anteriorly:* Posterior border of the medial malleolus.

*Posteriorly:* Medial tubercle of the calcaneum. Septa arising from the under surface of the retinaculum divides the area deep to it into 4 compartments. Following structures passes through each compartment from anterior to posterior.

1. Tibialis posterior tendon
2. Flexor digitorum longus tendon
3. Posterior tibial vessels and tibial nerve
4. Flexor hallucis longus tendon

The retinaculum is pierced by medial calcanean vessels and nerves supplying heel area.

## MUSCLES OF THE BACK OF THE LEG

The muscles of the back of the leg are often called the calf muscles. They are arranged in superficial and deep groups. They are all supplied by tibial nerve. They cause mainly plantar flexion at the ankle joint.

The attachments, nerve supply and actions of the muscles are explained in Table 10.13.

**Table 10.12:** Lateral compartment of leg (peroneal compartment) (Fig. 10.30)

| *Muscle* | *Origin* | *Insertion* | *Nerve supply* | *Actions* |
|---|---|---|---|---|
| **Peroneus longus** | Head of fibula<br>Upper 1/3rd and posterior half of middle 1/3rd of lateral surface of fibula | Passes deep to peroneal retinaculum, runs in the tunnel of cuboid and inserted to lateral side of base of first metatarsal adjoining medial cuneiform | Superficial peroneal nerve | Evertor of foot of the ground<br>Maintains the medial longitudinal and transverse arches of foot acting as a sling |
| **Peroneus brevis** | Anterior half of middle 1/3rd and lower 1/3rd of lateral surface of fibula | Passes deep to peroneal retinacula and is inserted to lateral side of base of 5th metatarsal | Superficial peroneal nerve | Evertor of foot |

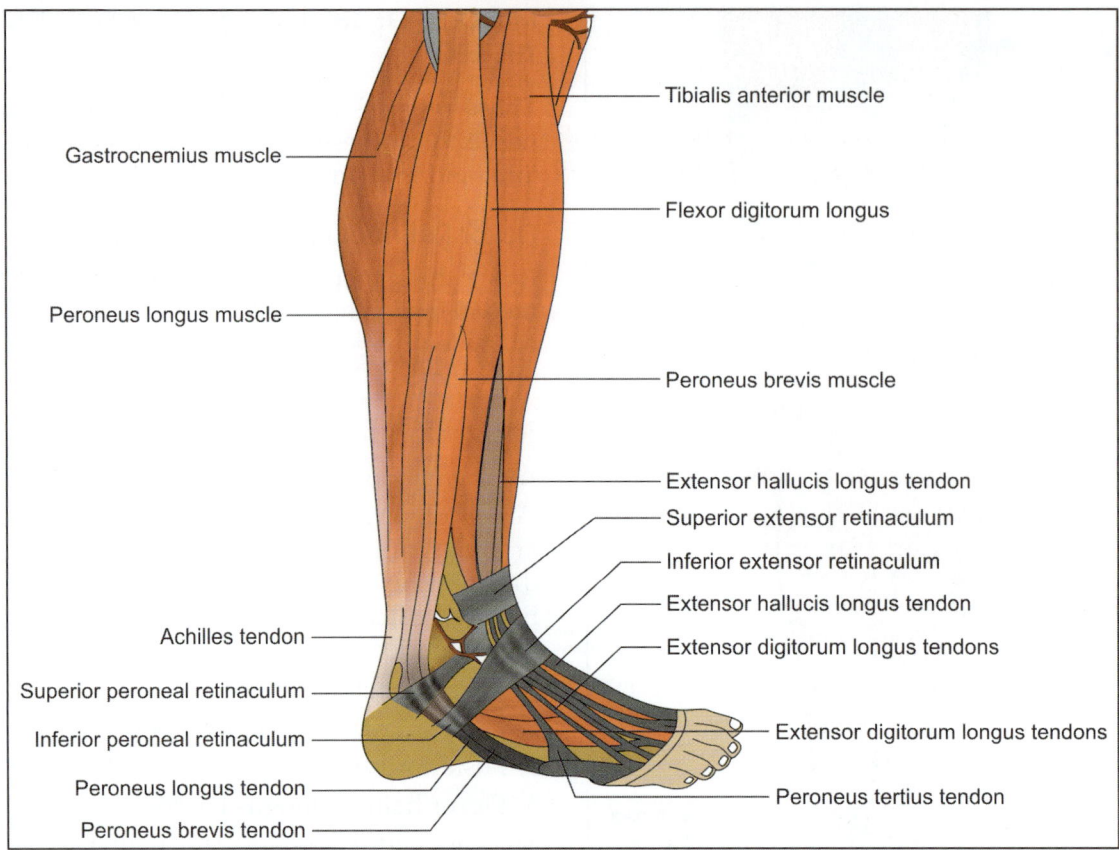

**Fig. 10.30:** Muscles of the lateral compartment of the leg

- Soleus and gastrocnemius together form a tendon called tendocalcaneus, which extends in the lower part of the posterior aspect of the leg. Inferiorly, it is attached to the middle one-third of the posterior surface of the calcaneus (Fig. 10.32).

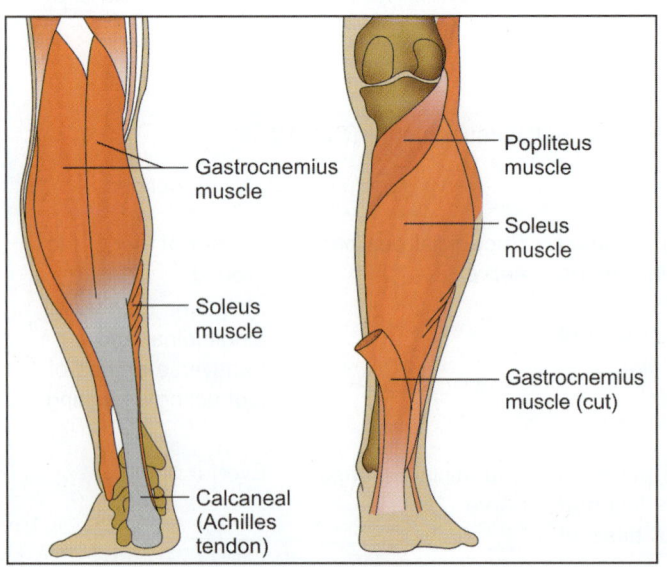

**Fig. 10.31:** Gastrocnemius muscle and soleus muscle

- Both soleus and gastrocnemius are involved in walking movement. The soleus overcomes the inertia of the body weight (initiates the walking movement). Gastrocnemius further increases the speed of walking.

- The substance of the soleus muscle presents many venous spaces. Contraction of the muscle helps in venous return. Hence soleus is called 'peripheral heart'.

The ankle jerk or Achillis tendon reflex is explained in Chapter 38.

## Popliteus Muscle

It takes origin by a tendon from the lateral condyle of the femur within the joint cavity. It passes through the knee joint cavity. The tendon passes downwards and medially between the fibular collateral ligament and the lateral meniscus. It comes out from the fibrous capsule of the joint and is inserted into popliteal surface of the tibia above the soleal line. It is supplied by tibial nerve. Popliteus initiates the flexion at knee joint (unlocking). Some of its fibers are attached to the lateral meniscus which pulls the lateral meniscus backward and prevents its injury during initiation of flexion.

**Table 10.13:** Muscles of anterior compartment of leg

| Muscle | Origin | Insertion | Nerve supply | Actions |
|---|---|---|---|---|
| **Gastrocnemius** | Medial head—arises as broad flat tendon-posterosuperior depression on medial condyle of femur behind adductor tubercle<br>Part of popliteal surface of femur<br>Capsule of knee joint<br>Lateral head—lateral surface of lateral condyle of femur<br>Lateral supracondylar line<br>Capsule of knee joint | Fuses with tendon of soleus to form tendo-Achilles and inserted to middle 1/3rd of posterior surface of calcaneum | Tibial nerve | Gastrocnemius and soleus are strong plantar flexors of foot at ankle joint along with soleus in running and walking<br>Gastrocnemius is also a flexor of knee joint<br>Soleus is more powerful than gastrocnemius while the latter is fast in action<br>Soleus acts as power-gear while gastrocnemius acts as top gear of a car |
| **Soleus** | Back of head of the fibula and upper 1/4 of posterior surface of shaft of fibula, soleal line and middle 1/3rd of medial border of shaft of tibia.<br>Tendinous soleal arch between tibia and fibula | Refer gastrocnemius insertion | Tibial nerve | Refer gastrocnemius |
| **Plantaris** | Lower part of lateral supracondylar line of femur | Tendon is thin, runs medial to tendo-Achilles and inserted to posterior surface of calcaneum<br>Plantar aponeurosis is its degenerated tendon | Tibial nerve | Rudimentary<br>Used in tendon transplants |

## Deep Muscles of the Back of the Leg

1. *Flexor digitorum longus:* It divides into four tendons for lateral four toes and inserted into base of the distal phalanx. It causes plantar flexion of lateral 4 toes.

2. *Flexor hallucis longus:* Its tendon passes into plantar surface of the great toe. It flexes the distal phalanx of great toe.

3. *Tibialis posterior:* It takes origin mainly from upper 2/3rd of the posterior surface of the tibia and posterior surface of the fibula. The tendon of the muscle passes behind the medial malleolus deep to the flexor retinaculum. It is inserted into tuberosity of the navicular bone. Apart from plantar flexion it causes inversion at subtalar joint and also maintain medial longitudinal arch.

## SOLE OF THE FOOT

Foot is an organ of support and locomotion. Accordingly, the muscles of the foot (sole) are modified to steady the toes and to maintain the arches of foot.

### Plantar Aponeurosis

The deep fascia of the sole is thick in the central part forming plantar aponeurosis. The plantar aponeurosis is triangular in shape with its apex directed proximally and the base distally. The apex is attached to the medial tubercle of the calcaneus. The base divides into 5 slips near the heads of the metatarsals (Fig. 10.33). The interval between the slips allows the passage of the digital nerves and vessels. Each slip divides into superficial and deep slip. The superficial slip is attached

10

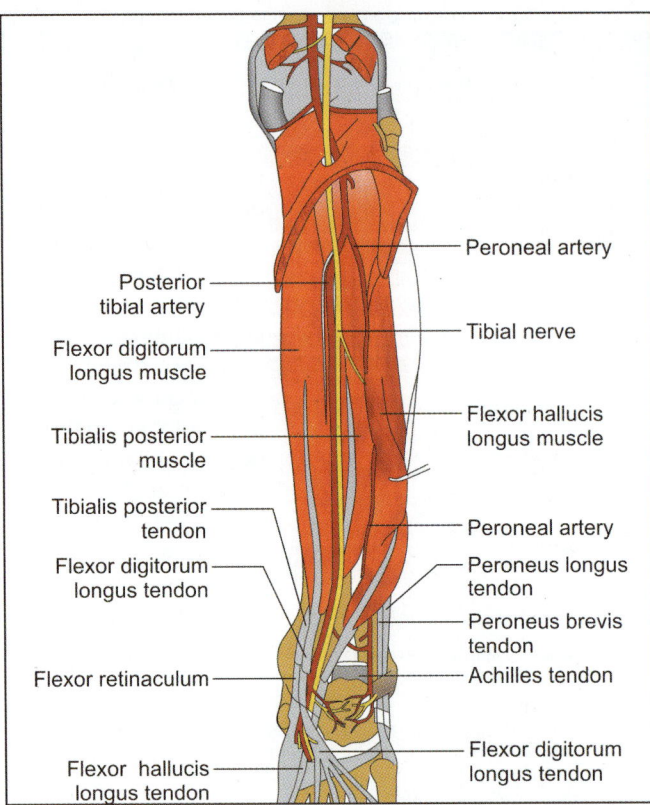

**Fig. 10.32:** Deep muscles of the back of the leg

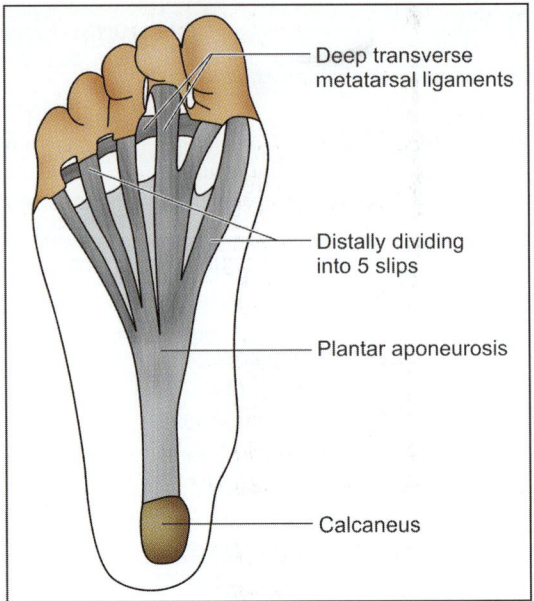

**Fig. 10.33:** Plantar aponeurosis

to the skin and the deep slip blends with fibrous flexor sheaths and also with deep transverse metatarsal ligaments. The plantar aponeurosis provides protection to the deeper structure. It also contributes to the maintenance of the arch.

> *Plantar fasciitis:* It occurs due to straining and inflammation of plantar aponeurosis. It is characterized by pain over heel and medial aspect of foot, which increases with passive extension of great toe and by dorsiflexion of ankle joint. It results from running and high-impact aerobics (most common hind-foot problem in runners).
>
> There are 18 intrinsic muscles in the sole. Structures of the sole are explained in many layers (Fig. 10.34).

*First layer* has 3 muscles
- Flexor digitorum brevis
- Abductor hallucis
- Abductor digiti minimi

*Second layer* has 5 muscles: Flexor digitorum accesorius, 4 lumbricals and also tendons of flexor digitorum longus and flexor hallucis longus.

*Third layer* has 3 muscles
- Flexor hallucis brevis
- Flexor digiti minimi
- Adductor hallucis

*Fourth layer* has 7 muscles:
- Three (3) plantar interossei
- Four (4) dorsal intereossei (and also tendons of tibialis posterior and peroneus longus)

These muscles are supplied by medial and lateral plantar nerves (terminal branches of tibial nerve) (Fig. 10.35).

## ARCHES OF FOOT

Human foot is designed to perform two basic functions:
- It acts as a pliable platform to support the body weight.
- It acts as a lever to propel the body forward during locomotion.
- To perform these functions the foot is designed in the form of elastic arches.

Elastic arches are classified into longitudinal and transverse arches.

### Longitudinal Arches

When the foot is on the ground only its anterior (heads of the metatarsals) and posterior (calcaneum) parts rest on the ground forming a convex arch directed upward. This longitudinal arch is further divided into medial and lateral arches. The medial arch is higher then lateral arch (Figs 10.36 and 10.37).

### Transverse Arch

Foot also presents anterior and posterior transverse arches.

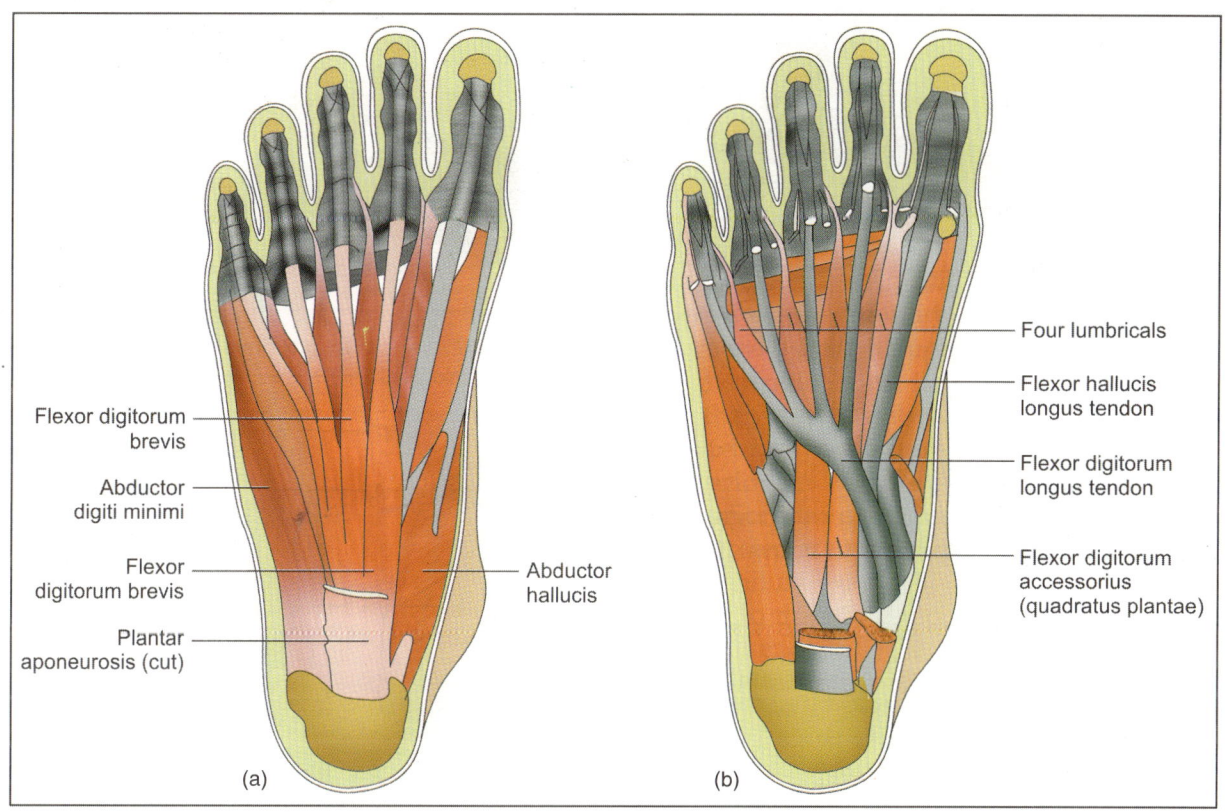

**Fig. 10.34a and b:** (a) Sole—first layer; (b) Sole—second layer

Flexor digitorum brevis

Abductor digiti minimi

Flexor digitorum brevis

Plantar aponeurosis (cut)

Abductor hallucis

Four lumbricals

Flexor hallucis longus tendon

Flexor digitorum longus tendon

Flexor digitorum accessorius (quadratus plantae)

(a)

(b)

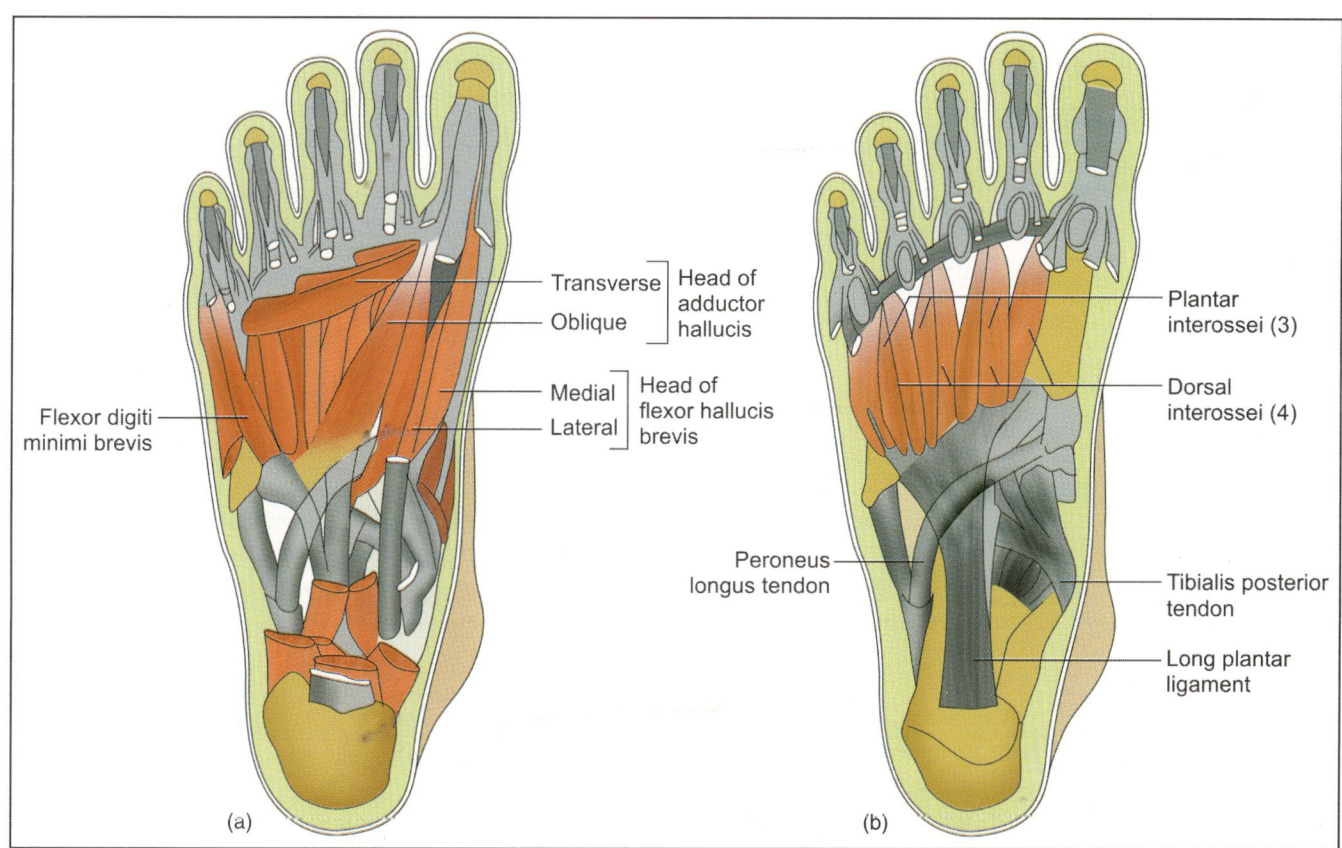

**Fig. 10.35a and b:** (a) Sole—third layer; (b) Sole—fourth layer

Transverse | Head of adductor hallucis

Oblique

Flexor digiti minimi brevis

Medial | Head of flexor hallucis brevis

Lateral

Peroneus longus tendon

Plantar interossei (3)

Dorsal interossei (4)

Tibialis posterior tendon

Long plantar ligament

(a)

(b)

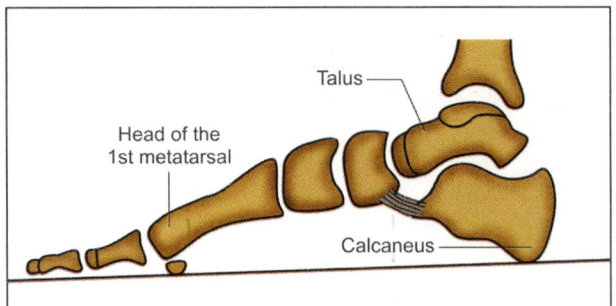

**Fig. 10.36:** Medial longitudinal arch—bones forming

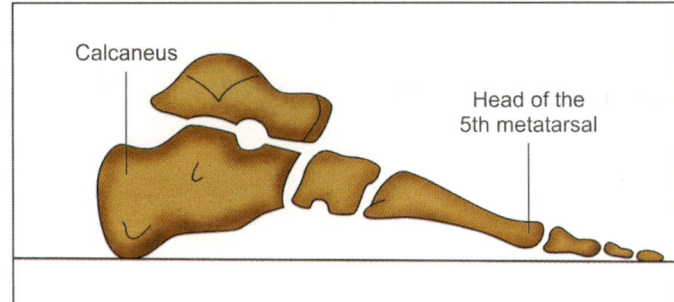

**Fig. 10.37:** Lateral longitudinal arch—bones forming

## Functions of Arches of Foot

- Proportional distribution of body weight.
- Arched foot acts as a segmented lever through series of joints, and thus made pliable to adapt itself to uneven surfaces.
- Plantar concavity of the arch protects the nerves and vessels of the sole.
- Arched foot acts as a shock absorber and helps in jumping movement (Tables 10.14 and 10.15).

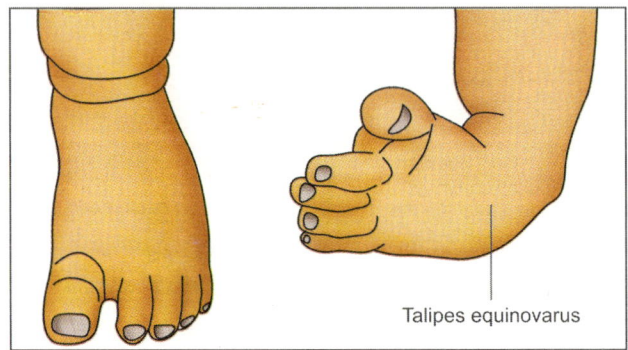

Talipes equinovarus

**Fig. 10.38:** Clubfoot

| Table 10.14: Formation of longitudinal arch | | |
|---|---|---|
| | *Medial longitudinal arch* | *Lateral longitudinal arch* |
| Anterior end | Heads of the medial 3 metatarsals | Heads of the 4th and 5th metatarsals |
| Posterior end | Medial tubercle of the calcaneus | Lateral tubercle of the calcaneus |
| Summit | Trochlear (upper) surface of the talus | Facet on the superior surface of the calcaneus |
| Anterior pillar | Shafts of the medial 3 metatarsals | Shafts of 4th and 5th metatarsals |
| Posterior pillar | Medial part of the calcaneus | Lateral part of the calcaneus |
| Main joint of the arch | Talo-calcaneonavicular joint | Calcaneocuboid joint |

| Table 10.15: Maintenance of arches of foot | | |
|---|---|---|
| *Factors responsible for maintenance* | *Medial longitudinal arch* | *Lateral longitudinal arch* |
| Shape of the bones | Sustentaculum tali hold up the talus. Rounded head of talus is 'key stone' | Calcanean angle of the cuboid |
| Intersegmental ties | Spring ligament, Long plantar ligament and dorsal ligaments | Long and short plantar ligaments, dorsal ligaments |
| Tie beams | Medial part of the plantar aponeurosis, medial part of the flexor digitorum brevis and longus, abductor hallucis, flexor hallucis longus and brevis | Lateral part of the plantar aponeurosis, lateral part of the flexor digitorum brevis and longus, abductor digiti minimi, flexor digiti minimi brevis |
| Sling support | Tibialis anterior, superficial fibers of deltoid ligament and, tibialis posterior muscles | Peroneus longus, brevis and tertius muscles |

## Summary

The thigh is divided into three compartments by intermuscular septa. Muscles of each compartment have a particular function and nerve supply. Muscles of the anterior compartment are supplied by femoral nerve and their main action is extension of the knee joint.

The muscles of the medial compartment are supplied by obturator nerve and they adduct the thigh at hip joint. The posterior compartment (hamstring) muscles are supplied by sciatic nerve. They extend the hip joint and flex the knee joint.

The leg is also divided into three compartments. The muscles of the anterior compartment are supplied by deep peroneal nerve. They bring dosiflexion at ankle joint. The muscles of the lateral compartment are supplied by superficial peroneal nerve and they bring about evertion at subtalar joint. Muscles of the posterior compartment of the leg are supplied by tibial nerve and they cause plantar flexion at ankle joint.

## Applied Anatomy

1. *Pes planus (flat foot):* Abnormal distribution of the body weight on to the arch causes flat foot.
2. *Pes cavus* is condition with exaggeration of arches of foot.
3. *Clawfoot:* In this condition toes are dorsiflexed at metatarsophalangeal joints and plantar flexed at interphalangeal joints.
4. *Hammer toe:* Metatarsophalangeal and distal interphalangeal joints are hyper extended but proximal interphalangeal joint is acutely flexed. It usually affects 2nd and 3rd toes due to involvement of lumbrical muscles.
5. *Talipes equinus:* In this condition the person walks on the forefoot with raised heel.
   a. Talipes equinovarus—foot is inverted and adducted (Fig. 10.38).
   b. Talipes equionovalgus—foot is everted and abducted.
6. *Talipes calcaneus:* In this condition the person walks on heel with raised forefoot. It can be again classified into talipes calcaneovarus and valgus.

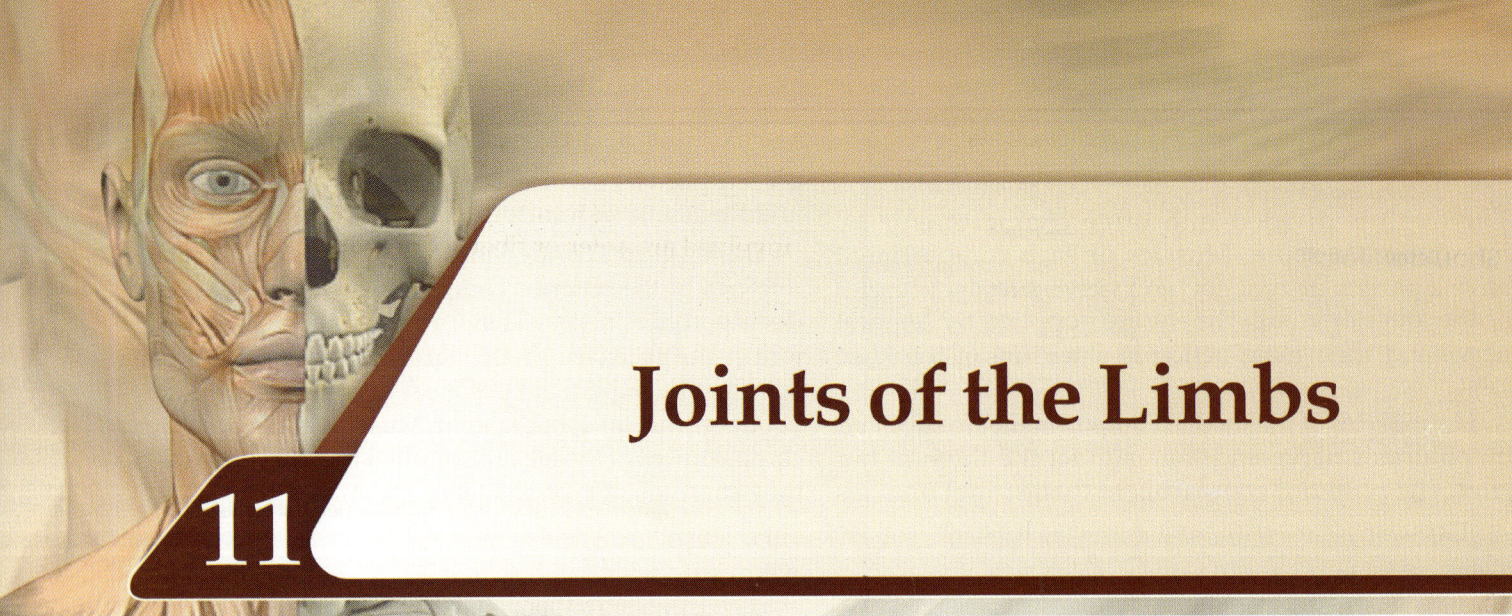

# Joints of the Limbs

**11**

Shoulder or pectoral girdle connects the bones of the upper limb with the axial skeleton. It consists of two joints:

a. Sternoclavicular joint
b. Acromioclavicular joint

## STERNOCLAVICULAR JOINT

*Type:* It is a saddle variety of synovial joint.

*Bones articulating:* Sternal end of the clavicle articulates with clavicular notch of sternum and also first costal cartilage.

An articular disc made of fibrocartilage intervenes between the articulating bones.

The joint is stabilized by capsular ligament, interclavicular ligament and costoclavicular ligament (Fig. 11.1).

## ACROMIOCLAVICULAR JOINT

*Type:* It is a plane synovial joint.

*Bones articulating:* Lateral end of the clavicle with medial margin of acromion process of scapula.

The joint is stabilized by fibrous capsular ligament and coracoclavicular ligament.

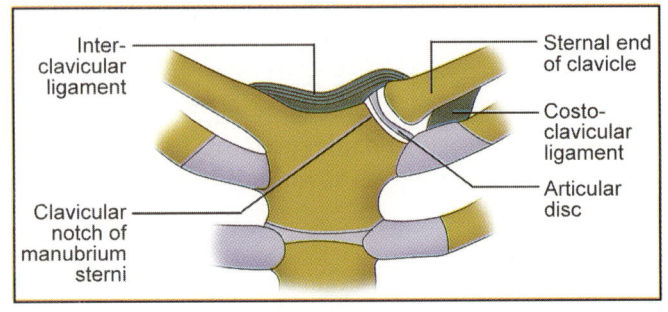

**Fig. 11.1:** Sternoclavicular joint

*Coracoclavicular ligament:* It forms the strong bond of union between the scapula and the clavicle. It consists of conoid and trapezoid parts. The conoid part stretches between conoid tubercle on the undersurface of the clavicle to the root of the coracoid process. The trapezoid part stretches between trapezoid ridge on the under surface of the clavicle to the upper surface of the coracoid process. The weight of the upper limb is transmitted through costoclavicular ligament. The acromioclavicular joint is prone for dislocation or shoulder separation, in which the coracoclavicular ligament is likely to be torn.

### Movements of the Shoulder Girdle

*Elevation of scapula:* The lateral end of the clavicle is elevated and medial end rotates downward.
Muscles involved—upper fibers of trapezius muscle and levator scapulae muscle.

*Depression of scapula:* The medial end of the clavicle is rotated upward by the weight of the upper limb and also by lower fibers of serratus anterior muscle.

*Forward movement of the scapula (pushing and punching movements):* The lateral end of the clavicle advances forward and medial end swings backward. This action is brought by serratus anterior and pectoralis minor muscle.

*Retraction of the scapula:* The medial end of the clavicle swings forward and the lateral end swings backwards. This action is brought by middle fibers of trapezius and rhomboideus muscles.

*Forward rotation of the scapula:* This movement occurs during abduction of the arm above the level of shoulder. The glenoid cavity is directed almost vertically upward and greater tuberosity of the humerus is accommodated in subacromial bursa. This action is produced by upper and lower fibers of trapezius with serratus anterior.

## Shoulder Joint

*Type:* It is a ball and socket variety of synovial joint.

*Bones articulating:* The head of the humerus covered by hyaline articular cartilage with glenoid cavity of the scapula, which is also covered by hyaline cartilage (Fig. 11.2a).

### Structures Stabilizing

1. *Capsular ligament (fibrous capsule):* It is made up of collagen and elastic fibers. Medially, it is attached to the peripheral margin of the glenoid cavity outside the labrum. The attachment encloses the origin of long head of biceps brachii. Laterally, it is attached to the anatomical neck of the humerus but extending a little below on the inferior medial aspect (Fig. 11.2b).

   Synovial membrane lines the capsule and also invests the tendon of the long head of biceps brachii.

2. *Glenohumeral ligaments* are three fibrous bands, which are derived from the thickening of the fibrous capsule.

3. *Glenoidal labrum:* It is a fibrocartilaginous rim attached to the peripheral part of the glenoid cavity. It deepens the glenoidal cavity.

4. *Coracohumeral ligament:* It extends from the root and lateral border of the coracoid process of scapula to anatomical neck of the humerus.

5. *Musculotendinous rotator cuff:* The tendons of the muscles around the shoulder joint on their way to their insertion blend with the fibrous capsule. It keeps the head of humerus in contact with glenoidal cavity. The tendons are:

   Subscapularis—infront
   Supraspinatus—above
   Infraspinatus—behind
   Teres minor—behind

6. *Coracoacromial arch:* It is formed by three structures— Coracoid process, acromion process and coraco-acromial ligament.

   It acts as a secondary synovial socket for the head of the humerus (Fig. 11.2c).

### Arterial supply

Shoulder joint is supplied by anterior and posterior circumflex humeral arteries.

### Nerve supply

Shoulder joint is supplied by axillary nerve, suprascapular nerve and lateral pectoral nerve.

## Movements and muscles producing them

*Flexion:* Arm moves forward and medially. Muscles involved are anterior fibers of deltoid, clavicular fibers of pectoralis major.

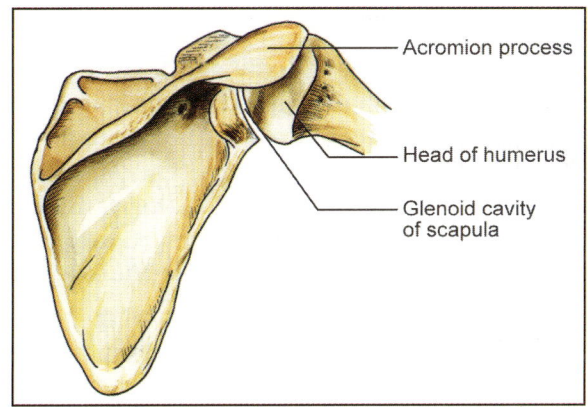

**Fig. 11.2a:** Shoulder joint—bones articulating

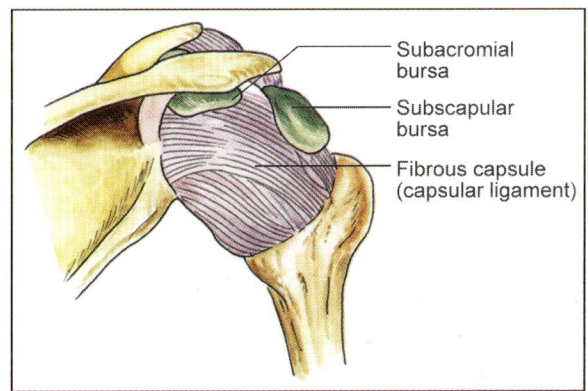

**Fig. 11.2b:** Shoulder joint capsule

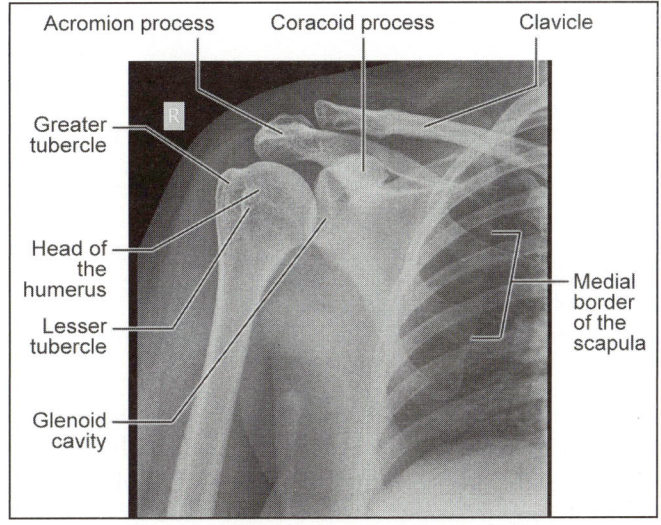

**Fig. 11.2c:** Radiograph of the should joint

11

*Extension:* Arm moves backward and laterally. Muscles involved are posterior fibers of deltoid, teres major latissimus dorsi muscle.

*Adduction:* Arm moves medially and backwards towards the trunk. Muscles involved are anterior fibers of deltoid, pectoralis major, teres major, and latissimus dorsi.

*Abduction:* Arm moves laterally and forward towards the trunk. Supraspinatus muscle abducts up to 15°. Then the middle fibers of deltoid abduct up to 90°.

Above the head (overhead abduction) occurs at both shoulder joint and shoulder girdle (forward rotation of the scapula). It is done by upper and lower fibers of trapezius acting with serratus anterior muscle.

*Medial rotation:* It carries the arm medially. Muscles involved are anterior fibers of deltoid, pectoralis major, teres major, subscapularis, and latissimus dorsi.

*Lateral rotation:* It carries the arm laterally. Muscles involved are posterior fibers of deltoid, infraspinatus and teres minor.

*Circumduction:* Combination of flexion, adduction, abduction and extension in succession.

## Applied Anatomy

**Dislocation of the shoulder:** The anterior dislocation can be sub-coracoid, sub-glenoid or sub-clavicular. The downward dislocation is more common in abducted position of arm. It can injure the axillary nerve, which is closely related to the lower part of the joint capsule. To reduce the dislocation, the elbow must be flexed under traction, humerus laterally rotated first, adducted and then rotated medially. An X-ray is taken to ensure proper reduction, and axillary nerve function is assessed by asking the patient to abduct the shoulder while supporting the arm.

**Frozen shoulder:** In this condition, shoulder movements are restricted due to tendinitis of the rotator cuff.

Aspiration of the fluid from the joint cavity is done by introducing the needle through the deltopectoral groove.

## Elbow Joint

*Type:* It is a hinge variety of synovial joint. It is also a compound joint since three bones are taking part in the joint.

*Bones articulating:* The lower end of the humerus presents trochlea and capitulum. The trochlea of the humerus articulates with trochlear notch of ulna and capitulum with upper surface of the head of the radius (Fig. 11.3a and b).

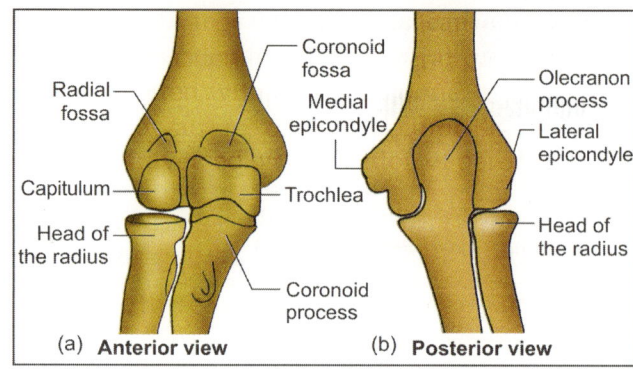

Fig. 11.3a and b: Bones articulating in the elbow joint

### Structures Stabilizing

1. *Capsular ligament (fibrous capsule):* It is attached to the lower end of the humerus in such a way that it encloses coronoid, radial fossae in front and olecranon fossa behind. However, the two epicondyles of the humerus are outside the attachment of fibrous capsule. Below it is attached to the margins of trochlear notch of ulna medially. Laterally, it blends with annular ligament of the superior radioulnar joint (Fig. 11.3c).

The fibrous capsule is lined by synovial membrane.

Inside the joint cavity there are three fat filled fossae. On the anterior aspect the coronoid fossa is present above the trochlea and radial fossa above the capitulum. On the posterior aspect there is an

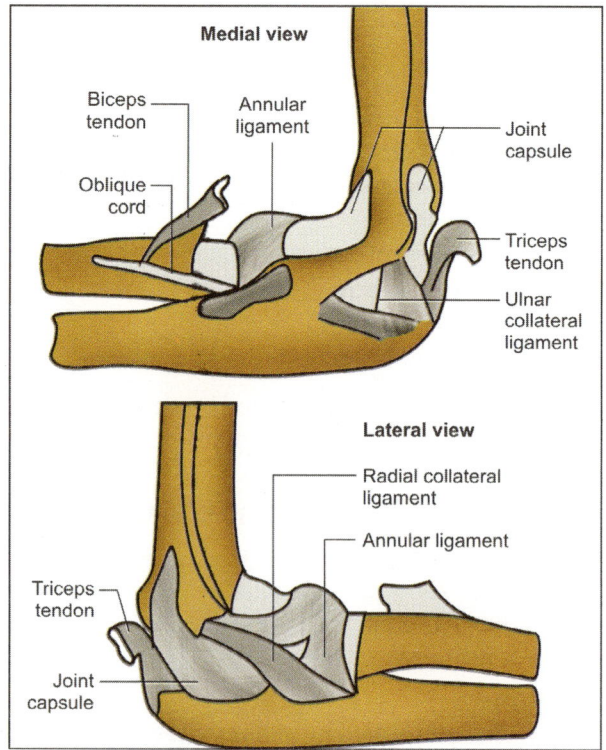

Fig. 11.3c: Ligaments of the elbow joint

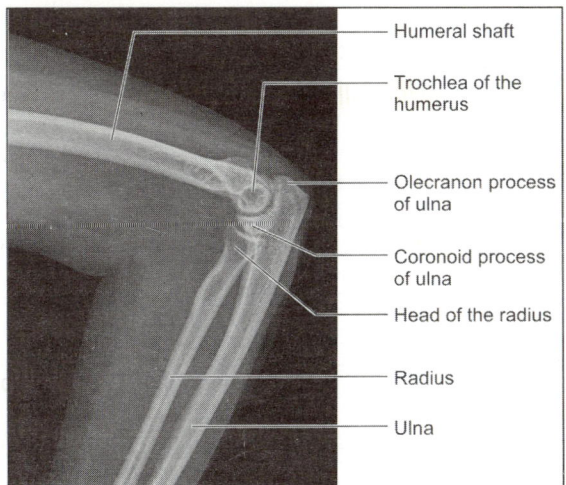

Humeral shaft

Trochlea of the humerus

Olecranon process of ulna

Coronoid process of ulna

Head of the radius

Radius

Ulna

**Fig. 11.3d:** Radiograph of elbow

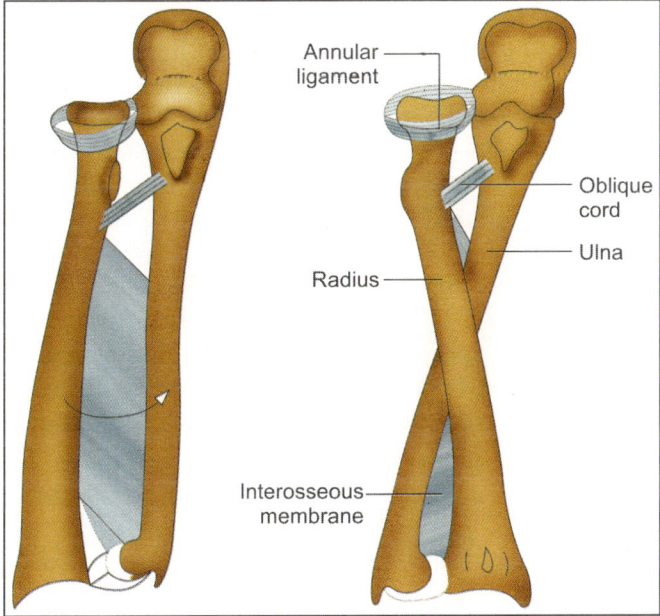

Annular ligament

Oblique cord

Ulna

Radius

Interosseous membrane

**Fig. 11.3e:** Pronation and supination

olecranon fossa. During flexion of the elbow joint, the coronoid and radial fossae are occupied by coronoid process of ulna and head of the radius respectively (Fig. 11.3d). During extension the olecranon fossa is occupied by olecranon process of the ulna.

2. *Ulnar collateral (medial ligament):* It is thickening of fibrous capsule on the medial side. It is triangular in shape with its apex attached to the medial epicondyle of the humerus and base to the medial margin of the trochlear notch of the ulna. It is closely related to ulnar nerve.

3. *Radial collateral (lateral) ligament:* It is the lateral thickening of the fibrous capsule. Above it is attached to the lateral, epicondyle of the humerus and below it blends with annular ligament.

## Arterial supply

Elbow joint is supplied by arterial anastomosis around the elbow. The anastomosis is formed by branches of brachial, ulnar, radial and profunda brachii arteries.

## Nerve supply

The elbow joint is supplied by branches of musculocutaneous, radial and ulnar nerves.

## Movements and muscles producing them

*Flexion:* Brachialis, biceps brachii, brachioradialis and superficial flexors of forearm

*Extension:* Triceps and anconeus

## Applied Anatomy

Examination of three important bony land marks around the elbow is a common practice to differentiate posterior dislocation of the elbow joint and supracondylar fracture of humerus. The 3 bony points are medial and lateral epicondyles on each side and olecranon process posteriorly. In extended elbow these three points lie in a straight horizontal line. When the elbow is flexed they form an equilateral triangle. In posterior dislocation this triangle is distorted with backward movement of the olecranon process. But in humeral head fracture the normal bony relation is retained since olecranon moves along with the lower end of the humerus.

The aspiration of the fluid from the joint is performed usually around the olecranon process.

**Tennis elbow:** It occurs due to the inflammation of the radial collateral ligament and periosteum around the lateral epicondyle. Inflammation or tearing of muscles attached to the lateral epicondyle especially extensor carpi radialis brevis results in pain around the lateral epicondyle. The common cause for this injury is abrupt pronation with fully extended elbow. It is characterized by severe pain and tenderness in the area of lateral epicondyle.

**Golfer's elbow:** It is a condition with inflammation at the medial epicondyle. It may be due to inflammation of the ulnar collateral ligament or involvement of muscles attached to the medial epicondyle.

**Carrying angle:** It is the angle of deviation of forearm from the axis of the arm when forearm is extended and supinated. The angle ranges from 10 to 15°. The carrying angle permits the arm to be swung without contacting the hips. The angle is slightly more in females. The angle is due to more downward projection of trochlea of humerus when compared to capitulum.

In **cubitus valgus**, the forearm is deviated more laterally than the normal with increase in the carrying angle. A childhood injury to the lateral epicondyle could cause cubitus valgus, which may gradually stretch the ulnar nerve behind the medial epicondyle (tardy ulnar palsy).

In **cubitus varus**, the forearm is deviated medially and the carrying angle is reduced.

Carrying angle may also be defined as an angle between the arm and forearm and is measured from lateral side, which ranges from 160 to 170°.

## Radioulnar Joints

The two bones of the forearm are connected at their proximal and distal ends by synovial joints. They are called superior and inferior radioulnar joints respectively. However, the shafts of radius and ulna are connected by a fibrous interosseous membrane (fibrous joint) (Fig. 11.3e).

### Superior Radioulnar Joint

*Type:* It is a pivot variety of synovial joint.

*Bones taking part:* The circumference of the head of the radius articulates with radial notch of ulna and annular ligament.

*Annular ligament:* It keeps the radial head in position and is attached to the anterior and posterior margins of radial notch of ulna. The annular ligament is continuous above with fibrous capsule of the elbow joint. The ligament enables the head of the radius to rotate during pronation and supination. The annular ligament is internally lined by synovial membrane which continues with synovial membrane of the elbow joint.

The annular ligament in the adult is 'cup-shaped' and is firmly attached to the neck of the radius which prevents downward displacement of the radial head. In children the annular ligament is tubular and the size of the head is smaller. This factor is responsible for downward displacement of radial head in children and is referred as "pulled elbow".

*Quadrate ligament:* It extends between the neck of the radius and the lower margin of the radial notch of the ulna.

### Inferior Radioulnar Joint

*Type:* It is a pivot variety of synovial joint.

*Bones taking part:* The head of the ulna articulates with ulnar notch of the radius.

The two articulating parts are enclosed in a fibrous capsule and are connected below by an articular disc.

*Articular disc:* It is a white fibrocartilagenous structure and is triangular in shape. It separates the head of the ulna from the wrist joint. (It is between the head of ulna and triquetral bone.)

*Middle radioulnar joint:* It is formed by the interosseous membrane which extends between the interosseous borders of the radius to ulna. Proximally the membrane begins about 2–3 cm below the radial tuberosity and distally up to the inferior radioulnar joint. The interosseous membrane transmits weight from radius to ulna. The membrane is taut at midprone position. It also provides attachments to many muscles.

*Oblique cord:* It extends from the lateral aspect of the ulnar tuberosity to the lower end of the radial tuberosity.

*Movements:* The radioulnar joint permits pronation and supination movements. During these movements the head of the radius and ulna rotate in their bony sockets.
- *Pronation:* The palmar aspect of the hand is turning to face downwards with semiflexed elbow. Pronation is brought by pronator teres and pronator quadratus.
- *Supination:* The palmar aspect of the hand turns to face upward (screwing movement) with semiflexed elbow. Supination is brought by biceps brachii and supinator muscle.

## Wrist Joint (Radiocarpal Joint)

*Type:* It is an ellipsoid variety of synovial joint.

*Bones taking part:* The inferior surface of the lower end of the radius and the articular disc of the inferior radioulnar joint, above.

Scaphoid, lunate and triquetral bones, (from lateral to medial side) below.

The joint is stabilised by a capsular ligament and its thickening on either side forming medial and lateral collateral ligaments (Fig. 11.4a and b).

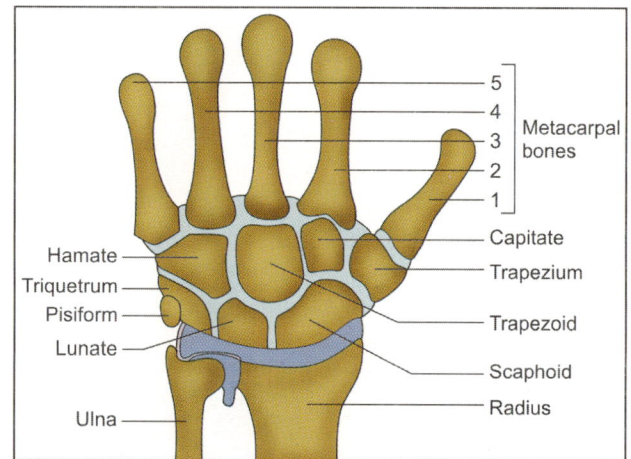

**Fig. 11.4a:** Wrist and inferior radioulnar joints

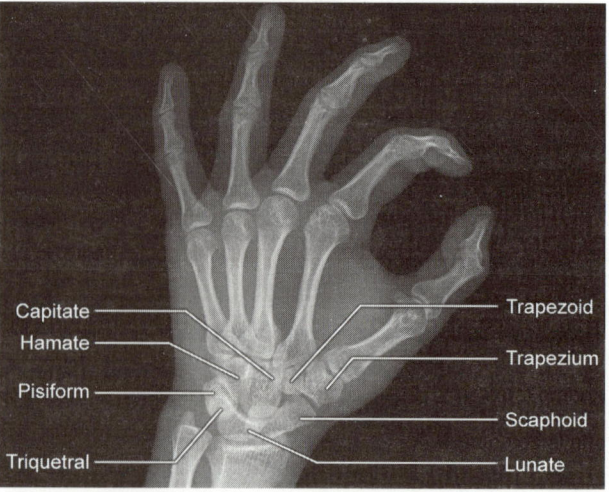

**Fig. 11.4b:** Radiograph of the hand

**Arterial supply:** Palmar and dorsal carpal arches.

**Nerve supply:** Anterior and posterior interosseous nerves.

**Movements and muscles producing them**

| | | |
|---|---|---|
| **Flexion** | : | Flexor carpi radialis and ulnaris |
| | | Flexor digitorum superficialis and profundus and palmaris longus |
| **Extension** | : | Extensor carpi radialis longus and brevis |
| | | Extensor carpi ulnaris |
| | | Extensor digitorum, extensor indicis |
| | | Extensor pollicis longus, extensor digiti minimi |
| **Adduction** | : | Flexor and extensor carpi ulnaris |
| **Abduction** | : | Abductor pollicis longus |
| | | Flexor carpi radialis, extensor carpi radialis longus and brevis. |

## Joints of the Hand

**Intercarpal joints**

The individual carpal bones are connected to each other by plane synovial joints.

**Midcarpal joint**

It is the joint between proximal and distal rows of carpal bones.

**First Carpometacarpal Joint (of the thumb)**

It is a saddle variety of synovial joint.

- It is the articulation between the trapezium and base of the first metacarpal bone.
- The joint permits flexion, extension, abduction, adduction and opposition movements.

*Flexion:* The palmar surface of the thumb moves across the palm towards the medial side, till the thumb comes in contact with the palm.

*Muscles involved in flexion:* Flexor pollicis brevis, opponens pollicis and flexor pollicis longus.

*Extension:* The thumb moves away from the palm so that its dorsal surface comes to face the dorsum of the hand.

*Muscles involved in extension:* Abductor pollicis longus, extensor pollicis brevis, extensor pollicis longus.

*Abduction:* The thumb moves away from the index finger at right angles to the plane of the palm (Fig.10.22).

*Muscles involved in abduction:* Abductor pollicis longus and abductor pollicis brevis.

*Adduction:* The thumb is brought back to the resting position (in contact with the index finger)

*Muscles involved in adduction:* Adductor pollicis and first palmar interossei.

*Opposition:* The tip of the thumb is brought in contact with the base or tip of other fingers.

*Muscles involved involved:* Opponens pollicis (**Note:** Median nerve is responsible for opposition).

*Metacarpophalangeal joints* are ellipsoid variety of synovial joints. They permit flexion, extension, abduction and adduction.

*Interphalangeal joints* are hinge variety of synovial joints permitting flexion and extension.

## LOWER LIMB

### HIP JOINT

*Type:* It is a ball and socket variety of synovial joint.

*Bones taking part:* Head of the femur articulating with lunate surface of the acetabulum (of hip bone). The articulating surfaces are covered by hyaline cartilage (Fig. 11.5a).

### Structures Stabilizing the Joint

1. **Capsular ligament (fibrous capsule):** Structurally, it is made of collagen and elastic fibers. Inferomedial part of the fibrous capsule is weakest and is stretched during abduction.

   **Attachment:**

   It is attached to the intertrochanteric line of the femur in front and medial to the intertrochanteric crest, behind. Hence the neck of the femur is intra capsular

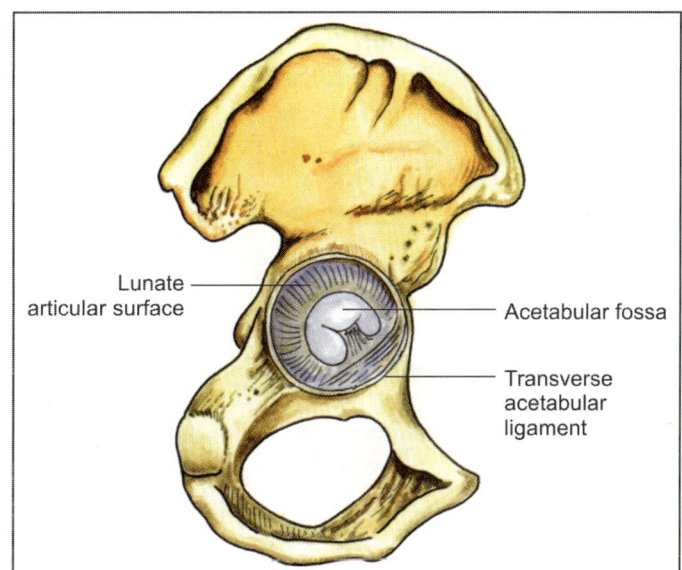

Lunate articular surface

Acetabular fossa

Transverse acetabular ligament

**11**

**Fig. 11.5a:** Acetabular fossa and transverse acetabular ligament

and is covered by synovial membrane. Some part of the fibrous capsule is reflected towards the neck as retinacular fibers, which carry blood vessels to the neck and head of the femur.

Medially the fibrous capsule is attached close to the acetabular margin and also blends with transverse acetabular ligament.

**Synovial membrane:**

It lines the inner surface of the fibrous capsule, acetabular labrum and intracapsular part of the neck of femur. The synovial membrane also invests the ligament of the head of the femur.

2. **Acetabular labrum**

It is a fibrocartilaginous rim attached to the acetabular margin. It deepens the socket and holds the femoral head tightly.

3. **Transverse acetabular ligament**

It extends across the acetabular notch. Thus, the acetabular notch is converted into a foramen through which blood vessels and nerves enter the joint.

4. **Ligament of the head of the femur**

It is triangular in shape with its apex attached to the fovea capitis of the femoral head and by its base to transverse acetabular ligament. This ligament is stretched in adduction of semiflexed hip. It transmits blood vessels into the head of femur.

5. **Iliofemoral ligament (ligament of Bigelow)**

It is one of the strongest ligaments of the body. It is triangular in shape with its apex attached to the anterior inferior iliac spine of the hip bone. The base is attached to the intertrochanteric line. It prevents the hyperextension of hip joint (Fig. 11.5b).

6. **Pubofemoral ligament**

It is the thickening of the fibrous capsule on inferomedial aspect. It is attached above to the iliopubic eminence and obturator crest. Below it blends with medial part of the iliofemoral ligament (Fig. 11.5b).

7. **Ischiofemoral ligament**

It covers the joint posteriorly. It is attached to the ischium close to the acetabular margin. The twisted fibers pass behind the neck and are attached to the greater trochanter of the femur but most of the fibers are continuous with the inner circular fibers of the fibrous capsule (zona orbicularis) (Fig. 11.5c).

**Arterial supply**

The hip joint is supplied by branches from medial and lateral circumflex femoral, obturator, superior and inferior gluteal arteries.

**Nerve supply**

The hip joint is supplied by femoral (branch supplying rectus femoris), anterior division of obturator nerve and nerve to quadratus femoris. Accessory obturator nerve if present can supply the hip joint.

### Movements and Muscles Producing them

*Flexion:* Psoas major and iliacus, pectineus, sartorius, rectus femoris.

*Extension:* Gluteus maximus and hamstring muscles. Gluteus maximus helps in raising the trunk from sitting position or in climbing upstairs. Hamstring muscles maintain extension in normal standing and walking.

*Adduction:* Adductor longus, brevis and magnus, gracilis and pectineus.

*Abduction:* Gluteus medius and minimus and tensor fasciae latae.

*Medial rotation:* Mainly by anterior fibers of gluteus medius and minimus with tensor fasciae latae.

*Lateral rotation:* Obturator internus and externus, superior and inferior gemelli, quadratus femoris, piriformis, gluteus maximus and sartorius.

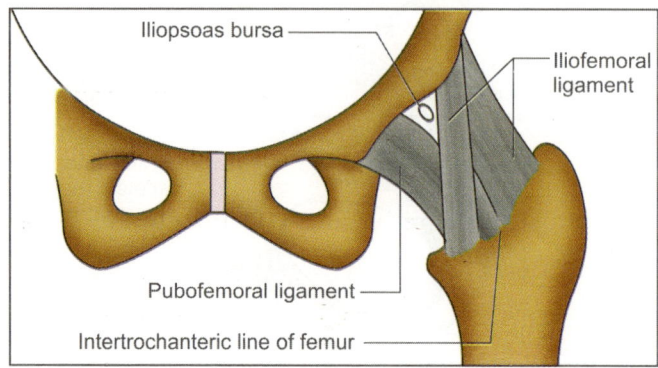

**Fig. 11.5b:** Pubofemoral and iliofemoral ligaments

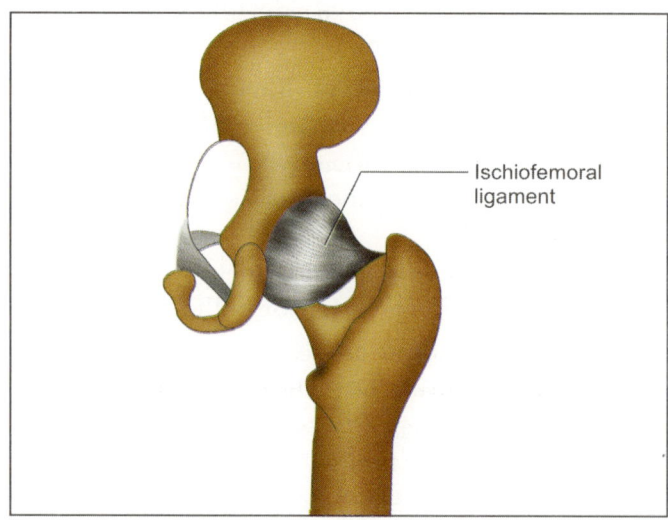

**Fig. 11.5c:** Ischiofemoral ligament

## Applied Anatomy

Dislocation of hip joint is more common on posterior aspect. The sciatic nerve may be injured in this dislocation.

*The fracture of the neck of femur:*

- It is very common in elderly due to osteoporotic changes in the neck.
- Postmenopausal women who develop osteoporosis, are more prone to this fracture on trauma. This fracture is of 2 types.

  1. **Intracapsular:** In this retinacular arteries are injured leading to delay in healing or non-union of fracture. Its serious complication is avascular necrosis of head of the femur with resultant loss of function of hip joint. In intracapsular fracture, the affected limb is shortened and held in characteristic laterally rotated position with toes pointing laterally. The anatomical explanation of this is as follows. Since the head of femur separates from the shaft (carrying the trochanter) in intracapsular fracture, the shaft can rotate independent of the head. The gluteus maximus and short lateral rotator muscles rotate the femur laterally. The psoas major becomes a lateral rotator after fracture due to the axis of action.

  2. **Extracapsular:** In the extracapsular fracture of neck (e.g. intertrochanteric fracture), the retinacular arteries are saved, hence healing is faster.

- Diseases of the hip may cause referred pain in the knee joint.

**Shenton's line:** By joining the medial margin of the femoral neck and the inferior margin of the superior ramus of pubis, a smoothly curved Shenton's line is demarcated. Fracture of neck or dislocation of hip joint distorts this line (Fig. 11.5d).

**Neck-shaft angle (angle of inclination):** The normal neck-shaft angle is 125° in adult and 160° in children. When there is increase in angle it is called **coxa valga**. It is found in congenital dislocation of the hip joint. **Coxa valga** limits the adduction movement of the hip joint.

If the angle is reduced it is called **coxa vara**. It is seen in fracture of neck of femur and it limits the abduction at the hip joint.

### Congenital Hip Dislocation

- Girls are affected more often than boys.
- About 60% of the affected children are first subling, suggesting unstretched uterine and abdominal walls that limit fetal movement.
- If it is not detected the child's hip may develop incorrectly and is evident when the child begins to walk.
- If one hip is affected the child will have a limp and lurch (sways on one side to clear the opposite foot of the ground) and if it is bilateral dislocation then there will be a waddling gait.

**Galeazzi test:** It is also known as the Alli's sign, is used in the diagnosis of congenital dislocation of the hip. It is performed by flexing an infant's knees in the supine position so that the ankles touch the buttocks. If the knees are not at same level then the test is positive, indicating a potential congenital hip malformation.

**Ortolani maneuver:** Gently abducting the infant's thigh with the examiner's thumb while placing anterior pressure on the greater trochanter using index finger. A distinctive 'clunk', is heard indicating the relocation of head anteriorly into the acetabulum. This test usually follows Barlow's maneuver.

**Barlow's maneuver:** Gently adducting the hip of infant and applying light pressure on the knee and directing the force posteriorly. If the hip is dislocatable—that is if the hip can be popped out of socket in this test then it is considered positive. This is an examination that is performed to screen out for hip dysplasia in newborn.

**Acquired dislocation:** Uncommon, in posterior dislocation the sciatic nerve may be injured.

Complications of hip dislocations include deep venous thrombosis (DVT), sciatic nerve injury, avascular necrosis, vascular injury, recurrent dislocation, arthritis and chronic pain.

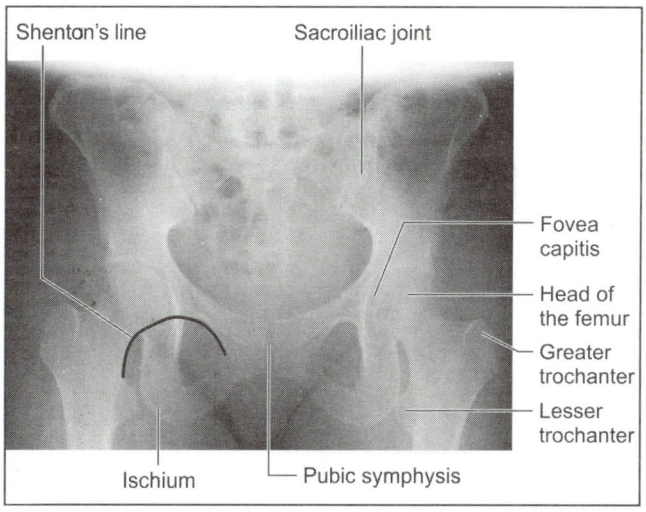

**Fig. 11.5d:** Normal radiograph of the hip joint: A Shenton's line

## KNEE JOINT

*Type:* It is a modified hinge variety of the synovial joint. It is also a complex (by the presence of menisci) and compound (more than two bones taking part) joint.

The articulation between the condyles of femur and tibia is a condylar variety of synovial joint. The articulation between femur and patella is a saddle variety of synovial joint (Fig. 11.6a and b).

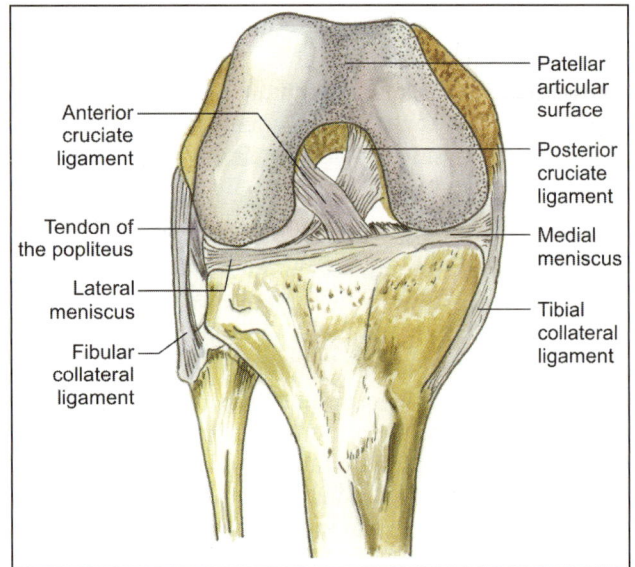

**Fig. 11.6a:** Knee joint—anterior view

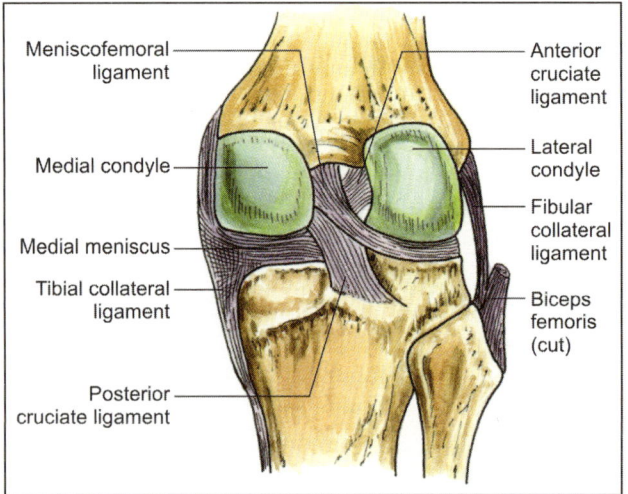

**Fig. 11.6b:** Knee joint—posterior view

**Bones taking part**

Condyles of the femur articulate with condyles of tibia. The patellar articular surface of the femur articulates with posterior surface of the patella.

**Structures stabilizing**

Structurally, knee joint is a weak joint, however, it is stabilised by number of factors of which cruciate and collateral ligaments are important.

1. **Capsular ligament (fibrous capsule)**

   The fibrous capsule is absent in the anterior aspect, where it is replaced by tendon of the quadriceps femoris muscle, patella and ligamentum patellae (from above downwards).

   *Femoral attachment:* It is attached to the articular margin of the femur (intercondylar line), however,

it is absent in the anterior aspect. The attachment encloses the origin of the popliteus muscle.

*Tibial attachment:* Anteriorly, it is attached to the margins of the condyles extending up to the tibial tuberosity. Posteriorly, it is attached to intercondylar ridge. The part of the fibrous capsule attached from the peripheral margins of the menisci to the articular margins of tibial condyle is called coronary ligament.

*Synovial membrane:* The investment of the synovial membrane is complex. It is absent on the inner aspect of the patella. Above the patella, it is prolonged upwards as 'suprapatellar bursa'. Below the patella it is separated from the ligamentum patellae by fat (infrapatellar pad of fat). Posteriorly, it is reflected forward by the cruciate ligaments (Fig. 11.6c).

2. **Ligamentum patellae**

   It is an extension of the tendon of quadriceps femoris muscle. It extends from the apex of patella to the tuberosity of tibia.

3. **Tibial collateral (medial) ligament**

   It is a strong ligament stabilizing the knee from medial side. Above it is attached to the medial epicondyle of the femur. Below it divides into superficial and deep parts. The superficial part is attached to the upper part of the medial surface and deep part into the medial condyle of the tibia.

4. **Fibular collateral (lateral) ligament**

   Above it is attached to the lateral epicondyle of the femur. Below it is attached to the apex of the fibula. It is separated from the lateral meniscus by the tendon of popliteus and part of the fibrous capsule.

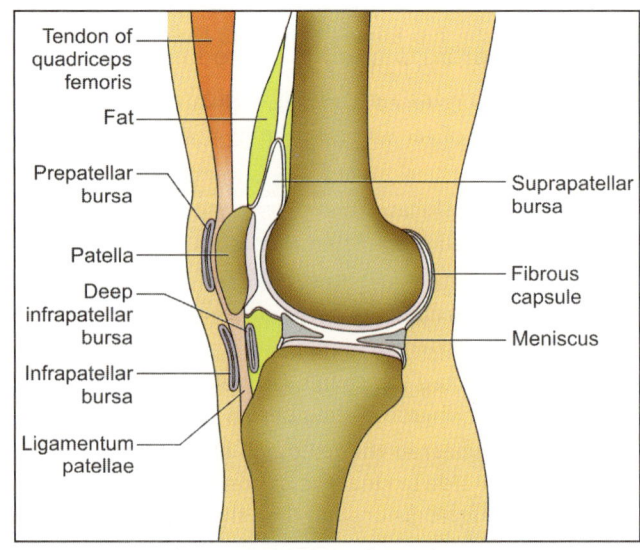

**Fig. 11.6c:** Knee—lateral view

5. **Oblique popliteal ligament**

   It is an extension from the tendon of semimembranosus muscle. It thickens the posterior aspect of the fibrous capsule and is attached to the lateral condyle of the femur. It is pierced by middle genicular nerve and vessels.

6. Arcuate popliteal ligament and short lateral ligaments are thickenings of the fibrous capsule.

   ### Intra-articular structures:

   The intra-articular structures include anterior and posterior cruciate ligaments, medial and lateral menisci, meniscofemoral ligament and tendon of popliteus.

7. **Cruciate ligaments**

   These are two strong fibrous ligaments connecting the femur and tibia (Fig. 11.6d and e).

   a. *Anterior cruciate ligament (ACL):* It extends from the anterior part of the intercondylar area of the tibia. It passes upwards, backwards and laterally and is attached to medial surface of lateral condyle of femur. It is stretched during extension of the knee joint. It prevents the forward displacement of tibial condyles.

   b. *Posterior cruciate ligament (PCL):* It extends from the posterior part of the intercondylar area of the tibia. It passes upwards, forwards and medially and is attached to the lateral surface of the medial condyle of femur. It is stretched during flexion of the knee joint. It prevents the backward displacement of tibial condyles.

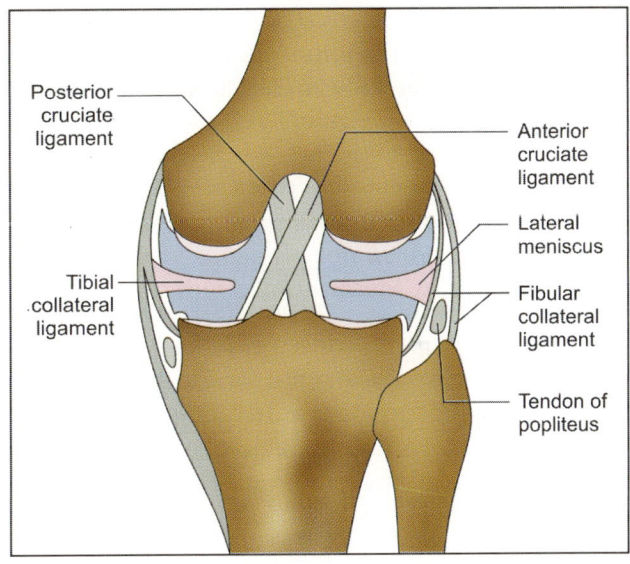

**Fig. 11.6d:** Cruciate ligaments and menisci of knee joint—anterior view

The two cruciate ligaments cross like the letter 'X', hence are called cruciate ligaments.

Both ligaments are covered by synovial membrane on their anterior aspect.

Anterior cruciate ligament is more prone for injury (in hyperextension or anterior dislocation of the tibia). It causes severe pain and the swelling of the knee joint.

**Drawer sign:** It is a test to evaluate the integrity of the cruciate ligaments. The person is in supine position with hip and knee in flexed position. The examiner firmly grasps the leg with

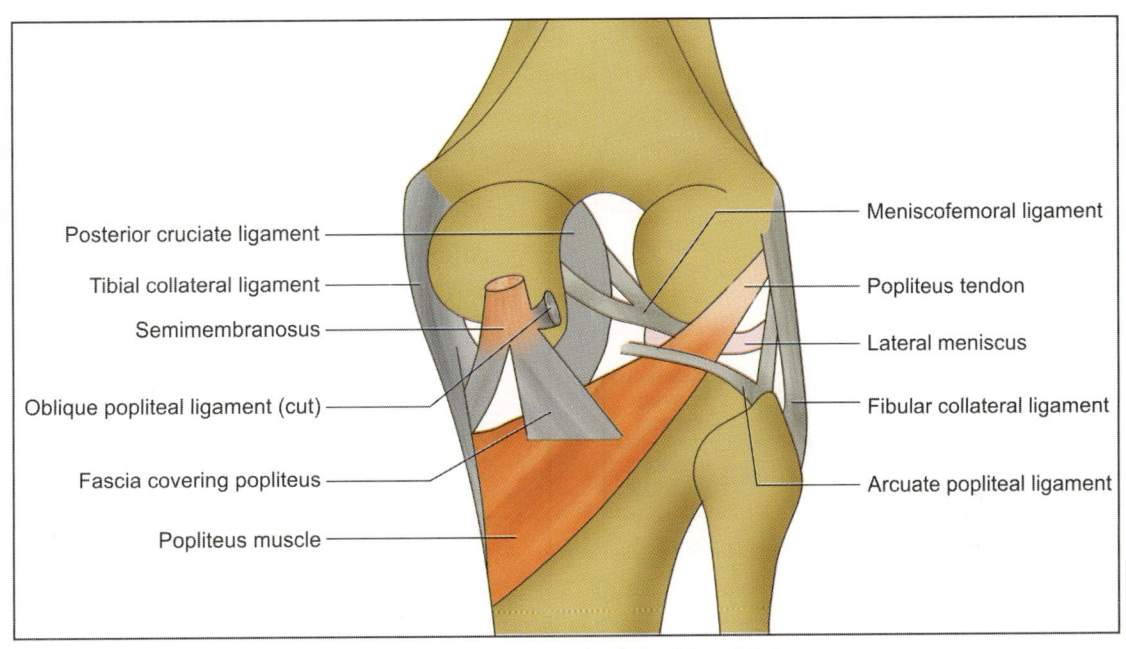

**Fig. 11.6e:** Ligaments of the knee joint

both hands with thumbs placed on the patella. If there is excessive forward (anterior) movement of the leg (tibia), it indicates injury to the anterior cruciate ligament and is called anterior drawer sign. If there is an excessive backward (posterior) movement of the leg, it indicates the injury to posterior cruciate ligament and is called posterior drawer sign (Fig. 11.6f)

8. **Menisci (Semilunar cartilages):**

Menisci are fibrocartilaginous structures, which deepen the articular surfaces of tibia.

Each meniscus presents anterior and posterior ends, upper and lower surfaces, medial and lateral margins.

The outer margin is thick and connected to the fibrous capsule and inner margin is free. The upper surface is concave for femur and lower surface is flat and articulates with the tibial condyles (Fig. 11.6g).

a. *Medial meniscus:* It is semilunar in shape. The anterior ends of the medial and lateral menisci are connected by 'transverse ligament'. The peripheral margin of the medial meniscus is attached to tibial collateral ligament. This makes the medial meniscus less mobile and more prone for injuries.

b. *Lateral meniscus:* It is circular in shape. The anterior and posterior ends of the lateral meniscus are attached to the intercondylar area of the tibia (Fig. 11.6h). The peripheral margin of the meniscus is not attached to the fibular

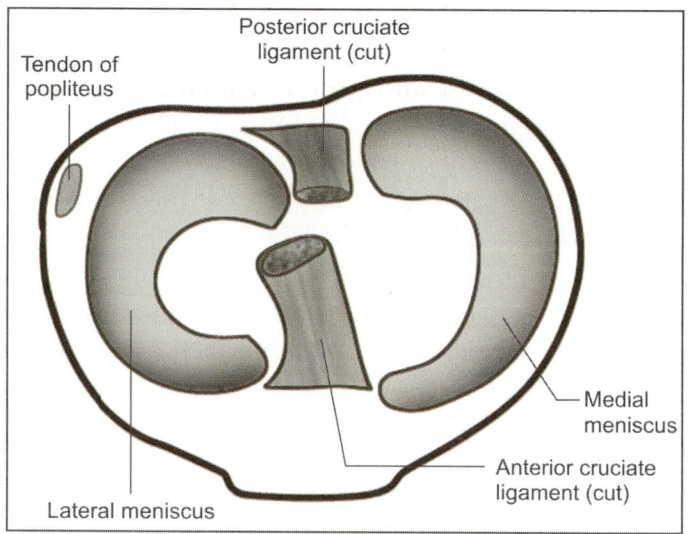

Fig. 11.6g: Menisci of the knee joint

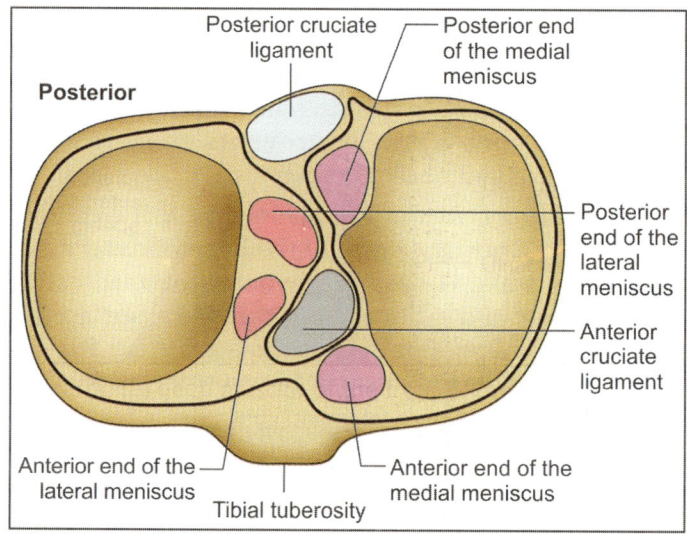

Fig. 11.6h: Intercondylar area

collateral ligament or fibrous capsule unlike medial meniscus. The tendon of the popliteus passes between the lateral meniscus and fibular collateral ligament. Some fibers of popliteus is attached to the posterior horn of the lateral meniscus, which pulls the meniscus backwards when femur is rotated laterally which prevents the crushing of meniscus during flexion of the knee joint. In this way popliteus protects the lateral meniscus.

The posterior end of the lateral meniscus is connected with medial condyle of the femur by two-meniscofemoral ligaments. The anterior and posterior meniscofemoral ligaments pass anterior and posterior to the posterior cruciate ligaments respectively. The tendon of the popliteus is

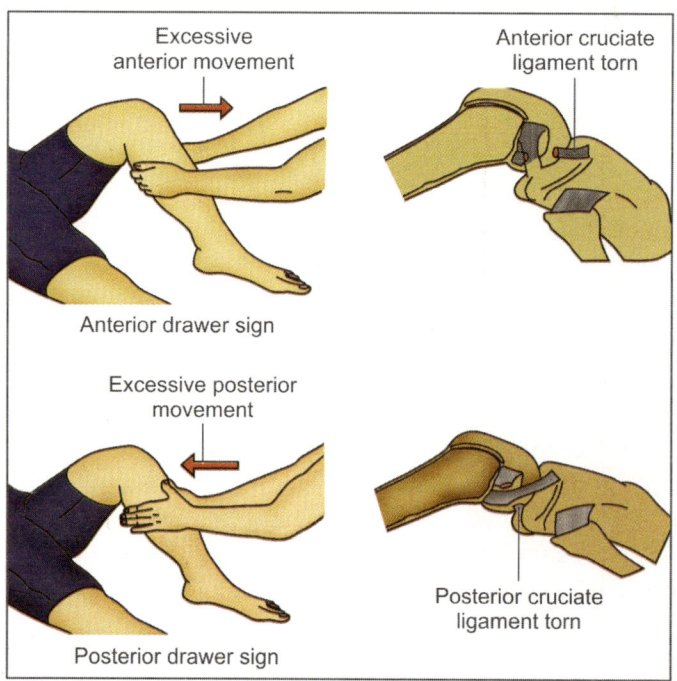

Fig. 11.6f: Anterior and posterior drawer signs

attached to the lateral meniscus, which pulls the meniscus backwards and prevents its injury.

The anterior and posterior meniscofemoral ligaments pass anterior and posterior to the posterior cruciate ligaments respectively. The tendon of the popliteus is attached to the lateral meniscus, which pulls the meniscus backwards and prevents its crushing-during flexion of the knee joint.

*Functions of Menisci*

- They deepen the tibial articular surfaces.
- They act as a shock absorbers to protect the articular cartilages.
- They flush the synovial fluid to provide nutrition to the articular cartilages.

## Arterial Supply

Knee joint is supplied by many genicular arteries derived from popliteal, femoral, anterior and posterior tibial arteries.

## Nerve Supply

a. Femoral nerve supplying vasti muscles also supply knee joint.

b. Genicular branches of tibial, common peroneal and posterior division of obturator nerves.

## Movements and Muscles Producing them

1. *Flexion:* Hamstring muscles (biceps femoris, semitendinosus, semimembranosus) and assisted by gracilis, sartorius and poplites muscle.

2. *Extension:* Quadriceps femoris and tensor fasciae latae.

3. Rotation of knee occurs below the menesci and the range of movement is very less.
   a. *Medial rotation:* Semitendinosus, semimembranosus and popliteus.
   b. *Lateral rotation:* Biceps femoris.

4. *Locking of the knee:* It is defined as medial rotation of femur on tibia during the final stages of extension of the knee, when the foot is on the ground. When the knee is locked, all the ligaments are stretched. It is an asset to the knee joint because knee can be held in extended position without any muscular contraction.

5. *Unlocking of the knee:* It is defined as 'lateral rotation' of femur on tibia during initial stages of flexion of the knee joint when the foot is on the ground. Popliteus muscle unlocks the knee by initiating flexion and further flexion is brought by hamstring muscles.

## Applied Anatomy

**Meniscal tears:**

- A sudden blow on the lateral side of a flexed weight-bearing knee can cause rupture of the tibial collateral ligament with a concomitant tear in the medial meniscus.
- The bucket handle rupture of the medial meniscus is common in football player.
- During extension of knee the femoral condyles first roll forwards and then spin forward on the upper surface of the menisci.
- The anterior horn of the medial meniscus is the last part to receive medial femoral condyle
- Since the anterior horn of the medial meniscus is the site of rotation of medial condyle of femur during locking and unlocking, it undergoes wear and tear.
- A sudden blow on the lateral side of a flexed weight-bearing knee can cause rupture of the tibial collateral ligament with a concomitant tear in the medial meniscus.
- On rupture of medial meniscus, the knee gets locked in the flexed position and swollen due to synovitis.
- Medial meniscus is less mobile (firmly fused with the tibial collateral ligament) and more prone to tear.
- Lateral miniscus is more mobile, since a few fibers of popliteus are attached to the posterior horn of lateral miniscus, the muscle pulls the meniscus back if the femur is rotated laterally.
- A combination of injury to the tibial collateral ligaments, medial meniscus and anterior cruciate ligament is called **'unhappy triad'** of knee joint.
- Rupture of anterior cruciate ligament may occur if the knee is forcibly hyperextended.

## ANKLE JOINT

*Type:* It is a hinge variety of synovial joint.

## Articulating Nones

*From above:* Inferior end of the tibia with medial malleolus, lateral malleolus of fibula and inferior transverse tibiofibular ligament.

*From below:* Superior surface of the body of the talus (Fig. 11.7).

## Structures Stabilizing

1. **Fibrous capsule (capsular ligament)**
   It is attached to articular margins but anteroinferiorly it extends upto the neck of the talus (for dorsiflexion). Synovial membrane lines the fibrous capsule.

2. **Deltoid (medial collateral) ligament**
   It is a strong triangular shaped ligament. Its apex is attached to the medial malleolus of tibia (Fig. 11.8a). It has a superficial and a deep part.

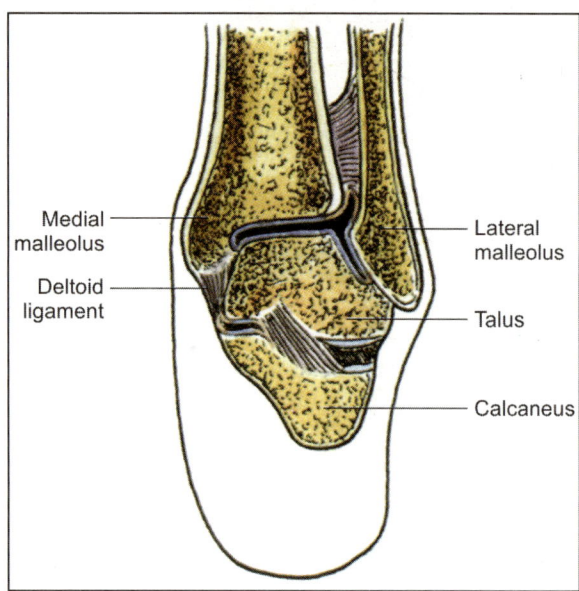

**Fig. 11.7:** Ankle joint—bones articulating

*Superficial part:* It consists of following ligaments:
i. *Tibionavicular:* To the tuberosity of the navicular bone.
ii. *Tibiocalcaneal:* To the whole length of the sustentaculum tali.
iii. *Posterior tibiotalar:* To the medial surface of the talus.

*Deep part:* It consists of anterior tibiotalar ligament which is attached to the anterior part of the medial surface of the talus.

3. **Lateral (fibular collateral) ligament**

It consists of three bands, which extend from the lateral malleolus to talus and calcaneum. It has been explained in three parts (Fig. 11.8b), namely:
• Anterior talofibular ligament: To the neck of the talus

• Posterior talofibular ligament: It extends from the lower part of the malleolar fossa of the fibula to the lateral tubercle of the talus.
• Calcaneofibular ligament: To the tubercle on the lateral surface of the calcaneus.

*Arterial supply:* Anterior and posterior tibial arteries.

*Nerve supply:* Deep peroneal and tibial nerves.

### Movements and Muscles Producing them

1. **Dorsiflexion:** The forefoot is raised and the angle between front of the leg and dorsum of the foot is diminished.

   *Muscles involved:* Tibialis anterior, extensor digitorum longus, extensor hallucis longus and peroneus tertius.

2. **Plantar flexion:** The forefoot is depressed and the angle between the leg and foot is increased.

   *Muscles involved:* Gastrocnemius, soleus, tibialis posterior, flexor hallucis longus, flexor digitorum longus, peroneus longus and peroneus brevis.

• Ankle joint is most frequently injured. Injury occurs in plantar flexed position of the foot. The lateral ligament is more often injured compared to the medial. **The anterior talofibular ligament is the most common of the lateral ligaments to be injured.** A sprained ankle results due to tear of anterior talofibular and calcaneofibular ligament, when the foot is twisted in lateral direction (inversion injury).

• In forcible eversion of foot the deltoid ligament may be torn. At times, the deltoid ligament pulls the medial malleolus thereby causing avulsion fracture of the medial malleolus.

• *Pott's fracture (fracture dislocation of ankle):* It is caused by forcible eversion leading to horizontal fracture of medial

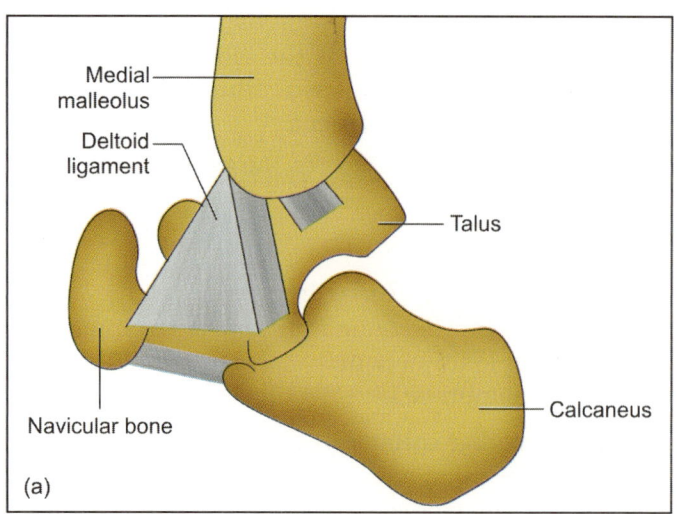

(a)

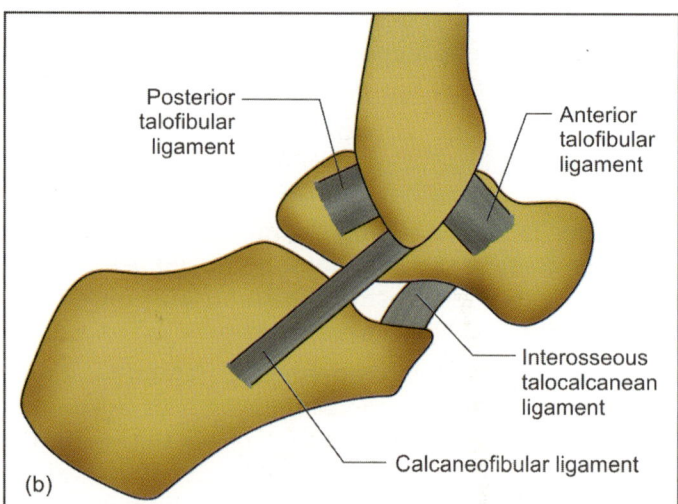

(b)

**Fig. 11.8a and b:** (a) Deltoid ligament of the ankle joint; (b) lateral ligament of the ankle joint

malleolus and oblique fracture of shaft of fibula and also lateral malleolus. It occurs when the foot is caught in the rabbit hole in the ground and the foot is forcibly everted. If the tibia is carried anteriorly, the posterior margin of the distal end of the tibia is also broken by the talus producing 'trimalleolar fracture'.

## Tibiofibular Joints

1. *Superior tibiofibular joint:* It is a plane synovial joint. The head of the fibula articulates with lateral condyle of tibia.

2. *Inferior tibiofibular joint:* It is a syndesmosis variety of fibrous joint. The lower ends of tibia and fibula are connected by a strong interosseous ligament.

## JOINTS OF THE FOOT

### SUBTALAR JOINT (TALOCALCANEAN JOINT)

The talus and calcaneum are connected by two strong joints.

a. **Talocalcanconavicular joint**

It is a ball and socket variety of synovial joint.

The head of the talus articulates with the calcaneo-navicular socket (formed by calcaneum and navicular bone)

The two bones are connected by fibrous capsule, interosseus talocalcaneal ligament, spring ligament and medial part of the bifurcate ligament.

b. **Talocalcanean joint**

It is a plane synovial joint

It is the articulation between the inferior surface of the talus and middle part of the superior surface of the calcaneum.

The joint is stabilized by fibrous capsule, interosseus talocalcaneal ligament and cervical ligament.

*Spring ligament (plantar calcaneonavicular ligament):* It extends from the anterior margin of the sustentaculum tali to the plantar surface of the navicular bone. The head of the talus directly rests on the upper surface of the spring ligament, separated by a fibrocartilage. This ligament is the key structure in maintaining the medial longitudinal arch.

### Movements and Muscles Producing them

1. *Inversion:* The medial border of the foot is elevated, so that the sole (plantar surface) faces medially. During this movement, the calcaneum and navicular with the forefoot move medially on the talus.

   *Muscles producing them:* Tibialis anterior, tibialis posterior and flexor hallucis longus

2. *Eversion:* The lateral border of the foot is elevated, so that the sole (plantar surface) faces laterally.

   *Muscles producing them:* Peroneus longus, peroneus brevis and peroneus tertius.

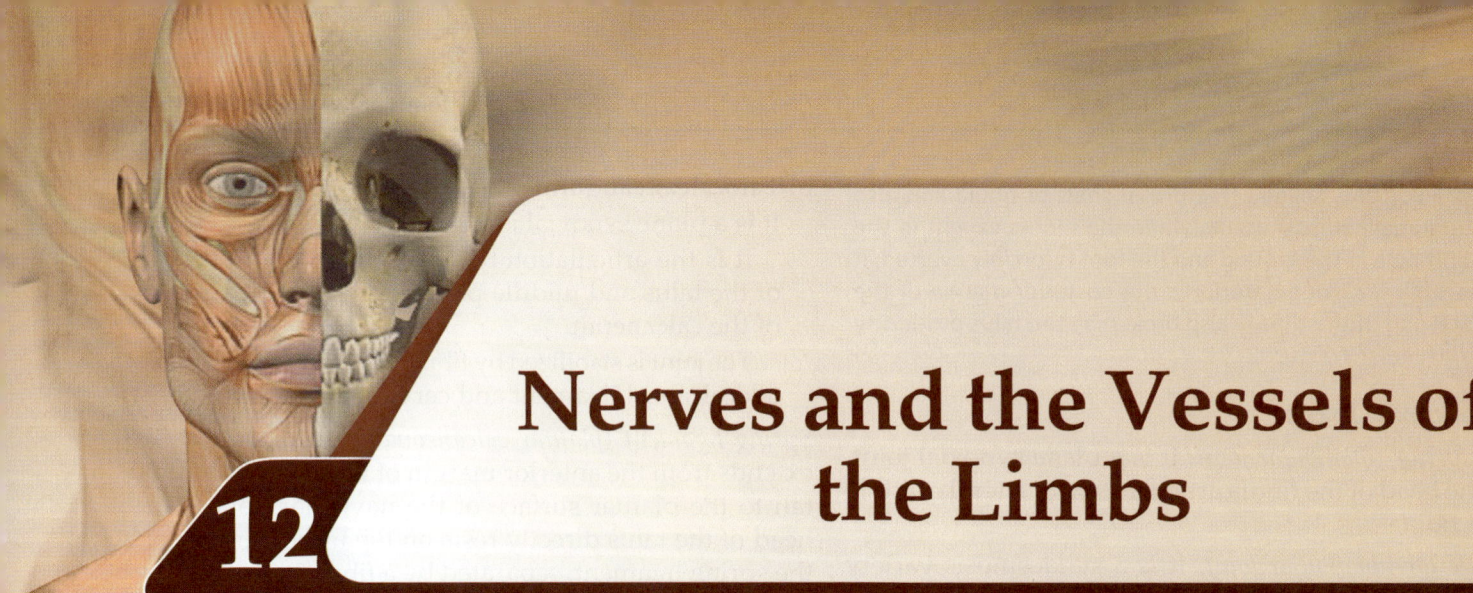

# Nerves and the Vessels of the Limbs

**12**

## BRACHIAL PLEXUS

Brachial plexus of nerves supply, upper limb (Figs 12.1 and 12.2).

### Formation

It is formed by ventral rami of lower four cervical and first thoracic nerves ($C_{5, 6, 7, 8}$ and $T_1$).

Contribution from $C_4$ nerve constitutes 'pre-fixed condition' of the brachial plexus and contribution from $T_2$ nerve constitutes post-fixed condition of the brachial plexus.

### Parts

The proximal part of the brachial plexus occupies the posterior triangle of the neck. This part is called 'supra-clavicular part'. The distal part of the plexus occupy the axilla (arm pit) and it is called 'infraclavicular part'.

Brachial plexus consists of roots, trunks, divisions and cords.

### Roots

- The ventral rami of $C_5$ and $C_6$ join to form 'upper trunk'.
- The ventral ramus of $C_7$ continue as 'middle trunk'.
- The ventral rami of $C_8$ and $T_1$ join to form 'lower trunk'.
  Each trunk divides into ventral and dorsal divisions.

### Cords

- The ventral divisions of upper and middle trunks join to form 'lateral cord'.
- The ventral division of lower trunk continues as 'medial cord'.
- The dorsal divisions of all the trunks (upper, middle and lower) join to form 'posterior cord'.

## Branches

### *Branches from the Roots*

1. Nerve to serratus anterior (long thoracic nerve) $C_{5, 6, 7}$
2. Nerve to rhomboideus (dorsal scapular nerve) $C_5$

### *Branches from the Upper Trunk*

1. Suprascapular nerve ($C_{5, 6}$)
2. Nerve to subclavius ($C_{5, 6}$)

### *Branches from the Lateral Cord*

1. Lateral pectoral nerve ($C_{5, 6, 7}$)
2. Musculocutaneous nerve ($C_{5, 6, 7}$)
3. Lateral root of the median nerve ($C_{5, 6, 7}$)

### *Branches from the Medial Cord*

1. Medial root of the median nerve ($C_8$, $T_1$)
2. Medial pectoral nerve ($C_8$, $T_1$)
3. Medial cutaneous nerve of the arm ($C_8$, $T_1$)
4. Medial cutaneous nerve of the forearm ($C_8$, $T_1$)
5. Ulnar nerve ($C_{7, 8}$, $T_1$)

### *Branches from the Posterior Cord*

1. Upper subscapular nerve ($C_{5, 6}$)
2. Lower subscapular nerve ($C_{5, 6}$)
3. Nerve to latissimus dorsi ($C_{6, 7, 8}$)
4. Axillary nerve ($C_{5, 6}$)
5. Radial nerve ($C_{5, 6, 7, 8}$, $T_1$)

### Applied Anatomy

**Brachial plexus injury**
Brachial plexus may be injured during labour (forceps delivery), automobile injury, stab injury, compression by enlarged lymph nodes or aneurysm of the axillary artery.

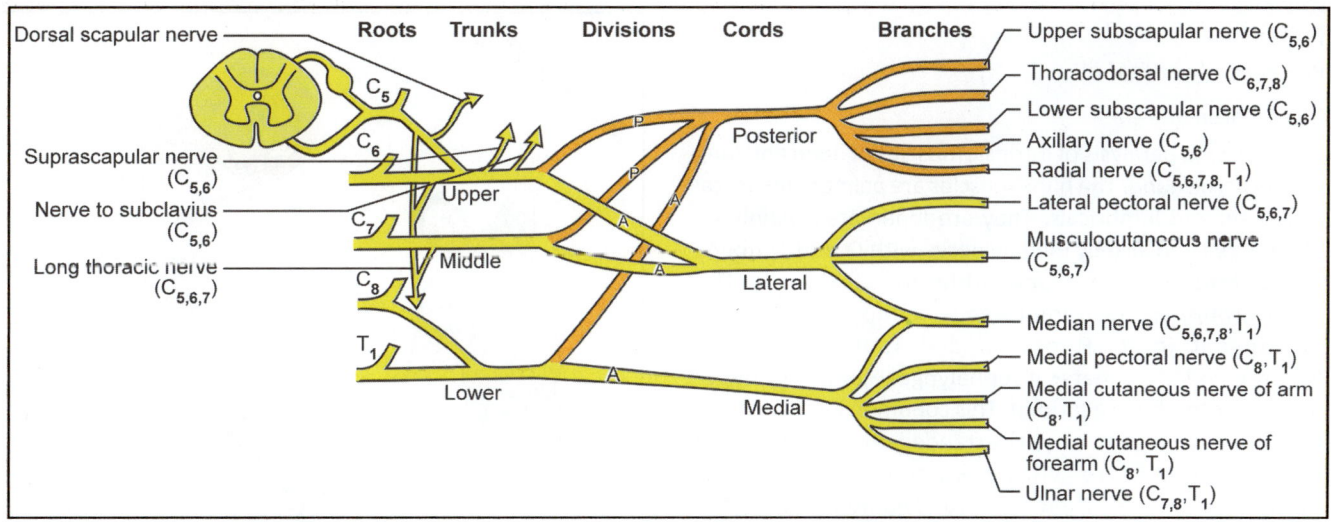

**Fig. 12.1:** Schematic representation of brachial plexus

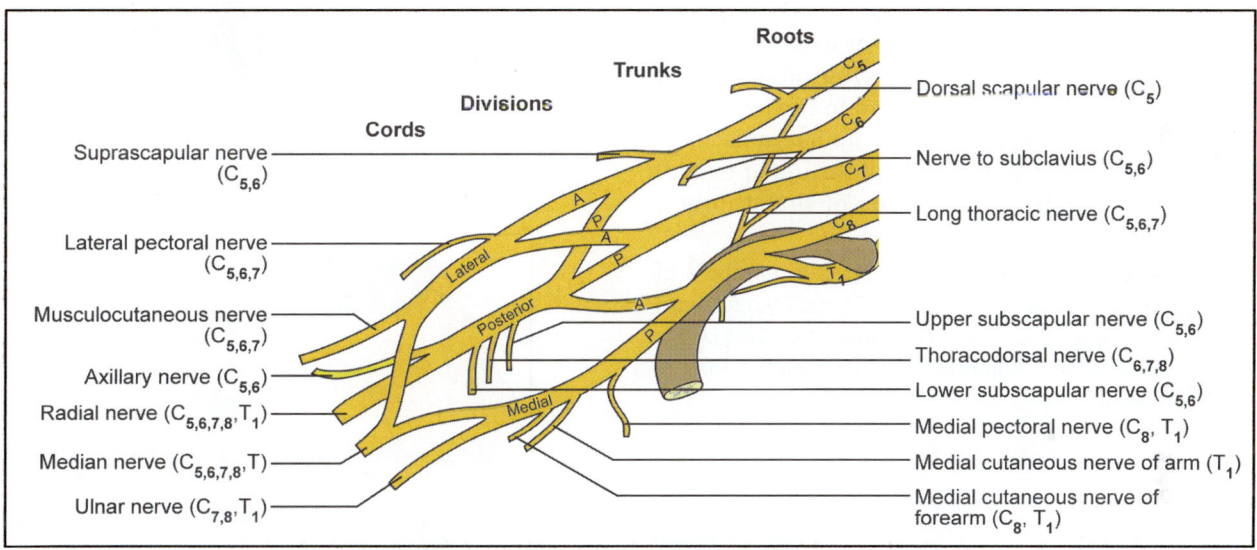

**Fig. 12.2:** Brachial plexus—position of trunks and cords

### Erb's paralysis

The upper trunk of the brachial plexus where six nerves ($C_5$ and C6 roots, nerve to subclavius and suprascapular nerve, anterior and posterior divisions of upper trunk) meet is called Erb's point. An injury to the Erb's point results in paralysis of muscles of the upper limb supplied by $C_5$ and $C_6$ fibers.

*Causes of injury* (Fig. 12.3):

Birth injury (excessive stretching of upper trunk)

Fall on the shoulder

During anesthesia (brachial plexus block)

*Clinical features:*

- The arm hangs by the side of the body and medially rotated. The arm cannot be abducted and laterally rotated.
- The elbow is extended and flexion is not possible.
- The forearm is pronated and supination is not possible.
- The wrist and fingers are flexed.

- This position of the upper limb is referred to as policeman's tip or waiter's tip hand.

*Muscles involved:*

- Deltoid (hence abduction at shoulder is not possible)
- Biceps, brachialis and brachioradialis (hence flexion at elbow is not possible)
- Supinator (hence supination of forearm is not possible)
- Supraspinatus (hence initiation of abduction is not possible)
- Teres minor (hence lateral rotation is not possible)
- Infraspinatus (hence lateral rotation is not possible)

### Klumpke's paralysis

It occurs due to injury to the lower trunk of the brachial plexus ($C_8$, $T_1$).

*Causes of injury* (Fig. 12.4):

- Undue abduction of arm (as in clutching something with hands while falling from a height.

- Birth injury
- Presence of cervical rib

*Clinical features:*

- This results in paralysis of intrinsic muscles of hand and long flexors of the hand. The hand muscles are palmar and dorsal interossei and lumbricals. They are innervated mainly by ulnar nerve and also by median nerve with $C_8$ and $T_1$ fibers. These muscles are responsible for flexion at the metacarpophalangeal joint and extention at the interphalangeal joint. Hence medial four fingers are hyperextended at metacarpophalyngeal joint and hyper flexed at interphalyngeal joint. This condition is called 'clawhand'. The wrist joint is hyper extended due to paralysis of wrist flexors. There will be wasting of thenar and hypothenar muscles. There is pain and numbness along the medial side of the arm, forearm and medial one and half finger.

- Involvement of ventral ramus of $T_1$ or its white ramus communicantes causes 'Horner's syndrome'. This is because the sympathetic innervation to the head area (sweat glands of the face, dilator pupillae muscle of the eye and superior tarsal muscle of the upper eyelid) is conveyed through ventral ramus of first thoracic nerve.

- *Injury to the long thoracic nerve:* It results in paralysis of Serratus anterior muscle, which is manifested by backward projection of scapula (winging of scapula) (Fig. 12.5). This nerve may be injured while removing the lymph nodes of the axilla as well.

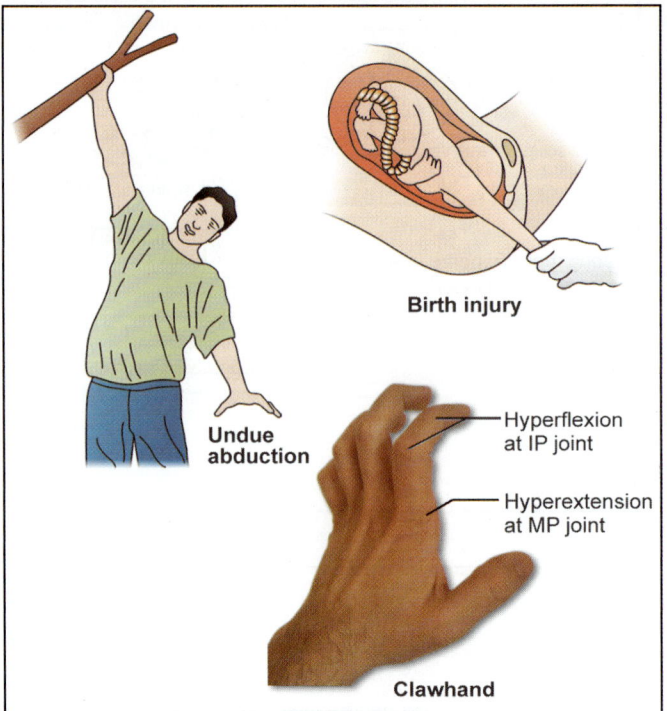

**Birth injury**

**Undue abduction**

Hyperflexion at IP joint

Hyperextension at MP joint

**Clawhand**

**Fig. 12.4:** Klumpke's paralysis

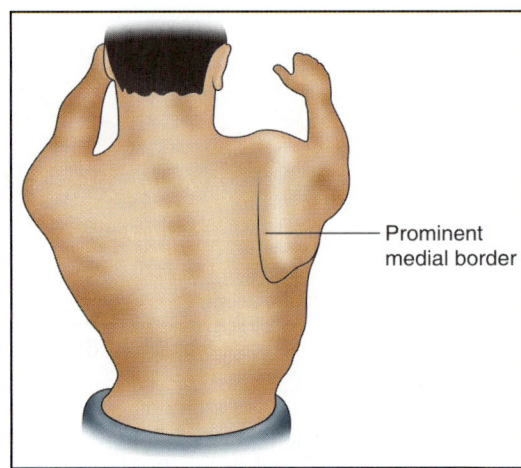

Prominent medial border

**Fig. 12.5:** Winging of scapula

## Musculocutaneous Nerve ($C_{5, 6, 7}$) (Fig. 12.6a)

- It has both muscular and cutaneous distribution.
- It arises from the lateral cord of the brachial plexus.
- It supplies three muscles in the front of the arm (coracobrachialis, biceps brachii and brachialis).
- It continues as lateral cutaneous nerve of the forearm.

## Axillary Nerve (Circumflex Nerve) ($C_{5, 6}$) (Fig. 12.6b)

- It arises from the posterior cord of the brachial plexus.
- It passes through the quadrangular space below the shoulder joint along with the posterior circumflex humeral artery.

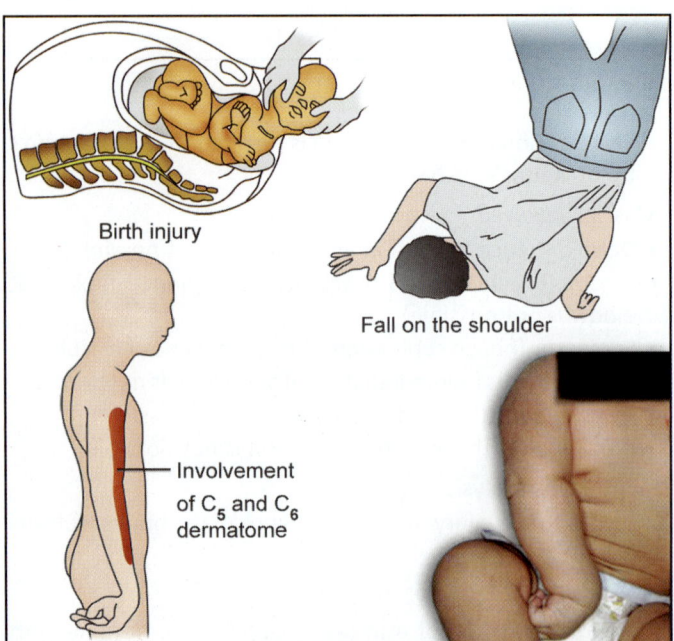

Birth injury

Fall on the shoulder

Involvement of $C_5$ and $C_6$ dermatome

**Fig. 12.3:** Erb's paralysis

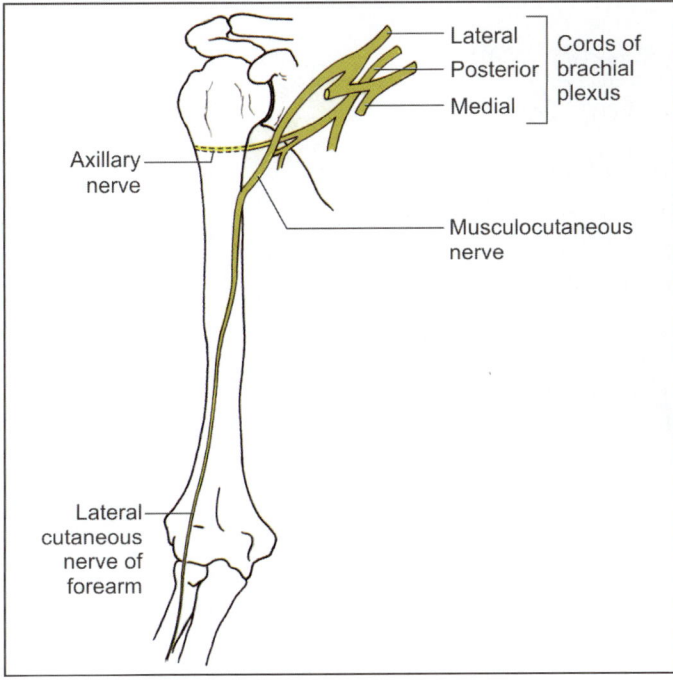

**Fig. 12.6a:** Musculocutaneous nerve

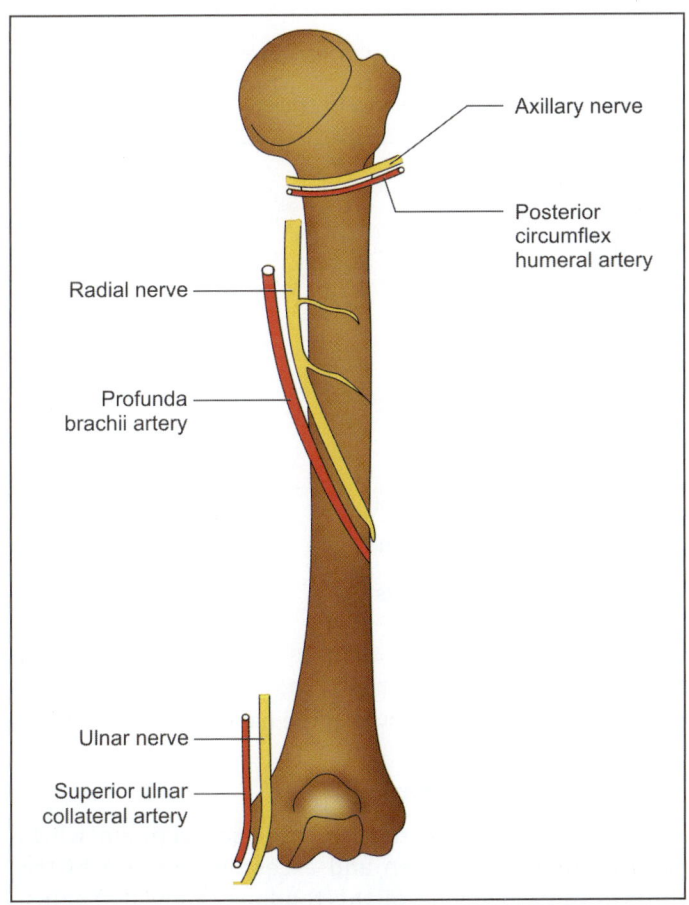

**Fig. 12.6b:** Nerves in contact with humerus

- It winds close to the surgical neck of the humerus.
- It supplies deltoid and teres minor muscle.
- It continues as upper lateral cutaneous nerve of the arm.
- Fracture of the surgical neck of the humerus can cause injury to the axillary nerve, which results in loss of power of abduction at shoulder joint. There is also a sensory loss on the skin over the deltoid muscle.

  In case of fracture of surgical neck or downward dislocation of the shoulder the axillary nerve function is tested by gently pricking on the skin over the deltoid.

### Median Nerve (C$_{5, 6, 7, 8}$, T$_1$)

*Formation*

Median nerve is formed by the union of two-nerve roots in the axilla (Figs 12.1 and 12.2).

a. Medial root from the medial cord of the brachial plexus (C$_8$ T$_1$)

b. Lateral root from the lateral cord of the brachial plexus (C$_{5, 6, 7}$)

*Course*

- It descends in the front of the arm and crosses the brachial artery from lateral to medial side and enters the cubital fossa.
- In the cubital fossa the median nerve occupies medial to the brachial artery.
- Median nerve descends between superficial and deep flexor muscles of forearm.
- It enters the palm by passing deep to the flexor retinaculum of the hand (through carpal tunnel).
- It terminates in the palm by dividing into medial and lateral branches.

*Branches and Distribution*

**In the forearm:**
- Muscular branches to pronator teres, flexor carpi radialis, flexor digitorum superficialis, and palmaris longus muscles.
- Anterior interosseous branch supplies: Lateral part of flexor digitorum profundus (tendons for the index and middle fingers), flexor pollicis longus, pronator quadratus.
- Palmar cutaneous branch supplies skin of the lateral part of the hand.
- It also give articular and vascular branches.
- **In the hand** it supplies skin of the lateral three and a half fingers, thenar muscles (abductor pollicis brevis,

12

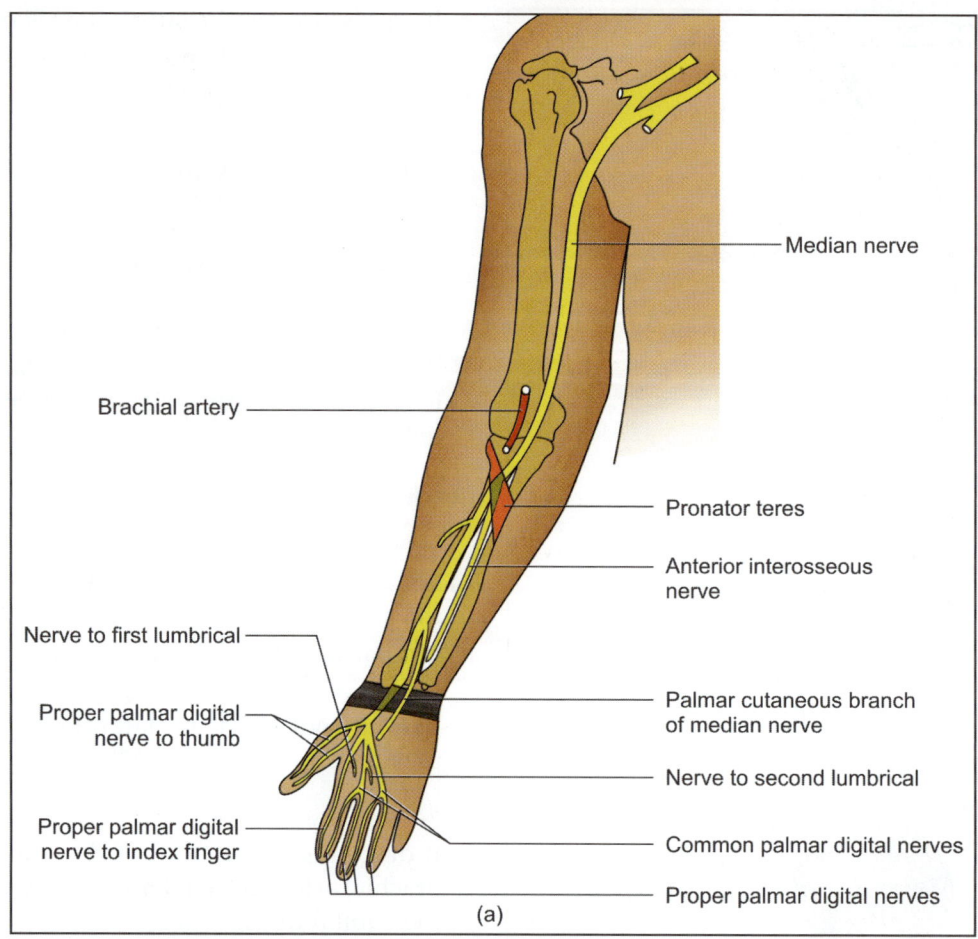

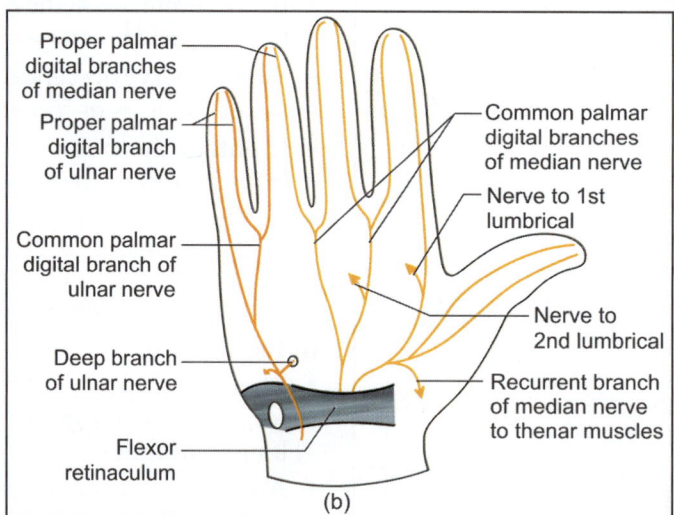

**Fig. 12.7a and b:** (a) Median nerve-schematic; (b) median and ulnar nerves in the hand

flexor pollicis brevis, opponens pollicis) and first and second lumbricals (Fig. 12.7a and b).

To summarise median nerve supplies mainly flexor muscles of the forearm and a few muscles of the hand acting on the thumb.

## Carpal Tunnel Syndrome

It occurs due to fluid retention in the carpal tunnel which may be due to infection and excessive exercise of the fingers cause swelling of the tendons/synovial sheaths. The myxedema, pregnancy or anterior dislocation of

12

lunate bone also causes fluid retention and results in carpal tunnel syndrome. The signs and symptoms are gradual in onset.

*Effects:*

- At first, it causes numbness, tingling and burning pain in lateral three and half fingers.
- Gradually there may be a loss of sensation in the same fingers in due course of time.
- Weakness of thenar muscles and flattening of thenar eminence, loss of motor function (loss of coordination and strength in the thumb—unable to oppose the thumb, difficulty in buttoning the shirt/blouse).
- Will lead to ape thumb deformity if left untreated.
- There is no sensory loss on the lateral part of the palm of the skin because this area is supplied by palmar cutaneous branch of the median nerve which arises in the forearm and enters the palm superficial to the flexor retinaculum.

  Surgical division of flexor retinaculum is one of the methods to relieve pressure on the median nerve in carpal tunnel.

## Ulnar Nerve ($C_{7, 8}$, $T_1$)

### Formation

Ulnar nerve is a branch of the medial cord of the brachial plexus. Occasionally ulnar nerve receives $C_7$ fibers from the lateral root of the median nerve, which is believed to supply flexor carpi ulnaris muscle and skin along the medial border of the ring finger (Fig. 12.8a).

### Course

1. Ulnar nerve descends in the front of the arm on the medial side.
2. At the middle of the arm it pierces the medial intermuscular septum and *passes posterior to the medial epicondyle of humerus*.
3. The nerve enters the anterior compartment of the forearm by piercing the flexor carpi ulnaris muscle.
4. In the forearm it is accompanied by ulnar vessels and together they enter the palm by passing superficial to the flexor retinaculum of the hand.
5. In the palm it terminates by dividing into superficial and deep branches.

### Branches and Distribution

1. Muscular branches in the forearm supply flexor carpi ulnaris and medial part of the flexor digitorum profundus (tendons for the ring and little fingers).
2. Palmar cutaneous branch arises in the forearm and enters the palm superficial to the flexor retinaculum. It supplies the skin of the palm on the medial side (Fig. 12.9a).

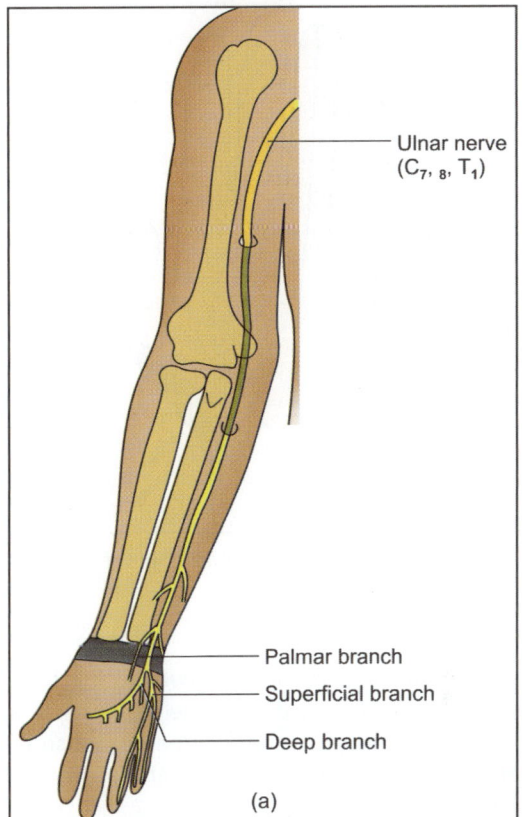

(a)

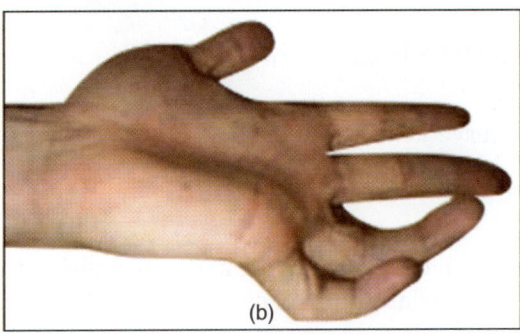

(b)

**Fig. 12.8a and b:** (a) Ulnar nerve-schematic; (b) ulnar clawhand

3. Dorsal branch supplies the skin of the medial side of the dorsum of the hand and medial one and a half fingers on the dorsal aspect (Fig. 12.9b).
4. The superficial terminal branch in the hand supplies palmaris brevis muscle and skin of the medial one and a half fingers, on the palmar aspects.
5. The deep branch supplies the following intrinsic muscles—abductor digiti minimi, flexor digiti minimi, opponens digiti minimi, adductor pollicis, third and fourth lumbricals, all the four palmar interossei, all the four dorsal interossei.
6. Ulnar nerve also gives articular and vascular branches.

   To summarise, the ulnar nerve mainly supplies intrinsic muscles of the hand and a few flexor muscles of the forearm.

In the figure: Ulnar nerve ($C_{7, 8}$, $T_1$); Palmar branch; Superficial branch; Deep branch.

12

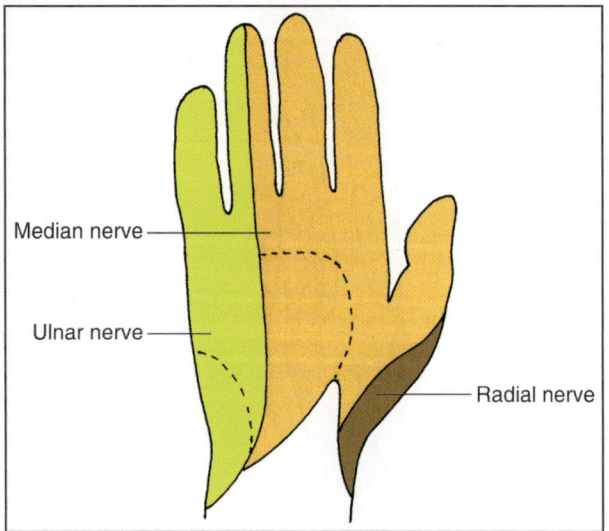

**Fig. 12.9a:** Palm—cutaneous innervation

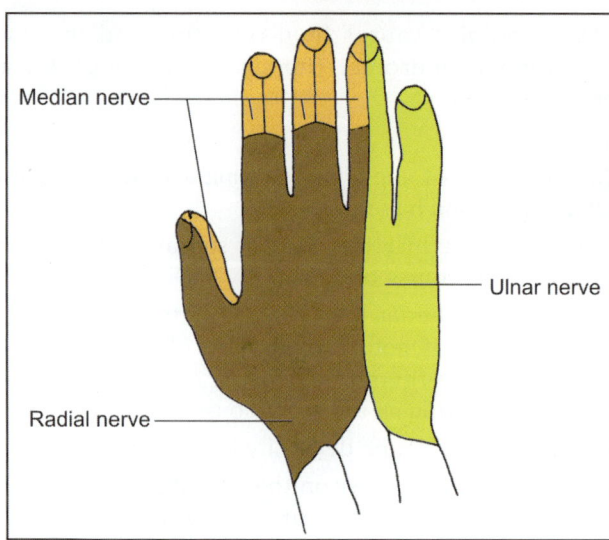

**Fig. 12.9b:** Dorsum of the hand—cutaneous innervation

## Applied Anatomy

Injury to the ulnar nerve produces **'clawhand'** involving mainly the ring and little fingers due to the paralysis of intrinsic muscles. In clawhand there is hyper extension at the metacarpophalangeal joint and flexion at the interphalangeal joints (Fig. 12.8b).

## Radial Nerve (C$_{5, 6, 7, 8}$, T$_1$)

### Origin

Radial nerve is a branch from the posterior cord of the brachial plexus (Fig. 12.10a and b).

### Course

1. The radial nerve leaves the axilla by passing through the lower triangular space and enters the back of the arm.
2. It *descends in the radial groove (spiral) on the posterior aspect of the humerus* between lateral and medial heads of the triceps muscle. It is accompanied by profunda brachii artery.
3. The radial nerve enters the front of the arm by piercing the lateral intermuscular septum and runs downwards between brachialis and brachioradialis muscles.
4. It terminates in front of the elbow by dividing into superficial and deep branches.
5. The superficial branch descends along the radial (lateral) side of the forearm and enters the dorsum of the hand.
6. The deep branch pierces the 'supinator muscle' and enters posterior compartment of the forearm as 'posterior interosseus nerve'.

### Branches and Distribution

**In the axilla**
1. Muscular branches to long and medial head of the triceps.
2. Cutaneous branch—posterior cutaneous nerve of the arm.

**In the spiral groove**
1. Muscular branches to lateral and medial head of the triceps.
2. Cutaneous branches—posterior cutaneous nerve of the forearm, and lower lateral cutaneous nerve of the arm.

**In the front of the arm**
It gives muscular branches to brachialis, brachioradialis and extensor carpi radialis longus.

**Terminal branches**
1. The superficial terminal branch supplies skin of the (lateral half) the dorsum of the hand and also dorsal aspect of the lateral three and a half fingers.
2. The deep terminal branch (posterior interosseus nerve) supplies muscles of the back of the forearm (extensor muscles). The muscles include:
   - Supinator
   - Extensor carpi radialis brevis
   - Extensor digitorum
   - Extensor digiti minimi
   - Extensor indicis
   - Extensor carpi ulnaris
   - Abductor pollicis longus
   - Extensor pollicis brevis

To summarise, the radial nerve supplies all extensor muscles of arm and forearm.

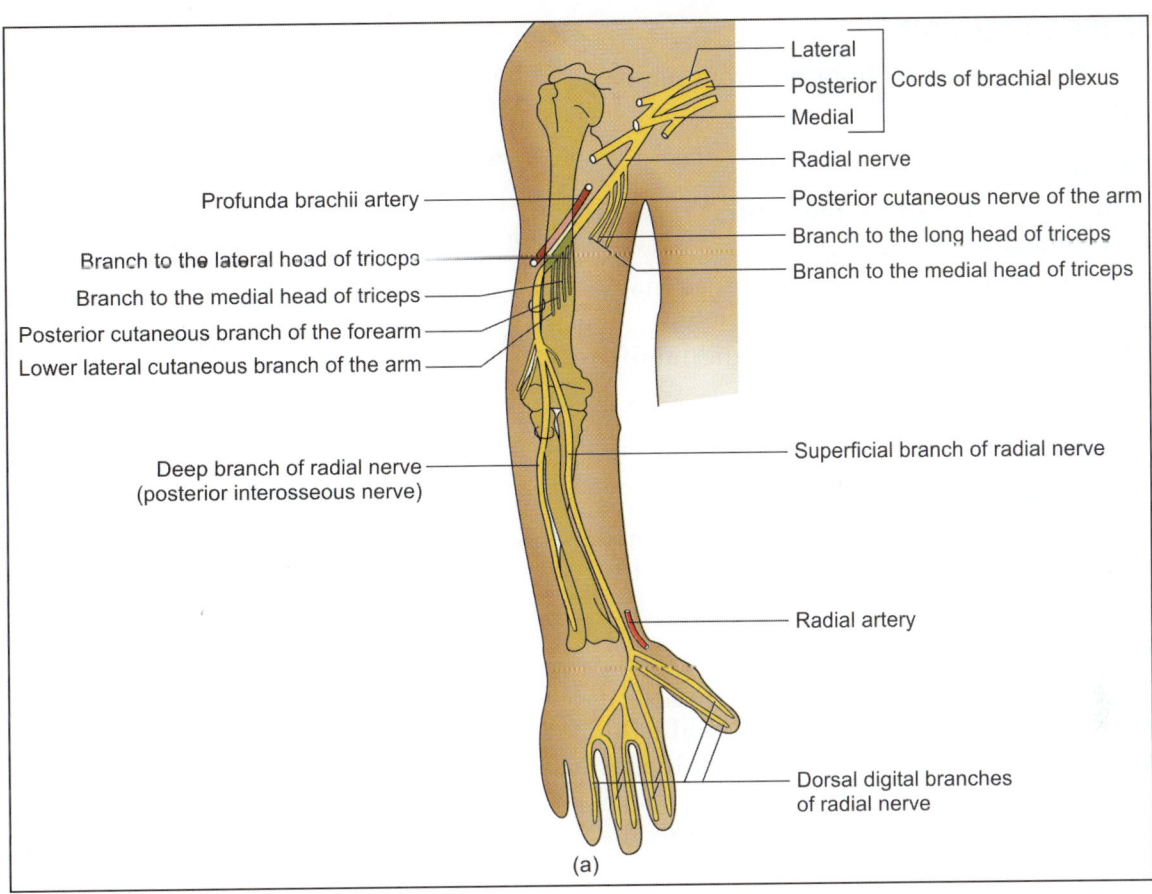

Lateral
Posterior ] Cords of brachial plexus
Medial
Radial nerve
Posterior cutaneous nerve of the arm
Branch to the long head of triceps
Branch to the medial head of triceps

Profunda brachii artery
Branch to the lateral head of triceps
Branch to the medial head of triceps
Posterior cutaneous branch of the forearm
Lower lateral cutaneous branch of the arm

Deep branch of radial nerve
(posterior interosseous nerve)

Superficial branch of radial nerve

Radial artery

Dorsal digital branches
of radial nerve

(a)

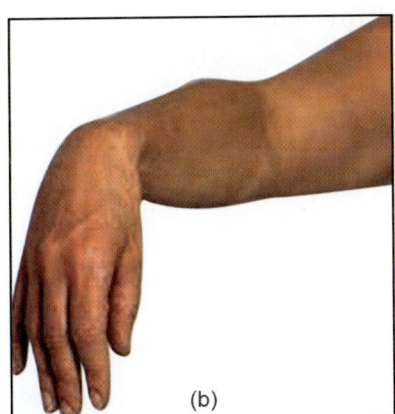

(b)

**Fig. 12.10a and b:** (a) Radial nerve-schematic; (b) wrist drop

## Applied Anatomy

- Radial nerve may be injured in fracture of the humerus in the region of the spiral groove, which results in **wrist drop** (Fig. 12.10b).
- Radial nerve may also be compressed by the pressure of a crutch in the axilla (crutch paralysis).
- Compression of the radial nerve against the spiral groove by placing the outstretched arm (as in sleeping) in an arm chair under drunken condition can lead to temporary 'Saturday night palsy'.

- *Injury to the radial nerve:* All the extensor muscles of the forearm are paralyzed and the patient will not able to extend the wrist. This condition is called 'wrist drop'. Extension of the elbow is lost when the triceps is paralyzed (when the nerve is injured in the axilla). The sensory loss depends on the site of injury. If injured in the axilla, there will be a loss of cutaneous sensation at the back of the arm, forearm and lateral aspect of the dorsum of the hand.

12

## NERVES OF THE LOWER LIMB

The lower limb is supplied by branches from lumbar and sacral plexus.

### Lumbar Plexus

- Lumbar plexus is formed by the ventral rami of upper four lumbar nerves ($L_1$–$L_4$).
- It is formed within the substance of psoas major muscle in the posterior abdominal wall.
- Following are the major branches of the lumbar plexus.

### Femoral Nerve ($L_{2, 3, 4}$)

*Origin:* Femoral nerve arises from the lumbar plexus within the substance of psoas major muscle. It is formed by the dorsal divisions of ventral rami of second to fourth lumbar spinal nerves (Fig. 12.11a).

### Course

1. After emerging from the psoas major muscle it descends in the posterior abdominal wall, the nerve lies in a groove between psoas and iliacus muscle.
2. The nerve enters, front of the thigh deep to the inguinal ligament lateral to the femoral vessels.
3. In the upper part of the thigh the nerve terminates by dividing into anterior and posterior divisions.

### Branches and Distribution

1. The main trunk in the abdomen gives muscular branches to iliacus and pectineus.
2. The anterior division provides one muscular and two cutaneous branches.
   - branch to sartorius muscle
   - medial cutaneous nerve of the thigh
   - intermediate cutaneous nerve of the thigh
3. The posterior division provides one cutaneous and four muscular branches.
   - Saphenous nerve—It supplies skin of the medial side of the leg and medial border of foot up to the ball of the big toe
   - Muscular branches supply rectus femoris, vastus medialis, and vastus intermedius and vastus lateralis muscles. The nerve supplying rectus femoris also supplies hip joint and the nerves supplying vasti muscle supply knee joint.

### Obturator Nerve ($L_{2, 3, 4}$)

Obturator nerve supplies muscles of the medial compartment of the thigh (Fig. 12.11b).

*Origin:* It is a branch from the lumbar plexus formed by the ventral divisions of ventral rami of second, third and fourth lumbar spinal nerves.

### Course

1. After emerging from the psoas major muscle, it descends in the lateral pelvic wall.
2. It enters the medial side of the thigh through obturator canal where it terminates by dividing into anterior and posterior divisions (Fig. 12.11).

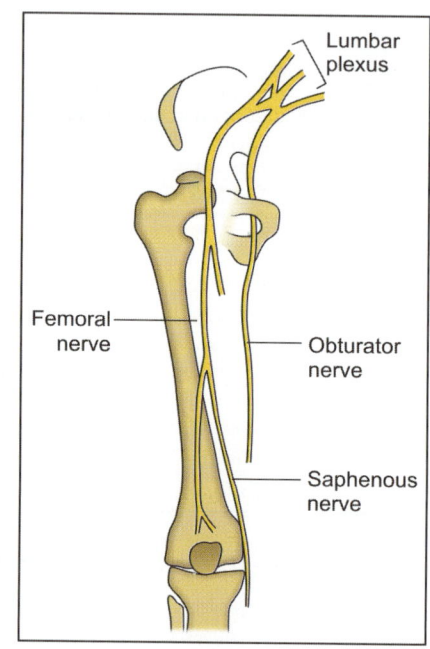

**Fig. 12.11a:** Femoral and obturator nerves

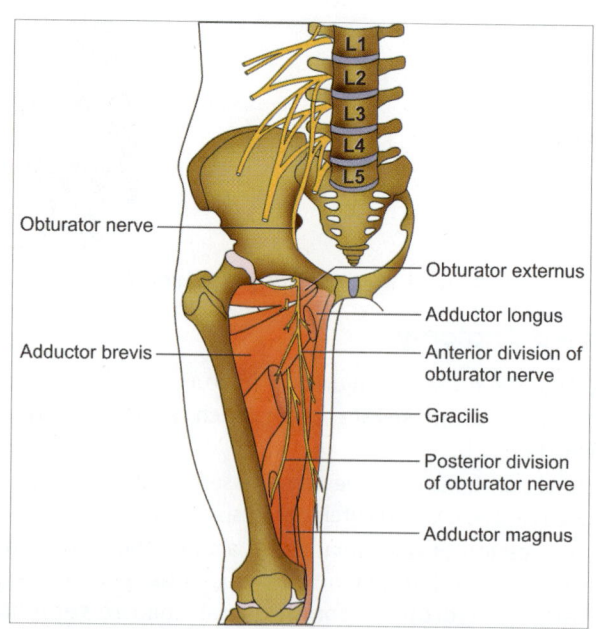

**Fig. 12.11b:** Obturator nerve

### Branches and Distribution

1. The anterior division supplies gracilis, adductor longus, adductor brevis and pectineus muscles.
2. The posterior division supplies obturator externus and part of the adductor magnus muscle. It terminates by supplying the knee joint.

## Sacral Plexus

Sacral plexus is formed by the ventral rami of last two lumbar nerves ($L_4$ and $L_5$) and upper four sacral nerves ($S_{1, 2, 3}$ and $S_4$).

The contribution from $L_4$ and $L_5$ is given by a common nerve trunk called 'lumbosacral trunk'.

Following are the branches of sacral plexus:

1. Sciatic nerve
2. Posterior cutaneous nerve of the thigh
3. Superior gluteal nerve
4. Inferior gluteal nerve
5. Nerve to piriformis
6. Perforating cutaneous nerves
7. Nerve to quadratus femoris
8. Nerve to obturator internus
9. Pudendal nerve
10. Pelvic splanchnic nerves
11. Muscular branches to levator ani, coccygeus and external anal sphincter

Most of these nerves leave the pelvic cavity and enters the gluteal region through the greater sciatic foramen.

## SCIATIC NERVE

It is the thickest nerve of the body, about 2 cm broad and supplies majority of the muscles of lower limb through its branches (Fig. 12.12).

*Origin:* It arises form the sacral plexus and it has tibial and peroneal components.

a. Tibial component is derived from ventral divisions of ventral rami of $L_4$, $L_5$, $S_1$, $S_2$ and $S_3$ nerves.
b. Peroneal component is derived from dorsal divisions of ventral rami of $L_4$, $L_5$, $S_1$ and $S_2$ nerves.

### Course

1. From the pelvis, the sciatic nerve enters the gluteal region through the greater sciatic foramen below the piriformis muscle.
2. In the gluteal region it passes deep to the gluteus maximus, mid-way between greater trochanter of the femur and the ischial tuberosity.
3. In the back of the thigh the nerve lies on adductor magnus muscle and is crossed superficially by the long head of the biceps femoris muscle.

4. Sciatic nerve terminates in the superior angle of the popliteal fossa by dividing into tibial and common peroneal nerves.

### Branches and Distribution

1. Muscular branches supply all the hamstring muscles: Semimembranosus, semitendinosus, long head of biceps femoris and adductor magnus (partly).

    These branches are derived from tibial component. The short head of the biceps femoris is supplied by the peroneal component of the sciatic nerve.
2. Articular branches to the hip joint.

## Applied Anatomy

1. Injury to the sciatic nerve as in dislocation or fracture of the hip, causes paralysis of all the muscles below the knee (with foot drop).
2. Stretching of the sciatic nerve or its compression after sitting for a long time, may give rise to 'sleeping foot'.
3. Sciatica—shooting pain over the back of the thigh, lateral side of the leg and dorsum of the foot. This occurs mainly due to compression of nerve roots forming sciatic nerve. The compression can be due to lumbar disc prolapse or osteoarthritis.
4. The disc prolapsed between $L_4$ and $L_5$ vertebrae involves $L_5$ nerve which is manifested by numbness in the medial 3 toes and difficulty in dorsiflexion. The disc prolapsed between $L_5$ and $S_1$ vertebrae involves $S_1$ nerve which is manifested by numbness in the lateral border of the foot and difficulty in plantar flexion.

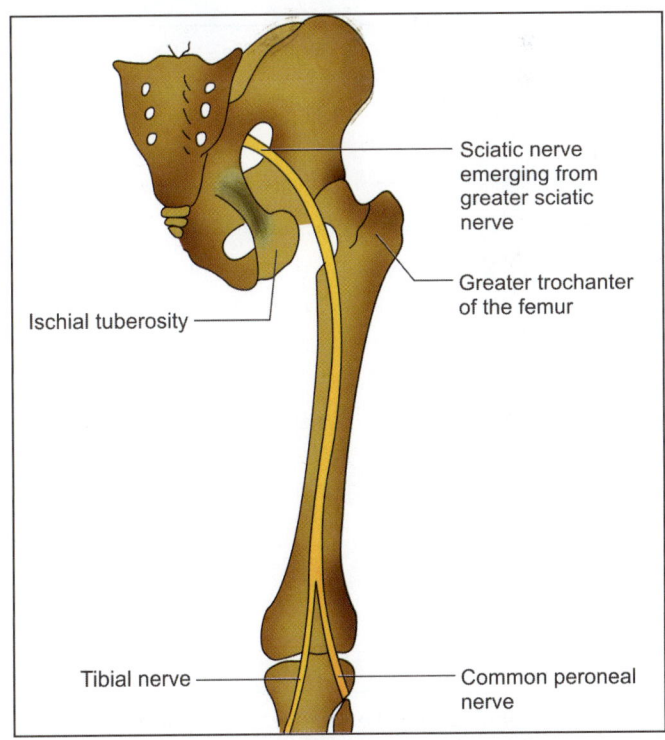

**Fig. 12.12:** Sciatic nerve—schematic

## Tibial Nerve (L$_{4, 5}$, S$_{1, 2}$ and S$_3$)

- It is the terminal branch of the sciatic nerve arising at the superior angle of the popliteal fossa.
- The never descends in the popliteal fossa and enters the back of the leg.
- In the leg it descends deep to gastrocnemius and soleus muscle.
- It enters the sole by passing deep to the flexor retinaculum of the ankle.

  It terminates in the sole by dividing into medial and lateral plantar nerves.

### Distribution

1. Muscular branches

   In the popliteal fossa to gastrocnemius, soleus, plantaris and popliteus

   In the back of the leg-tibialis posterior, flexor digitorum longus and flexor hallucis longus.

   The terminal branches (medial and lateral plantar nerves) of tibial nerve supply all the muscles of the sole.
2. Cutaneous branch called 'sural nerve', is given in the popliteal fossa. It supplies skin of the lower part of the back of the leg and lateral border of the foot.
3. Articular branches supply knee and other distal joints.

Injury to the tibial nerve is rare due to its safe position. However injury to the tibial nerve results in dorsiflexion of the ankle joint and inversion at the subtalar joint. This deformity is referred as 'talipes calcaneovalgus'. There will also be a sensory loss in sural area and heel.

## Common Peroneal Nerve (L$_{4, 5}$, S$_{1, 2}$)

- It is the terminal branch of the sciatic nerve arising at the superior angle of the popliteal fossa.
- The nerve descends obliquely along the tendon of the biceps femoris muscle.
- **It winds around the neck of fibula** and enters the substance of peroneus longus muscle.
- Within the peroneus longus muscle the nerve terminates by dividing into superficial and deep peroneal nerves (Fig. 12.13a).

## Superficial Peroneal Nerve

It descends between peroneus longus and brevis muscles in the lateral compartment of the leg. The nerve becomes superficial and descend superficial to the extensor retinaculum of the ankle and terminates on the dorsum of the foot (Fig. 12.13b).

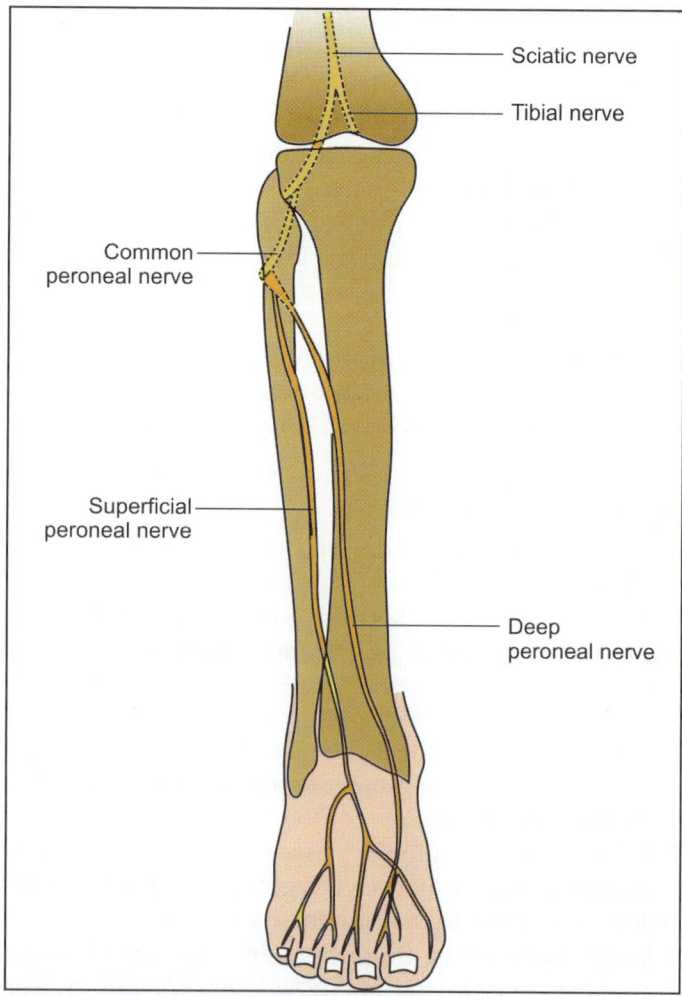

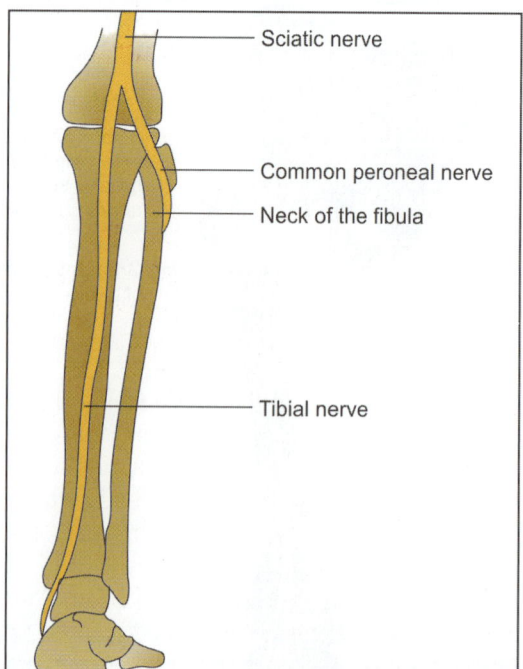

**Fig. 12.13a:** Common peroneal nerve winding around the neck of the fibula

**Fig. 12.13b:** Superficial and deep peroneal nerve

12

## Deep Peroneal Nerve

It appears in the anterior compartment of the leg after piercing the anterior intermuscular septum. It enters the dorsum of the foot deep to the extensor retinaculum of the ankle. At the dorsum of the foot, it divides into medial and lateral terminal branches. The lateral terminal branch passes laterally deep to extensor digitorum brevis and ends in pseudoganglion (Fig. 12.13).

### Branches and Distribution

### I. Common peroneal nerve
- Two cutaneous branches—sural communicating nerve and lateral cutaneous nerve of leg (calf).
- Genicular branches supplying the knee joint.

### II. Superficial peroneal nerve
- Muscular branches to peroneus longus and brevis.
- Cutaneous branches supply dorsum of the foot and digits except the area supplied by saphenous, sural and deep peroneal nerves.

### III. Deep peroneal nerve
- Muscular branches to muscles of the anterior compartment of the leg-tibialis anterior, extensor hallucis longus, extensor digitorum longus, peroneus tertius, and extensor digitorum brevis (on the dorsum of the foot).
- Cutaneous branch supplies adjacent sides of the first and second toes
- Articular branches supply ankle joint, and other distal joints.

## Applied Anatomy

**Injury to the common peroneal nerve:** It is more vulnerable to injury compared to the tibial nerve as it lies superficial against the head of the fibula before winding around the neck of the fibula. A tight plaster cast can also compress the common peroneal nerve.

*Motor manifestation:* Injury to the common peroneal nerve results in paralysis of dorsiflexors of the ankle joint (muscles of the anterior compartment through its deep peroneal nerve) and evertors of the foot (peroneus longus and brevis through superficial peroneal nerve). This results in **foot drop**. In this deformity the foot is inverted and plantar flexed. This deformity is referred as **talipes equinovarus** and the patient walks on toes.

*Sensory loss:* The sensory manifestation depends on site of nerve injury. The common site of nerve injury is at the level of the neck of the fibula. Hence lateral cutaneous nerve of the leg and peroneal communicating nerves are spared. There will be a sensory loss on most of the dorsum of the foot except at the medial border up to the ball of the great toes (saphenous nerve), lateral border of the foot (sural branch of the tibial nerve).

**Deep peroneal nerve entrapment:** Injury or compression of the deep peroneal nerve results from anterior compartment syndrome. It is common in runners and dancers. Excessive use of the anterior compartment muscles results in swelling of the muscle which interferes with venous return causing edema in the anterior compartment. The pressure is released by an incision to the deep fascia along the whole length of the anterior compartment.

*Motor manifestation:* The muscles of the anterior compartment are paralyzed with disability to dorsiflex at the ankle joint. This results in foot drop. The patient walks on tips of the toes on the affected side.

*Sensory manifestation:* Loss of cutaneous sensation in the first interdigital cleft.

**Superficial peroneal nerve entrapment:** It can occur in chronic ankle sprain.

*Motor manifestation:* It results in weakness in eversion of the foot.

*Sensory manifestation:* It involves the lower part of the anterior aspect of the leg, major portion of the dorsum of the foot except for saphenous and sural areas.

**Disc prolapsed and nerve injury of the lower limb:** The major part of the lower limb is supplied by sciatic nerve with its terminal branches—tibial and common peroneal branches.

Sciatic nerve is a composite of $L_4$, $L_5$, $S_1$, $S_2$ and $S_3$ spinal nerves. A herniated intervertebral disc (disc prolapsed) can involve some of these nerve roots and have manifestation in the lower limb. The disc prolapsed is common in lower lumbar region. A disc prolapsed between $L_4$ and $L_5$ vertebrae can compress 5th lumbar spinal nerve. Similarly a disc prolapsed between $L_5$ and $S_1$ vertebrae can compress 1st sacral spinal nerve (Fig. 12.14).

Remember the intervertebral foramen between $L_4$ and $L_5$ vertebra allow the passage of $L_4$ spinal nerve and the intervertebral foramen between $L_5$ and $S_1$ vertebrae allow the passage of $L_5$ spinal nerve. The nerve emerging between the vertebrae and the nerve likely to be injured is different. This is because the vertical length of the intervertebral foramen in the lumbar region increases lower down, hence the $L_4$ and $L_5$ nerves pass through the upper part of the intervertebral foramen and escapes from injury.

The 2 nerve roots commonly involved in disc prolapsed and their clinical manifestations are explained in Table 12.1. This knowledge is important is assessing the nerve roots involved in disc prolapsed.

**Table 12.1:** Disc prolapsed and their clinical manifestations

| | |
|---|---|
| A herniated disc between $L_4$ and $L_5$ would compress 5th lumbar spinal nerve root | A herniated disc between $L_5$ and $S_1$ would compress 1st sacral spinal nerve root |
| Pain over the hip, lateral part of the thigh and leg | Pain over the hip, posterolateral part of the thigh and leg to heel |
| Numbness in the medial 3 toes | Numbness in the posterior part of the calf and lateral border of the heel |
| Difficulty in dorsiflexion at the ankle, difficulty in walking on heel and foot drop may occur | Difficulty in plantar flexion at the ankle, difficulty in walking on toes |
| Muscular atrophy is minor | Muscular atrophy of gastrocnemius and soleus and ankle jerk diminished or absent |

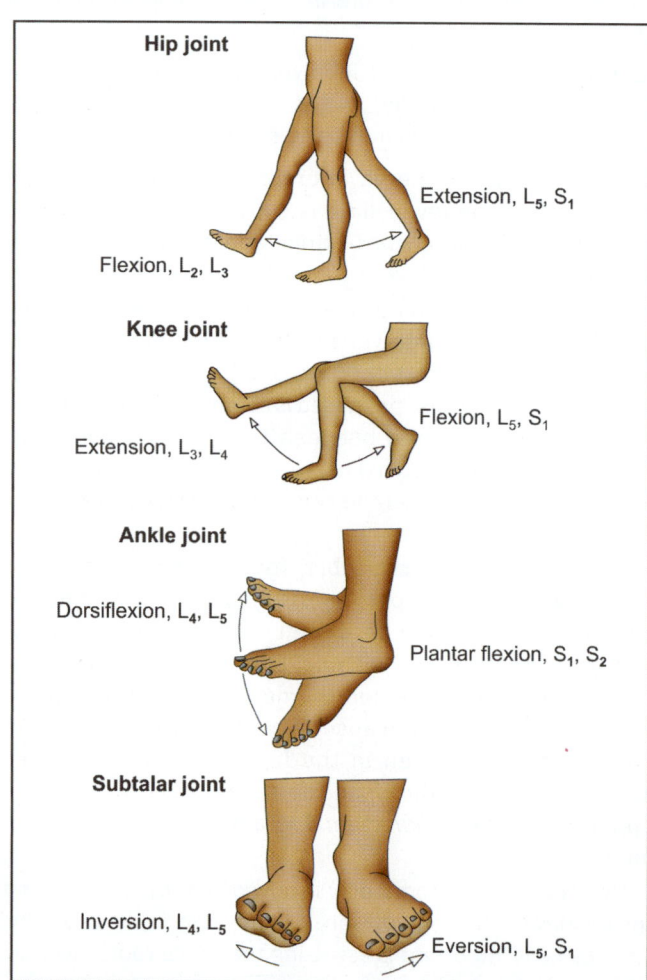

**Fig. 12.14:** Lower limb joint movement and neuronal control

## ARTERIES OF THE UPPER LIMB

### Axillary Artery

- It is the continuation of the subclavian artery and is present in the axilla.
- It extends from the outer border of the first rib to the lower border of the teres major muscle and it has been divided into three parts by pectoralis minor muscle.
- It gives the following branches (Fig. 12.11).
  - i. Superior thoracic artery
  - ii. Lateral thoracic artery
  - iii. Acromiothoracic artery
  - iv. Subscapular artery—it gives circumflex scapular branch
  - v. Anterior circumflex humeral artery
  - vi. Posterior circumflex humeral artery—these circumflex humeral arteries anastomose around the surgical neck of the humerus.

### Brachial Artery

- Brachial artery is the continuation of the axillary artery, and is present in the arm.
- It extends from the lower border of the teres major muscle up to the neck of the radius in the cubital fossa where it divides into radial and ulnar arteries.
- The brachial artery gives many named and unnamed branches (Fig. 12.15). The important branches include.
  1. Profunda brachii artery, which accompanies the radial nerve in the back of the humerus.
  2. Superior and inferior ulnar collateral arteries.

### Applied Anatomy

- Arterial pulsations are felt or ausculated in front of the elbow just medial to the tendon of the biceps while recording the blood pressure.
- Compression of the brachial artery is possible with tight plaster cast or tourniquet to the arm. Injury to the artery is also possible in supracondylar fracture of the humerus, where the proximal fractured segment of the bone is displaced anteriorly and can compressing or injuring the brachial artery. Compression of the brachial artery reduces the blood flow to the forearm and the hand. It is clinically manifested by 5 Ps (**p**allor, **p**ain, **p**uffiness, **p**ulselessness and eventually **p**aralysis of muscle). Impaired blood supply to the muscle for a prolonged period leads to necrosis and fibrosis of the muscle, which leads to Volkman's ischemic contracture, in which there is flexion contracture of the metacarpophalangeal and interphalangeal joints.

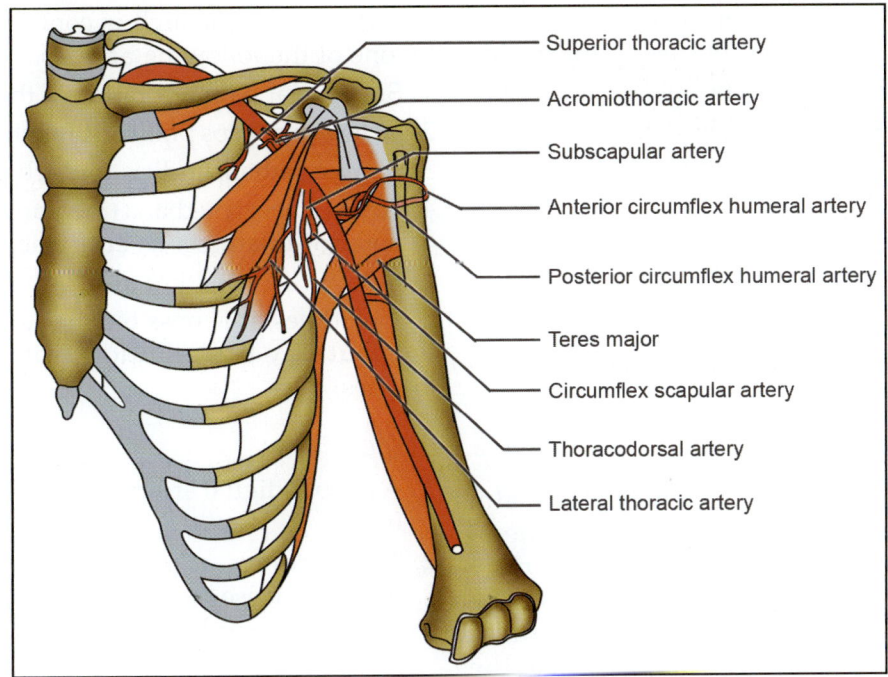

**Fig. 12.15:** Axillary and brachial arteries

- Superior thoracic artery
- Acromiothoracic artery
- Subscapular artery
- Anterior circumflex humeral artery
- Posterior circumflex humeral artery
- Teres major
- Circumflex scapular artery
- Thoracodorsal artery
- Lateral thoracic artery

## Radial Artery

- It is one of the terminal branches of the brachial artery given at the neck of the radius in the cubital fossa.
- It descends superficially in the forearm along the lateral border. It leaves the forearm by turning posteriorly to enter the anatomical snuffbox.
- The terminal part of the radial artery appears in the hand where it forms deep palmar arch (Fig. 12.16).
- The radial artery gives radial recurrent, muscular, palmar carpal, dorsal carpal and superficial palmar branches, arteria princeps pollicis and arterial radialis indicis.

*Radial pulse:* It is felt against the anterior surface of the lower end of the radius, lateral to the tendon of the flexor carpi radialis muscle.

Being most superficial the artery is punctured for blood gas analysis and also used for coronary angiogram procedures where special catheter is introduced through this artery.

## Ulnar Artery

- It is the larger terminal branch of brachial artery in the cubital fossa (i.e. at the neck of radius).
- It descends deep to the muscles of the forearm. It enters the palm, superficial to the flexor retinaculum along with the ulnar nerve. In the palm, the ulnar artery divides into superficial and deep branches.

- The ulnar artery gives anterior and posterior ulnar recurrent branches, common interosseous artery (which gives anterior and posterior interosseous arteries).
- The superficial branch continues to form **superficial palmar arch**, which is joined on the lateral side by branches of the radial artery.

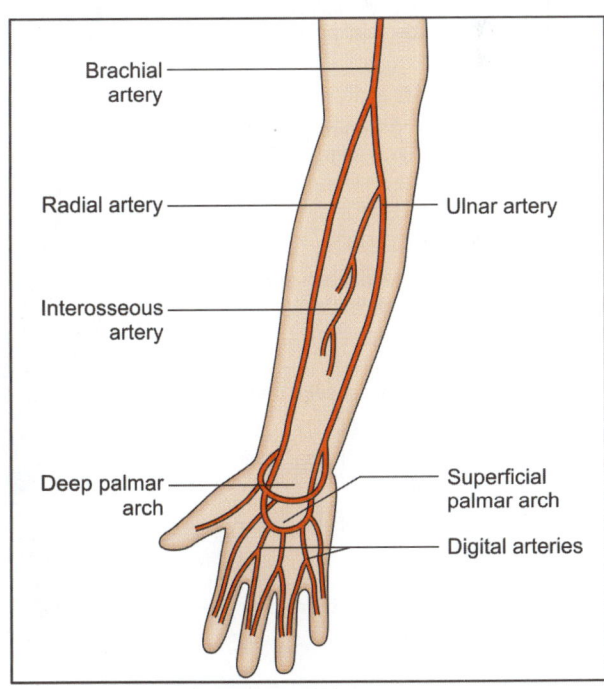

- Brachial artery
- Radial artery
- Ulnar artery
- Interosseous artery
- Deep palmar arch
- Superficial palmar arch
- Digital arteries

**Fig. 12.16:** Radial and ulnar arteries

- The deep branch of ulnar artery joins the terminal part of the radial artery to form the **deep palmar arch**.
- Hence the two terminal branches of brachial artery anastomose with each other and help in collateral circulation in case of any thrombosis of any one of the arteries (Fig. 12.16).

### Superficial Palmar Arch

It is an arterial arch present on the superficial aspect of the palm.

*Relations:* It is present superficial to long flexor tendons and deep to the palmar aponeurosis.

### Formation

*On medial side:* The ulnar artery enters the palm superficial to the flexor retinaculum on the lateral side of the pisiform bone. Immediately the artery divides into superficial and deep branches. The superficial branch is the direct continuation of ulnar artery, which continues laterally to form the superficial palmar arch (contributing the arch on its medial 2/3rd).

*On lateral side:* The arch is contributed (lateral 1/3rd) by one of the following arteries:
1. Superficial palmar branch of the radial artery.
2. Arteria princeps pollicis (branch of the radial artery).
3. Arteria radialis indicis (branch of the radial artery).
4. Arterial nervi mediana (median artery—branch from anterior interosseous artery accompanying median nerve).

Sometimes, it is possible that the arch is incomplete without any contribution from above mentioned arteries.

### Branches

1. A proper digital artery to the medial side of the little finger.
2. Three common palmar digital arteries: These branches arise from the convexity of the arch and proceed towards the second, third and the fourth web spaces where they divide into proper digital branches to the adjacent fingers.
3. Recurrent branch to palmar carpal arch.

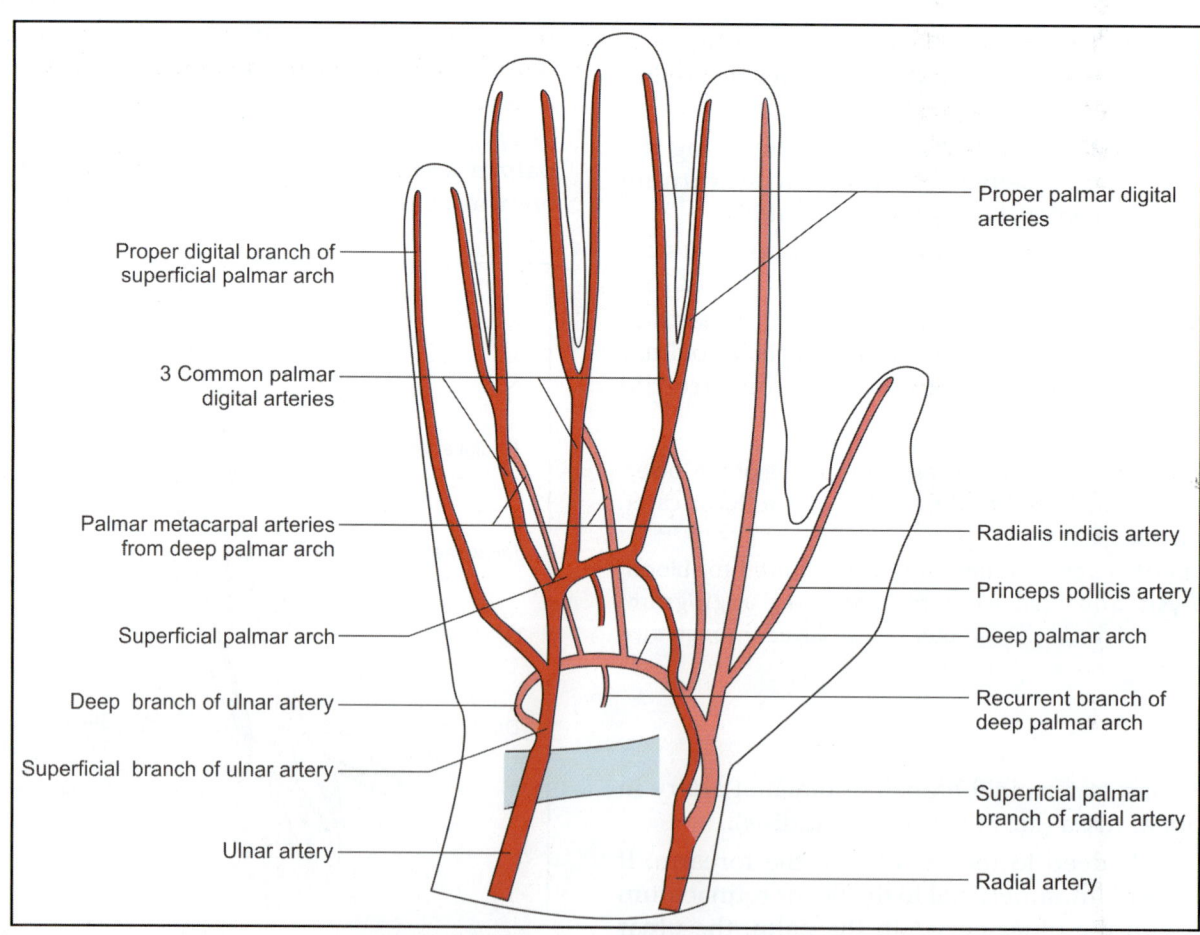

**Fig. 12.17:** Palmar arches

All these branches receives blood from palmar metacarpal arteries which are branches of deep palmar arch near the web space. In this way the superficial palmar arch is also connected with the deep palmar arch.

The superficial palmar arch does not supplies thumb and radial side of the index finger.

## Deep Palmar Arch

It is an arterial arch present deep to the long flexor tendons of the palm and proximal to the level of superficial palmar arch.

### *Formation*

*On the lateral side:* The radial artery after traversing the anatomical snuff box, enters the hand between the two heads of the first dorsal interossei muscle. It lies between the oblique and transverse head of the adductor pollicis muscle, where it continues to form deep palmar arch (contribution on the lateral 2/3rd).

*On the medial side:* The deep branch of the ulnar artery accompanied by the deep branch of the ulnar nerve passes between the abductor and flexor digiti minimi and then turns laterally below the hook of the hamate to join the radial artery to complete the deep palmar arch (*see* Fig.10.17d).

### *Branches*

1. Three palmar metacarpal arteries which join the common palmar metacarpal arteries of the superficial palmar arch.
2. Three perforating branches pass backwards through 2nd to 4th interosseous space to anastomose with the dorsal metacarpal arteries.
3. Recurrent branch proceed backwards and take part in formation of palmar carpal arch.

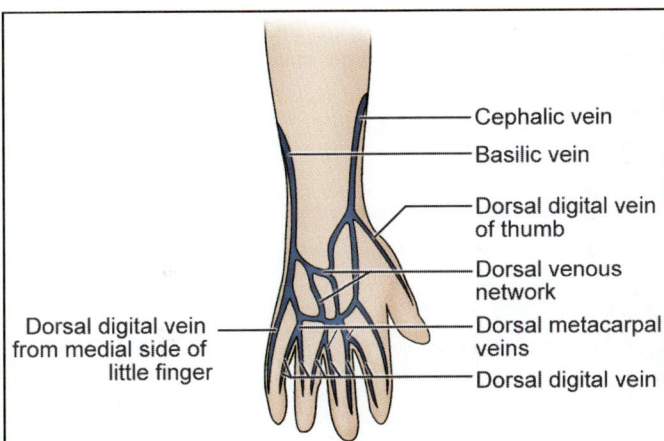

**Fig. 12.18a:** Dorsal venous arch

## VEINS OF THE UPPER LIMB

**Dorsal venous arch:** It is an irregular network of veins on the dorsum of the hand.

**Cephalic vein:** It begins from the lateral end of the dorsal venous arch. It ascends superficial to the anatomical snuffbox and then along the lateral border of the forearm. The cephalic vein ascends superficially in the arm to join the axillary vein. At the elbow, the greater part of the blood from the cephalic vein is drained into the basilic vein through the median cubital vein (Fig. 12.18a).

## Basilic Vein

It begins from the medial end of the dorsal venous arch. It ascends in the forearm in the superficial fascia and pierces the deep fascia in the middle of the arm. It continues as the axillary vein at the lower border of the teres major muscle.

## Median Cubital Vein

- It is a large communicating vein between cephalic and the basilic vein.
- It begins from the cephalic vein below the elbow and ends in the basilic vein (Fig. 12.18b and c).

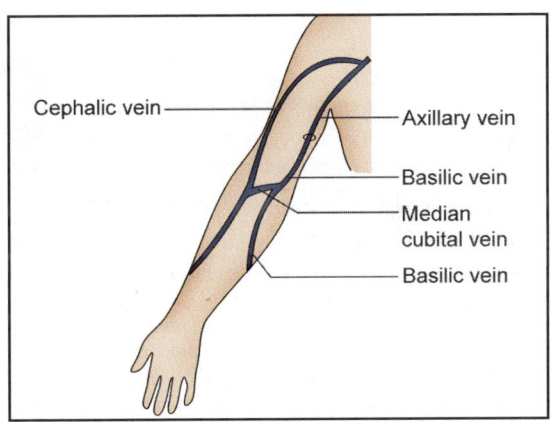

**Fig. 12.18b:** Median cubital vein

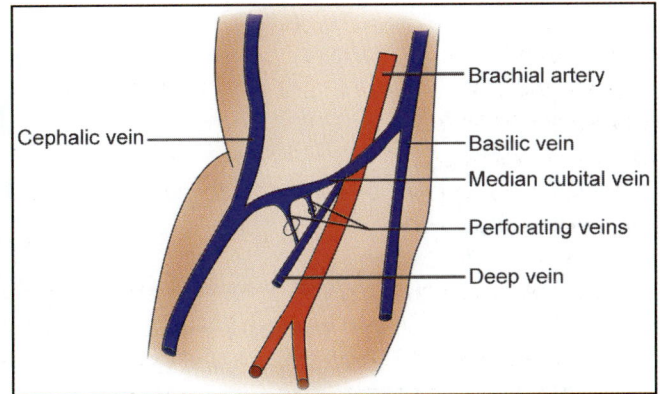

**Fig. 12.18c:** Perforating veins of median cubital vein

12

- It receives tributaries from the front of the forearm.
- From its under surface few perforating vein perforates bicipital aponeurosis to join veins accompanying brachial artery. This makes the median cubital vein more fixed and hence often used for intravenous injections.
- The median cubital vein is separated from deeply placed brachial artery by bicipital aponeurosis.

## BLOOD VESSELS OF THE LOWER LIMB

### ARTERIES OF THE LOWER LIMB

### Femoral Artery

- It is the chief artery of the lower limb.
- Femoral artery is the continuation of the external iliac artery. It enters the thigh from behind the midinguinal point superficial to the tendon of psoas major muscle (Fig. 12.19a).
- It descends from base to apex of the femoral triangle and then enters adductor canal. Finally it emerges from the adductor canal by passing through hiatus magnus (last opening in the adductor magnus muscle) to enter the popliteal fossa.
- Femoral artery gives three superficial and three deep branches. The superficial branches are:
  - i. Superficial epigastric artery
  - ii. Superficial circumflex iliac artery
  - iii. Superficial external pudendal artery.

  The deep branches include:
  - i. Profunda femoris artery
  - ii. Deep external pudendal artery
  - iii. Muscular branches

### Profunda Femoris Artery

It is the largest branch of the femoral artery, which gives medial and lateral circumflex femoral arteries. They form an anastamosing circle around the neck of the femur. The perforating branches of the profunda femoris artery pass through openings present in the adductor magnus muscle to enter the posterior compartment.

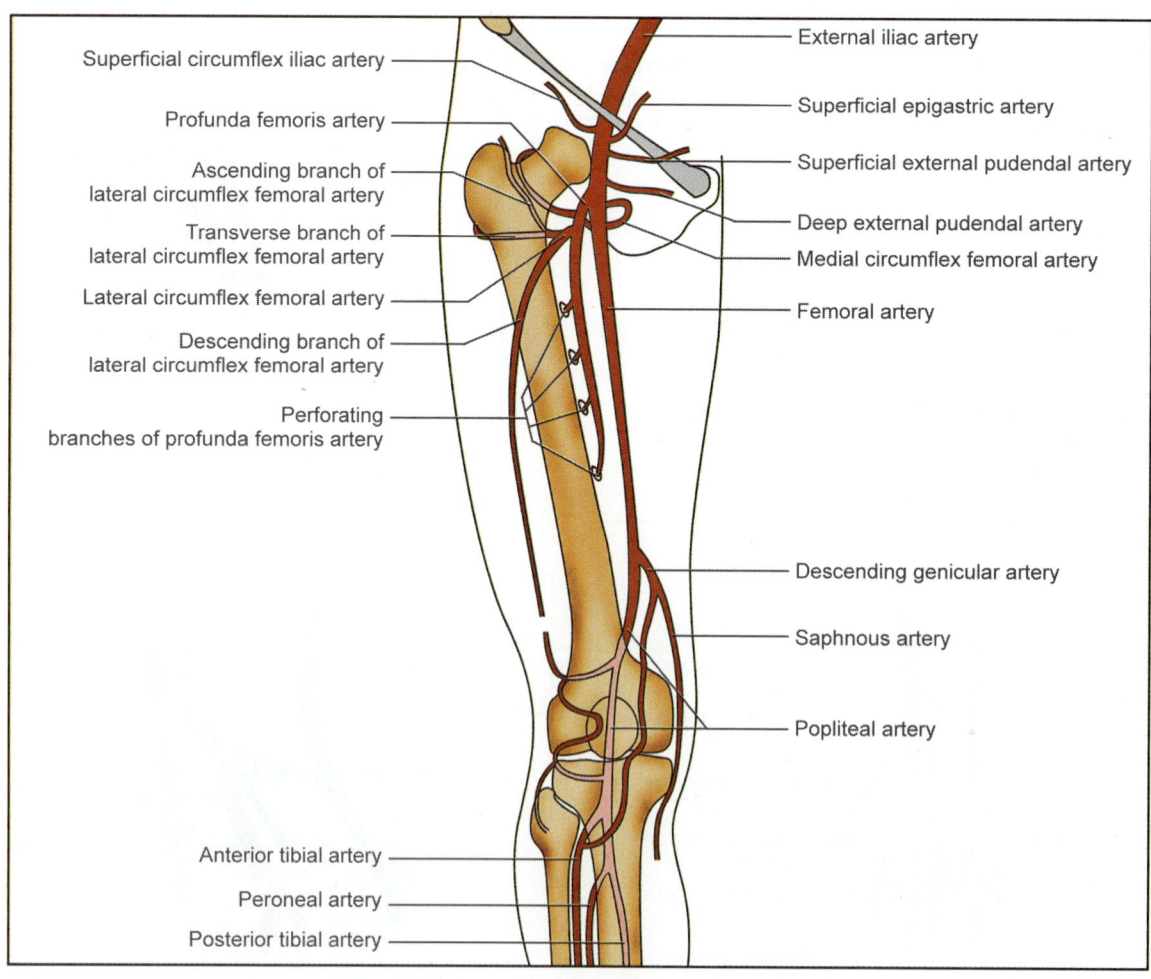

Fig. 12.19a: Femoral artery and its branches

*Femoral pulse:* The pulsation of the femoral artery is felt at the midinguinal point (mid-point between the anterior superior iliac spine and the pubic symphysis) where the artery is against the tendon of psoas major muscle.

Femoral artery is superficial in position in the upper part of the thigh and often selected for various procedures like angiographic studies (by injecting radiopaque dye through a catheter inserted to femoral artery) of abdominal, lower limb arteries and even coronary arteries.

*Popliteal pulse:* Among the arteries of the lower limb, it is difficult to feel the pulse of the popliteal artery as it is the deepest content of the fossa. However, the pulse can be felt when the knee is flexed and the finger tips of both hands are placed in the fossa firmly with the thumbs resting on the patella.

Popliteal aneurysm can compress the popliteal vein which results in edema of the leg. The aneurysm presents as a midline swelling in the fossa with prominent pulse.

## Popliteal Artery

- This is the continuation of femoral artery present in the popliteal fossa.
- It is about 20 cm in length and deepest structure in the fossa present close to the knee joint.
- It is accompanied by popliteal vein and tibial nerve.
- It terminates at the lower border of the popliteus muscle by dividing into anterior and posterior tibial arteries.
- Popliteal artery gives many muscular and genicular branches (to knee joint) (Fig. 12.19b).

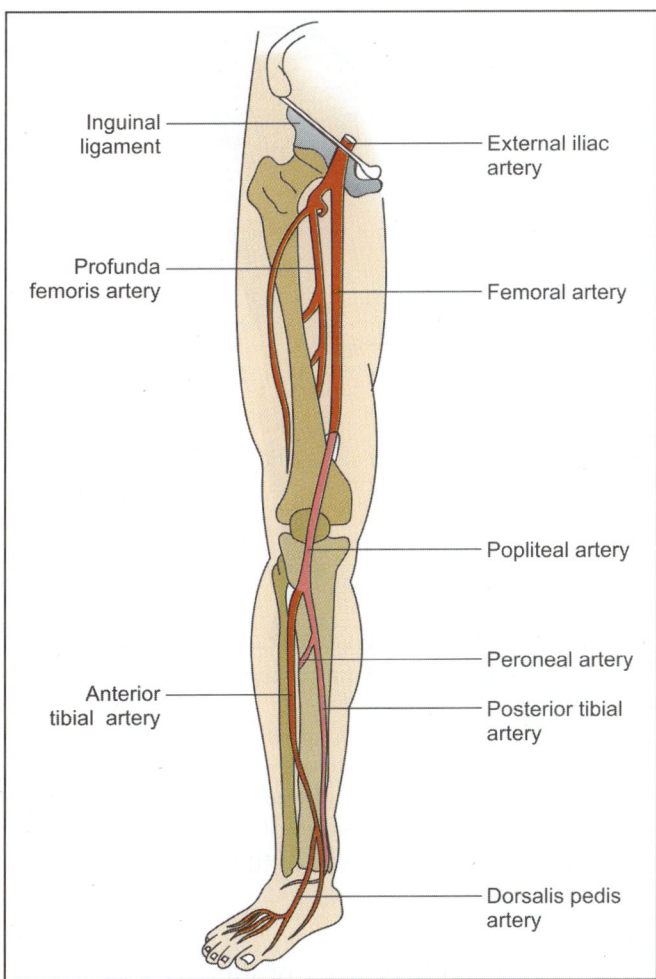

**Fig. 12.19b:** Arteries of the lower limb

*(labels: Inguinal ligament; External iliac artery; Profunda femoris artery; Femoral artery; Popliteal artery; Peroneal artery; Anterior tibial artery; Posterior tibial artery; Dorsalis pedis artery)*

## Anterior Tibial Artery

It is one of the terminal branches of the popliteal artery. It descends in the anterior compartment of the leg with deep peroneal nerve.

It continues as the dorsalis pedis artery on the dorsum of the foot (Fig. 12.20a).

## Dorasils Pedis Artery

- It is the main artery present on the dorsum of the foot.
- It terminates in the proximal part of the first interosseous space by dipping downwards into the sole where it completes the plantar arch.
- Dorsalis pedis artery gives many branches including arcuate artery.

The dorsalis pedis artery is superficial and lies on the trasal bones. Hence its pulsation can be felt. The absence of this pulse indicates that the blood supply to the leg is inadequate. Checking the pedal pulse is routine in patients known to have impaired circulation to the legs and after surgery to the leg or groin (Fig. 12.20a and b).

## Posterior Tibial Artery

It is the larger terminal branch of popliteal artery. Begins at the lower border of popliteus and enters the back of leg. It is accompanied by tibial nerve.

The artery terminates deep to flexor retinaculum of the ankle by dividing into a lateral and a medial plantar arteries. The posterior tibial artery gives many branches including peroneal artery.

## Peroneal Artery

It is the largest branch of the posterior tibial artery, which supplies the posterior and lateral compartments of leg.

## Plantar Arch

Formed by the direct continuation of the lateral plantar artery and is completed medially by the dorsalis pedis

12

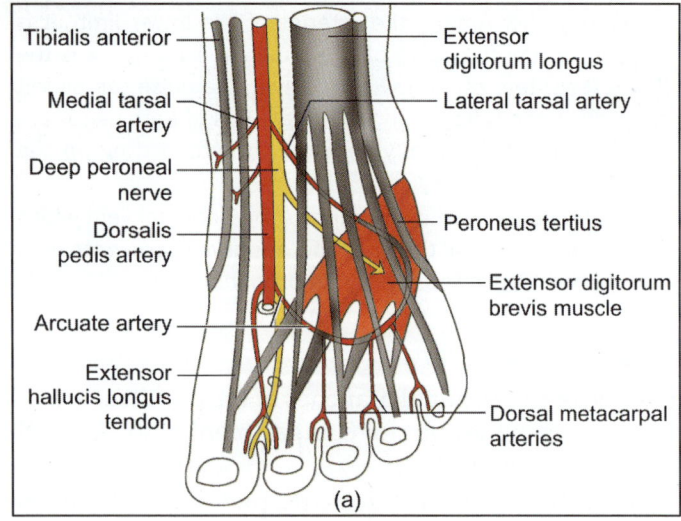

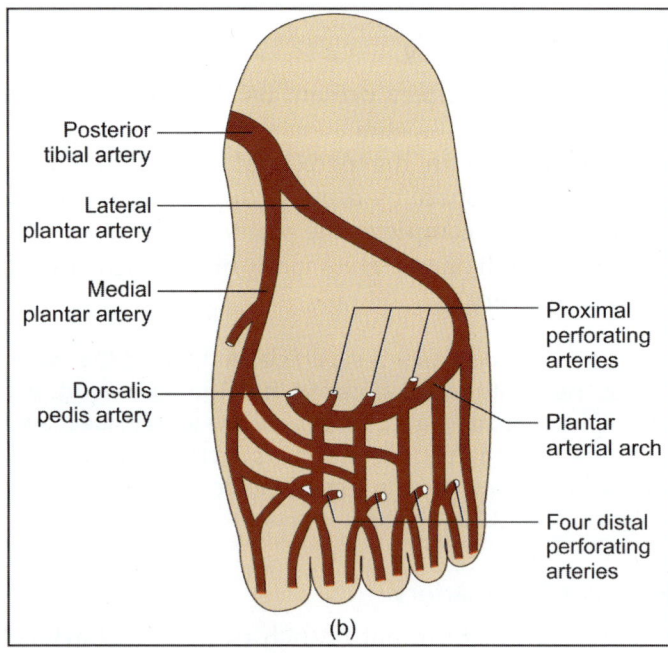

**Fig. 12.20a and b:** (a) Dorsum of the foot and dorsalis pedis artery; (b) arteries of the sole

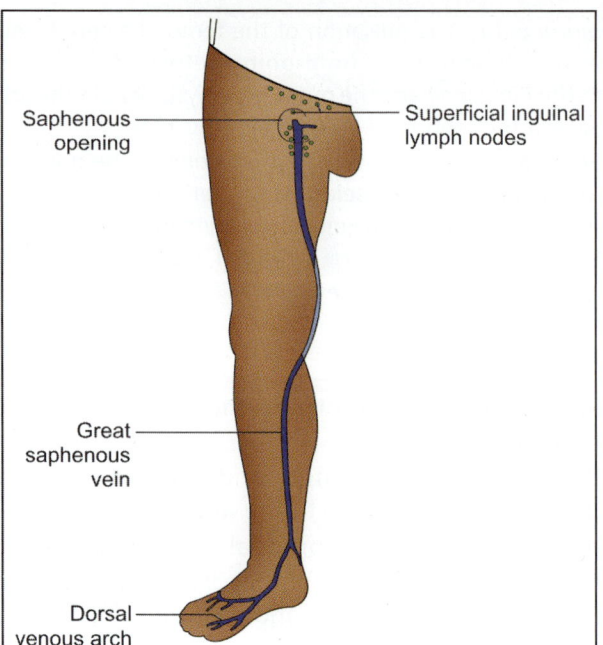

**Fig. 12.21a:** Great saphenous vein

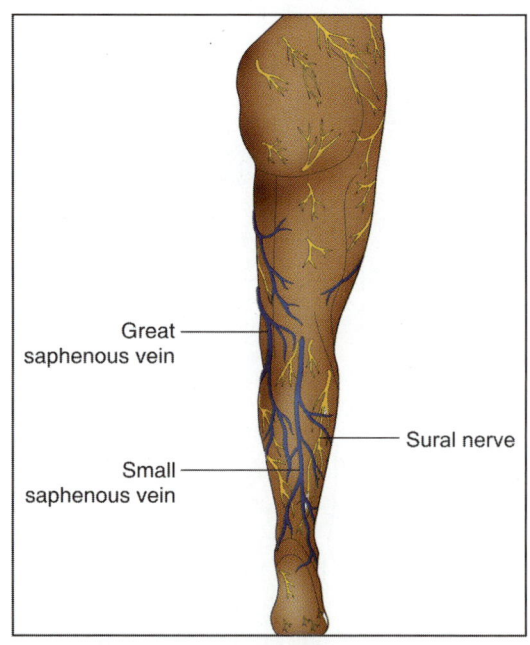

**Fig. 12.21b:** Small saphenous vein

artery. This arch connects the terminal part of the anterior and posterior tibial arteries and helps in collateral circulation.

## VEINS OF THE LOWER LIMB

The veins of the lower limb may be classified into three groups, the superficial, deep and perforating. The superficial veins include great saphaneous and small saphenous veins (Fig. 12.21a and b).

### Great Saphaneous Vein

It is the longest superficial vein in the body.

### Formation

It is formed by the union of medial end of the dorsal venous arch (on the dorsum of the foot) and a vein arising from the medial side of the great toe.

### Course

• The vein ascends in front of the medial malleolus and medial subcutaneous surface of the tibia.

12

- It passes behind the knee and then ascends along the medial side of the thigh.
- It passes through saphenous opening (Fig. 12.21a).

## Termination

It terminates by joining the femoral vein.

The great saphenous vein has many tributaries. Perforating veins connect the great saphenous vein with deeper veins. Blood from this superficial vein passes into the deeper veins. The vein has many valves and incompetence of these valves or thrombosis of the deeper veins causes 'varicose veins'.

## Applied Anatomy

**Venesection:** In case of an emergency, when all the superficial veins are collapsed, venous cut down is performed through great saphenous vein just in front of the medial malleolus. The position of the vein is constant at this site, but care has to be taken to avoid damage to the saphenous nerve.

**Varicose veins:** Varicosity of the superficial veins of the lower limb is common in those who have to work in standing position for long periods. Age related structural changes in the valve are also responsible for varicosity. The varicose veins can cause inflammation of the affected part of the vein with pain, swelling and redness. The stagnation of venous blood causes change in the skin color and leads to ulcers which can bleed.

Incompetence of the valves of the perforating veins or saphenofemoral vein cause varicosity of the great saphenous vein. A Trendelenburg test is performed to test whether valves of the perforating veins or the saphenofemoral valve are incompetent.

**Testing:** The patient is asked to lie down in supine position and the affected leg was raised to empty the blood in it. A tourniquet is applied in the upper part of the thigh to occlude the saphenous vein. The terminal part of the great saphenous vein can also be occluded manually by applying pressure through thumb (3 cm below and lateral to the pubic tubercle). Now the patient is asked to stand up. A slow filling of the great saphenous vein from below without releasing the pressure indicates the incompetency of valves of perforating vein. If the great saphenous vein is filled from above immediately after releasing the pressure at saphenofemoral junction indicates incompetency of saphenofemoral valve.

Great saphenous vein is often selected for coronary bypass surgeries in case of obstruction in coronary arteries. Due to the presence of valves, the vein has to be reversed while placing the graft.

## Small Saphenous Vein

- It begins from the lateral end of the dorsal venous arch.
- It ascends behind the lateral malleolus along with sural nerve.
- It terminates by joining the popliteal vein.

## Deep Veins

Include the veins accompanying the arteries.

## Perforating Veins

They connect the superficial veins with the deep veins. Their valves permit only one way flow of the blood from the superficial to the deep veins.

*Venous pump of the leg:* In standing position the venous return is against the gravity. Though the valves present in the superficial and deep veins allow unidirectional blood flow, the muscle contraction especially the calf muscles help this cause. When the calf muscles contract the deep veins are compressed and the valves open up and the blood is propelled in upward direction. The soleus muscle contains many endothelial lined venous spaces and the contraction of this muscle squeeze the blood in upward direction. Hence soleus is often referred as peripheral heart. All the calf muscles together called 'venous pump'.

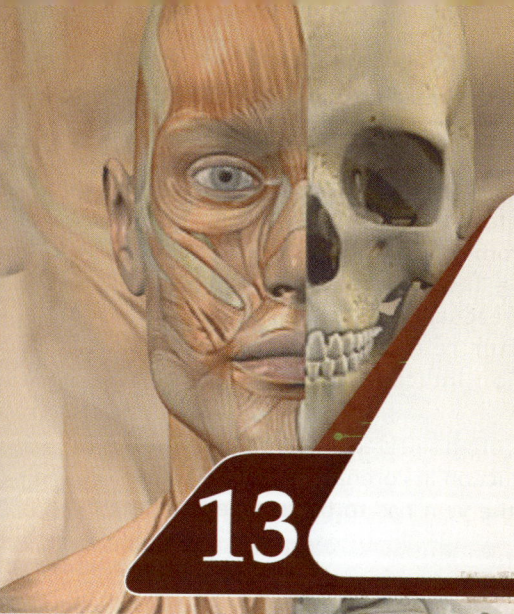

# Axial Skeleton and their Joints

## 13

## VERTEBRAL COLUMN

- It is a skeletal framework that supports the body.
- It transmits its weight to the pelvis and lower extremities.
- It protects the spinal cord and its membranes. The vertebral column extends from the base of the skull to the coccyx. It is made up of 33 vertebrae. Intervertebral discs further increase the length of the column (Fig. 13.1).

  The length of the adult vertebral column is about 70 cm in male and 60 cm in female.

The vertebral column is subdivided into the following parts:

- Cervical part: Consists of 7 vertebrae
- Thoracic part: Consists of 12 vertebrae
- Lumbar part: Consists of 5 vertebrae
- **Sacrum** (formed by the fusion of 5 sacral vertebrae)
- Coccyx (formed by the fusion of 4 coccygeal pieces)

### Typical Vertebra

A typical vertebra consists of two parts—body and vertebral arch.

a. *Body:* It is the anterior part of the vertebra. Its upper and lower surfaces are connected to intervertebral discs.

b. *Vertebral arch:* It consists of a pair of pedicles, a pair of laminae and many processes.

*Pedicle:* On each side it extends backwards from the body. Between the adjacent pedicles is a narrow space called intervertebral foramen through which spinal nerve emerges.

*Laminae:* These are backward extensions of pedicles and they join in the posterior aspect.

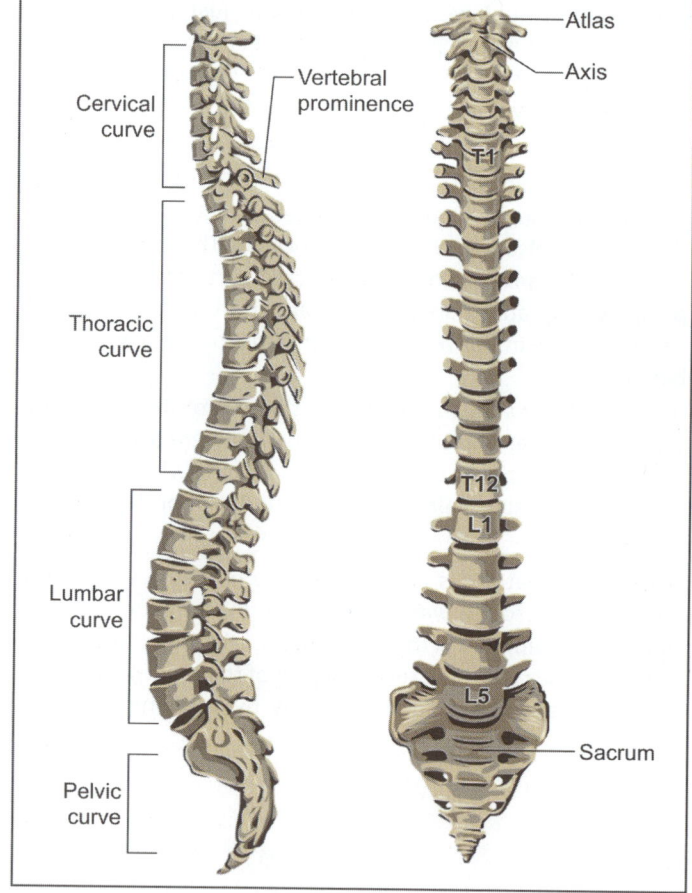

**Fig. 13.1:** Vertebral column—lateral view and anterior view

The body, pedicles and laminae enclose the vertebral foramen.

*Articular processes:* There are four articular processes. A pair of superior articular processes and a pair of inferior articular processes arise at the junction of pedicles and laminae. The superior articular facets articulate with inferior articular facets of the vertebra above. The inferior with superior articular facets of the vertebra below.

*Transverse process:* It projects laterally from the junction of pedicle and lamina.

*Spinous process (spine):* It projects backwards in the midline from the meeting point of laminae.

## Distinguishing Features among Different Regional Vertebrae

1. Cervical vertebrae are identified by the presence of a foramen in their transverse process.
2. Thoracic vertebrae are identified by the presence of facets on their bodies for the ribs.
3. Lumbar vertebrae are larger in size and lack the above said features.

   Cervical, thoracic and lumbar parts of the vertebral column show following movements:

   | Flexion | : | Forward bending |
   |---|---|---|
   | Extension | : | Backward bending |
   | Lateral flexion | : | Side bending |
   | Rotation | : | Twisting of trunk |

## Normal Curvature of the Vertebral Column

The adult vertebral column presents four curvatures when viewed from the side (Fig. 13.1).
1. The cervical curve
2. The thoracic curve
3. The lumbar curve
4. The pelvic curve

The thoracic and pelvic curves are called primary curves because they retain the anterior concave shape of the fetus.

The cervical and lumbar curves are called secondary curves, which appears when the infant learns to sit up and walk. This is anterior convex curvature.

## Applied Anatomy

Clinically there are three major types of abnormal curvatures of vertebral column (Fig. 13.2). These are due to failure of segmentation of vertebrae.

1. **Kyphosis:** It is an accentuated flexion (forward bending) of the thoracic curvature. In cervical and lumbar regions the convexity is reduced. In old age, due to osteoporosis of the vertebrae, poor posture and degeneration of the discs, the forward convexity is reduced in lumbar and cervical region.

2. **Lordosis:** It is an accentuated extension (backward bending) of lumbar spine. Weak trunk muscles, late pregnancy, obesity are the cause for lordosis.

3. **Scoliosis:** It is an accentuated extension (backward bending) of lumbar spine. The causes includes genetic and trauma. It occurs in adolescent girls more than boys. It may be failure in segmentation on the lateral part of the vertebral column.

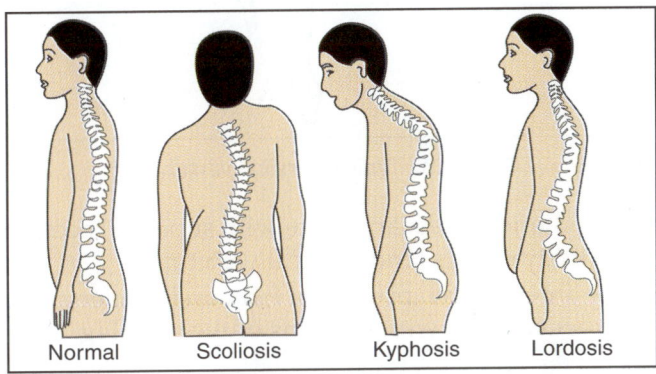

**Fig. 13.2:** Vertebral column deformities

## Cervical Vertebrae

They are 7 in number. The first, second and seventh cervical vertebrae are atypical. The remaining are typical.

The cervical vertebra presents a foramen—(foramen transversarium)—in its transverse process.

The first cervical vertebra is called *atlas.*

The second cervical vertebra is called the *axis.*

### Typical Cervical Vertebra

- The transverse diameter of the body is more than anteroposterior diameter.
- Vertebral foramen is triangular in shape.
- The pedicles are short and directed backwards and laterally.
- Superior articular facets directed upwards and backwards and inferior facet is directed downwards and forwards.
- Transverse process presents an anterior root and tubercle and a posterior root and tubercle and a foramen between them (foramen transversarium). Vertebral vessels pass through them.
- Spinous process is small and a bifid (Fig. 13.3).

### Atlas—First Cervical Vertebra

- It has no body and spinous process.
- It has an anterior and a posterior arch connected to the lateral masses.
- The lateral mass presents a concave superior articular facet for condyles of the occipital bone (of skull).

13

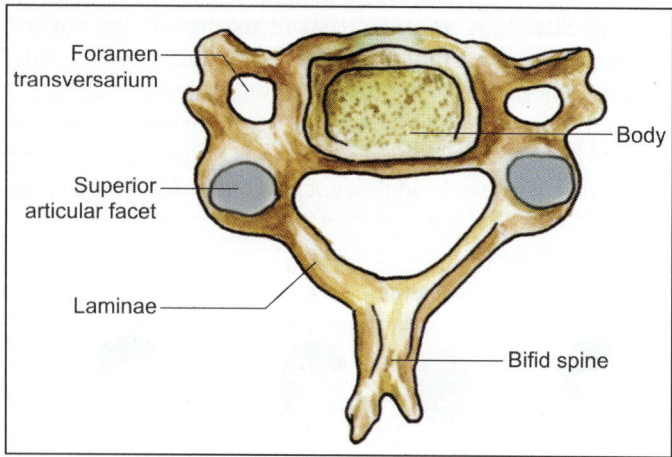

**Fig. 13.3:** Typical cervical vertebra

- The inferior facets articulate with superior facets on the body of axis (2nd cervical vertebra).
- The anterior arch presents a facet on its inner aspect for articulation with the dens of the axis (Fig. 13.4).

### Axis—Second Cervical Vertebra

- The body presents a strong bony projection on the upper part called dens (odontoid process).
- Anterior surface of the dens articulates with anterior arch of the atlas and posterior surface is related to transverse ligament of atlas.
- Transverse process is very small and presents posterior tubercles only.
- Spinous process is short, thick and bifid (Fig. 13.5).

## Thoracic Vertebrae

Thoracic vertebrae are 12 in number of which 2nd to 8th thoracic vertebrae are typical, while 1st and 9th to 12th thoracic vertebrae are atypical (Fig. 13.6a and b).

### Typical Thoracic Vertebra

- The body is heart shaped.
- Vertebral foramen is circular.

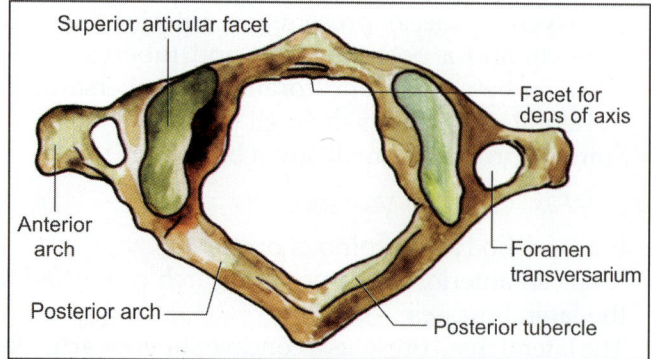

**Fig. 13.4:** Atlas vertebra

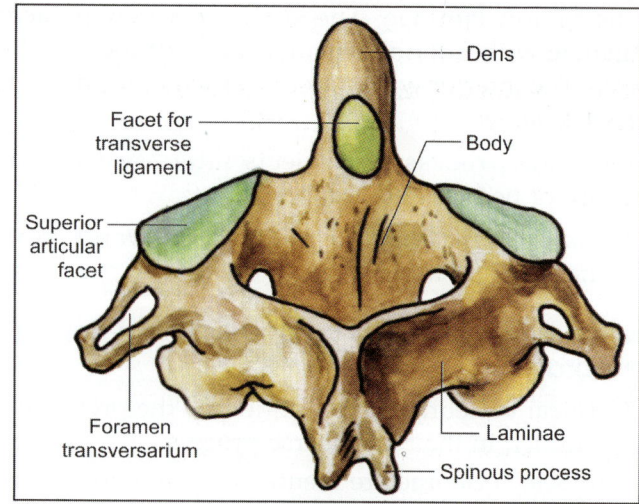

**Fig. 13.5:** Axis vertebra

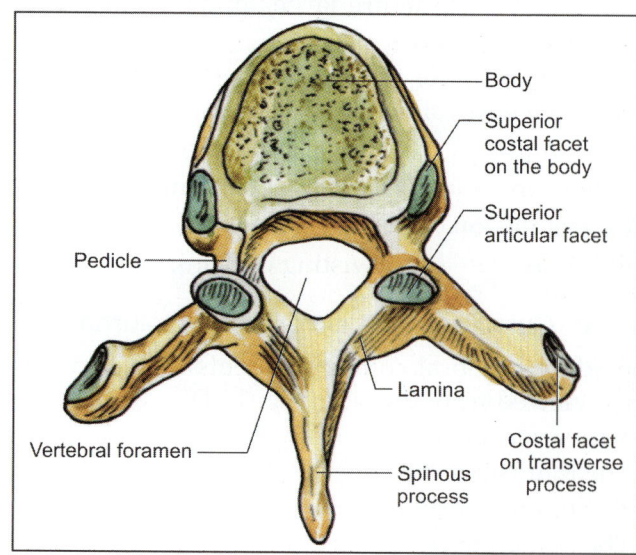

**Fig. 13.6a:** Typical thoracic vertebra (superior view)

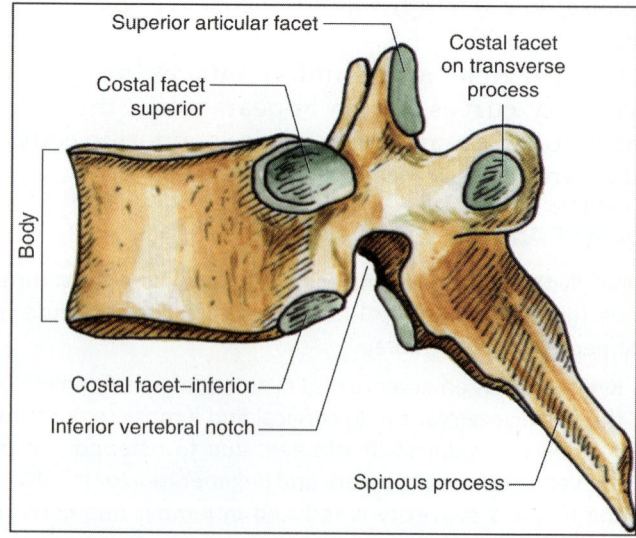

**Fig. 13.6b:** Typical thoracic vertebra (lateral view)

13

- The pedicles arises from the lower part of the body and are directed backwards.
- The superior articular facets are directed backwards and laterally and the inferior downwards and medially.
- Transverse process projects backwards and laterally and presents a facet for articulation with the tubercle of the corresponding rib.
- Spinous process is pointed and directed downwards.
- The body presents two superior costal facets close to the upper border and two small inferior costal facets close to the lower border (posterolaterally).

## Lumbar Vertebrae

There are 5 lumbar vertebrae of which the fifth lumbar vertebra is atypical. Remaining are typical.

### Typical Lumbar Vertebra

- The body is large with its transverse diameter more than anteroposterior diameter.
- The vertebral foramen is triangular.
- Pedicles are short and strong directed backwards.
- The superior articular facet faces medially while inferior articular facet is directed laterally.
- The distance between the superior articular facets is more than the distance between inferior articular facets.
- The spinous process is quadrilateral in shape.
- Accessory process is a rough elevation at the posteroinferior aspect of each transverse process at its root.

- Mamillary process is a rough elevation along the posterior border of superior articular process (Fig. 13.7a and b).

## Sacrum

- The sacrum is a large, flattened, triangular bone formed by the fusion of five sacral vertebrae.
- It forms the posterior wall of the bony pelvis.
- It has a base and an apex. The base articulates with the body of the 5th lumbar vertebra, and the apex with the coccyx.
- The base presents a central portion called **promontory** (anterior border of the body) and two lateral parts called ala .
- The sacrum presents a pelvic and a dorsal surface.
- The pelvic surface presents four pairs of ventral sacral foramina (through which ventral rami of upper 4 sacral nerves and branches of lateral sacral arteries pass).
- The dorsal surface is rough and presents many vertical crests. It also presents four pairs of dorsal sacral foramina for dorsal rami of upper four sacral nerves.
- The sacrum presents sacral canal (part of the vertebral canal) and it opens below at sacral hiatus.
- It has a lateral surface, which is broader above and narrow below. The upper part of the lateral surface presents an articular (auricular) surface, which articulates with the ilium of the hip bone to form the sacroiliac joint.
- The sacral canal is occupied by terminal part of the cauda equina, filum terminale, spinal meninges and blood vessels.

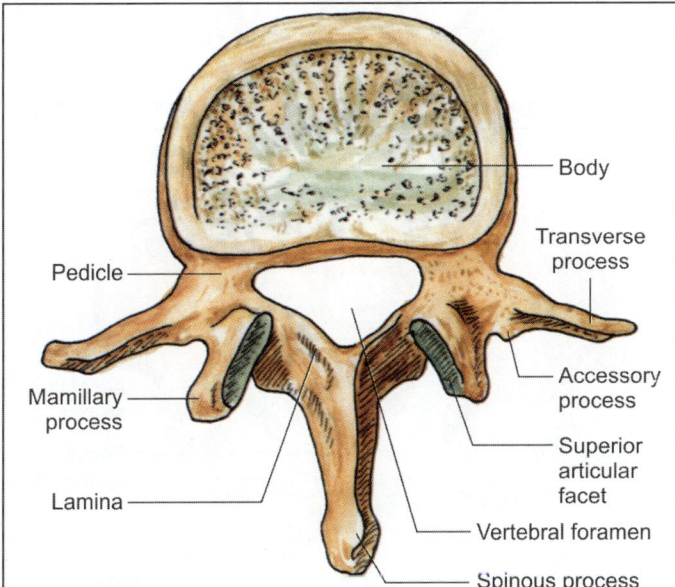

**Fig. 13.7a:** Typical lumbar vertebra (superior view)

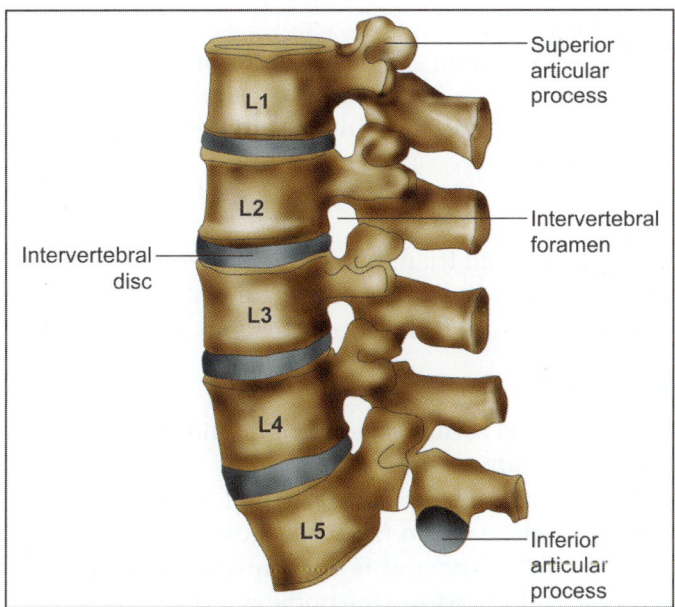

**Fig. 13.7b:** Typical lumbar vertebra (lateral view)

13

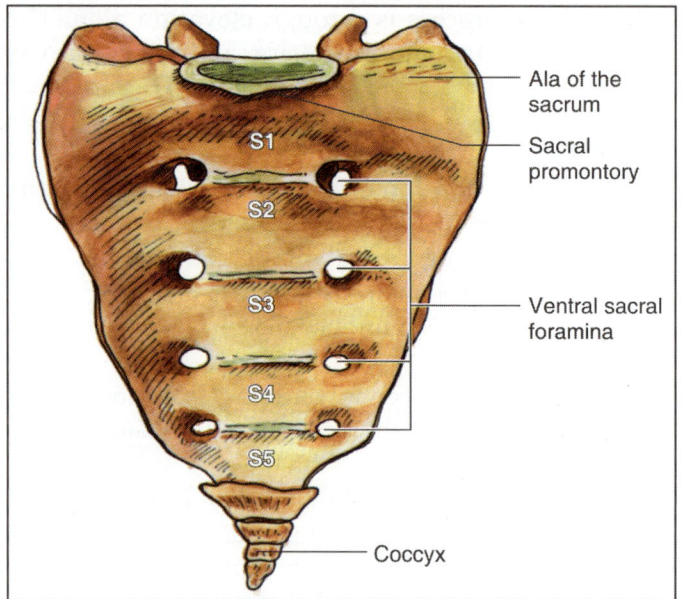

**Fig. 13.8a:** Sacrum—anterior view

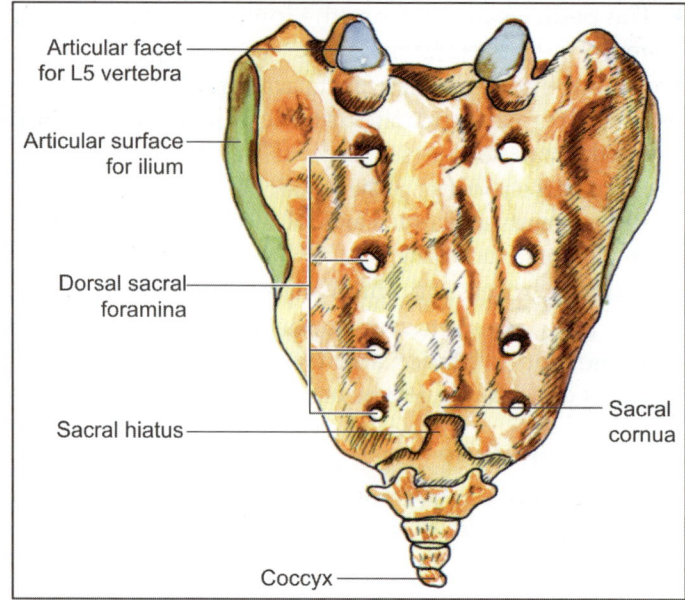

**Fig. 13.8b:** Sacrum—posterior view

- The sacral hiatus transmits 5th sacral nerve, coccygeal nerve and filum terminale (Fig. 13.8a and b).

### Counting of Individual Vertebra

1. Spine of the 7th cervical vertebra is very prominent and is an important landmark to count the spines.
2. The line joining the medial ends of the spinous processes of scapulae corresponds to 3rd thoracic spine.
3. The inferior angle of the scapula corresponds to 7th thoracic spine.
4. The line joining highest points of the iliac crest corresponds to $L_4$ vertebra (transtubercular plane), which is important in procedures like lumbar puncture.

## Coccyx

Coccyx is a small triangular bone formed by the fusion of usually 4 rudimentary coccygeal vertebrae.

In lower animals the coccyx extends into the tail.

## Bony Pelvis

Bony pelvis is formed by the right and left hip bones and the sacrum.

The ilium of the hip bone articulates with the lateral margin of the sacrum (sacroiliac joint) posteriorly.

Anteriorly, the pubis (of hip bone) articulates with each other, to form the pubic symphysis (Fig. 13.9a and b).

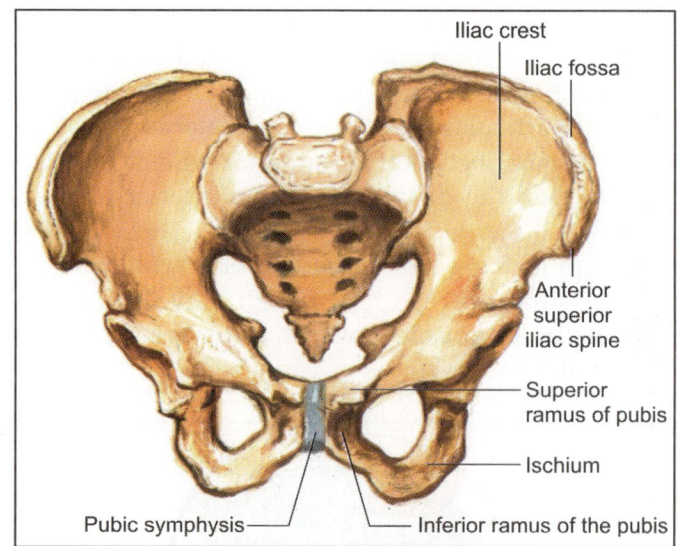

**Fig. 13.9a:** Male pelvis

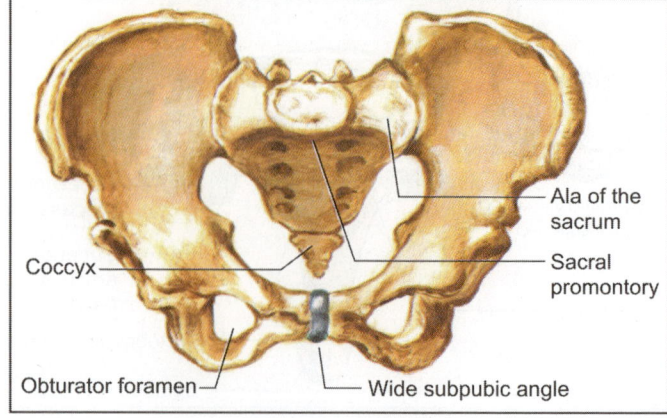

**Fig. 13.9b:** Female pelvis

**13**

## THORACIC CAGE

The vital organs of the thorax (heart and lungs) are well protected inside the bony thoracic cage. It is formed anteriorly by the sternum. On either sides, by the ribs and their costal cartilages and posteriorly, by the thoracic vertebral bodies (Fig. 13.10a and b).

### Sternum

Sternum is a flat bone, present in front of the thoracic cage. It presents the following parts:

Manubrium, body and xiphoid process (Fig. 13.10a).

The **manubrium** is the upper part of the sternum. It articulates with the medial ends of clavicles and first costal cartilages.

Sternal angle (joint between manubrium and body) is an important landmark for counting the ribs. The 2nd costal cartilage can be felt at the sides of this angle.

The **body** is larger part of the sternum: On each side, it receives ribs through their costal cartilages (3rd to 6th ribs).

The **xiphoid process:** It is the most variable part of the sternum. It is a cartilaginous structure in adults. It ossifies in the later part of life (Fig. 13.10c).

The 7th costal cartilage articulates with the sternum at the junction of the body of the sternum and xiphoid process.

### Ribs (Costae)

There are 12 pairs of ribs in the body. Each rib anteriorly articulates with the sternum, through its costal cartilages (1st to 7th). The lower ribs articulate anteriorly with the higher costal cartilages (8th to 10th). The anterior ends of the last two ribs are free. Posteriorly each rib articulates with the thoracic vertebrae.

The 3rd to 9th ribs present almost the same features, hence are referred as 'typical ribs'. The 1st, 2nd, 10th, 11th and 12th ribs are atypical.

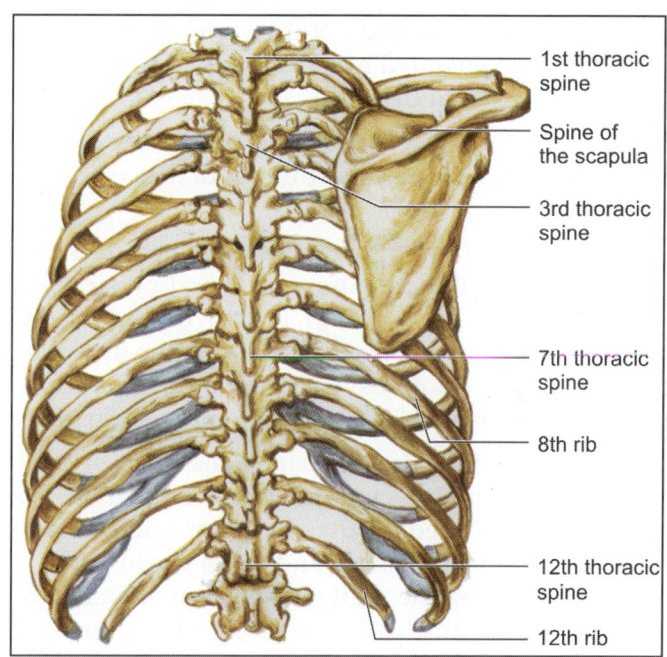

1st thoracic spine

Spine of the scapula

3rd thoracic spine

7th thoracic spine

8th rib

12th thoracic spine

12th rib

**Fig. 13.10b:** Thoracic cage—posterior view

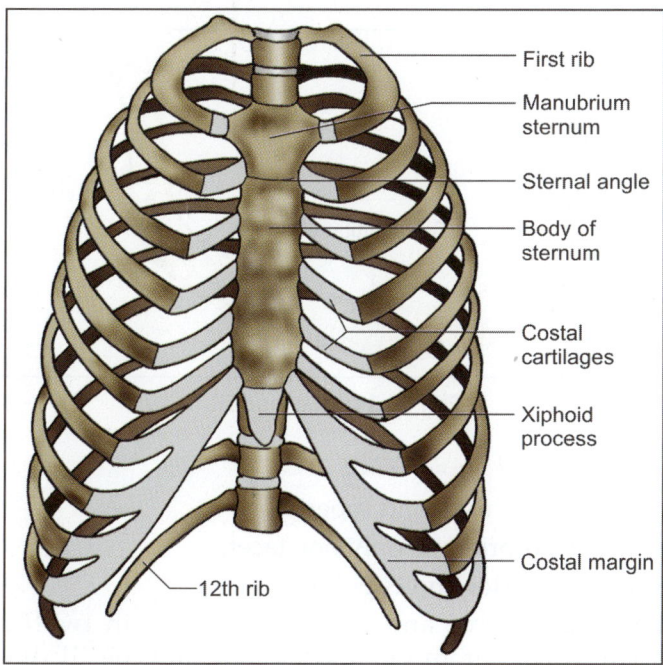

First rib

Manubrium sternum

Sternal angle

Body of sternum

Costal cartilages

Xiphoid process

Costal margin

12th rib

**Fig. 13.10a:** Thoracic cage—anterior view

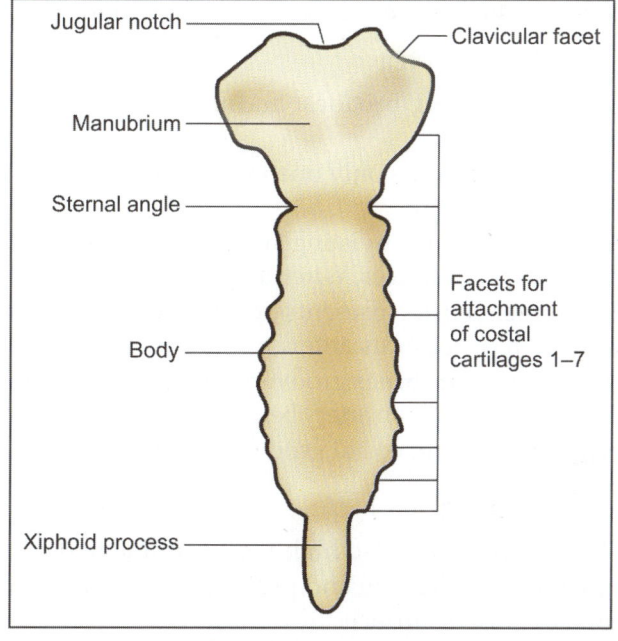

Jugular notch

Clavicular facet

Manubrium

Sternal angle

Body

Facets for attachment of costal cartilages 1–7

Xiphoid process

**Fig. 13.10c:** Sternum

13

### Typical Rib

Each typical rib has an anterior end, shaft and posterior end (Fig. 13.11a).

a. Anterior end: It joins the corresponding costal cartilage by primary cartilaginous joint

b. Posterior end presents head, neck and tubercle.

**Head:** It comprises two facets. The lower facet of the head articulates with body of the corresponding vertebra (plane synovial joint). The upper facet of the head articulates with body of the vertebra above. The two facets are separated by a crest, which corresponds to the intervertebral disc.

**Neck:** It is the narrow succeeding part of the head. It lies in front of the transverse process of the corresponding vertebra.

**Tubercle:** It is the rough portion between neck and shaft. It has medial articular and lateral nonarticular parts. The medial articular part articulates with transverse process of corresponding vertebra by a plane synovial joint (costotransverse joint). The lateral part provides attachment to lateral costotransverse ligament.

**Shaft:** It is the elongated flat part of the rib. It presents angulation about 5–6 cm lateral to the tubercle. The shaft is also twisted so that its inner surface faces upwards behind the angle and faces downwards in front of the angle. The shaft presents upper and lower borders, outer and inner surfaces. They provide attachments to mainly intercostal muscles.

**Costal groove:** The lower part of the inner surface presents costal groove, which is occupied by posterior intercostal vein, artery and intercostal nerve from above downwards.

### First Rib (Fig. 13.11b)

- It is the shortest, broadest and most curved among the ribs.
- The head presents only one facet for the body of 1st thoracic vertebra.
- The shaft has no twisting hence presents superior and inferior surfaces, outer and inner borders.
- The inner border presents scalene tubercle for the insertion of scalenus anterior muscle.
- Its superior surface is grooved by subclavian vein in front and subclavian artery behind the scalene tubercle.
- The shaft has no costal groove.

### Second Rib (Fig. 13.11c)

- The second rib is also highly curved like first rib.
- Shaft has no twisting and presents outer convex and inner concave surface.
- The head presents two articular facets.

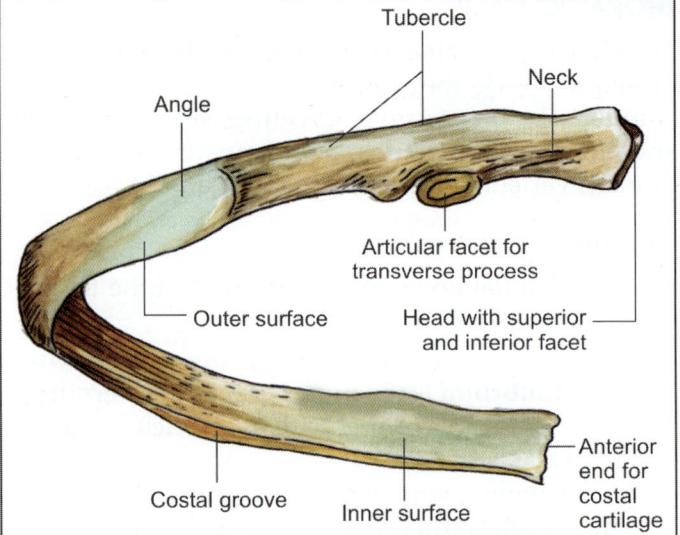

**Fig. 13.11a:** Typical rib

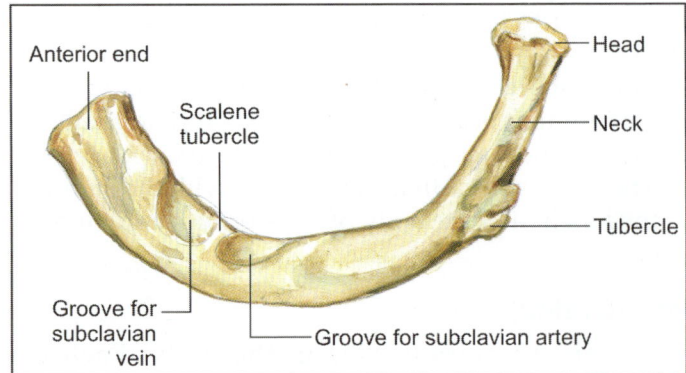

**Fig. 13.11b:** First rib

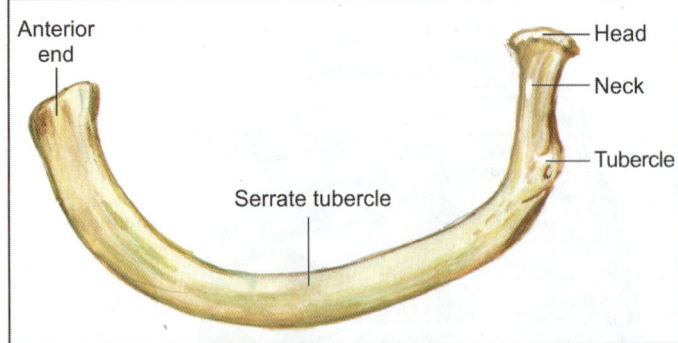

**Fig. 13.11c:** Second rib

### Eleventh and Twelfth Ribs

- There is no neck and tubercle.
- The head presents only one facet.
- Their anterior end is pointed.
- Costal groove and angle are absent in twelfth rib, however in eleventh rib it may be ill defined.

## Applied Anatomy

- The weak point of the rib is near its angle. Fracture involving this site can penetrate the lungs.
- Ribs may be fractured occasionally during muscular strains (coughing).
- In coarctation of aorta, X-rays shows notching of the ribs due to pressure by posterior intercostals arteries.

## SKULL

The skeleton of the head is called skull. It consists of several bones that are joined together to form the cranium. The skull includes the mandible (lower jaw) which is a separate bone.

Skull consists of **22 bones** and 6 ear ossicles (total 28+ hyoid bone = 29). Twenty-one bones are connected to each other by sutures and are immobile. The only movable bone is the mandible.

The bones are classified into paired and unpaired.

| *Paired* | *Unpaired* |
|---|---|
| Parietal | Frontal |
| Temporal | Occipital |
| Maxilla | Sphenoid |
| Zygomatic | Ethmoid |
| Nasal | Mandible |
| Lacrimal | Vomer |
| Palatine | |
| Inferior nasal concha | |

The important features of the skull can be described by viewing the skull from different sides.

1. Norma verticalis : Superior view
2. Norma occipitalis : Posterior view
3. Norma frontalis : Anterior view
4. Norma lateralis : Lateral view
5. Norma basalis : Inferior view

The important parts of the skull are mentioned here and the students are expected to identify these structures.

## Norma Verticalis

Identify the following sutures (Fig. 13.12) are:

i. *Coronal suture:* It is between frontal and two parietal bones.

ii. *Sagittal suture:* It is between the two parietal bones.

iii. *Lambdoid suture:* It is between the occipital and the two parietal bones.

iv. *Metopic suture:* It is present in only 3 to 8% individuals. It lies between the two halves of the frontal bone.

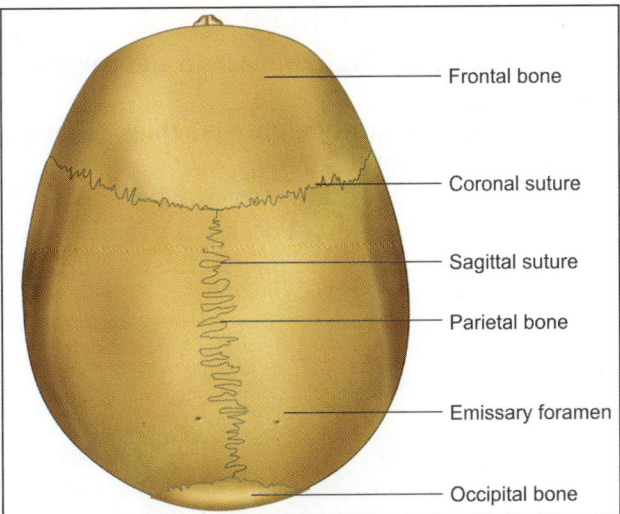

**Fig. 13.12:** Norma verticalis

## Other Features

- *Bregma:* It is the meeting point between the coronal and sagittal sutures. In the fetal life bregma presents a membranous gap called 'anterior fontanelle'. It closes by 12–18 months.
- *Lambda:* It is the meeting point between the sagittal and lambdoid sutures. In the fetal life lambda presents a membranous gap called 'posterior fontanelle'. It closes by 2–3 months.
- *Vertex* is the highest point on sagittal suture.

**Fontanelles** are the membranous gaps between the skull bones. Functionally they allow the brain to grow. A bulge in the fontanelle indicates increased intracranial pressure. An early fusion of sutures in infants can be diagnosed through these fontanelles. Such early fusion craniosynostosis can retard the growth of the brain The anterior fontanelles normally close by 18 months (Fig. 13.13).

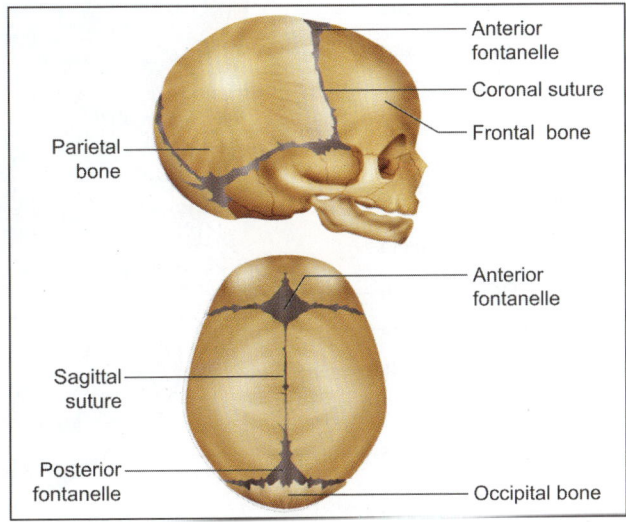

**Fig. 13.13:** Fetal skull

## Norma Occipitalis (Fig. 13.14)

- It shows lambdoid, occipitomastoid and parietomastoid sutures.
- External occipital protuberance is a thick ridge in the midline of the occipital bone.
- Superior nuchal lines are curved ridges extending laterally from the external occipital protuberance.

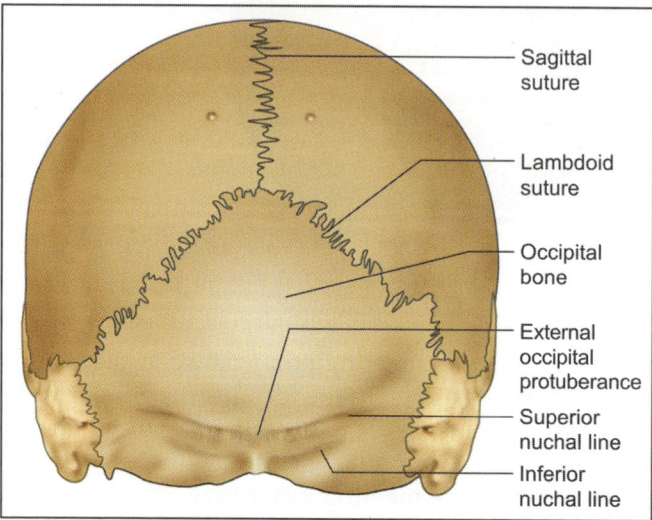

**Fig. 13.14:** Norma occipitalis

## Norma Frontalis (Fig. 13.15)

- It presents 2 orbital and one nasal apertures.
- The base of the bony orbit is bounded

  Above     : frontal bone

  Below     : maxilla

  Laterally : zygomatic bone

  Medially : nasal bone above frontal process of maxilla below.

- Superciliary arch: A curved elevation above the medial part of the orbit.
- Glabella is the median elevation between the two superciliary arches.

  The maxilla presents incisive fossa above the incisor teeth and canine fossa above and lateral to the canine tooth.

## Norma Lateralis (Fig. 13.16)

- *Superior and inferior temporal lines:* The temporal line commences at frontal process of zygomatic bone, arches upwards and backwards and divides into superior and inferior temporal lines in front of coronal suture. Then the two lines run backwards across the parietal bone.

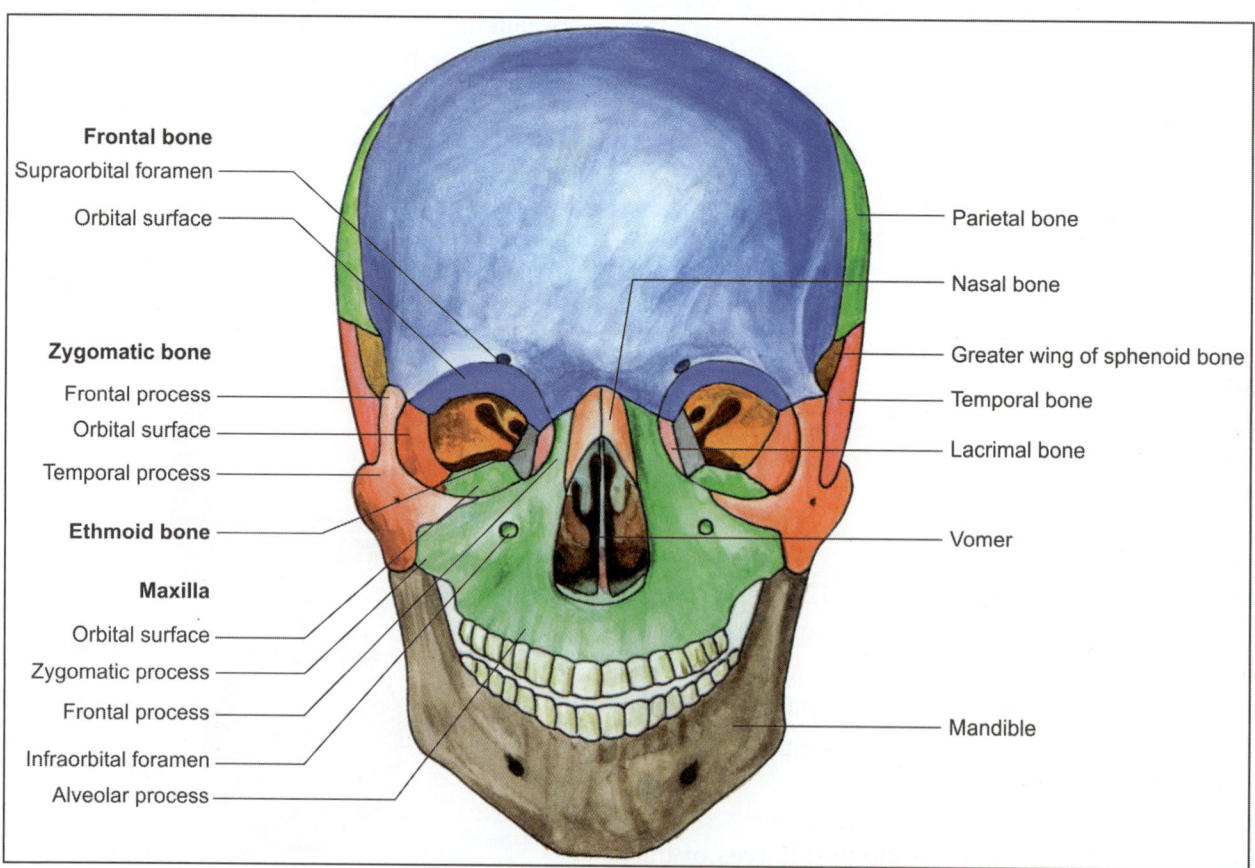

**Fig. 13.15:** Norma frontalis

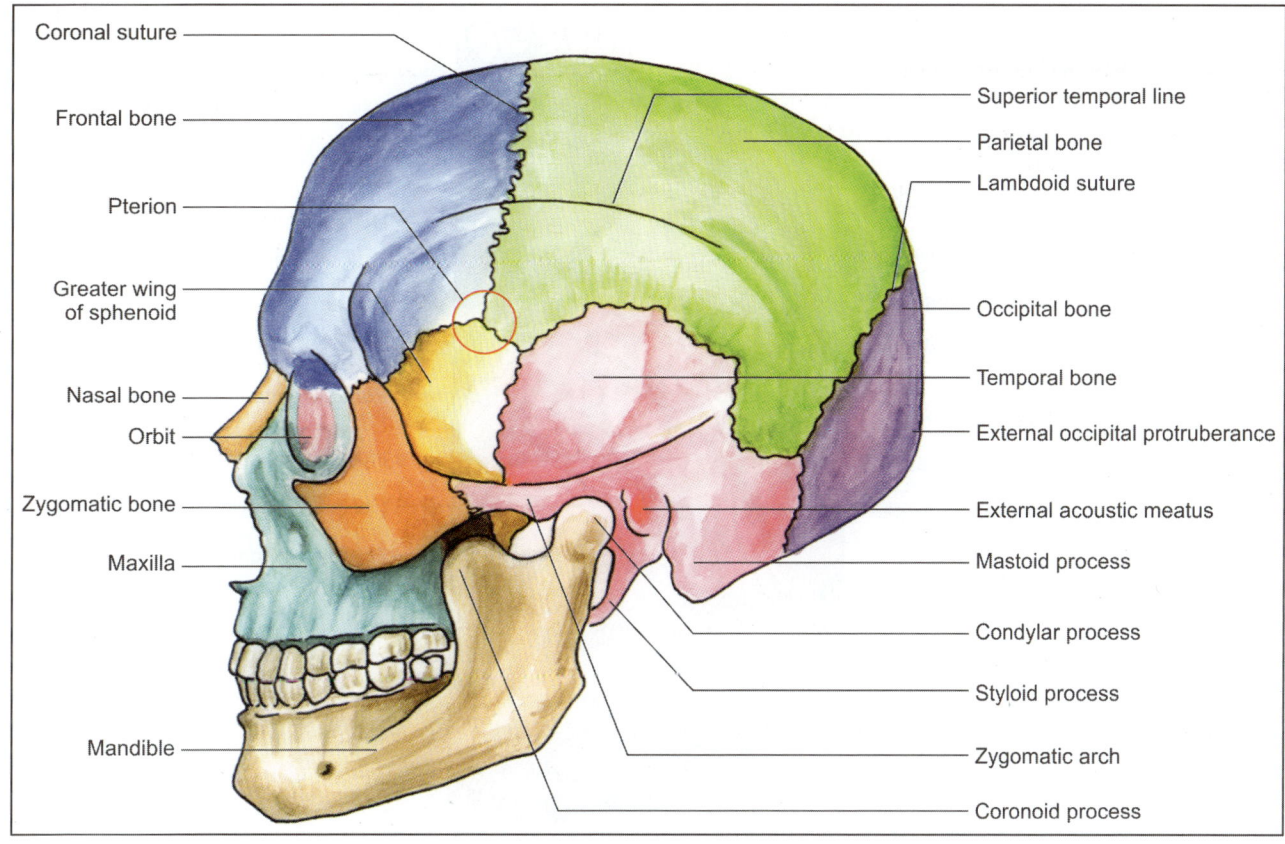

**Fig. 13.16:** Norma lateralis

- *Zygomatic arch:* It is formed by temporal process of zygomatic bone and zygomatic process of temporal bone. The area above the zygomatic arch is the temporal fossa and below is the infratemporal fossa.
- *External acoustic meatus:* It is the opening of external ear at the posterior end of the zygomatic process.
- *Suprameatal triangle:* A triangular area situated posterosuperior to external acoustic meatus. Mastoid antrum is situated deep to it.
- *Mastoid process:* A thick bony projection from temporal bone.
- *Styloid process:* An elongated bony projection from the temporal bone.
- Pterygomaxillary fissure communicates infratemporal fossa with pterygopalatine fossa.
- Inferior orbital fissure communicates infratemporal fossa with bony orbit.
- Pterion is an area where four bones (frontal, parietal, sphenoid and temporal) meet at 'H' shaped suture. Anterior division of middle meningeal artery lies deep to it (inside the skull). Further deep it is related to motor speech area of the cerebrum.

## Norma Basalis (Fig. 13.17)

### Anterior Part

- Hard palate formed by palatine processes of maxillae and horizontal plates of palatine bone.
- Greater and lesser palatine foramina along postero-lateral aspect of hard palate.
- Alveolar arch possesses sockets for the roots of upper teeth.

### Middle Part

- Medial and lateral pterygoid plates descends from the junction of body and greater wing of sphenoid.
- The greater wing of the sphenoid presents two important foramina.
- Foramen ovale transmits mandibular nerve, accessory meningeal artery, lesser petrosal nerve and emissary vein.
- **Foramen spinosum** transmits middle meningeal artery and meningeal branch of the mandibular nerve.
- Spine of the sphenoid is a projection from greater wing of the sphenoid.
- Sulcus tubae: It is a groove between the greater wing of the sphenoid and petrous part of the temporal

**13**

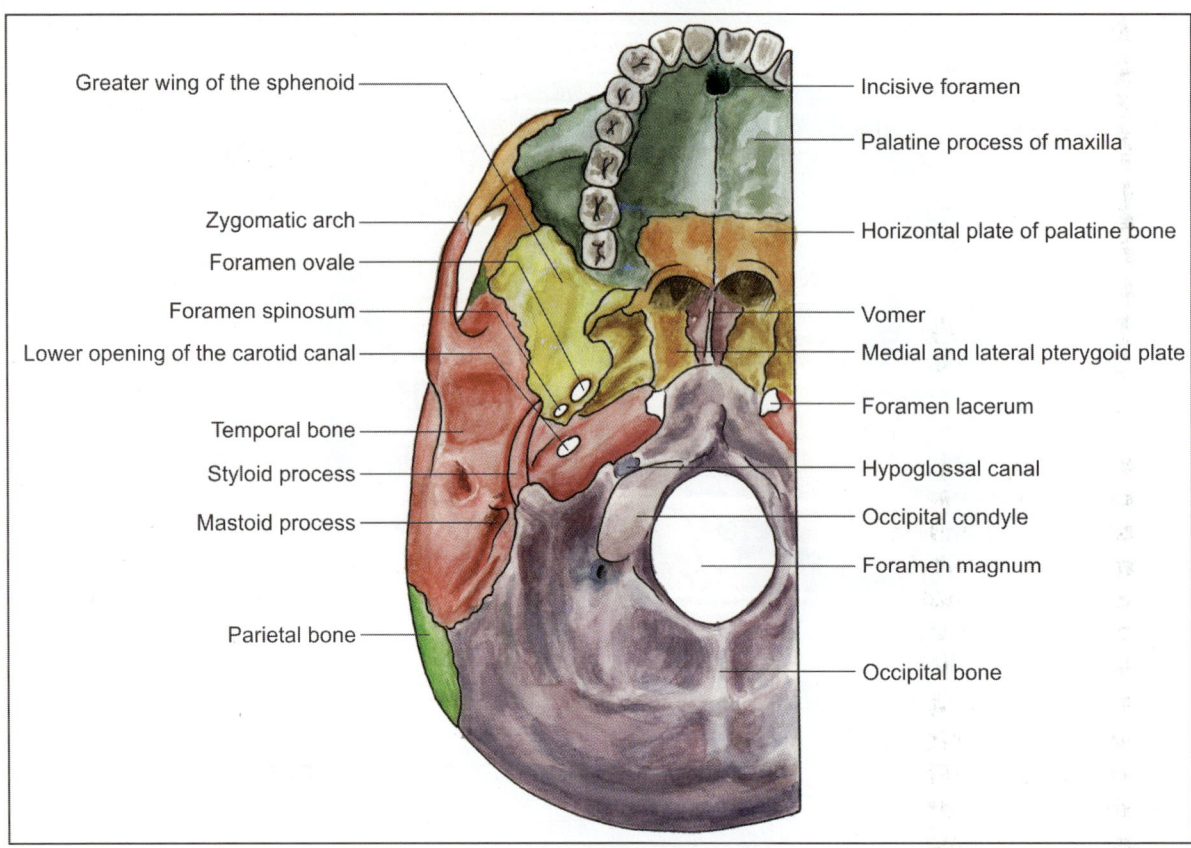

**Fig. 13.17:** Norma basalis

bone. Cartilaginous part of the auditory tube occupies this sulcus.

- Inferior surface of the petrous part of the temporal bone presents lower opening of carotid canal. Its upper opening is located in the posterior wall of the foramen lacerum. The internal carotid artery enters the cranial cavity through it.
- Foramen lacerum is located between sphenoid and apex of petrous temporal bone. Its upper part is traversed by internal carotid artery.

*Posterior Part*

- **Foramen magnum** is the largest foramen in the skull. Medulla oblongata of the brainstem passes through this foramen and continues as spinal cord. The right and left vertebral arteries enter the cranial cavity through it.
- Occipital condyles are convex articular surfaces located lateral to the anterior part of the foramen magnum. They articulate with superior articular facets of atlas to form atlanto-occipital joints.
- Hypoglossal canal is located lateral to anterior part of the condyle. It transmits hypoglossal nerve.

- Jugular foramen is located at the junction of petrous part of the temporal bone and occipital bone. The 9th, 10th and 11th cranial nerves pass through this foramen. The sigmoid sinus continues as internal jugular vein through this foramen.
- Styloid process is a conical projection from temporal bone.
- Stylomastoid foramen between styloid process and mastoid process transmits facial nerve.

## Interior of the Skull (Base of the Skull)

After removal of brain the cranial cavity (cranial fossa) can be studied. It is subdivided into three parts: Anterior, middle and posterior cranial fossae (Fig.13.18).

**Anterior cranial fossa:** It presents the following important features

- Orbital part of the frontal bone forming roof of the bony orbit on each side
- Cribriform plate of the ethmoid bone is in the middle part. It has many small openings for the transmission of olfactory nerve fibers from the roof of the nasal cavity. A bony projection from it, called 'crista galli' provides attachment to anterior end of the falx cerebri.

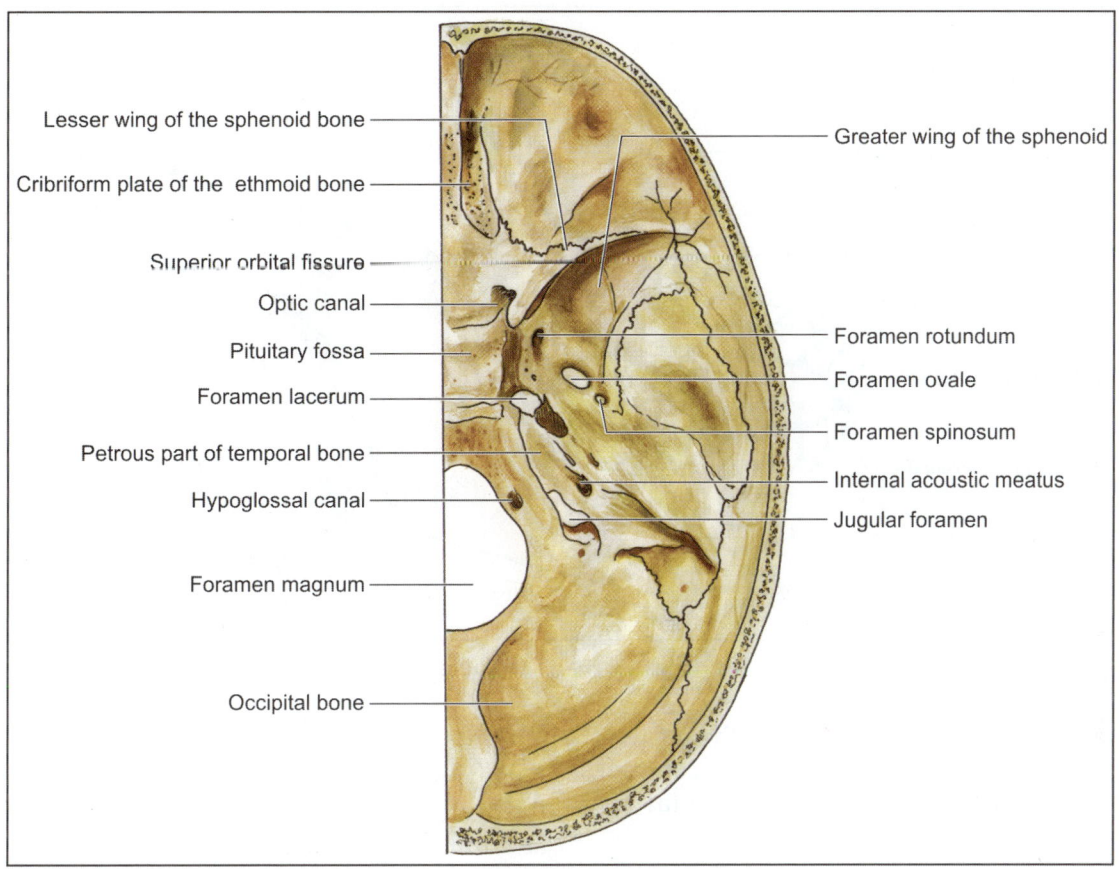

**Fig. 13.18:** Cranial cavity

- Lesser wing of the sphenoid extends from the body of sphenoid and passes laterally. It is the posterior limit of the anterior cranial fossa.

**Middle cranial fossa:** It shows the following important features.

- **Sella turcica (hypophyseal fossa)** is present in the middle part. Anteriorly it is bounded by a bony ridge called 'tuberculum sellae' and similar ridge on the posterior aspect is called 'dorsum sellae'. The pituitary gland is located in this fossa. Sphenoidal air sinus is present below the floor of the hyophyseal fossa.

- *Optic canal:* The two roots of lesser wing of the sphenoid arising form the body of the sphenoid enclose optic canal. It connects the middle cranial fossa with the orbit. Optic nerve and ophthalmic artery pass through it.

- *Superior orbital fissure:* It is an elongated fissure connecting the middle cranial fossa and orbit. It is bounded above by lesser wing and below by greater wing of the sphenoid. It transmits three terminal branches of ophthalmic nerve (frontal, nasociliary and lacrimal), oculomotor, trochlear and abducent nerves.

- Foramen rotundum is present in the greater wing of the sphenoid. Anteriorly it opens into pterygopalatine fossa. It transmits maxillary nerve.

- The other foramina of the middle cranial fossa (foramen ovale, spinosum and lacerum) are explained in the norma basalis.

**Posterior cranial fossa:** It lodges the cerebellum, pons and medulla oblongata. It shows the following important features.

- Clivus is the sloping surface in front of the foramen magnum. It is formed by the body of the sphenoid and basilar part of the occipital bone.

- Foramen magnum (explained in norma basalis)

- Internal occipital protuberance is situated opposite the external occipital protuberance.

- Transverse sulcus is a shallow groove, which extends laterally from internal occipital protuberance. It lodges the transverse sinus.

- *Sigmoid sulcus:* It is the downward continuation of transverse sulcus and ends at jugular foramen. It lodges sigmoid sinus.

- Jugular foramen and hypoglossal canal (explained in the norma basalis)

13

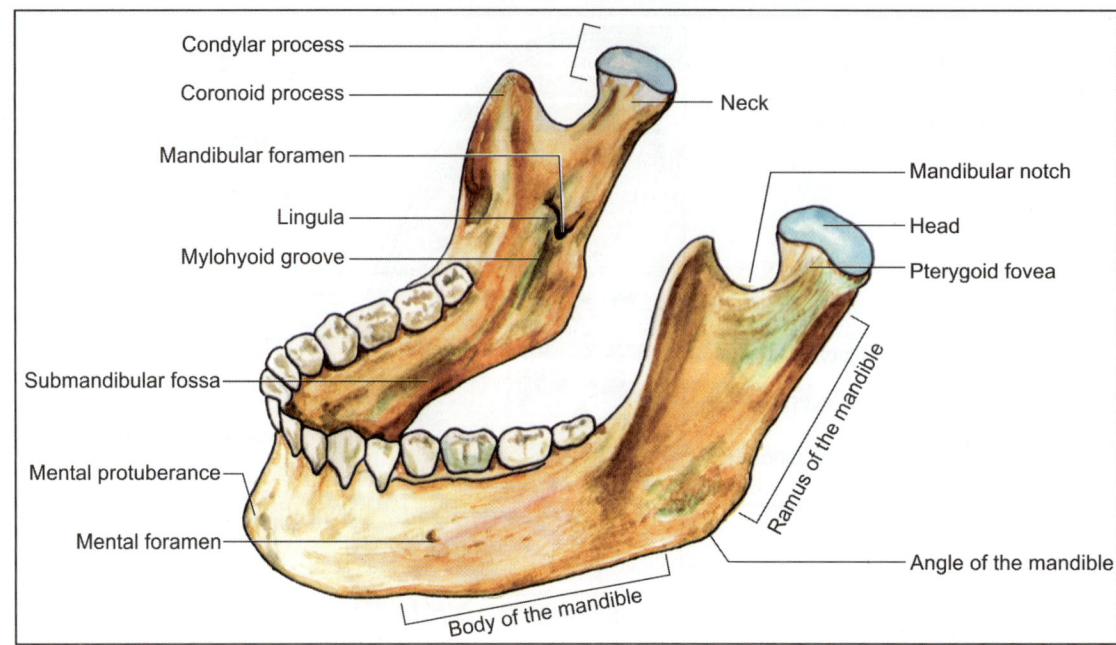

**Fig. 13.19a:** Mandible

- *Internal acoustic meatus:* It is located on the posterior surface of the petrous temporal bone. It continues into the internal ear. It transmits facial and vestibulocochlear nerves.

## Mandible

- The mandible forms the lower jaw and is the only movable bone of skull.
- It articulates with temporal bone by a synovial joint.
- Mandible consists of body and ramus in each half (Figs 13.19a and b).

### Body

a. Symphysis menti: It is a faint ridge in the midline. It indicates the fusion of two halves of mandible.
b. The body has upper alveolar border containing sockets for the roots of the teeth of lower jaw. The lower border continues backward and meet the posterior border of ramus at an angle (angle of mandible).
c. The inner surface of body lodges submandibular salivary gland.
d. The inner surface also presents mylohyoid line for the attachment of the mylohyoid muscle.
e. The inner aspect of the symphysis menti presents a pair of superior and a pair of inferior genial tubercles.
f. The body is traversed inside by mandibular canal. This canal opens externally through mental foramen on the side of symphysis menti. The bony canal transmits inferior alveolar nerve and vessels.

### Ramus

Each ramus is a flattened plate, which extends from the posterior part of the body. The ramus presents outer and inner surfaces.

- *Coronoid process:* It is a triangular projection from the anterosuperior part of the ramus. It receives the insertion of temporalis muscle.
- *Condylar process:* It is an upward projection from the posterosuperior part of the ramus. It consists of head and neck.
- Head is the upper expanded part, which articulates with temporal bone to form temporomandibular joint.

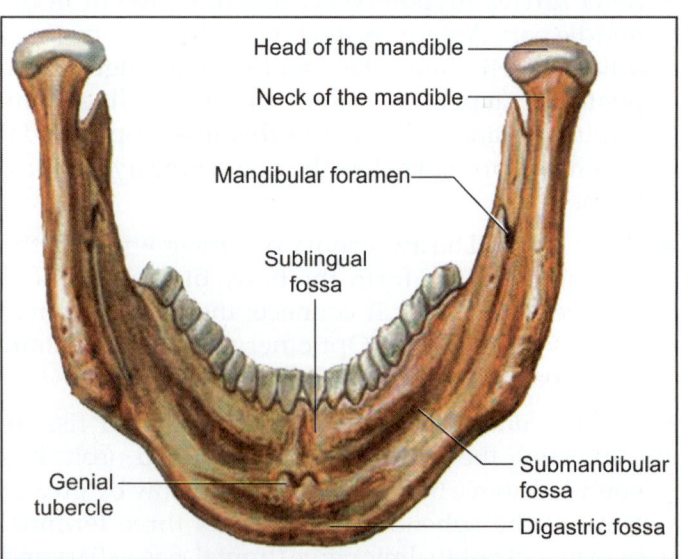

**Fig. 13.19b:** Mandible—inner view

- Neck is the lower constricted part below the head. The anterior aspect of the neck presents a depression called pterygoid fovea, which receives the insertion of lateral pterygoid muscle.
- The outer surface of the ramus receives the insertion of masseter muscle
- The inner surface presents mandibular foramen. The inferior alveolar vessels and nerve enter the mandibular canal through mandibular foramen.
- A rough area below and behind the mandibular foramen provides insertion to medial pterygoid muscle.

## JOINTS OF THE AXIAL SKELETON

### Joints of the Thorax

#### Manubriosternal Joint

Between the body and the manubrium of the sternum. It is a secondary cartilaginous joint.

#### Costovertebral Joint

The head of a typical rib articulates with the numerically corresponding vertebra and the vertebra above. It is a plane synovial joint.

#### Costotransverse Joint

The tubercle of a typical rib articulates with the transverse process of the corresponding vertebra. It is a synovial joint.

#### Costochondral Joint

Each rib continues anteriorly with its cartilage. It is a primary cartilaginous joint.

#### Chondrosternal Joint
(between costal cartilages and sternum)

The first chondrosternal joint is primary cartilaginous, and it does not permit any movement. The remaining 2nd to 7th costal cartilages articulate with the sternum by synovial joints.

### Intervertebral Joints

Adjoining vertebrae are connected to each other at three joints.

One joint is between the vertebral bodies. It is secondary cartilaginous joint and is separated by intervertebral disc.

The other two joints are between the articular processes. They are synovial joints.

*Intervertebral disc:* These are fibrocartilaginous discs present between the bodies of the vertebrae (Fig. 13.20). Each disc is made up of:

a. *Nucleus pulposus:* In the central part, it is a remnant of notochord. Nucleus pulposus a gelatinous mass

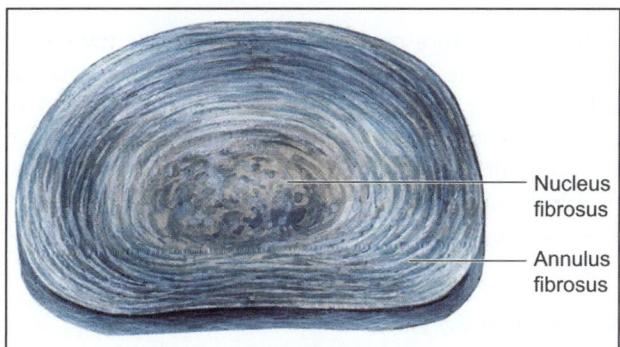

Nucleus fibrosus

Annulus fibrosus

**Fig. 13.20:** Intervertebral disc

containing mucopolysaccharides with large amount of water. It is normally under pressure. Because it is gelatinous it allows changing its shape and permitting the movement of the vertebra one over the other. In old age the nucleus pulposus loses it water content and reduces the elasticity of the vertebral column.

b. *Annulus fibrosus:* In the peripheral part, which is a fibrocartilage.

Intervertebral discs act as shock absorbers. Because of their elasticity, they allow slight movement of vertebral bodies over each other.

*Disc prolapse:* Severe or sudden physical trauma to the spine for example, from lifting heavy object may results in herniation of one or more discs. A herniated disc is also called prolapsed disc or, in common terms, a slipped disc. The most common sites for disc prolapse are between $L_4$ and $L_5$ and $S_1$ or $C_5$ and $C_6$ or $C_6$ and $C_7$. It occurs due to peripheral tears of annulus fibrosus will allow the herniation of gelatinous nucleus pulposus. As age advances, nucleus pulposus get dehydrated. Most disc herniation occurs in posterolateral direction. Thus, the rupture precedes posterolaterally towards the spinal nerve roots. The resulting pressure on these nerve roots leads to pain or numbness.

Herniated discs are treated with bedrest, traction and pain killers. If this treatment fails, the protruding disc may have to be surgically removed. Most herniated discs occur in the lumbar region, because these vertebrae continually experience the largest compressive stresses.

The involvement of $L_5$ and $S_1$ spinal nerve roots and related clinical manifestations are discussed in Chapter 12.

Severe or sudden physical trauma to the spine, for example, from lifting a heavy object—may results in herniation of one or more discs. A herniated disc is also called prolapsed disc or, in common terms, a slipped disc. It usually involves the rupture of the nucleus pulposus through the annulus fibrosus. The annulus is thinnest posteriorly, so the nucleus usually herniates in that direction. Actually, the posterior longitudinal ligament prevents the herniations from proceeding directly posteriorly.

13

Thus, the rupture proceeds posterolaterally towards the spinal nerve roots. The resulting pressure on these nerve roots leads to pain or numbness. Herniated discs are treated with bedrest, traction and pain killers. If this treatment fails, the protruding disc may have to be surgically removed. Most herniated discs occur in the lumbar region, because these vertebrae continually experience the largest compressive stresses.

## Joints of the Pelvis

### Lumbosacral Joint

Between the 5th lumbar vertebra and base of sacrum. It is stabilized by strong iliolumbar ligaments.

### Sacrococcygeal Joint

This is between the apex of the sacrum, and the base of the coccyx. It is a secondary cartilaginous joint.

### Sacroiliac Joint

It is between the sacrum and the articular surface of the ilium. It is a synovial joint.

### Pubic Symphysis

Secondary cartilaginous joint, between the bodies of the pubic bones.

## Joints of the Neck

**Atlanto-occipital joints**

They are synovial joints. The occipital condyles of the skull articulate with first the cervical vertebra (Atlas).

The joints permit flexion and extension movements ('yes' movement).

**Atlantoaxial joints:** They are three in numbers—one median atlantoaxial and two lateral atlantoaxial joints.

- The median atlantoaxial joint is a pivot type of synovial joint. It is between the anterior arch of the atlas and the dens of the axis. The main ligament is transverse ligament of the atlas.
- The lateral atlantoaxial joints are between the lateral masses of the atlas and the body of the axis (superior articular facets on the body of the axis). They are enclosed in a loose fibrous capsule. These joints permit rotatory movements ('no' movements).

Most of the bones in the skull are joined by fibrous (sutural) joints and are immobile.

### Temporomandibular Joint

**Type:** It is a condylar variety of synovial joint.

**Bones articulating**

The head of the mandible articulates with mandibular fossa of the skull (of temporal bone) (Fig. 13.21).

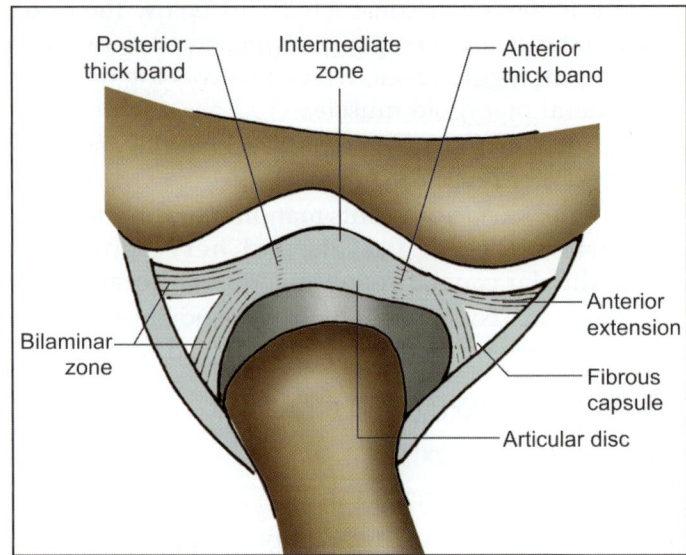

**Fig. 13.21:** TMJ ligaments and articular disc

The articulating surfaces are separated by an articular disc.

**Articular disc:** Structurally, it is fibrocartilage which divides the joint completely into two compartments.

a. Upper meniscotemporal compartment: It permits gliding movement (protrusion, retraction and chewing).

b. Lower meniscomandibular compartment: It permits roatory movement (elevation, depression and side to side movement).

### Structures Stabilizing

The joint is strengthened by a fibrous capsule, lateral ligament. The sphenomandibular and stylomandibular ligaments are accessory ligaments.

### Movements and Muscles Involved

The joint permits depression, elevation, protrusion, retraction and side to side movements. These movements occur during mastication.

1. *Protrusion:* Action of lateral and medial pterygoid muscles of both sides simultaneously.

2. *Retraction:* Posterior fibers of the temporalis muscle.

3. *Depression:* Lateral pterygoids assisted by geniohyoid and mylohyoid and digastric muscles. During depression head of the mandible and the articular disc together glide forward.

4. *Elevation:* Masseter, temporalis and medial pterygoid muscles.

5. *Side to side movement:* Lateral and medial pterygoid muscles of one side acting alternatively with other side.

Dislocation of mandible takes place in forward direction. The head of the mandible slips into infratemporal fossa during wide opening of mouth by lateral pterygoid muscle.

## Applied Anatomy

**Spondylolysis:** It is the medical term meaning degeneration of the vertebra, especially a fusion and immobilization of the vertebral bones. Its symptoms include pain and restriction of movement.

**Spondylolisthesis:** It is the forward slippage of one vertebra on another. This most commonly occurs at the lumbosacral junction with $L_5$ slipping over $S_1$, but it can occur at higher levels as well. It can be congenital or acquired. The causes for acquired are trauma, degenerative changes and bone diseases.

**Spondylitis:** It is an inflammation of the vertebral joint causing back and neck pain.

**Back pain associated with intervertebral joints:** It is often associated with degeneration of articular cartilage and osteophyte (bony outgrowth) of the facet articular process.

**Hangman fracture:** During judicial hanging, the odontoid process usually breaks to hit the medulla oblongata. It is the pedicle fracture of the axis. It can be unilateral or bilateral. It can be associated with anterior dislocation of the body of axis vertebra. It results from severe extension injury (in automobile accident where the face forcibly strikes the dashboard) or from hanging.

**Jefferson fracture:** It is a burst fracture of atlas affecting anterior or posterior arches (unilateral or bilateral). This results from an axial loading injury to the head with compressive force on atlas (typically from diving).

**Whiplash injury (cervical hyperextension injury):** Relaxed neck is thrown backwards, as vehicle accelerates rapidly forward. Rapid recoil of the neck into extreme flexion occurs next. This abnormal motion causes damage to the soft tissues that hold the cervical vertebrae together (ligaments, capsules and muscles) and will not involve fracture.

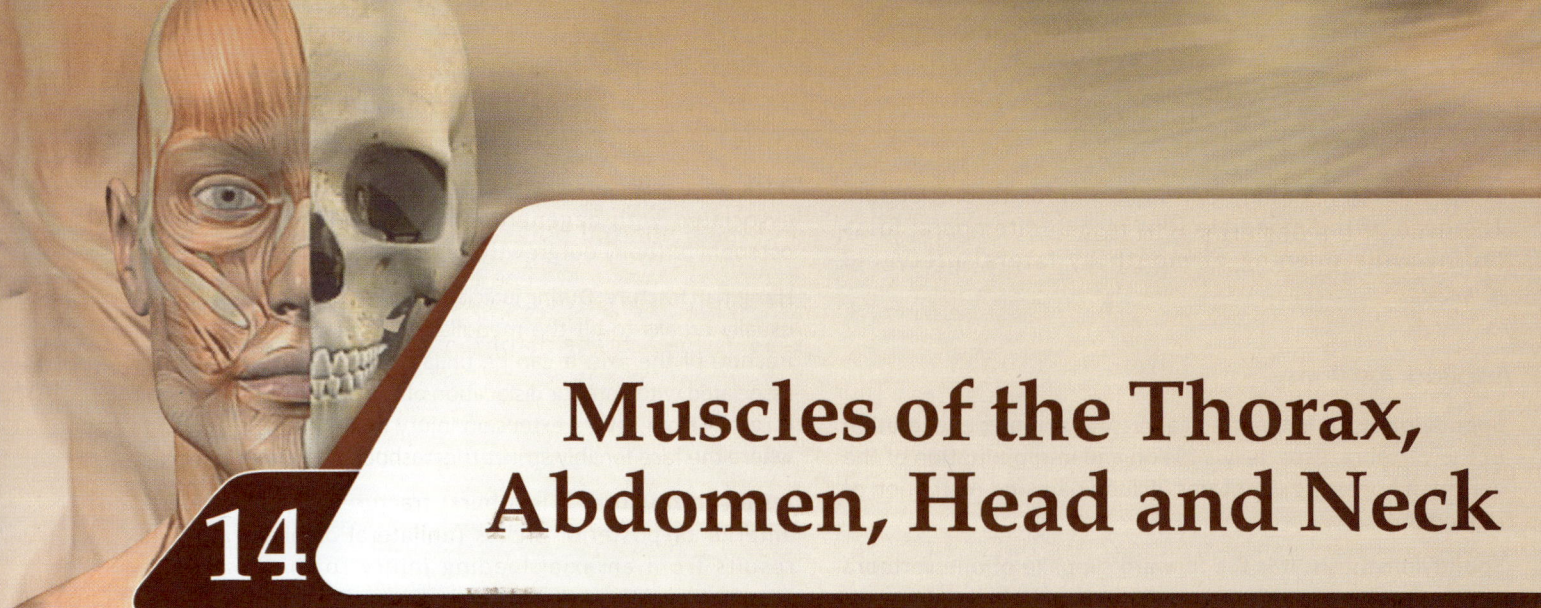

# Muscles of the Thorax, Abdomen, Head and Neck

**14**

## MUSCLES OF THE THORACIC WALL

The thoracic cage forms the skeletal framework of the walls of the thorax. The gaps between the ribs are called intercostal spaces, which are filled up by intercostal muscles (Fig. 14.1a). They are:

1. External intercostal
2. Internal intercostal
3. Transverse thoracis with three parts: Subcostalis, sternocostalis and intercostalis intimi.

All these muscles are supplied by the intercostal nerves (thoracic spinal nerves).

The main action of the intercostal muscles is to prevent retraction of the intercostal spaces during inspiration, and bulging during expiration. Such movements are an indication of the paralysis of the intercostal muscles.

The external intercostal elevates the rib during inspiration. Internal intercostal may depress the ribs during expiration (Fig. 14.1b).

### Typical Intercostal Space

The spaces between the typical ribs and traversed by intercostal nerves supplying only thorax are known as 'typical intercostal spaces'. The 3rd, 4th, 5th and 6th intercostal spaces are typical.

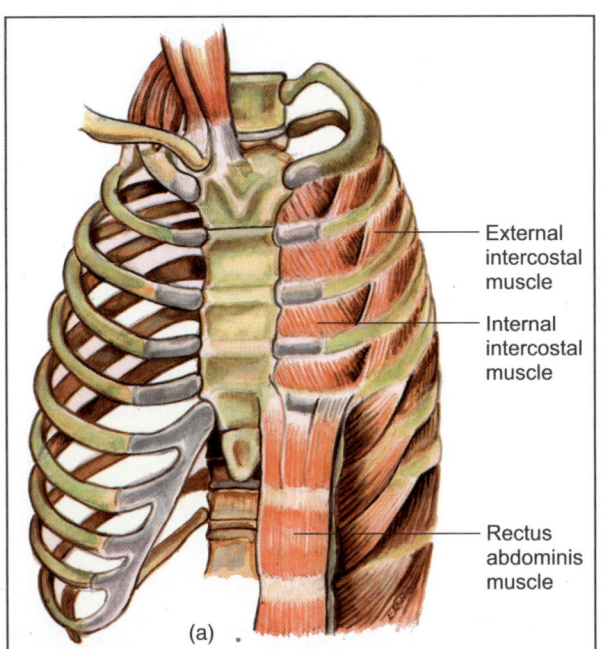

External intercostal muscle

Internal intercostal muscle

Rectus abdominis muscle

(a)

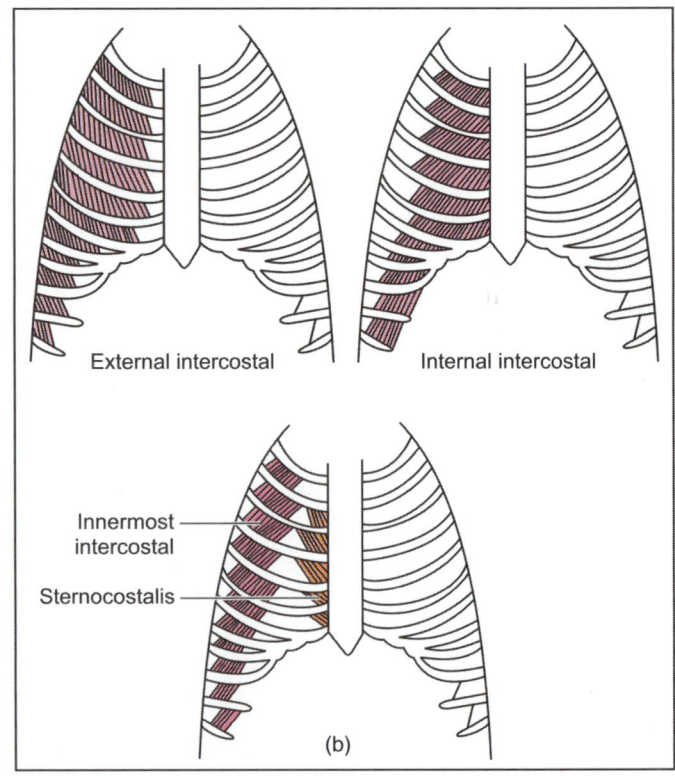

External intercostal

Internal intercostal

Innermost intercostal

Sternocostalis

(b)

**Fig. 14.1a and b:** Intercostal muscles

Each space is directed downwards and forwards. It is narrow at the posterior part (towards vertebra) and wider at the anterior part (towards sternum).

## Contents

Each typical intercostals space contains intercostals muscles, nerves and vessels. The course and distrtibution of a typical intercostal nerve is explaincd in Chapter 35.

## Intercostal Muscles (Fig. 14.1a and b)

*External intercostal muscles:* They extend from angle of the ribs posteriorly to costochondral junction anteriorly. The direction of the muscle fibers are downwards and medially.

*Internal intercostal muscles:* They are present deep to the external intercostal, extend from the angle of the ribs posteriorly to lateral border of the sternum. Its fibers are directed right angle to the direction of external intercostal muscles.

*Innermost intercostal (intercostalis intimi):* Thcy are present deep to the internal intercostal muscle in the middle and lateral part of the intercostal spaces. The directions of the muscle fibers are similar to that of internal intercostal muscles. However they are separated by intercostal vessels and nerves.

*Sternocostalis:* It arises from the posterior surface of the lower part of the sternum. It extends to inner surface of 2nd to 6th costal cartilages.

## Respiratory Movements

*Inspiratory movement:* Increase in thoracic volume (decrease in intrapulmonary pressure) is achieved by movement of thoracic wall and diaphragm. The increase in anteroposterior diameter of the thorax is due to contraction of intercostal muscles. Movement of the ribs (2nd to 6th) at the costovertebral joints around an axis passing through necks of the ribs causes anterior ends of the ribs to rise. Since anterior ends of the ribs are directed downwards, their elevation results in anteroposterior movement of the sternum. This is called **'pump handle movement'**. The increase in transverse diameter of the thorax is also due to contraction of intercostal muscles. Movements of lower ribs rises the middle part of the ribs, thus increasing transverse diameter. This is called **'bucket handle movement'**.

Increase in vertical diameter is due to contraction of the diaphragm. When diaphragm contracts, it descends, which leads to increase in vertical diameter of the thorax.

With increase in the thoracic volume, the pressure inside the lung is reduced. So air is drawn into the lungs through, nose, mouth, larynx and trachea.

*Chief muscles of inspiration:* Diaphragm, external intercostal and Interchondral portion of the internal intercostal.

*Expiratory movement:* The air is expelled out from the lung, due to elastic recoiling tendency of the lungs. It is a passive act. The diaphragm and intercostal muscle relax, thus decreasing the thoracic volume and increasing the prcssure inside the lungs.

*Chief muscles of expiration:* Interosseous part of the internal intercostal muscle.

## The Diaphragm

It is a musculoaponeurotic partition between thorax and abdomen.

Its upper surface (facing thoracic cavity) is convex on right and left sides (right and left domes) and depressed in the middle. The right dome is slightly higher than left due to presence of liver.

The muscle takes origin from the peripheral part and is inscrted into a central tendon (Fig. 14.2a).

## Origin

It has sternal, costal and lumbar parts.

1. *Sternal origin:* By two fleshy slips from posterior aspect of the xyphoid process.

2. *Costal origin:* From the inner surfaces of the lower six ribs and adjoining costal cartilages.

3. *Lumbar origin:* It is the strongest attachment of the diaphragm on the posterior side. The lumbar origin is from lumbar vertebrae and lumbocostal ligaments.

   a. From the lumbar vertebral bodies by a pair of crura (right and left). The right crus is longer and arises from anterolateral aspects of upper three lumbar vertebrae and intervening intervertebral discs. The left crus arises from the corresponding parts of upper two lumbar vertebrae. The two crura are connected by a tendinous arch in front of the aorta is called 'median arcuate ligament'.

   b. Lumbocostal ligaments: There are two lumbocostal ligaments.

**Medial lumbocostal ligament** (medial arcuate ligament): It extends from the side of body of $L_1$ vertebra to its transverse process. This tendinous arch is the thickening of the fascia covering the upper part of psoas major muscle.

**Lateral lumbocostal ligament** (lateral arcuate ligament): It extends from transverse process of $L_1$ vertebra to lower border of 12th rib. This tendinous arch is the thickening of the fascia covering the upper part of quadratus lumborum muscle.

14

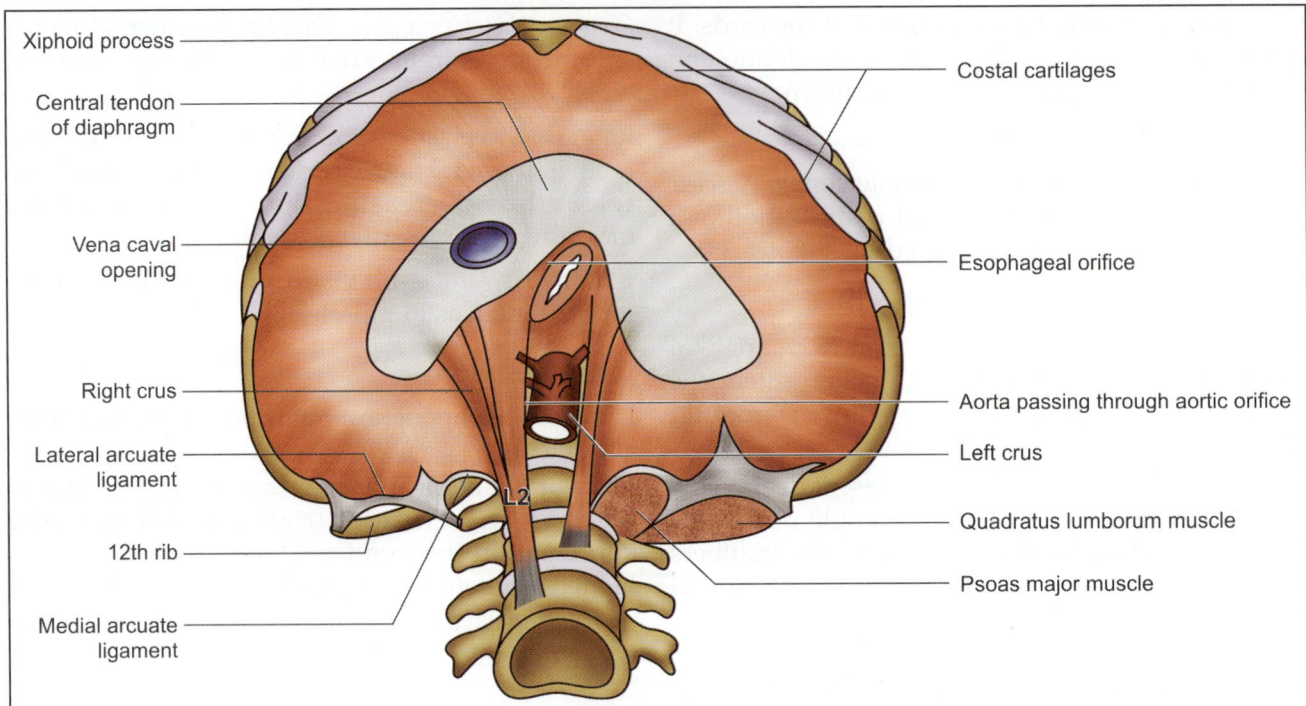

**Fig. 14.2a:** Abdominal surface of the diaphragm

### Insertion

All fibers are inserted into the central tendon, which is situated in the median depressed part close to the sternum. It is trilobar in shape.

### Openings of the Diaphragm

*Major Openings* (Fig. 14.2b)

1. *Vena caval opening:* It is situated at the central tendon of the diaphragm at the level of $T_8$ vertebra (Fig. 14.2c).

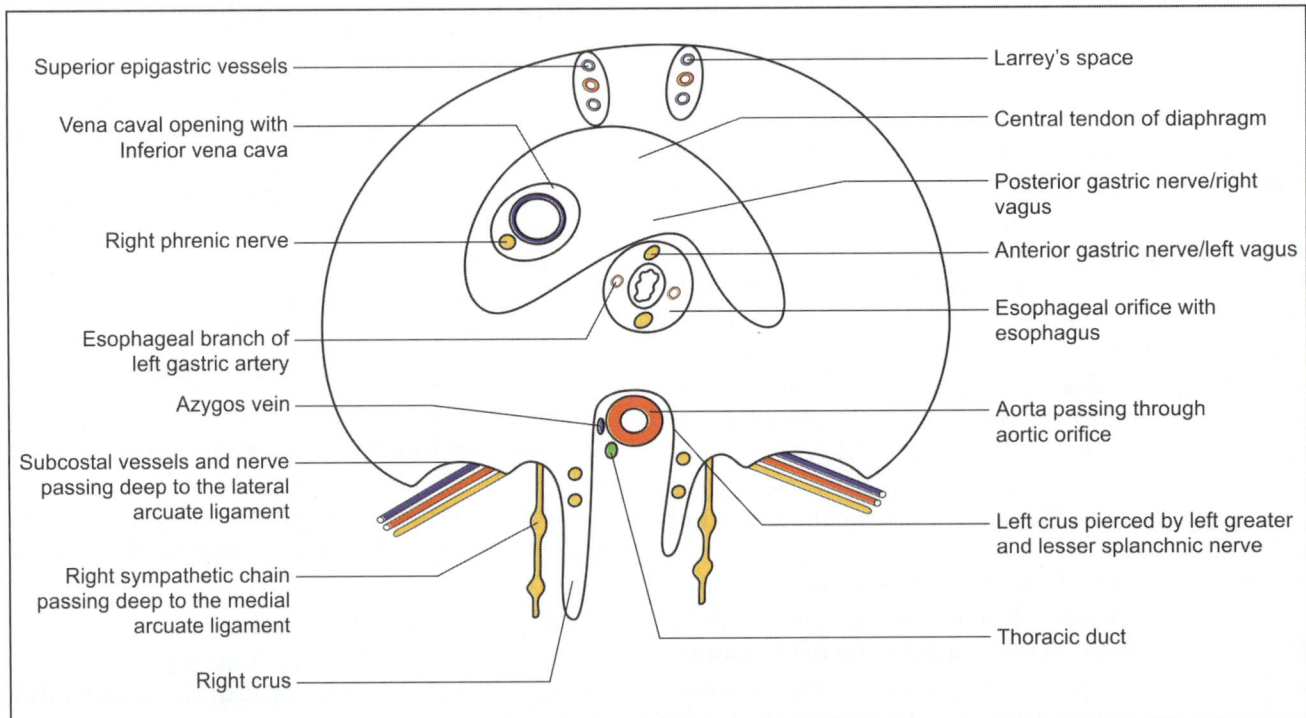

**Fig. 14.2b:** Major and minor openings of the diaphragm

14

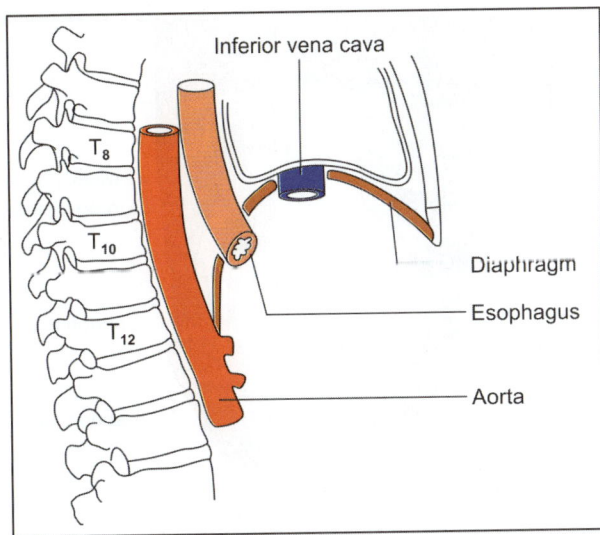

**Fig. 14.2c:** Openings of the diaphragm

*Structures passing through it:*

a. Inferior vena cava from the abdomen enters the right atrium through it

b. Right phrenic nerve

When the diaphragm contracts in inspiration, the vena caval opening dilates and more blood enters the right atrium.

2. *Esophageal opening:* It is situated in the muscular part of the diaphragm at the level of $T_{10}$ vertebra.

*Structures passing through it:*

a. Esophagus.

b. Right and left vagus nerves.

c. Esophageal branch of the left gastric artery.

When the diaphragm contracts this opening is constricted and prevents regurgitation of food from the stomach to the esophagus.

3. *Aortic opening:* It is situated behind the diaphragm and in front of the body of 12th thoracic vertebra.

*Structures passing through it:*

a. Abdominal aorta

b. Thoracic duct

c. Azygos vein

### Minor Openings

1. Larrey's space (foramen of Morgagni): It is the gap between the xiphoid and costal (7th costal cartilage) origins of diaphragm. It transmits superior epigastric vessels.

2. Behind the lateral arcuate ligament—subcostal vessels and nerve

3. Behind the medial arcuate ligament—sympathetic chain

4. Right crus is pierced by greater and lesser splanchnic nerves (from thoracic sympathetic ganglia).

### Nerve Supply

1. The motor nerve supply is from phrenic nerves $(C_{3, 4, 5})$.

2. The proprioceptive sensation is carried by phrenic and lower interostal nerves.

### Actions

It is a muscle of inspiration, when the diaphragm contracts it descends, so that the vertical diameter of the thorax is increased (lower ribs are fixed).

On further contraction it descends further downwards and the transverse diameter of thorax is increased (lower ribs are elevated).

When the diaphragm moves down it compresses the abdominal viscera and increases the intra-abdominal pressure (as in vomiting, micturition or defaecation).

### Applied Anatomy

**Congenital Diaphragmatic Hernia**

Due to defect in the formation of diaphragm, the abdominal viscera herniate into the thorax, which can compress the lung. It requires immediate surgical intervention.

**Hiatal Hernia**

Hernia occurs through the dilated esophageal opening of diaphragm. It can cause regurgitation of stomach contents into esophagus (gastroesophageal reflux/GR).

### MUSCLES OF ABDOMEN

Muscles of the abdomen are classified into anterior and posterior abdominal wall muscles (Fig. 14.3).

### ANTERIOR ABDOMINAL WALL MUSCLES

This group includes six muscles on each side.

*Four of them are large:*

1. **External oblique muscle of the abdomen (obliquus externus abdominis):** This is the outermost muscle of the anterior abdominal wall. Its fibers are directed downwards forwards and medially.

2. **Internal oblique muscle of the abdomen (obliquus internus abdominis):** Its fibers (those from inguinal ligament) are directed upwards and medially opposite to the direction of external oblique.

3. **Transversus abdominis:** It occupies deep to the internal oblique abdominis and majority of its fibers are horizontal in direction.

14

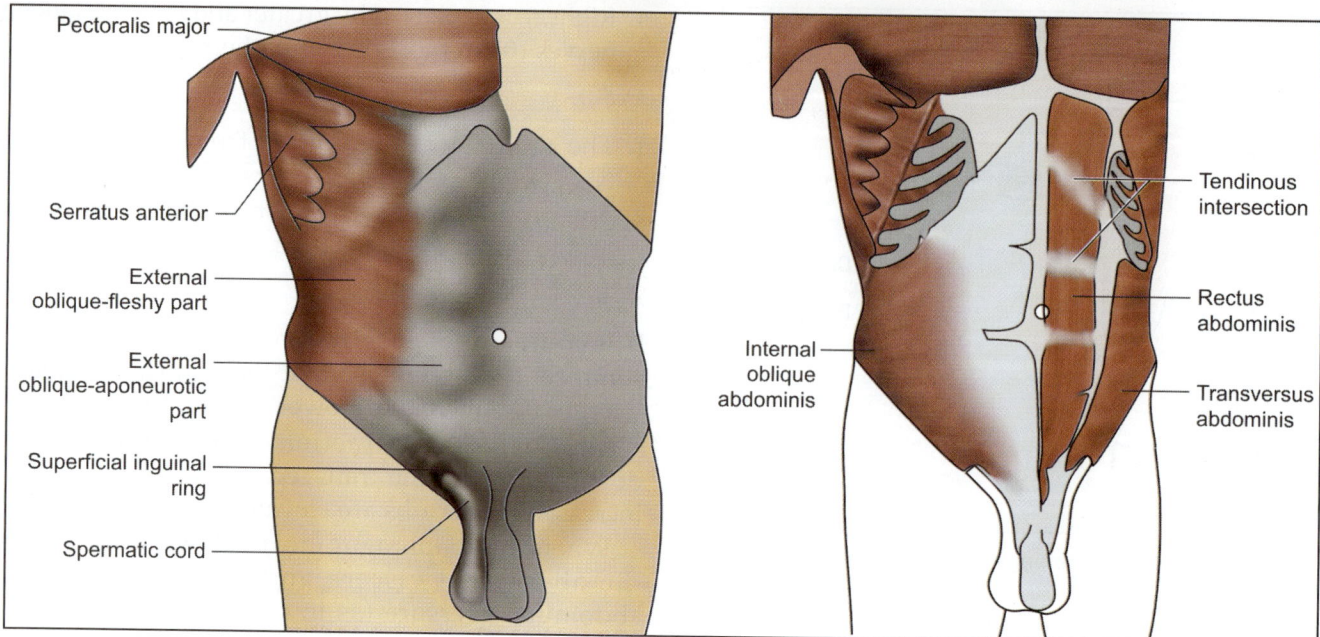

**Fig. 14.3:** Muscles of the anterior abdominal wall

4. **Rectus abdominis:** It is vertically placed muscle on either side of the linea alba.

The other two small muscles include: Cremaster and pyramidalis.

The lower thoracic and upper lumbar nerves supply these muscles.

### Actions

1. Support the abdominal viscera
2. Help in all expulsive acts like micturition, defecation, parturition, vomiting, etc.
3. They also help in forceful expiratory acts.
4. These muscles cause the movement of the trunk.
5. Cremaster helps to suspend the testis.

### Rectus Sheath

It is an aponeurotic sheath covering the rectus abdominis muscle (also pyramidalis in the lower part). Functionally, it checks the bowing of the rectus abdominis muscle while flexing the trunk. It provides strength to the anterior adominal wall muscles.

The composition of the aponeurotic sheath varies on the anterior aspect but it is uniform on the posterior aspect (Fig. 14.4).

### Contents

1. Rectus abdominis muscle and pyramidalis
2. Superior and inferior epigastric vessels
3. Lower six thoracic nerves.

The anterior wall of the rectus sheath presents tendinous intersections.

*Linea alba:* It is formed by decussating aponeurotic fibers of the anterior abdominal wall muscles. It extends from the pubic symphysis to xiphoid process in the anterior midline.

### Inguinal Ligament

It is the lower part of the aponeurosis of external oblique muscle and extends from the anterior superior iliac spine to pubic tubercle. It is the ligament demarcating the thigh from the anterior abdominal wall (Fig. 14.4).

### Inguinal Canal

The arrangement of the anterior abdominal wall muscles makes a canal in the lower part. This musculo-aponeurotic canal is about 4 cm in length (Fig. 14.5).

### Extension

It extends from deep inguinal ring to superficial inguinal ring. The canal is placed above and parallel to the medial half of the inguinal ligament.

1. *Deep inguinal ring:* It is an oval gap in the fascia trasversalis about 1.25 cm above the midinguinal point and lateral to the inferior epigastric artery.
2. *Superficial inguinal ring:* It is a triangular opening in the aponeurosis of external oblique muscle. It is placed above and lateral to the pubic crest.

**14**

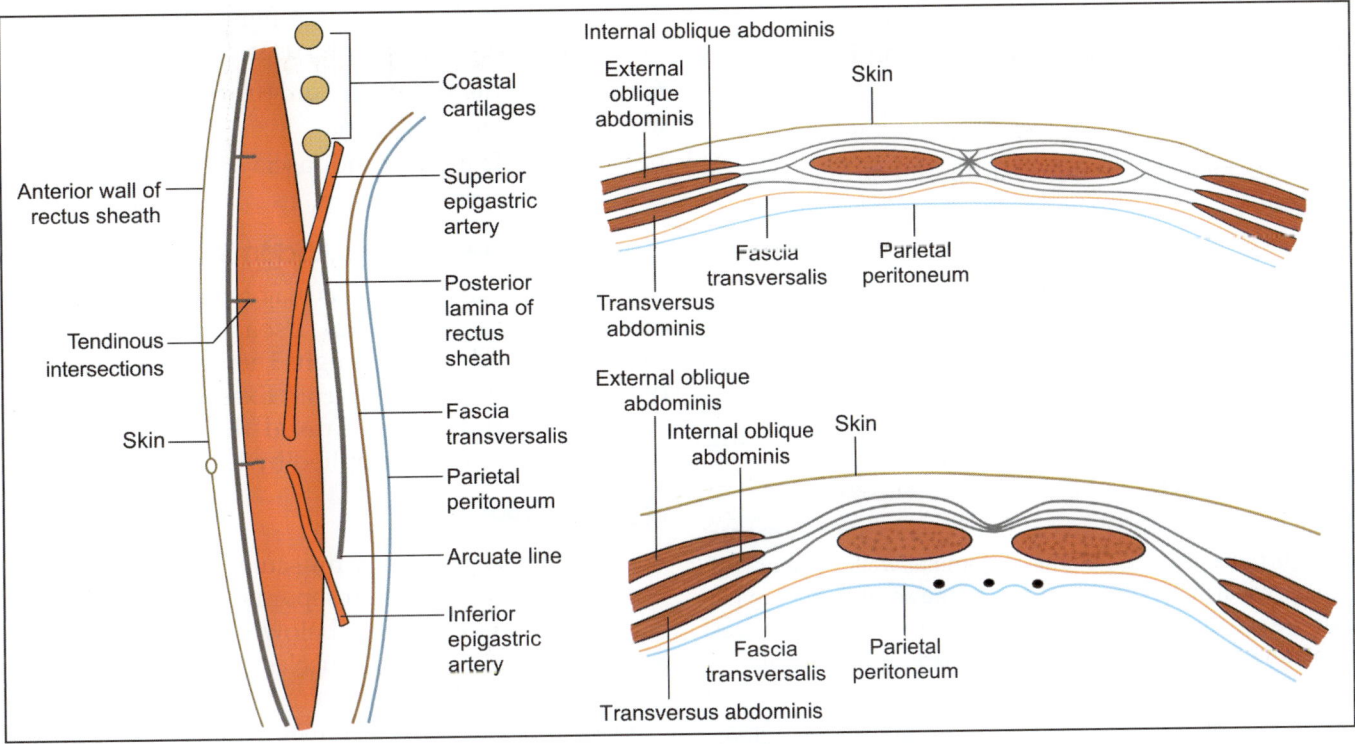

**Fig. 14.4:** Rectus sheath and its formation

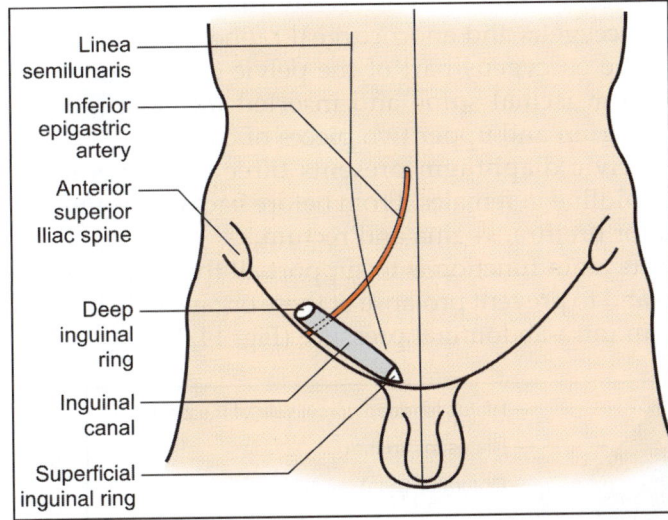

**Fig. 14.5:** Extent of inguinal canal

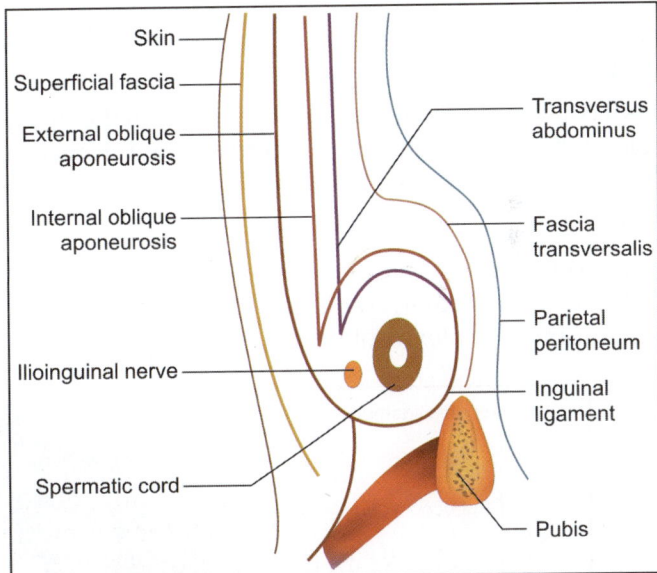

**Fig. 14.6:** Boundaries of the inguinal canal (lateral view)

## Boundaries of the Inguinal Canal

The canal presents anterior and posterior wall, roof and floor (Fig. 14.6).

### Anterior Wall

1. Skin
2. Superficial fascia
3. Aponeurosis of the external oblique muscle
4. Fleshy fibers of internal oblique muscle in lateral 1/3.

### Posterior Wall

1. Parietal peritoneum
2. Extraperitoneal connective tissue
3. Fascia transversalis
4. Conjoint tendon in the middle half
5. Reflected part of the inguinal ligament in the medial 1/4th.

14

### Roof

Arched fibers of the internal oblique and transversus abdominis muscle

### Floor

Upper surface of the inguinal ligament and lacunar ligament.

### Contents

1. Spermatic cord in males, or round ligament of uterus in females
2. Ilio-inguinal nerve (in both sexes) pierces the internal oblique muscle and traverses the medial part of the canal and emerges from the superficial inguinal ring.

## Inguinal Hernia

Hernia is an abnormal protrusion of abdominal contents through the weak area of the abdominal wall. Presence of inguinal canal makes the lower part of the anterior abdominal wall weak. Increased intra-abdominal pressure causes herniation through this area and is called inguinal hernia.

Inguinal herniae are of two types

a. Indirect inguinal hernia: Hernia occurs through deep inguinal ring, traverses the canal. It is often congenital.
b. Direct inguinal hernia: Hernia occurs through the posterior wall of the inguinal canal. It occurs in adults.

## Spermatic Cord

It is a collection of structures extending from the upper pole of the testes to the deep inguinal ring. It traverses the inguinal canal.

### Contents

1. Vas deferens
2. Arteries—testicular, cremasteric and artery to the vas
3. Pampiniform plexus of veins

4. Genital branch of the genitofemoral nerve
5. Nerve and lymphatic plexuses.

**Coverings of the spermatic cord** (from within outwards):
a. Internal spermatic fascia
b. Cremasteric muscle and fascia
c. External spermatic fascia.

## Muscles of the Posterior Abdominal Wall

These muscles include psoas major, psoas minor, iliacus and quadratus lumborum. Psoas major and iliacus together extend into the thigh. They help in the flexion of thigh. Quadratus lumborum fixes the last rib during inspiration and causes lateral flexion of vertebral column. They are all supplied by $L_1$–$L_4$ spinal nerves.

## PELVIC DIAPHRAGM

- Pelvic diaphragm is a muscular structure forming the floor of the pelvis. It separates pelvic cavity from perineal region present below.
- It is made up of two muscles on each side namely levatorani and coocygeus
- **Levator ani** has two parts—pubococcygeus and iliococcygeus. They arise anteriorly from pubic bone and fascia covering (tendinous arch) the obturator internus muscle. Posteriorly they are attached to coccygeus and anococcygeal raphe.
- The coccygeus part of the pelvic diaphragm arises from ischial spine and inserted into last piece of sacrum and upper two pieces of coccyx.
- Pelvic diaphragm presents three apertures in the midline in females. From before backwards they are for urethra, vagina and rectum.
- Its main function is to support all the pelviv organs and to prevent prolapse of these organs with increase in intra-abdominal pressure (Fig. 14.7).

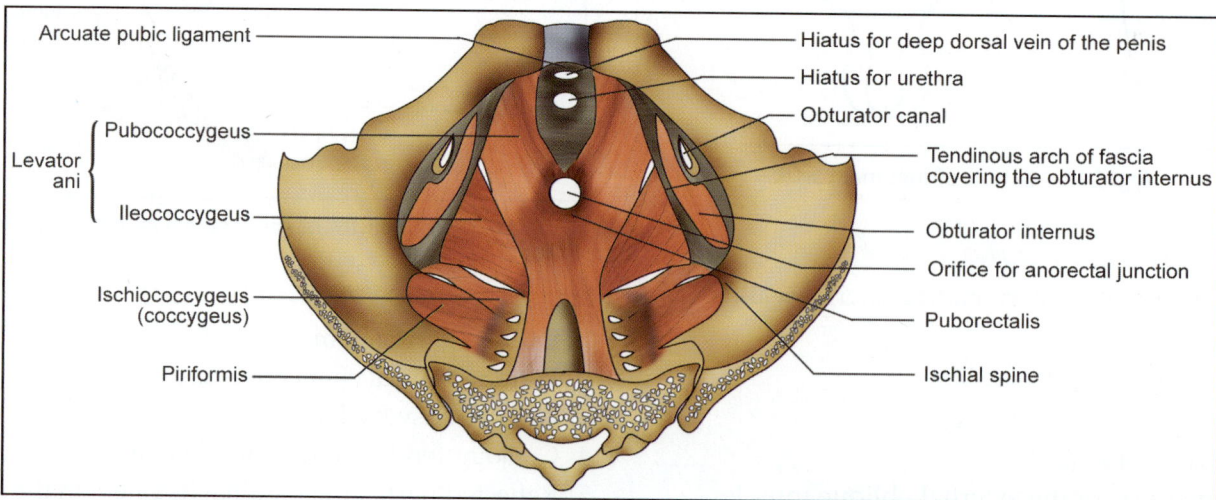

**Fig. 14.7:** Pelvic diaphragm—male (superior view)

### SCALP

The dense connective tissue covering the cranial vault is called the scalp. It is a five layered structure (Fig. 14.8a). The three superficial layers are closely adherent to each other. The layers are:

1. **Skin**
2. **Connective tissue of the superficial fascia**
3. **Aponeurotic layer of occipitofrontalis muscle**
4. **Loose areolar tissue (subaponeurotic layer)**
5. **Pericranium (outer surface of the skull)**

The connective tissue of the superficial fascia is dense. It has many cutaneous nerves and vessels. The walls of the vessels are adherent to the thick connective tissue.

The aponeurotic layer is made up of epicranial aponeurosis (galea aponeurotica) in the central part. In the anterior and posterior quadrants of the scalp it presents a pair of **frontalis** and a pair of **occipitalis** muscles respectively. Both these muscles are supplied by **facial nerve**.

The fourth layer of the scalp is made of loose areolar tissue. It is a potential space over which all the three superficial layers move. This space is traversed by emissary veins. These emissary veins connect the veins out side the skull with intra-cranial veins. These veins are devoid of valves. Hence infection from the scalp may spread into the cranial cavity. This layer of the scalp is called dangerous area of the scalp. Injuries of the scalp can rupture the blood vessels and the blood will accumulate in this area. It can extend up to upper eyelid causing black eye. Blood from the cranial cavity can also spread into this area in accidental injuries involving the fracture of the skull (Fig. 14.8a and b).

### Nerve Supply

The anterior quadrant is supplied by ophthalmic, maxillary and mandibular divisions of the trigeminal nerve. The posterior quadrant is supplied by cervical spinal nerves ($C_2$ to $C_3$).

### Arterial Supply

Scalp is highly vascular and supplied by branches of ophthalmic artery, superficial temporal artery, posterior auricular artery and occipital artery.

### FACE

The muscles of facial expression are subcutaneous muscles. They bring about different facial expressions.

These muscles regulate the three openings situated on the face, namely the palpebral fissure (around eye), the nostrils and the oral fissure (around mouth). Each opening has a sphincter and many dilators (Fig. 14.9a).

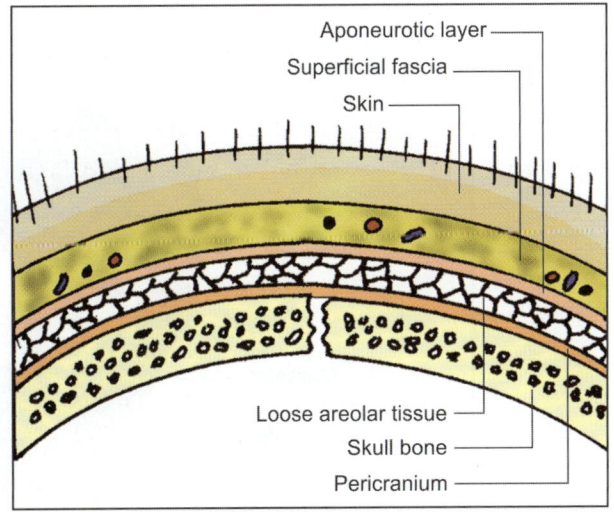

**Fig. 14.8a:** Layers of the scalp

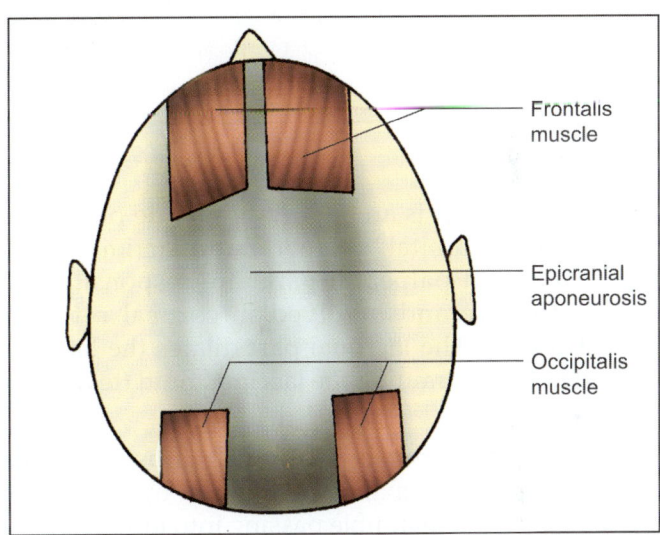

**Fig. 14.8b:** Superior view showing the muscles

### Muscles

| | | |
|---|---|---|
| 1. Palpebral fissure | : | Orbicularis oculi |
| | | Levator palpebrae superioris |
| | | Occipitofrontalis |
| 2. Oral fissure | : | Orbicularis oris |
| | | Levator labii superioris alaeque nasi |
| | | Levator labii superioris |
| | | Levator anguli oris |
| | | Zygomaticus minor and major |
| | | Depressor anguli oris |
| | | Depressor labii inferioris |
| | | Mentalis |
| | | Risorius |
| | | Buccinator (blowing muscle) |
| 3. Nostrils | : | Compressor naris and dilator naris |

14

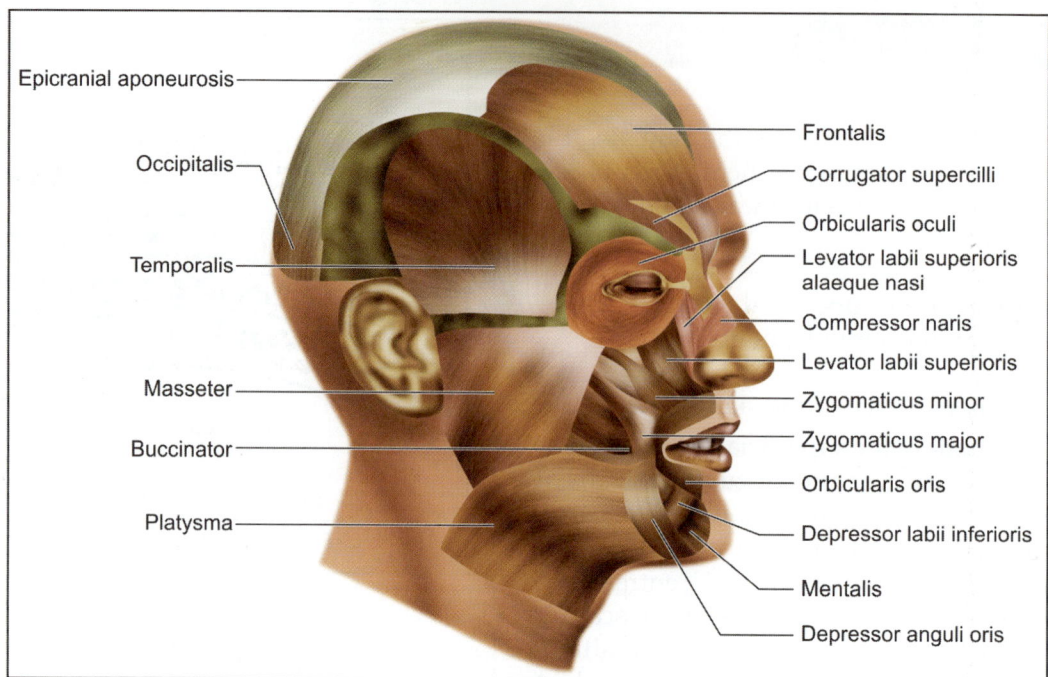

**Fig. 14.9a:** Muscles of the face—lateral view

*Orbicularis oculi:* It is an important muscle protecting the eye. It has orbital, palpebral and lacrimal parts. The orbital and palpebral parts are responsible for closing the eye and involved in corneal reflex to protect cornea. The lacrimal part dilates the lacrimal sac and helps in draining the lacrimal fluid (tears) into the nasal cavity.

*Buccinator muscle:* It is a blowing muscle. It has upper fibers from maxilla passing into upper lip and lower fibers from mandible passing into lower lip. The middle fibers decussate at the angle of the mouth and extend into both upper and lower lips. Externally the muscle is pierced by parotid duct and internally lined by mucous membrane.

All these muscles are supplied by the facial nerve: Injury to this nerve causes Bell's palsy. The corresponding half of the face is paralysed. The face becomes asymmetrical and is drawn up to the normal side. The affected side is motionless. Further details about Bell's palsy is explained in the chapter—cranial nerves.

## SIDE OF THE NECK

The quadrilateral side of the neck is divided into anterior and posterior triangles by the sternocleidomastoid muscle (Fig. 14.9b).

### Posterior Triangle

It is bounded (Fig. 14.10a).

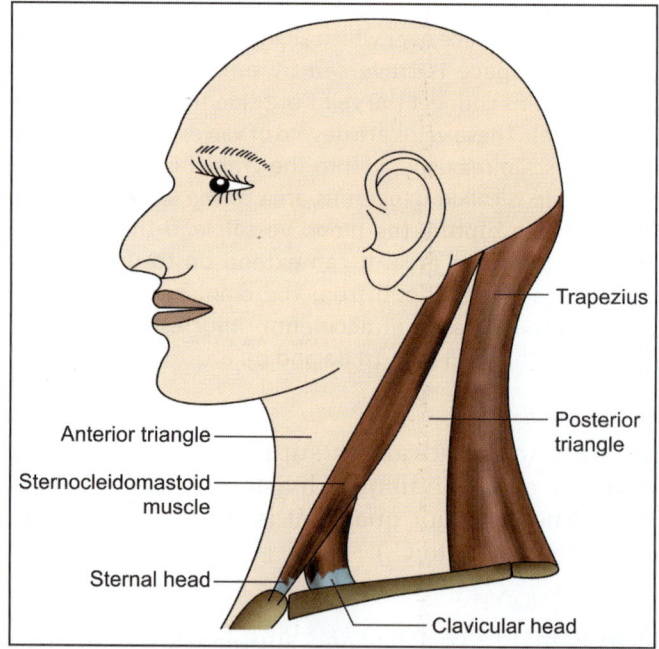

**Fig. 14.9b:** Sternocleidomastoid muscle and boundaries of posterior triangle

*Anteriorly:* Posterior border of sternocleidomastoid muscle.

*Posteriorly:* Anterior border of trapezius muscle

*Inferiorly:* Middle 1/3rd of the clavicle.

*Roof:* It is formed by skin, platysma and **investing layer of deep cervical fascia**. Between platysma and the deep fascia, there are nerves (great auricular nerve, lesser

**14**

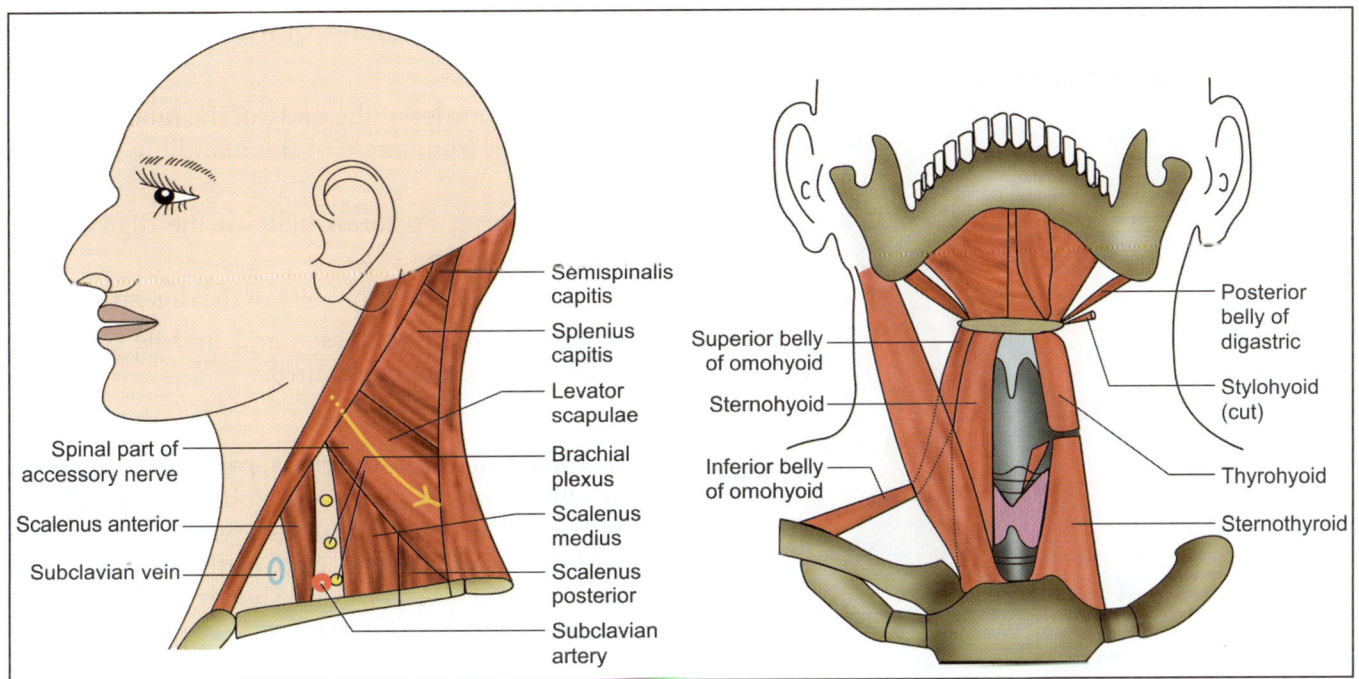

**Fig. 14.10a:** Floor and contents of posterior triangle; Supra and infrahyoid muscles

occipital nerve, transverse cutaneous nerve of the neck and supraclavicular nerve) and external jugular vein.

*Floor:* It presents following muscles:
Splenius capitis
Levator scapulae
Scalenus posterior
Scalenus medius
All these muscles are covered by **prevertebral fascia**.

Inferior belly of omohyoid, further divides the posterior triangle into an upper **occipital triangle** and lower **subclavian (supraclavicular) triangle**.

## Contents

The main contents of the triangle are:
1. Spinal part of the accessory nerve
2. Third part of the subclavian artery
3. Upper trunk of the brachial plexus.

## Sternocleidomastoid Muscle

It is a muscle present on the side of the neck, which divides the neck into an anterior and posterior triangles (Fig. 14.9b).

*Origin:* It takes origin from the upper part of manubrium sternum and medial 1/3rd of the clavicle.

*Insertion:* It is inserted into outer aspect of the mastoid process of the temporal bone and partly extending into superior nuchal line of the occipital bone.

*Nerve supply:* Spinal part of the accessory nerve.

*Actions:* Muscle acting unilaterally (one side) turns the face to the opposite side. Acting bilaterally (of both sides) draw the head forward.

*Torticollis (wryneck):* A condition in which the head is bent to the affected side while the face (or chin) turns to the opposite side. (If the right sternomastoid is paralysed, the face is turned towards the left side and head is tilted towards right side.)

*Congenital torticollis:* It is due to a fibrous tissue tumor in the sternocleidomastoid muscle before or shortly after birth. When torticollis occurs prenatally, the abnormal position of the infant's head requires a breech delivery. The muscle is also injured during child birth by tearing its fibers. A hematoma resulting from the ruptured blood vessels during child birth may develop into a fibrotic mass which entraps spinal accessory nerve. The stiffness and twisting of the neck results from fibrosis and shortening of the sternomastoid muscle.

## Anterior Triangle

It is present in front of the posterior triangle (Fig. 14.10b).

This triangle is further divided into four other triangles (submental triangle, digastric triangle, carotid triangle and muscular triangle).

## Boundaries and Contents of the Carotid Triangle

### Boundaries

*In front and above (anterosuperior):* Posterior belly of the digastric and stylohyoid muscles.

*In front and below (anteroinferior):* Superior belly of the omohyoid.

**14**

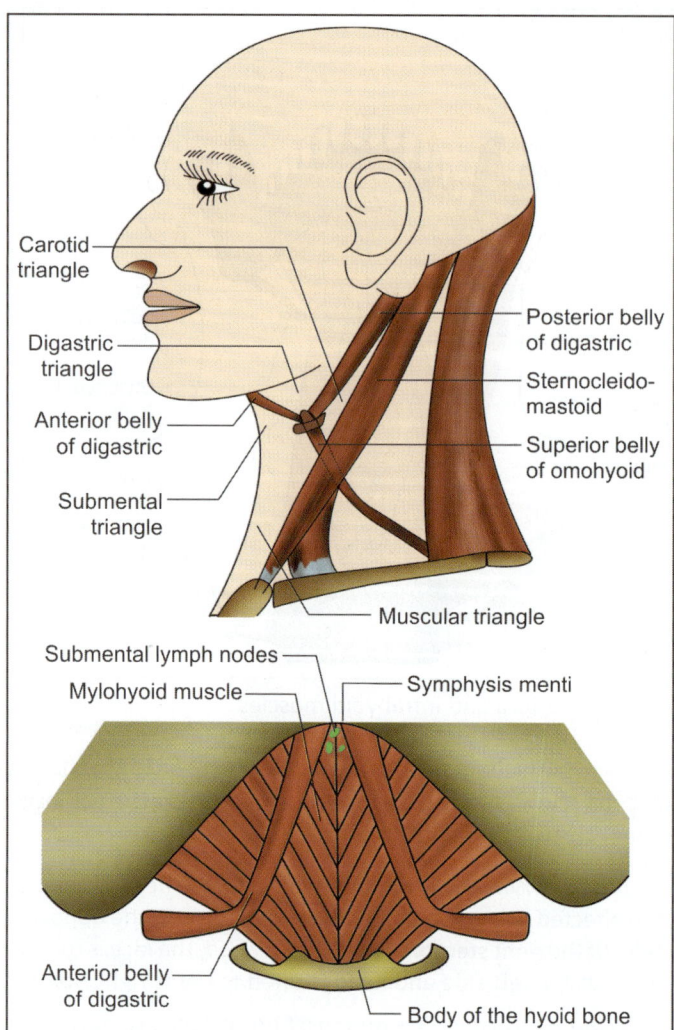

Carotid triangle

Digastric triangle

Anterior belly of digastric

Submental triangle

Posterior belly of digastric

Sternocleido-mastoid

Superior belly of omohyoid

Muscular triangle

Submental lymph nodes

Mylohyoid muscle

Symphysis menti

Anterior belly of digastric

Body of the hyoid bone

**Fig. 14.10b:** Subdivision of anterior triangle; Submental triangle

*Behind (posterior):* Anterior border of the sternomastoid muscle.

*Roof:* Skin, superficial fascia with platysma, investing layer of deep cervical fascia.

*Floor:* Four muscles contribute to the floor. Hyoglossus and thyrohyoid in the anterior part, middle and inferior constrictor muscles of pharynx in the posterior part.

### Contents

1. Common carotid artery and its bifurcation
2. Internal carotid artery
3. External carotid artery and its few branches
4. Internal jugular vein
5. Vagus nerve and its branches
6. Ansa cervicalis
7. Spinal accessory nerve
8. Hypoglossal nerve
9. Deep cervical lymph nodes

## Boundaries and Contents of the Digastric Triangle

### Boundaries

*Above:* Lower border of the body of the mandible and a line extending from angle of the mandible to mastoid process.

*Below and behind:* Posterior belly of the digastric and stylohyoid muscles.

*Below and in front:* Anterior belly of the digastric muscle.

*Floor:* Mylohyoid, hyoglossus and middle constrictor muscles from before backwards.

### Contents

The contents includes superficial part of the submandibular salivary gland, facial vein, submandibular lymph nodes, facial artery, mylohyoid vessels and nerve, hypoglossal nerve, lower part of the parotid gland, external carotid artery, carotid sheath with its contents and glossopharyngeal nerve.

### Infrahyoid Muscles

Following are the infrahyoid muscles: Sternohyoid, sternothyroid, thyrohyoid and omohyoid.

These muscles are also called strap muscles of the neck or extrinsic muscles of the larynx.

They are all supplied by ansa cervicalis (ventral rami of $C_{1, 2, 3}$).

The digastric triangle (of anterior triangle) presents following muscles (suprahyoid muscles) The muscles include digastric, stylohyoid, mylohyoid, geniohyoid and hyoglossus.

The **digastric muscle** presents two bellies. The anterior belly is attached to the mandible. It is supplied by mylohyoid nerve. The posterior belly is attached to the inner aspect of the mastoid process of the skull. It is supplied by facial nerve. The two bellies are connected by an intermediate tendon, which is attached to the hyoid bone.

**Stylohyoid muscle** extends between styloid process of the skull and hyoid bone. It presents two fleshy slips, which encloses the intermediate tendon of the digastric muscle. It is supplied by facial nerve.

**Mylohyoid muscle** of the two sides meet in the midline by a raphae. The right and left mylohyoid muscle together forms the floor of the mouth. It is supplied by mylohyoid nerve (mandibular nerve).

**Muscles of the back of the neck**

This region is called suboccipital region. The following muscles are present in this region:

Trapezius (superficial), splenius capitis, semispinalis capitis, rectus capitis posterior major, rectus capitis posterior minor, obliqus capitis superior and obliqus capitis inferior (deep).

## EXTRAOCULAR MUSCLES

These muscles are present inside the bony orbit. They are attached to the outer covering of the eyeball (sclera), thus being able to move the eyeball (Fig. 14.11a and b).

The muscles are superior and inferior oblique and 4 recti muscles, namely, superior, inferior, medial and lateral rectus (Fig. 14.11c and Table 14.1).

The **recti muscles** arise from a common tendinous ring, which is placed close to the apex of the orbit. The muscles extend forward and are inserted into the sclera in front of the equator of the eyeball.

The **superior oblique** muscle arises from the body of the sphenoid bone. Its tendon passes through a fibrous pulley and then extends backwards to be inserted into the sclera behind the equator of the eyeball.

The **inferior oblique** arises from the infraorbital margin of the maxilla on the medial side. It passes backward and is inserted into the sclera behind the equator.

The levator palpebrae superioris elevates the upper eyelid.

### Applied Anatomy

Paralysis or weakness of the extraocular muscles causes squint eye or strabismus (deviation of the eye to opposite side). It appears that two eyes are looking at different directions. This results in diplopia or double vision
- In congenital squint there is no diplopia.
- Paralysis of lateral rectus muscle produces internal strabismus or medial squint and diplopia on turning the eye laterally.

- Paralysis of medial rectus causes external strabismus or lateral squint and diplopia on turning the eye medially.
- In paralysis of superior oblique, there is no obvious squint, but diplopia occurs on looking down (for example, while coming down the staircase).
- Paralysis of inferior oblique produces diplopia on looking up.
- Paralysis of superior rectus produces diplopia on looking up and inferior rectus produce diplopia on looking down.

**Nystagmus:** It is the rhythmic oscillatory involuntary movement of the eye due to incordination of extraocular muscle.

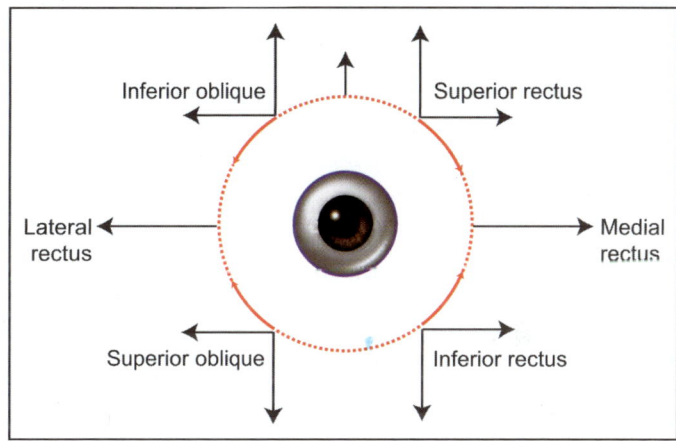

**Fig. 14.11c:** Actions of extraocular muscles

### Intraocular Muscles (Nonstriated Muscles)

1. *Ciliaris:* This muscle is present in the ciliary body of the eyeball. This muscle makes the lens thick while looking at the nearer objects. It is supplied by parasympathetic fibers through oculomotor nerve.

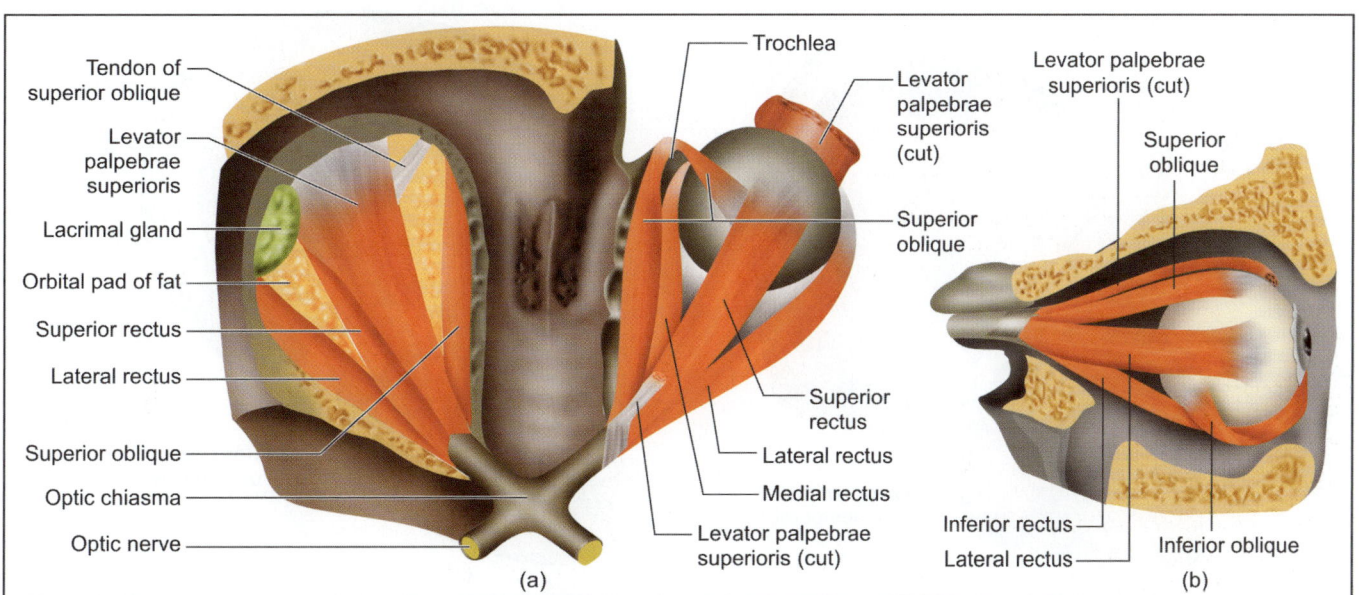

(a)      (b)

**Fig. 14.11a and b:** Extraocular muscles: (a) Superior view; (b) lateral view

14

**Table 14.1:** Nerve supply and actions of the muscle

| Name of the muscle | Nerve supply | Actions of the muscle |
|---|---|---|
| Superior oblique | Trochlear nerve (4th cranial nerve) | Depression of the eyeball Lateral rotation of the eyeball and intorsion |
| Inferior oblique | Oculomotor nerve (3rd cranial nerve) | Elevation of the eyeball Lateral rotation of the eyeball and extorsion |
| Superior rectus | Oculomotor nerve (3rd cranial nerve) | Elevation of the eyeball Medial rotation and intorsion |
| Inferior rectus | Oculomotor nerve (3rd cranial nerve) | Depression of the eyeball Medial rotation of the eyeball and extorsion |
| Medial rectus | Oculomotor nerve (3rd cranial nerve) | Medial rotation of the eyeball (adduction) |
| Lateral rectus | Abducent nerve (6th cranial nerve) | Lateral rotation of the eyeball (abduction) |

2. *Sphincter pupillae:* This muscle is present in the iris of the eyeball. It constricts the pupil when bright light falls on the eye. The muscle is supplied by parasympathetic fibers through oculomotor nerve.

3. *Dilator pupillae:* This muscle is also present in the iris of the eye. It is supplied by sympathetic fibers and it dilates the pupil.

## MUSCLES OF MASTICATION

The main muscles of mastication occupy the temporal and infratemporal fossae. All these muscles act on temporomandibular joint. They are all supplied by the mandibular nerve.

The muscles are—masseter, temporalis, lateral pterygoid and medial pterygoid (Fig. 14.12a to c).

1. *Masseter:* It takes origin from the zygomatic arch and is inserted into the outer surface of the ramus of the mandible. It elevates the mandible.

2. *Temporalis:* It arises from the temporal fossa of the skull and is inserted into coronoid process and anterior border of the ramus of the mandible. It elevates the mandible and its posterior fibers retract the protruded mandible.

3. *Lateral pterygoid:* It has two heads. The upper head arises from crest and infratemporal surface of the greater wing of the sphenoid bone. The lower head arises from lateral surface of the lateral pterygoid

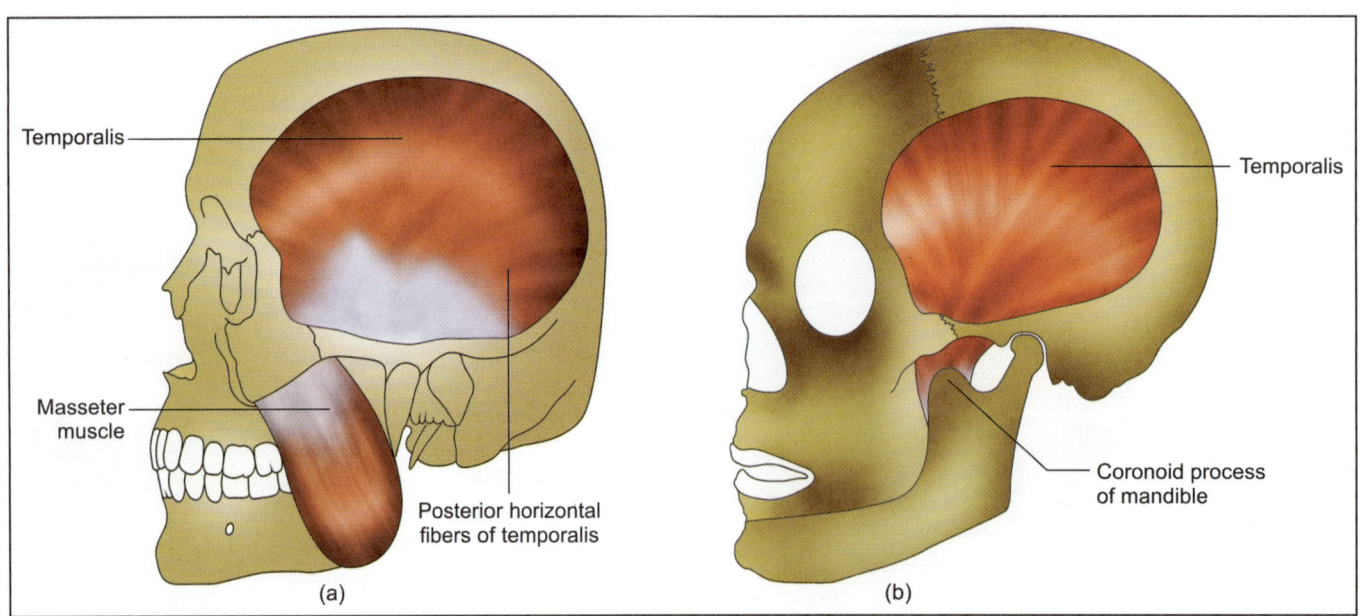

**Fig. 14.12a and b:** (a) Masseter muscle; (b) temporalis muscle

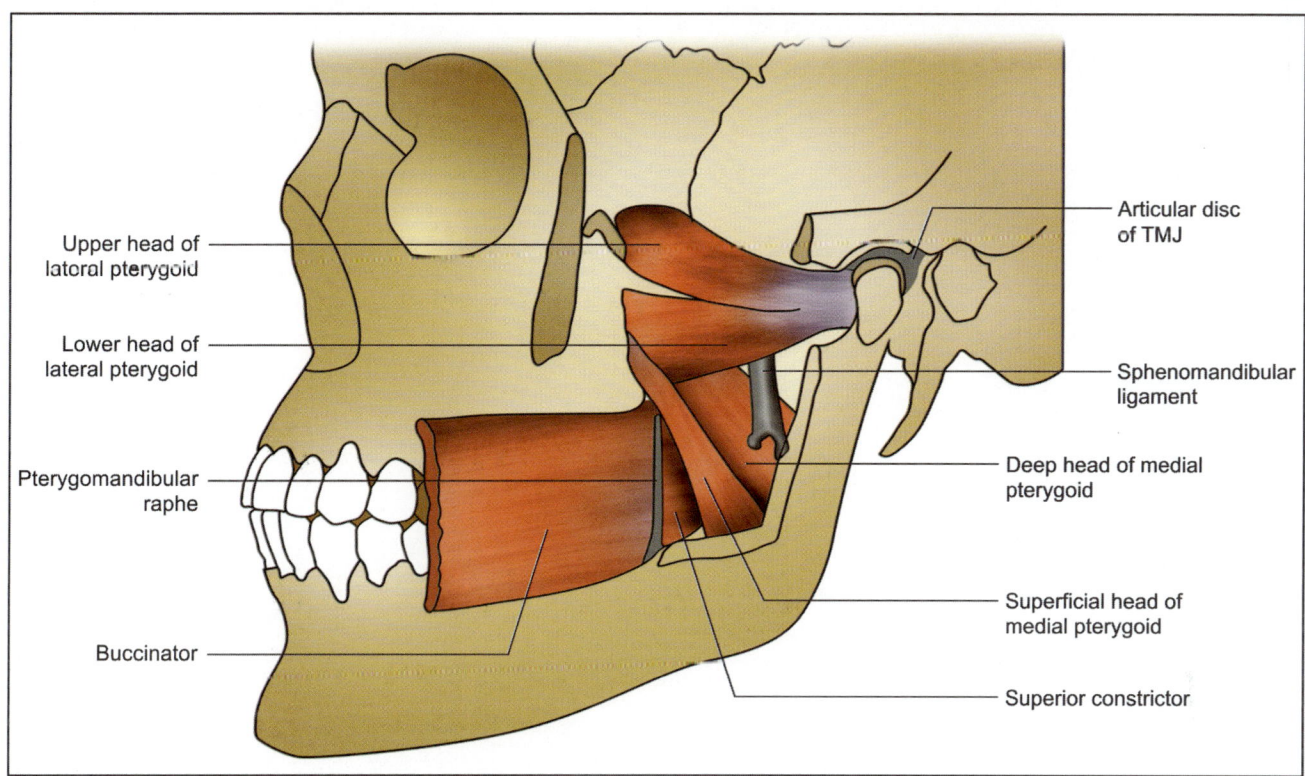

**Fig. 14.12c:** Lateral pterygoid and medial pterygoid muscles

plate. It is inserted into pterygoid fovea of the mandible and capsule and articular disc of the temporomandibular joint (Fig. 14.12c). It depresses the mandible.

4. *Medial pterygoid:* It has two heads. The superficial head arises from maxillary tuberosity and deep head from medial surface of the lateral pterygoid plate. It elevates the mandible.

## Prevertebral Muscles

The following muscles lie in front of the cervical vertebral bodies. Main action of these muscles is flexion of head. The muscles are:

1. Longus colli
2. Longus capitis
3. Rectus capitis anterior
4. Rectus capitis posterior
5. Rectus capitis lateralis

## Soft Palate

It is a muscular fold separating the nasopharynx from the orophanynx. The muscles present in it are explained in Chapter 19.

*Muscles of tongue:* It is explained in Chapter 19.

## Muscles of the Pharynx

The muscular wall of the pharynx consists of an outer circular (constrictors), and an inner longitudinal layer. They are all explained in Chapter 20.

## Muscle of the Larynx

It is explained under Chapter 15.

## Erector Spinae (Sacro-spinalis)

It is an elongated muscle present on the back which extend from the sacrum to the skull. It helps in extension of the vertebral column.

# Self-Assessment Exercise

☞ Select the Single Best Response Questions

☞ Short Note Questions

☞ Brief Essays

☞ Major Questions

## Select the Single Best Response

1. Which of the following statements is correct regarding the clavicle?
   A. It is the only long bone to ossify in membrane
   B. It is the first bone to ossify in the body
   C. It is the only long bone with two primary centers of ossification
   D. All of the above

2. Following are the parts of scapula *except*:
   A. Conoid tubercle    B. Coracoid process
   C. Acromion process  D. Spinous process

3. Which of these nerves is not in direct contact with humerus?
   A. Ulnar nerve        B. Axillary nerve
   C. Median nerve       D. Radial nerve

4. The lesser tubercle of the humerus receives the insertion of:
   A. Supraspinatus      B. Subscapularis
   C. Pectoralis minor   D. Teres minor

5. The axillary nerve winds around:
   A. Morphological neck of the humerus
   B. Surgical neck of the humerus
   C. Anatomical neck of the humerus
   D. Spiral groove of the humerus

6. The capitulum of the humerus articulates with:
   A. Head of the ulna
   B. Head of the radius
   C. Coronoid process of the ulna
   D. Olecranon process of the ulna

7. The tuberosity of the radius receives the insertion of:
   A. Brachialis         B. Brachioradialis
   C. Biceps brachii     D. Coracobrachialis

8. Which of the following bones is involved in Colles' fracture:
   A. Ulna               B. Humerus
   C. Scapula            D. Radius

9. The tuberosity of the ulna is a part of:
   A. Coronoid process
   B. Head of the ulna
   C. Olecranon process
   D. Styloid process

10. The ulnar tuberosity receives the insertion of:
    A. Brachioradialis   B. Brachialis
    C. Biceps brachii    D. Coracobrachialis

11. Which of the following carpal bones is more prone for fracture?
    A. Lunate            B. Trapezoid
    C. Scaphoid          D. Trapezium

12. Which of these carpal bones is a sesamoid bone?
    A. Hamate            B. Triquetral
    C. Pisiform          D. Capitate

13. Bennett's fracture involves
    A. Distal end of the 5th metacarpal bone
    B. Lower end of the radius
    C. Lower end of the ulna
    D. Base of the 1st metacarpal bone

14. Pubic tubercle is the:
    A. Medial end of the pubic crest
    B. Lateral end of the pubic crest
    C. Midpoint of the pubic symphysis
    D. Lateral end of the obturator crest

15. The highest point of the iliac crest is situated at the level of the interval between the spines of:
    A. $L_1$ and $L_2$ vertebrae
    B. $L_2$ and $L_3$ vertebrae
    C. $L_3$ and $L_4$ vertebrae
    D. $L_4$ and $L_5$ vertebrae

16. The anterior inferior iliac spine provides attachments to the:
    A. Reflected head of the rectus femoris muscle
    B. Sartorius
    C. Iliofemoral ligament
    D. Inguinal ligament

17. Which of these muscles is not attached to the ischial tuberosity?
    A. Semitendinosus
    B. Short head of the biceps femoris
    C. Adductor magnus
    D. Semimembranosus

18. Following muscles are inserted to greater trochanter of the femur *except*:
    A. Piriformis
    B. Gluteus minimus
    C. Obturator internus
    D. Quadriceps femoris

19. Which of these bones does not articulate with femur?
    A. Tibia             B. Fibula
    C. Patella           D. Hip bone

20. **A groove on the posterior aspect of the medial condyle of the tibia receives the insertion of:**
    A. Semimembranosus
    B. Semitendinosus
    C. Sartorius
    D. Gracilis

21. **The tibial tuberosity receives the attachment of:**
    A. Tibial collateral ligament
    B. Fibular collateral ligament
    C. Ligamentum patellae
    D. Anterior cruciate ligament

22. **Which of these muscles is inserted into fibula?**
    A. Peroneus brevis
    B. Peroneus longus
    C. Biceps femoris
    D. Adductor magnus

23. **The lateral malleolus articulates with:**
    A. Cuboid
    B. Tibia
    C. Talus
    D. Calcaneum

24. **Which of these nerves winds round the neck of the fibula?**
    A. Tibial nerve
    B. Common peroneal nerve
    C. Deep peroneal nerve
    D. Superficial peroneal nerve

25. **Following are the tarsal bones, *except*:**
    A. Cuboid
    B. Navicular
    C. Talus
    D. Trapezoid

26. **Sustentaculum tali is a part of:**
    A. Talus bone
    B. Calcaneum bone
    C. Cuboid bone
    D. Medial cuneiform bone

27. **Talus articulates with following bones except:**
    A. Tibia
    B. Fibula
    C. Navicular
    D. Cuboid

28. **Tuberosity of the navicular bone receives the insertion of:**
    A. Tibialis anterior
    B. Tibialis posterior
    C. Peroneus longus
    D. Tendocalcaneus

29. **The groove on the plantar surface of the cuboid is traversed by:**
    A. Tendon of the peroneus longus
    B. Tendon of the peroneus brevis
    C. Plantar arterial arch
    D. Medial plantar nerve

30. **The medial cuneiform bone receives the insertion of:**
    A. Tibialis anterior
    B. Peroneus brevis
    C. Peroneus tertius
    D. Tibialis posterior

31. **Following are the movements brought by pectoralis major muscle at shoulder joint *except*:**
    A. Medial rotation
    B. Flexion
    C. Abduction
    D. Adduction

32. **'Winging of the scapula' is due to the paralysis of:**
    A. Latissimus dorsi muscle
    B. Teres major muscle
    C. Trapezius muscle
    D. Serratus anterior muscle

33. **Which of the following statements is incorrect regarding the female breast?**
    A. It is a modified sebaceous gland
    B. It lies in the deep fascia
    C. Its suspensory ligaments extend between the skin and the pectoral fascia
    D. Unilateral cancer of the breast may become bilateral through lymphatics

34. **Following are the movements brought by latissimus dorsi muscle at shoulder joint *except*:**
    A. Abduction
    B. Adduction
    C. Medial rotation
    D. Extension

35. **Which of these muscles is not inserted into the greater tuberosity of the humerus?**
    A. Teres minor
    B. Infraspinatus
    C. Supraspinatus
    D. Subscapularis

36. **Branches from the posterior cord of the brachial plexus supply following muscles *except*:**
    A. Latissimus dorsi
    B. Subscapularis
    C. Teres major
    D. Coracobrachialis

37. **Which of the following statements is incorrect regarding the deltoid muscle?**
    A. It is supplied by axillary nerve
    B. Its middle fibers are multipennate
    C. Its middle fibers bring adduction at the shoulder joint
    D. It is inserted into the deltoid tuberosity of the humerus

38. **Which of these structures enter the axilla from the neck region?**
    A. Axillary vein
    B. Brachial plexus
    C. Cephalic vein
    D. Axillary lymph nodes

39. **Which of the following statements is correct regarding the biceps brachii muscle?**
    A. Its long head arises from coracoid process of scapula
    B. It is inserted into ulnar tuberosity
    C. It is supplied by the ulnar nerve
    D. It brings about supination of the forearm

40. **Which of the following statements is incorrect regarding the triceps muscle?**
    A. Its long head arises from supraglenoid tubercle of the humerus
    B. It is supplied by radial nerve
    C. It is inserted into the olecranon process of ulna
    D. It causes extension at the elbow joint

41. **Following are the contents of the cubital fossa** *except*:
    A. Median nerve
    B. Ulnar nerve
    C. Tendon of biceps brachii
    D. Brachial artery

42. **The ulnar nerve supplies:**
    A. Flexor digitorum superficialis
    B. Pronator teres
    C. Flexor carpi ulnaris
    D. None of the above

43. **Which of these muscles is not supplied by the posterior interosseous nerve?**
    A. Extensor digitorum
    B. Extensor carpi ulnaris
    C. Extensor carpi radialis longus
    D. Extensor digiti minimi

44. **Which of these muscles is not supplied by the deep terminal branch of the ulnar nerve?**
    A. Adductor pollicis
    B. Abductor pollicis brevis
    C. Third lumbrical
    D. First palmar interosseous

45. **Which of the following muscles is not acting on both hip joint and knee joint?**
    A. Biceps femoris
    B. Sartorius
    C. Adductor magnus
    D. Rectus femoris

46. **Which of these movements at hip joint is brought about by sartorius?**
    A. Flexion
    B. Lateral rotation
    C. Abduction
    D. All of the above

47. **Following muscles are supplied by femoral nerve** *except*:
    A. Sartorius
    B. Iliacus
    C. Quadratus femoris
    D. Pectineus

48. **Femoral canal is the:**
    A. Lateral compartment of the femoral sheath
    B. Intermediate compartment of the femoral sheath
    C. Medial compartment of the femoral sheath
    D. Apex of the femoral triangle

49. **Which of these structures bounds the adductor canal?**
    A. Vastus medialis
    B. Vastus intermedius
    C. Vastus lateralis
    D. Rectus femoris

50. **Following are the contents of adductor canal** *except*:
    A. Nerve to vastus medialis
    B. Nerve to vastus lateralis
    C. Saphenous nerve
    D. Posterior division of the obturator nerve

51. **Which of the following statements is incorrect regarding the hamstring muscles?**
    A. They extend the hip joint
    B. They are all supplied by sciatic nerve
    C. They are all inserted into tibia
    D. They take origin from ischial tuberosity

52. **The superior gluteal nerve supplies following** *except*:
    A. Gluteus medius    B. Gluteus minimus
    C. Gluteus maximus   D. Tensor fascia lata

53. **The hamstring part of the adductor magnus muscle is inserted into:**
    A. Tibia        B. Femur
    C. Fibula       D. Patella

54. **Hiatus magnus connects:**
    A. Femoral triangle and adductor canal
    B. Femoral triangle and popliteal fossa
    C. Adductor canal and popliteal fossa
    D. Popliteal fossa and back of the leg

55. **Which of these muscles is not supplied by deep peroneal nerve?**
    A. Tibialis anterior
    B. Extensor hallucis longus
    C. Extensor digitorum longus
    D. Peroneus brevis

56. **Which of the following statements is incorrect?**
    A. 'Hammer toe' results due to paralysis of lumbricals
    B. 'Flat foot' occurs when medial longitudinal arch drops
    C. In 'talipes equinus' patient walks on the heel with raised forefoot
    D. 'Footdrop' results from damage of common peroneal nerve

57. **Sternoclavicular joint is an example for:**
    A. Saddle variety of synovial joint
    B. Condylar variety of synovial joint
    C. Ellipsoid variety of synovial joint
    D. Hinge variety of synovial joint

58. **Which of these structures is present inside the shoulder joint cavity?**
    A. Coracohumeral ligament
    B. Tendon of the long head of the biceps
    C. Tendon of the long head of the triceps
    D. None of the above

59. **Following muscles contribute to the rotator cuff around shoulder joint, *except*:**
    A. Supraspinatus       B. Subscapularis
    C. Teres major         D. Infraspinatus

60. **Downward dislocation of humerus at the shoulder joint can damage:**
    A. Radial nerve        B. Axillary nerve
    C. Median nerve        D. Ulnar nerve

61. **Which of these ligaments is involved in 'tennis elbow'?**
    A. Radial collateral ligament
    B. Ulnar collateral ligament
    C. Annular ligament
    D. Quadrate ligament

62. **Which of these bones does not take part in radiocarpal joint?**
    A. Scaphoid            B. Lunate
    C. Triquetral          D. Ulna

63. **Which of the following statements is incorrect regarding the knee joint?**
    A. Tibial collateral ligament is separated from the medial meniscus by tendon of popliteus
    B. Ligamentum patellae is attached to tibial tuberosity
    C. The fibrous capsule is absent in the anterior aspect
    D. The medial meniscus is semilunar in shape

64. **Which of the following statements is incorrect regarding the cruciate ligaments of the knee joint?**
    A. Posterior cruciate ligament is attached to medial condyle of femur
    B. Anterior cruciate ligament is stretched during extension
    C. Anterior cruciate ligament is more prone for injury
    D. Posterior cruciate ligament prevents the forward displacement of the tibial condyles.

65. **The knee joint is unlocked by:**
    A. Quadriceps femoris
    B. Semimembranosus
    C. Popliteus
    D. Gastrocnemius

66. **The inferior tibiofibular joint is an example for:**
    A. Synovial jont
    B. Primary cartilaginous joint
    C. Secondary cartilaginous joint
    D. Fibrous joint

67. **The upper trunk of the brachial plexus gives:**
    A. Musculocutaneous nerve
    B. Nerve to serratus anterior
    C. Nerve to subclavius
    D. Long thoracic nerve

68. **Which of these nerves is not a branch from the posterior cord of the brachial plexus?**
    A. Dorsal scapular nerve
    B. Subscapular nerve
    C. Thoracodorsal nerve
    D. Axillary nerve

69. **An injury to the $C_8$ and $T_1$ nerve roots results in:**
    A. Erb's paralysis
    B. Klumpke's paralysis
    C. Winging of scapula
    D. Wrist drop

70. **Musculocutaneous nerve supplies following muscles:**
    A. Brachialis          B. Biceps brachii
    C. Coracobrachialis    D. All of the above

71. **Which of the following nerves supply only one muscle:**
    A. Nerve to rhomboideus
    B. Lower subscapular nerve
    C. Thoracodorsal nerve
    D. Axillary nerve

72. Which of the following statements is **incorrect** regarding median nerve?
    A. The lateral cord of the brachial plexus provides $C_8$ and $T_1$ fibers
    B. In the cubital fossa it lies medial to the brachial artery
    C. It enters the palm by passing deep to the flexor retinaculum
    D. It does not give any muscular branches in the arm

73. Which of the following statements is **incorrect** regarding the ulnar nerve?
    A. It is a branch from the medial cord of the brachial plexus
    B. It passes behind the medial epicondyle of the humerus
    C. It enters the palm by passing superficial to the flexor retinaculum
    D. Injury to the ulnar nerve results in carpal tunnel syndrome

74. Which of the following statements is **incorrect** regarding the radial nerve?
    A. It is a branch from the posterior cord of the brachial plexus
    B. It supplies all the extensor muscles of the arm and forearm
    C. Injury to the radial nerve results in 'wrist drop'
    D. In the spiral groove, it is accompanied by posterior circumflex humeral artery

75. Saphenous nerve is a branch of:
    A. Femoral nerve
    B. Obturator nerve
    C. Sciatic nerve
    D. Tibial nerve

76. Following are the muscles supplied by obturator nerve **except**:
    A. Gracilis          B. Obturator internus
    C. Adductor longus   D. Adductor brevis

77. Which of the following statements is **incorrect** regarding the sciatic nerve?
    A. Its peroneal component is derived from ventral rami of $L_4$, $L_5$, $S_1$ and $S_2$
    B. It enters the gluteal region through greater sciatic foramen
    C. All the hamstring muscles are supplied by its peroneal component
    D. At the back of the thigh, it is crossed superficially by long head of biceps femoris muscle.

78. All the muscles of back of the leg are supplied by:
    A. Deep peroneal nerve
    B. Common peroneal nerve
    C. Superficial peroneal nerve
    D. None of the above

79. Sural nerve is a branch of:
    A. Tibial nerve
    B. Common peroneal nerve
    C. Superficial peroneal nerve
    D. Deep peroneal nerve

80. Axillary artery is the continuation of:
    A. Brachial artery
    B. Subclavian artery
    C. Arch of aorta
    D. Ulnar artery

81. Following are the branches of axillary artery **except**:
    A. Posterior circumflex humeral artery
    B. Lateral thoracic artery
    C. Profunda brachii artery
    D. Thoracoacromial artery

82. Peroneal artery is a branch of:
    A. Popliteal artery
    B. Anterior tibial artery
    C. Posterior tibial artery
    D. Femoral artery

83. Blood in the median cubital vein passes from:
    A. Cephalic to basilic vein
    B. Basilic to cephalic vein
    C. Basilic to axillary vein
    D. Cephalic to axillary vein

84. Which of the following statements is **incorrect**?
    A. Femoral artery traverses both adductor and femoral canals
    B. Popliteal artery is the continuation of femoral artery
    C. Plantar arch is the continuation of lateral plantar artery
    D. Dorsalis pedis artery contributes to the plantar arch

85. Which of the following statements is **incorrect**?
    A. Great saphenous vein terminates into femoral vein
    B. Small saphenous vein terminates into popliteal vein
    C. Blood in the perforating veins passes from deep veins to superficial veins
    D. Femoral vein is enclosed in femoral sheath

86. Cervical vertebrae are characterised by the:
    A. Presence of mamillary and accessory processes
    B. Presence of facets on their body
    C. Presence of foramina in their transverse processes
    D. Quadrangular spinous process

87. Which of these vertebra does not have the body?
    A. First lumbar vertebra
    B. Fifth lumbar vertebra
    C. All the sacral vertebrae
    D. First cervical vertebra

88. Which of the following statements is incorrect regarding the typical thoracic vertebrae?
    A. The vertebral foramen is circular
    B. Its inferior articular facet is directed laterally
    C. The body presents four costal facets
    D. The body is heart shaped

89. The sacral canal contains the following structures *execept*:
    A. Cauda equina      B. Conus medullaris
    C. Spinal menings    D. All of the above

90. A condition in which the vertebral column is laterally flexed is called?
    A. Kyphosis          B. Lordosis
    C. Scoliosis         D. None of the above

91. Which of these bones is not an unpaired bone of the skull?
    A. Palatine bone     B. Vomer
    C. Ethmoid           D. Mandible

92. The suture between the occipital and the two parietal bone is:
    A. Coronal           B. Sagittal
    C. Lambdoid          D. Metopic

93. Anterior fontanelle of the skull is located at:
    A. Bregma            B. Lambda
    C. Vertex            D. Pterion

94. The meeting point of frontal, parietal, sphenoid and temporal bone is:
    A. Bregma            B. Pterion
    C. Asterion          D. Vertex

95. Foramen ovale of the skull transmits:
    A. Ophthalmic nerve  B. Maxillary nerve
    C. Mandibular nerve  D. Facial nerve

96. Jugular foramen of the skull transmits the following structures *except*:
    A. Glossopharyngeal nerve
    B. Vagus nerve

    C. Hypoglossal nerve
    D. Sigmoid sinus

97. The air sinus below the pituitary fossa of skull is:
    A. Sphenoidal air sinus
    B. Maxillary air sinus
    C. Ethmoidal air sinus
    D. Mastoid air cells

98. Foramen rotundum transmits:
    A. Ophthalmic nerve  B. Maxillary nerve
    C. Mandibular nerve  D. Facial nerve

99. The mandibular canal is traversed by:
    A. Mandibular nerve
    B. Mylohyoid nerve
    C. Inferior alveolar nerve
    D. Lingual nerve

100. The pterygoid fovea of the mandible receives the insertion of:
    A. Masseter musle
    B. Temporalis muscle
    C. Lateral pterygoid muscle
    D. Medial pterygoid muscle

101. The coronoid process of the mandible receives the insertion of:
    A. Masseter muscle
    B. Temporalis muscle
    C. Lateral pterygoid muscle
    D. Medial pterygoid muscle

102. The sternal angle corresponds to:
    A. First costal cartilage
    B. Medial end of the clavicle
    C. Second costal cartilage
    D. Third costal cartilage

103. The upper facet on the head of the typical rib articulates with:
    A. Body of the vertebra above
    B. Body of corresponding vertebra
    C. Transverse process of the vertebra above
    D. Transverse process of the corresponding vertebra

104. Which of the following statements is incorrect regarding the first rib?
    A. The head presents only one facet
    B. It is the most curved rib
    C. It has an outer and inner surface
    D. The shaft has no costal groove

**105. The central tendon of the diaphragm presents:**
A. Vena caval opening
B. Aortic opening
C. Esophageal opening
D. Foramen of Morgagni

**106. Following structures pass through the esophageal opening** *except*:
A. Vagus nerve
B. Esophagus
C. Esophageal branch of the left gastric artery
D. Greater splanchnic nerve

**107. The aortic opening of the diaphragm is situated at the level of:**
A. 12th thoracic vertebra
B. 10th thoracic vertebra
C. 8th thoracic vertebra
D. 6th thoracic vertebra

**108. The sternocleidomastoid muscle is supplied by:**
A. Cranial part of the accessory nerve
B. Spinal part of the accessory nerve
C. Hypoglossal nerve
D. Facial nerve

**109. The lateral rectus muscle of the eye is supplied by:**
A. Oculomotor nerve
B. Trochlear nerve
C. Abducent nerve
D. Nasociliary nerve

**110. The pituitary fossa is present in:**
A. Temporal bone
B. Sphenoid bone
C. Parietal bone
D. Frontal bone

**111. The foramen spinosum of the skull transmits:**
A. Mandibular nerve
B. Middle meningeal artery
C. Accessory meningeal artery
D. Maxillary nerve

**112. Which of these nerves provides motor fibers to diaphragm?**
A. Intercostal nerve
B. Vagus nerve
C. Phrenic nerve
D. Sympathetic nerve

**113. Inguinal ligament is a part of:**
A. Rectus abdominis
B. External oblique muscle of abdomen
C. Deep fascia of the abdomen
D. Transversus abdominis muscle

**114. Deep inguinal ring is an opening present in the:**
A. Aponeurosis of the external oblique muscle of abdomen
B. Fascia transversalis
C. Rectus sheath
D. Deep fascia of the abdomen

**115. The internal oblique muscle of the abdomen contributes to the following walls of the inguinal canal** *except*:
A. Anterior wall
B. Posterior wall
C. Roof
D. Floor

**116. Following are the contents of spermatic cord** *except*:
A. Testicular artery
B. Cremastric artery
C. Ilioinguinal nerve
D. Genital branch of the genitofemoral nerve

**117. The dangerous layer of the scalp is:**
A. First layer
B. Second layer
C. Third layer
D. Fourth layer

**118. The muscles of the scalp are supplied by:**
A. Ophthalmic nerve
B. Facial nerve
C. Mandibular nerve
D. Maxillary nerve

**119. Which of the following structures is not a content of the posterior triangle?**
A. Subclavian vein
B. Subclavian artery
C. Upper trunk of the brachial plexus
D. Spinal part of the accessory nerve

**120. Following are the suprahyoid muscles** *except*:
A. Stylohyoid
B. Mylohyoid
C. Thyrohyoid
D. Geniohyoid

**121. Which of the following statements is incorrect regarding the superior oblique muscle of the orbit?**
A. It is inserted into the sclera of the eyeball behind the equator
B. It depresses the eyeball
C. It is supplied by trochlear nerve
D. It rotates the eye medially

**122. Which of the following muscles is required for near vision?**
A. Ciliaris
B. Dilator pupillae
C. Superior oblique
D. Inferior oblique

123. **Which of these muscles depresses the mandible?**
    A. Masseter        B. Temporalis
    C. Lateral pterygoid   D. Medial pterygoid

124. **The superficial peroneal nerve supplies:**
    A. Tibialis anterior    B. Tibialis posterior
    C. Peroneus longus    D. Peroneus tertius

125. **The nerve to popliteus is a branch of:**
    A. Common peroneal nerve
    B. Deep peroneal nerve
    C. Tibial nerve
    D. Superficial peroneal nerve

126. **The median atlantoaxial joint is an example for:**
    A. Pivot synovial joint
    B. Ellipsoid synovial joint
    C. Fibrous joint
    D. Secondary cartilaginous joint

127. **The articular disc of the temporomandibular joint is made up of:**
    A. Fibrous tissue       B. Fibrocartilage
    C. Compact bone       D. Loose connective tissue

## Short Note Questions (3 marks)

1. Pecularities of the clavicle
2. Carpal bones
3. Hip bone
4. Greater trochanter of the femur
5. Patella
6. Calcaneum
7. Talus
8. Biceps brachii muscle
9. Deltoid
10. Triceps
11. Flexor retinaculum of the hand
12. Axillary artery
13. Brachial artery
14. Lower end of the humerus
15. Radius
16. Ulna
17. Upper end of the tibia
18. Fibula
19. Lumbrical muscles of the hand
20. Interosseous muscles of the hand
21. Cephalic vein
22. Median cubital vein
23. Quadriceps femoris
24. Gluteus maximus
25. Gluteus medius and minimus muscles
26. Adductor magnus muscle
27. Femoral artery
28. Dorsalis pedis artery
29. Great saphenous vein
30. Subtalar joint
31. Femoral nerve
32. Obturator nerve
33. Vertebral column deformities
34. Thoracic cage
35. Sternocleidomostoid muscle
36. Rectus sheath
37. Inguinal ligament
38. Minor openings of the diaphragm
39. Intercostal muscles
40. Spermatic cord
41. Atlantoaxial joint
42. Intervertebral joint
43. Femoral sheath
44. Sternoclavicular joint
45. Articulation of wrist joint
46. Cruciate ligaments of the knee joint
47. Menisci of the knee joint
48. Axillary nerve
49. Musculocutaneous nerve
50. Atlas
51. Normal curvature of the vertebral column
52. Sternum
53. First rib
54. Pituitary fossa
55. Intervertebral disc
56. Articular disc of the temporomandibular joint
57. Radioulnar joints
58. Typical cervical vertebrae
59. Typical thoracic vertebrae
60. Typical lumbar vertebrae
61. Sacrum
62. Typical rib

## Brief Essays (5 or 6 marks)

1. Enumerate the boundaries and contents of femoral triangle.
2. Enumerate the boundaries and contents of posterior triangle of the neck.
3. Enumerate the boundaries and contents of the popliteal fossA.
4. Give a brief account of the temporomandibular joint.

5. Give a brief account of the origin, insertion, actions and nerve supply of extraocular muscles.
6. Write briefly about elbow joint.
7. Write briefly about arches of foot. List the major foot deformities.
8. Give an account of the superficial veins of the upper limB. Give their clinical significance.
9. Give an account of the superficial veins of the lower limB. Give their clinical significance.
10. Given an account of the attachments, actions and nerve supply of hamstring muscles.
11. Enumerate the boundaries and contents of the adductor canal.
12. Enumerate the boundaries and contents of the cubital fossa.
13. Write briefly about the articulation, movements and muscles involved in radioulnar joints.
14. Enumerate the boundaries and contents of axilla
15. Give an account of the layers of the scalp.
16. Give an account of the boundaries and contents of the inguinal canal. Add a note on inguinal herniA.
17. Define a typical intercostal space. Enumerate the contents of the space in brief.
18. Discuss briefly about the ankle joint.
19. Give an account of the attachment, nerve supply and actions of gluteus maximus. List the structrues present deep to it.
20. Discuss the different movemernts of the scapulA.
21. Give an account of the origin, root value, course and distribution of femoral nerve
22. Give an account of the origin, root value, course and distribution of obturator nerve.
23. Name the extraocular muscles of the eye. Give their nerve supply and actions.
24. Give an account of attachment, nerve supply and actions of muscles of mastication.
25. Discuss the temporomandibular joint under—
   A. Type
   B. Bones articulating
   C. Structures stabilising
   D. Movements and muscles producing them.

## Major Questions (10 marks)

1. Name the bones of the upper limB. Give their specific articulation mentioning the names of the joint. (3+7)
2. Name the bones of the lower limB. Give their specific articulation mentioning the names of the joint. (3+7)

3. Discuss the shoulder joint under—
   A. Bones articulating
   B. Structures stabilising
   C. Movements and muscles producing them
   (1+4+5)
4. Discuss the hip joint under—
   A. Bones articulating
   B. Structures stabilizing
   C. Movements and muscles producing them
   (1+3+6)
5. Discuss the knee joint under—
   A. Bones articulating
   B. Structures stabilising
   C. Movements and muscles producing them
   (1+6+3)
6. With the help of a diagram, give an account of the formation and branches of brachial plexus.
7. Give an account of the origin, course, branches and distribution of median nerve. Add a note on its applied aspect. (1+3+5+1)
8. Give an account of the origin, course, branches and distribution of ulnar nerve. Add a note on its applied aspect. (1+3+5+1)
9. Give an account of the origin, course, branches and distribution of radial nerve. Add a note on its applied aspect. (1+3+5+1)
10. Give an account of the origin, course, branches and distribution of sciatic nerve. Add a note on its applied aspect. (1+3+5+1)
11. Give an account of the origin, course, branches and distribution of common peroneal nerve. Add a note on its applied aspect. (1+3+5+1)
12. Give an account of the attachment, major openings, nerve supply and functions of the diaphragm.
   (5+3+1+1)

## Answers to Single Best Response Questions

| | | | | | |
|---|---|---|---|---|---|
| 1. D | 2. A | 3. C | 4. B | 5. B | 6. B |
| 7. C | 8. D | 9. A | 10. B | 11. C | 12. C |
| 13. D | 14. B | 15. C | 16. C | 17. B | 18. D |
| 19. B | 20. A | 21. C | 22. C | 23. C | 24. B |
| 25. D | 26. B | 27. D | 28. B | 29. A | 30. A |
| 31. C | 32. D | 33. B | 34. A | 35. D | 36. D |
| 37. C | 38. B | 39. D | 40. A | 41. B | 42. C |
| 43. C | 44. B | 45. C | 46. D | 47. C | 48. C |
| 49. A | 50. B | 51. C | 52. C | 53. B | 54. C |
| 55. D | 56. C | 57. A | 58. B | 59. C | 60. B |
| 61. A | 62. D | 63. A | 64. D | 65. C | 66. D |
| 67. C | 68. A | 69. B | 70. D | 71. C | 72. A |

| | | | | | | | | | | | |
|---|---|---|---|---|---|---|---|---|---|---|---|
| 73. D | 74. D | 75. A | 76. B | 77. C | 78. D | 103. A | 104. C | 105. A | 106. D | 107. A | 108. B |
| 79. A | 80. B | 81. C | 82. C | 83. A | 84. A | 109. C | 110. B | 111. B | 112. C | 113. B | 114. B |
| 85. C | 86. C | 87. D | 88. B | 89. B | 90. C | 115. D | 116. C | 117. D | 118. B | 119. A | 120. C |
| 91. A | 92. C | 93. A | 94. B | 95. C | 96. C | 121. D | 122. A | 123. C | 124. C | 125. C | 126. A |
| 97. A | 98. B | 99. C | 100. C | 101. B | 102. C | 127. B | | | | | |

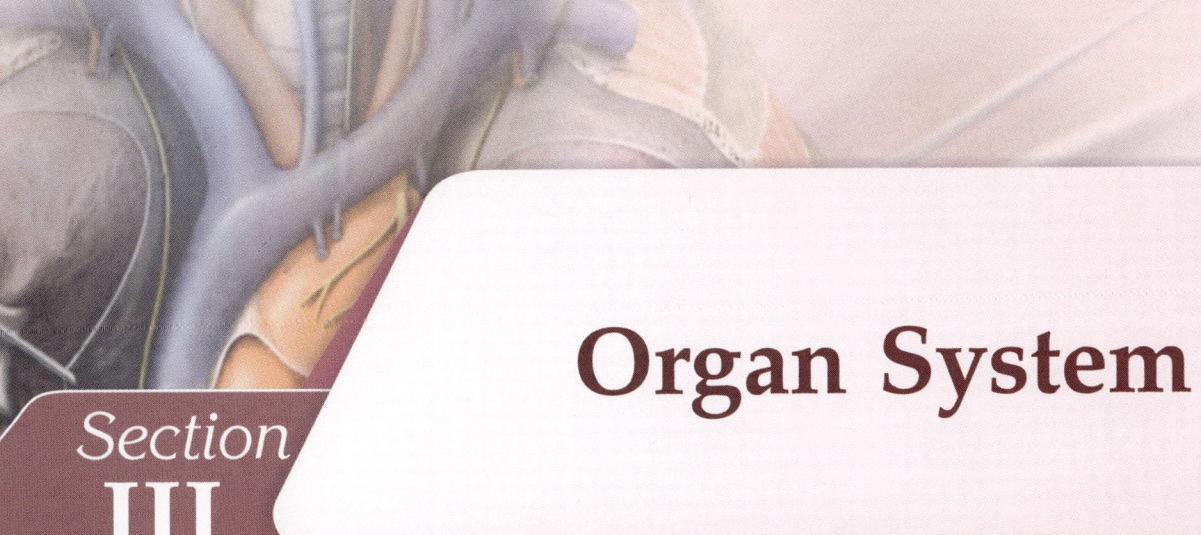

# Organg System

**Section III**

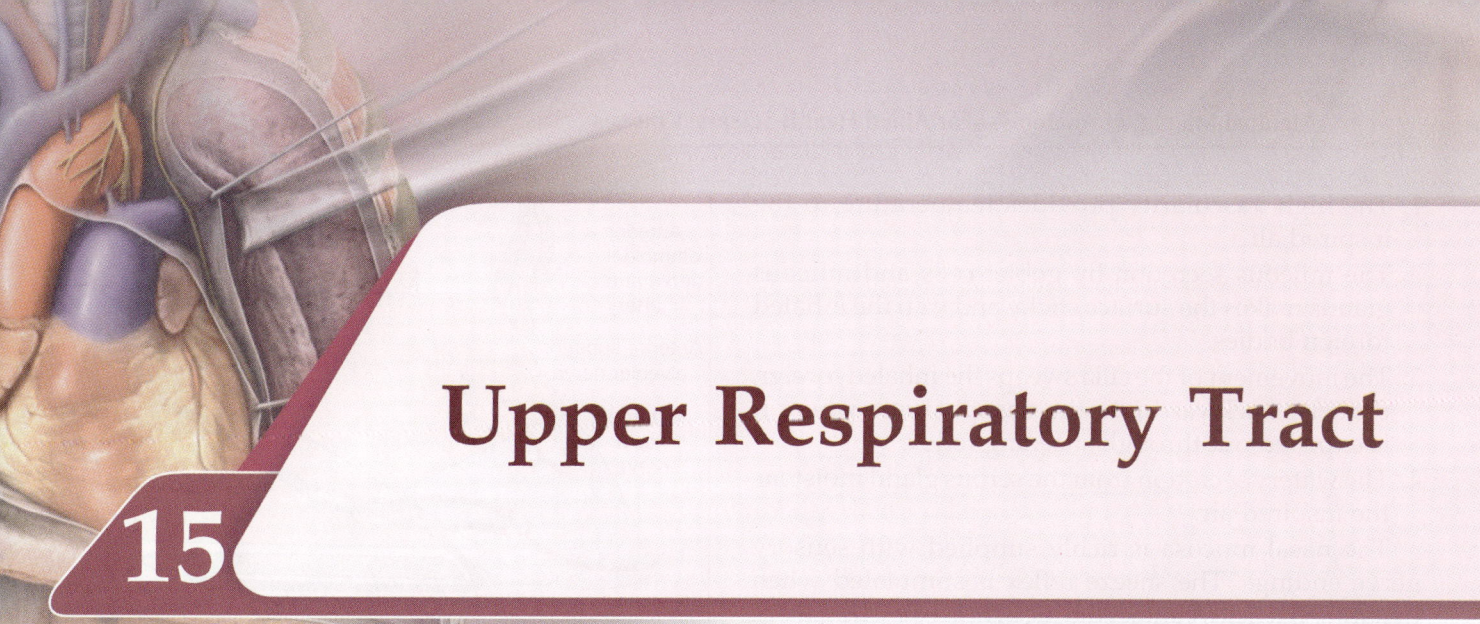

# Upper Respiratory Tract

## 15

Respiratory system is mainly involved in providing oxygen and removing carbon dioxide from the blood. Some part of this system is also involved in smell (nasal cavity) and speech (larynx) functions. The respiratory tract is divided into two parts (Fig. 15.1a):

1. *Conducting part:* It includes, nasal cavity, pharynx, larynx, trachea, bronchus and terminal bronchiole.

2. *Respiratory part:* It includes respiratory bronchiole, alveolar ducts, air saccules and pulmonary alveoli.

The conducting part provides humidity and temperature to the inhaled air. The respiratory part is involved in gaseous exchange.

### NASAL CAVITY

### INTRODUCTION

The nasal cavity extends from the nostrils and continues as the nasopharynx at choana. The nasal cavity is divided into right and left halves by the nasal septum. The nasal cavity presents roof, floor, medial wall and lateral wall.

Each half of the nasal cavity measures about 5 cm in height, 7 cm in length, 1.5 cm in width (floor).

The roof of the nasal cavity is lined by a specialized mucous membrane called the olfactory mucosa, concerned with the smell sensation. The remaining area is covered by respiratory mucosa. The respiratory mucosa is lined by pseudostratified ciliated columnar epithelium with many goblet cells. Deep to the mucous membrane there are many mucous and serous glands.

The floor of the nasal cavity is formed by hard palate. (Fig. 15.1b).

The respiratory mucosa makes the nasal cavity as an air-conditioning chamber.

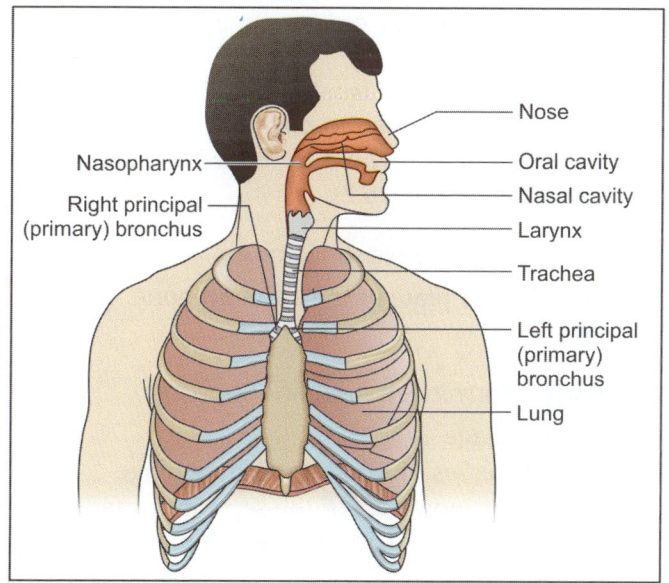

**Fig. 15.1a:** Parts of the respiratory system

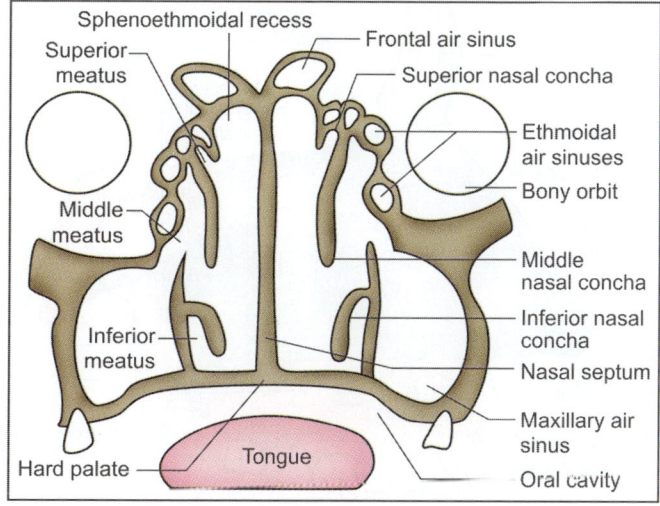

**Fig. 15.1b:** Nasal cavity

1. The high vascularity provides temperature to the inspired air.
2. The mucous secretion by goblet cells and mucous glands makes the surface sticky and trap the inhaled foreign bodies.
3. The movement of the cilia sweeps the inhaled foreign particles backward into the nasopharynx, where it is expelled out through sneezing reflex.
4. The watery secretion from the serous gland moistens the inspired air.

The nasal mucosa is richly supplied with sensory nerve endings. The sneeze reflex is stimulated when irritating particles contact the nasal mucosa. The sneeze forces air outward expelling the irritant from the nose.

## MEDIAL WALL OF THE NASAL CAVITY (NASAL SEPTUM)

Nasal septum forms the common medial wall for right and left nasal cavities.

The nasal septum is usually deflected to one or the other side, rarely median in position.

Nasal septum is formed by bones, cartilages and fibro-fatty tissue (Fig. 15.2).

### Bones Forming the Nasal Septum

1. Perpendicular plate of the ethmoid bone
2. Vomer

### Cartilages Forming the Nasal Septum

1. Septal cartilage
2. Septal processes of inferior nasal cartilage

The anterior most part of the septum is made up of fibro-fatty tissue and is mobile. This part is called 'columella'.

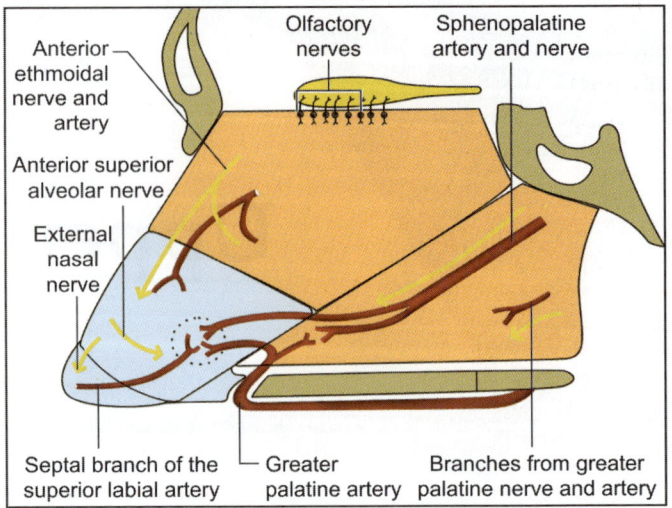

**Fig. 15.2b:** Blood and nerve supply to nasal septum

### Deviated Nasal Septum (DNS)

Condition in which the nasal septum takes a more lateral course than normal and may obstruct breathing. Deviated septum often manifests in old age.

### Little's Area of Epistaxis (Kiesselbach)

It is an area on the anteroinferior part of the nasal septum, which is highly vascular. Branches from facial, greater palatine and sphenopalatine arteries anastomose here. Small ulcer affecting the area produces arterial hemorrhage.

## LATERAL WALL OF THE NASAL CAVITY

The lateral wall of the nasal cavity is also formed by fibro-fatty tissue, cartilages, and irregular bones (Fig. 15.3).

### Bones Contributing to the Formation of the Lateral Wall

1. Nasal bone
2. Frontal process of maxilla
3. Lacrimal bone
4. Labyrinth of ethmoid with superior and middle cochae
5. Inferior nasal conchae
6. Perpendicular plate of palatine bone
7. Medial pterygoid plate

### Cartilages Contributing to the Formation of the Lateral Wall

Upper and lower nasal cartilages with few small cartilages.

The fibro-fatty tissue is present at the anterior most mobile part called 'ala'.

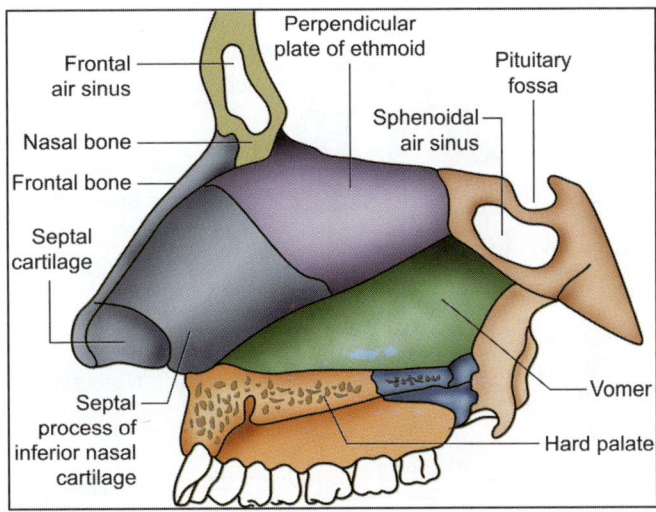

**Fig. 15.2a:** Nasal septum

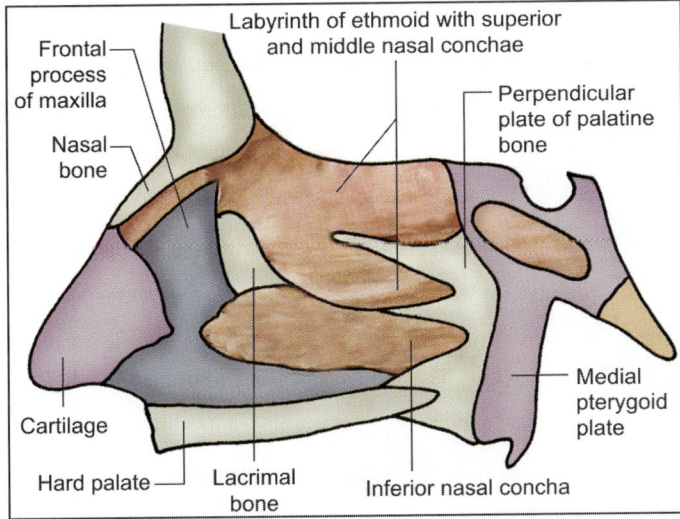

**Fig. 15.3:** Lateral wall of the nose-bones and cartilages

The lateral wall can be subdivided into three parts. (Figs 15.4 and 15.5).

1. Vestibule
2. Atrium of the middle meatus
3. Conchae with meatuses

1. *Vestibule:* A small depressed area in the anterior part. It is lined by modified skin containing short, stiff curved hairs called vibrissae.

2. *The atrium of the middle meatus:* It is the middle part just in front of the middle meatus and above the vestibule.

3. Conchae are irregular bony shelves in the posterior part.

The lateral wall presents irregular bony projections called the conchae. They increase the surface area.

There are three conchae
- Superior concha
- Middle concha
- Inferior concha, which is an independent bone

Meatuses are passages beneath the overhanging conchae. These meatuses receive the openings of the paranasal air sinuses (Fig. 15.5a and b).

1. **Inferior meatus**
   - Lies beneath the inferior concha
   - The nasolacrimal duct opens into it

2. **Middle meatus**
   - Lies underneath the middle concha
   - It presents a rounded elevation called ethmoidal bulla, which is formed, by the underlying middle ethmoidal air sinus.
   - The middle ethmoidal air sinus opens on or above the bulla ethmoidalis.
   - A deep semicircular sulcus lies below the bulla, called the hiatus semilunaris.
   - The anterior part of the hiatus semilunaris is a small passage called the infundibulum.
   - The following openings are seen in hiatus semilunaris:
     - Frontal air sinus (through frontonasal duct)
     - Anterior ethmoidal air sinus
     - Maxillary air sinus

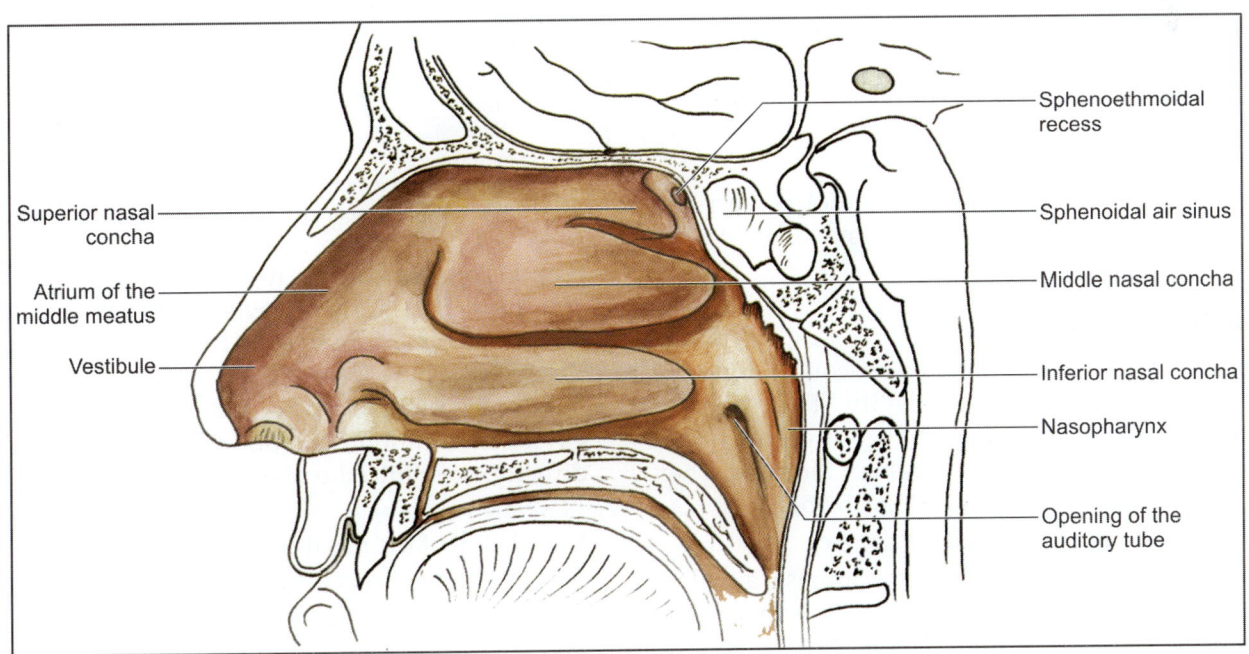

**Fig. 15.4:** Lateral wall with projections of conchae

15

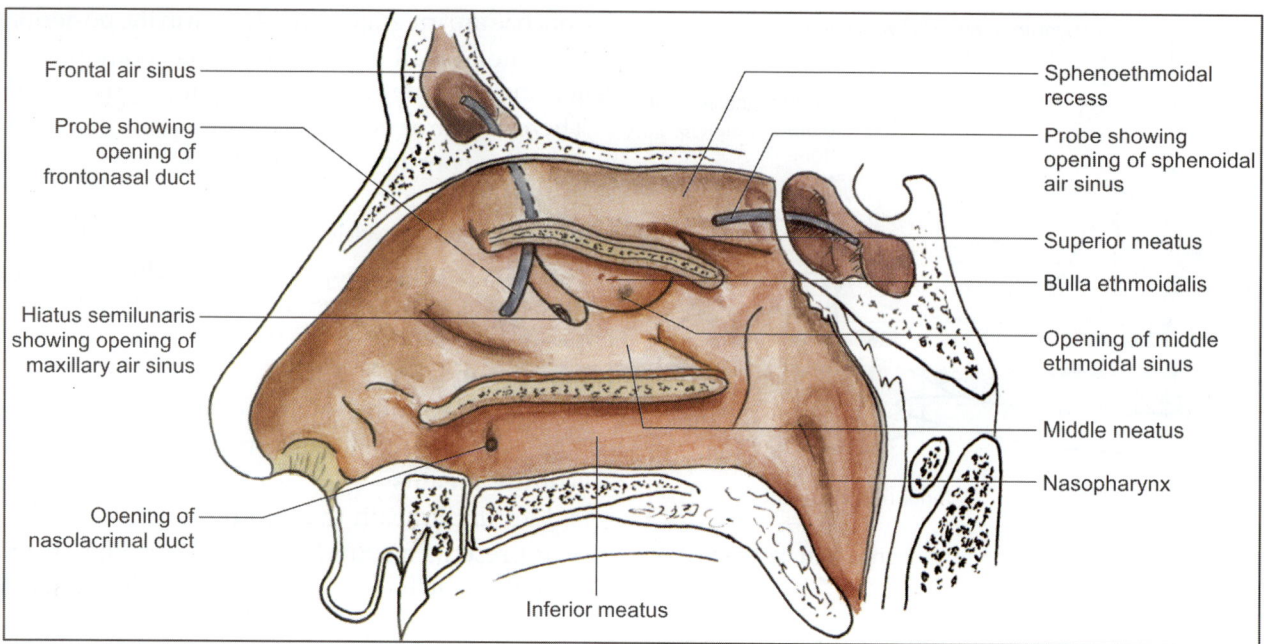

**Fig. 15.5a:** Lateral wall showing meatuses

3. **Superior meatus**
   - Lies below the superior conchae
   - It receives the opening of the posterior ethmoidal air sinus
4. **Sphenoethmoidal recess**
   - It is a triangular fossa above the superior concha.
   - It receives the opening of the sphenoidal air sinus.

## Arterial Supply

The arterial supply to the lateral wall of the nasal cavity is derived from branches of ophthalmic, facial and maxillary arteries (Fig. 15.6a).

## Nerve Supply

The sensory nerve (mucous membrane) is supplied by branches of the ophthalmic and maxillary nerves (Fig. 15.6a).

## PARANASAL AIR SINUSES

These are air filled spaces lined by mucous membrane and communicate with nasal cavity. They help in conditioning the inspired air by giving additional surface area. They reduce the weight of the skull. They also add resonance to the voice (Fig. 15.6b).

Following are the paranasal air sinuses.

1. *Maxillary air sinus:* It is the largest paranasal air sinus situated inside the body of maxilla. It is pyramidal in shape with its apex directed towards the zygomatic bone and base towards the nasal cavity.

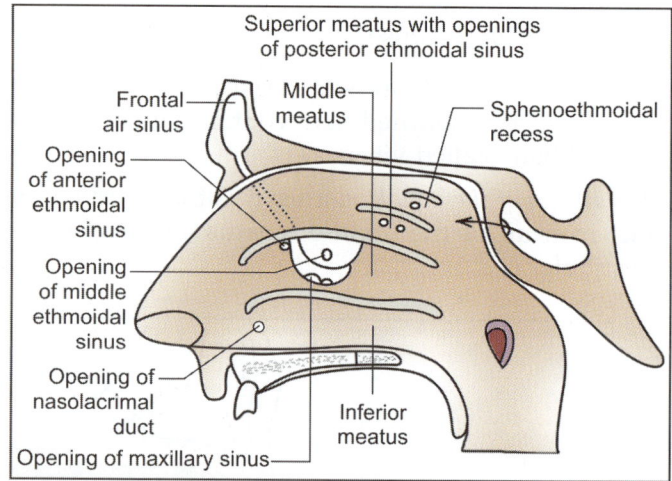

**Fig. 15.5b:** Lateral wall showing meatuses (schematic)

It opens into the middle meatus of the nose at hiatus semilunaris by one or two openings within the ethmoidal bone. The floor of the maxillar air sinus is placed below the level of the floor of the nasal cavity, hence drainage from maxillary sinus is against gavity. In addition, secretion from frontal sinus may directly enter into the maxillar sinus (Fig. 15.6c).

2. *Ethmoidal air sinuses:* They are placed between the lateral wall of the nasal cavity and medial wall of the orbit. There are three groups of ethmoidal air sinuses.
   Anterior—which opens into middle meatus.
   Middle—which opens into middle meatus above the bulla.
   Posterior—opens into superior meatus.

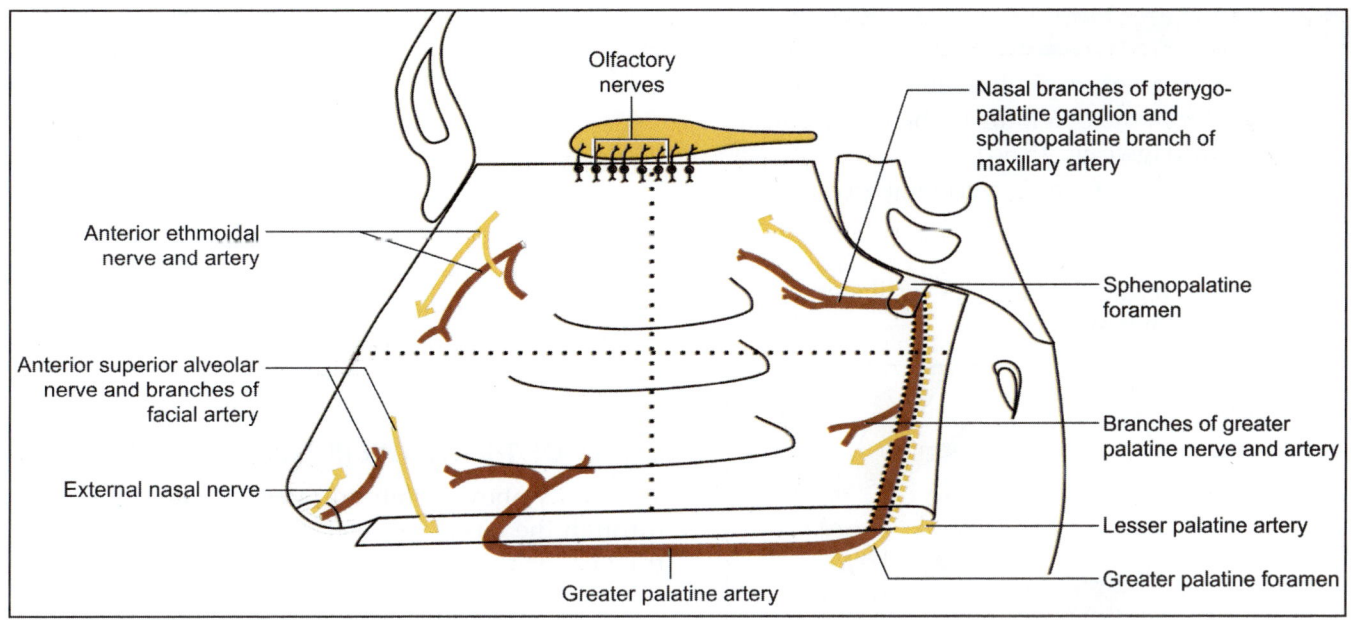

**Fig. 15.6a:** Blood and nerve supply to the lateral wall

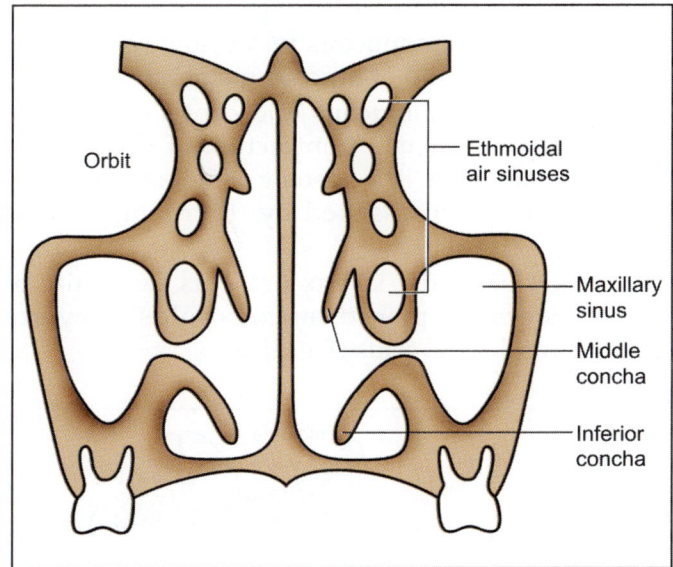

**Fig. 15.6b:** Paranasal air sinuses

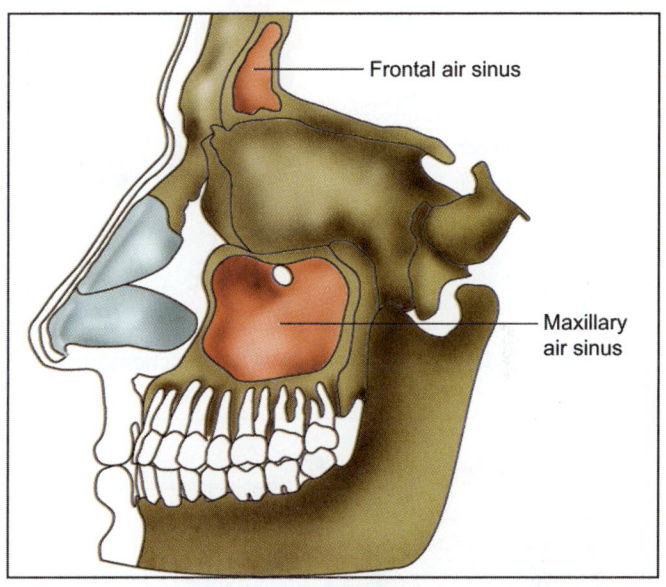

**Fig. 15.6c:** Maxillary sinus with its opening

3. *Sphenoidal air sinus:* It is present in the body of the sphenoid bone, just below the pituitary gland. It opens into sphenoehmoidal recess.

4. *Frontal air sinus:* It is present in the frontal bone. Frontal air sinus opens into anterior part of the hiatus semilunaris (infundibulum) through frontonasal duct.

**Rhinitis:** Inflammation in the nasal cavity due to viruses, bacteria or allergens. This inflammation of the nasal mucosa is accompanied by an excessive production of mucous. The mucous secretion results in nasal congestion and a running nose.

**Sinusitis:** Infection and inflammation of the paranasal air sinuses.

Nasopharynx and oropharynx will be considered in pharynx (Chapter 19).

15

## LARYNX

Larynx is an organ of respiration and phonation.

It extends from the epiglottis to the lower border of the cricoid cartilage (Fig. 15.6d).

It lies opposite the $C_3$ to $C_6$ vertebrae in adults.

### SKELETON OF THE LARYNX

The wall of the larynx is made up of cartilages, muscles, membranes and ligaments.

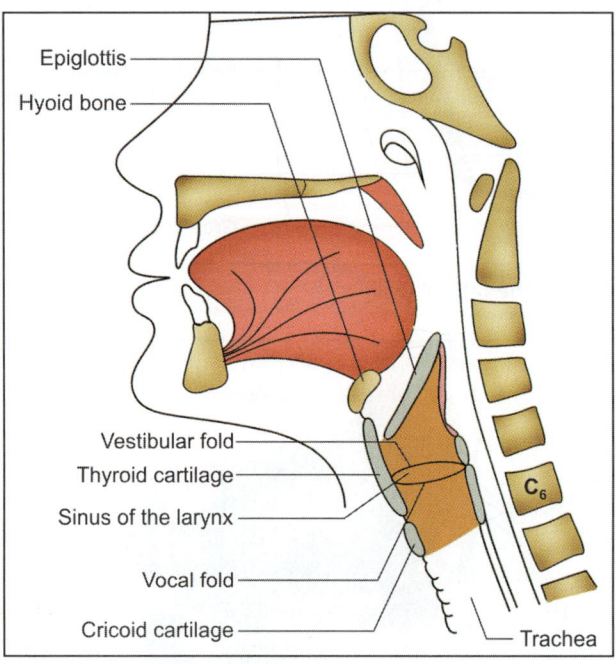

**Fig. 15.6d:** Sagittal section of larynx—schematic

Cartilages are 9 in number (Fig. 15.7)

| | |
|---|---|
| Three paired | Arytenoid |
| | Corniculate |
| | Cuneiform |
| Three unpaired | Thyroid cartilage |
| | Cricoid cartilage |
| | Epiglottis |

The membrane includes cricovocal membrane and quadrate membrane.

The ligaments include vestibular ligament and vocal ligament.

### CAVITY OF THE LARYNX (INTERIOR OF THE LARYNX)

The cavity above communicates with laryngopharynx through the laryngeal inlet. Below, it continues as the trachea, at the lower border of the cricoid cartilage (Fig. 15.7).

### Inlet of the Larynx

It is bounded above and in front by epiglottis, on each side by aryepiglottic mucous fold below and behind by interarytenoid fold of mucous membrane.

The aryepiglottic mucous fold contains a muscle called 'aryepiglotticus'. Contraction of this muscle closes laryngeal inlet. The opening of the laryngeal inlet is a passive action assisted by 'thyroepiglotticus muscle'.

The interior of the larynx presents two pairs of anteroposteriorly placed mucous folds, they are vestibular and vocal folds (Fig. 15.8).

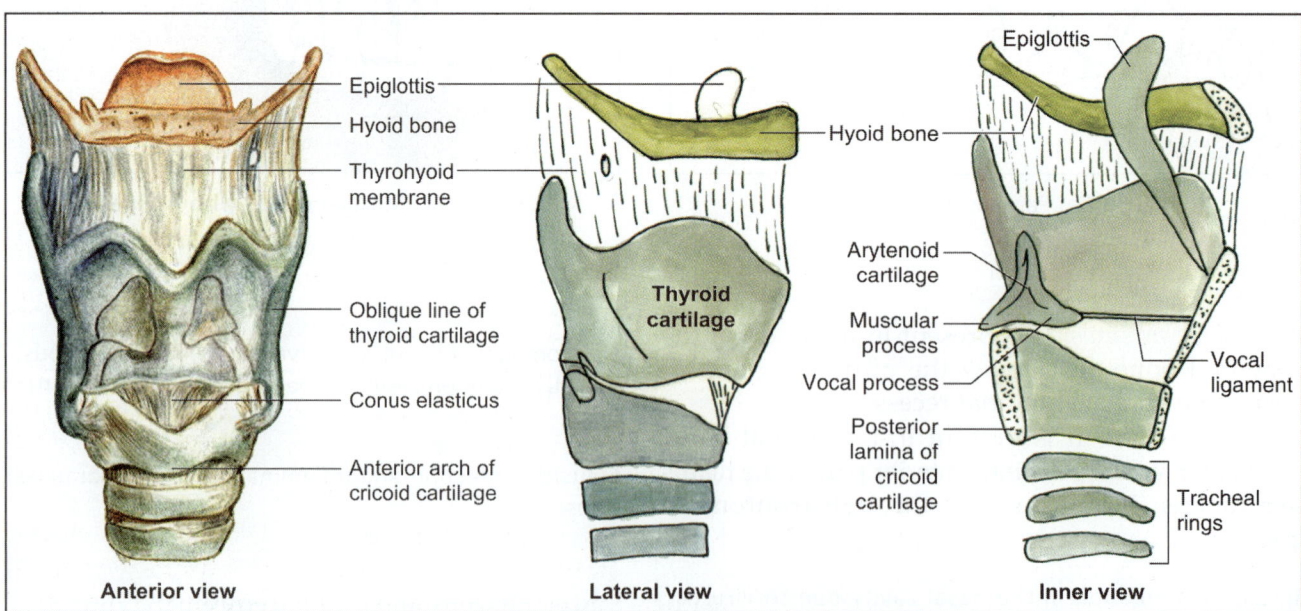

**Fig. 15.7:** Cartilages of the larynx

15

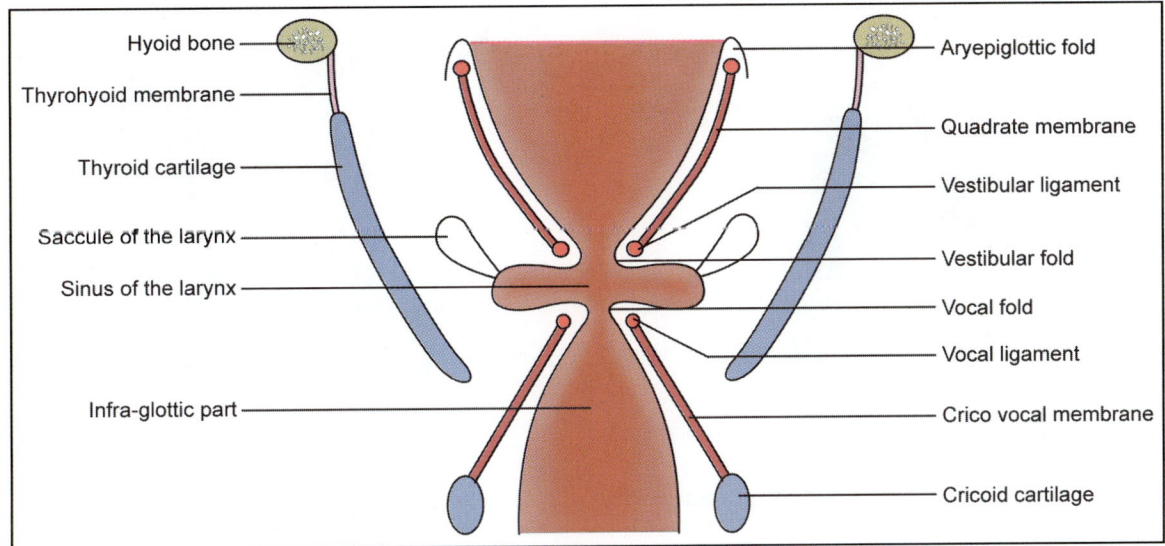

**Fig. 15.8:** Coronal section showing vocal and vestibular folds

Vestibular fold is the mucous fold with vestibular ligament deep to it. The thickening of the lower free margin of the quadrate membrane forms the vestibular ligament. The space between the two vestibular folds is called **'rima vestibuli'**.

Functionally, rima vestibuli permits air entry in inspiration and prevents air exit in expiration.

### VOCAL CORDS (VOCAL FOLDS)

Vocal folds (cords) are the mucous folds with vocal ligaments and vocalis muscles deep to them. The thickening of the upper free margin of the cricovocal membrane forms the vocal ligament. They extends from inner aspect of the lamina of thyroid cartilage to vocal processes of arytenoid cartilage. The vocal cords are lined by stratified squamous non-keratinized epithelium.

The space between the two vocal folds is called **'rima glottidis'**. Rima glottidis consists of two parts:

a. Anterior intermembranous part between the vocal folds.

b. Posterior intercartilaginous part between the vocal processes of arytenoid cartilages.

Shape of the rima glottides changes during phonation.

### Movements of the Vocal Cord

1. Abduction of the vocal cord widens the rima glottidis. It is due to the action of posterior cricoarytenoid muscle.

2. Adduction of vocal cord narrows the glottidis due to the action of lateral cricoarytenoid muscle.

3. Elongation (tension) of the vocal cord is done by cricothyroid muscle.

4. Relaxation (shortening) is mainly done by the thyro-arytenoid and vocalis muscles.

The interior of the larynx is divided into three parts:

1. *Vestibule or upper part:* It extends from inlet to the vestibular folds.

2. *Sinus of the larynx:* It intervenes between the vestibular folds above and vocal folds below. The cricovocal and quadrate membrane are absent in this region. Hence, the mucous membrane bulges outwards towards the lamina of thyroid cartilage. This tubular mucous diverticulum is called saccule of the larynx, projects upwards from the anterior part of the sinus of the larynx. The saccule presents many mucous glands, which provide additional lubrication to the vocal folds.

3. *Infra-glottic part:* It lies below the vocal folds.

### Nerve Supply

1. To the mucous membrane (sensory): Above the level of the vocal fold, it is supplied by internal laryngeal branch of vagus nerve. Below the vocal fold, it is supplied by recurrent laryngeal nerve.

2. To the muscles: All the muscles of the larynx are supplied by recurrent laryngeal nerve except cricothyroid, which is by external laryngeal nerve.

### The Muscles of the Larynx

The intrinsic muscles of the larynx are attached to the cartilages of the larynx. These muscles alter the shape of the inlet of larynx, rima vestibuli and rima glottidis. (Fig. 15.9a to d and Table 15.1).

15

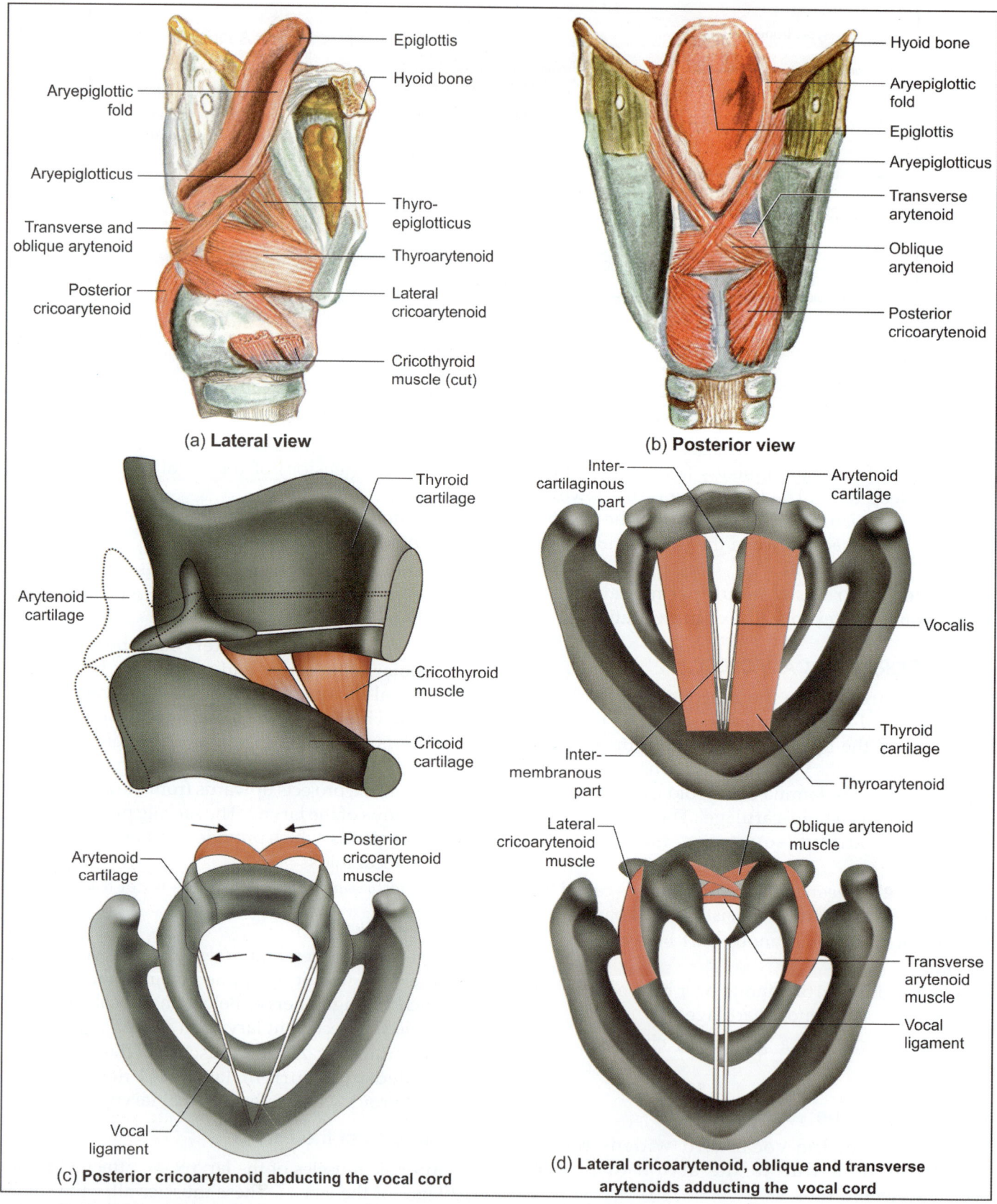

(a) **Lateral view**

(b) **Posterior view**

(c) **Posterior cricoarytenoid abducting the vocal cord**

(d) **Lateral cricoarytenoid, oblique and transverse arytenoids adducting the vocal cord**

**Fig. 15.9a to d:** (a) Muscles of larynx (lateral view); (b) Muscles of larynx (posterior view); (c) Cricothyroid tensing the vocal fold and vocalis and thyroarytenoid relaxing the vocal fold; (d) Actions of the laryngeal muscles

**Table 15.1:** Muscles of the larynx

| Name of the muscles | Origin | Insertion | Actions |
|---|---|---|---|
| **Cricothyroid** It is the only intrinsic muscle present on the external aspect of the larynx | Anterior arch of the cricoid cartilage | Lower border of the thyroid lamina | It lengthens (tenses) the vocal folds by tilting the cricoid lamina backward and pulling the thyroid cartilage forward |
| **Posterior cricoarytenoid** It is the sole abductor of the vocal folds, hence bilateral paralysis of this muscle can obstruct the airway | From the posterior surface of the cricoid lamina | Muscular process (posterior aspect) of the arytenoid cartilage | It pulls the muscular process towards the midline so that vocal processes move apart, thus abducting the vocal folds (widening the rima glottidis) |
| **Lateral cricoarytenoid** | Arch of the cricoid cartilage | Muscular process (anterior aspect) of the arytenoid cartilage | It pulls the muscular process laterally so that the vocal processes move towards each other causing adduction of the vocal folds (narrowing the rima glottidis) |
| **Transverse arytenoid** It is the only unpaired laryngeal muscle | Posterior surface of the arytenoid cartilage | Posterior surface of the other arytenoid cartilage | Adduction of vocal cords (narrowing of the inter cartilaginous part) |
| **Oblique arytenoid** | Vocal process of one arytenoids cartilage | Apex of the other arytenoid cartilage | Adduction of vocal cords (narrowing of the intercartilaginous part) |
| **Vocalis** | Vocal ligament | Vocal processes of arytenoid cartilage | Pulls the vocal process forward, thus shortens the vocal folds |
| **Thyroarytenoid** | Posterior surface of the thyroid angle | Anterolateral surface of the arytenoid cartilage | Pulls the vocal process forward, thus shortens the vocal folds |
| **Aryepiglotticus** | It is derived from oblique arytenoids | It ascends in the aryepiglottic fold and inserted into epiglottis | It closes the laryngeal inlet by approximating the aryepiglottic folds |
| **Thyroepiglotticus** | The upper lateral fibres of the thyro-arytenoid muscle | It is present within the aryepiglottic fold and inserted into epiglottis (opposite to the direction of aryepiglotticus) | It assists the opening of the inlet of the larynx |

Damage to the recurrent laryngeal nerve immobilizes one vocal cord, producing a degree of hoarseness. However, the other vocal cord can compensate and speech remains almost normal. If both nerves are transected speech is lost entirely (except whispering) Damage to recurrent laryngeal nerves is possible during thyroid surgeries.

## TRACHEA (WINDPIPE)

- Trachea is a part of the respiratory tract.
- It extends from the lower border of the cricoid cartilage (opposite $C_6$) to the lower border of $T_6$ in the living, and in the standing position.
- The length of the trachea is about 10 to 11 cm.
- The trachea bifurcates into right and left principal bronchi, and enters the hilum of the corresponding lungs.
- Carnia is hook like ridge present inside the trachea at the level of its bifurcation and is highly sensitive.

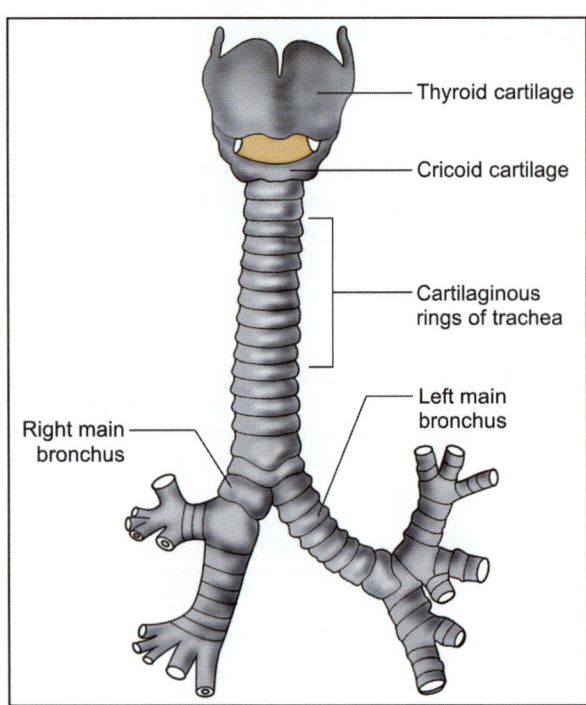

**Fig. 15.10:** Trachea

- The bronchus divides successively to give secondary bronchi, tertiary bronchi and bronchioles.
- Bronchioles also divide successively, to end in alveoli, where gaseous exchange takes place.
- The esophagus descends posterior to the trachea.

## Arterial Supply

Trachea is supplied by branches of inferior thyroid and bronchial arteries.

## Structure of the Trachea

Trachea is lined by ciliated pseudo-stratified columnar epithelium with numerous goblet cells. The submucous coat contains many mucous and serous glands. The anterior part of the trachea is composed of C shaped cartilaginous rings (16 to 20 in numbers). Posteriorly, it is replaced by a fibrous membrane containing smooth muscle fibers (trachealis) which allows the expansion of esophagus during the passage of food substances.

## Applied Anatomy

- Tracheal compressions cause difficulty in breathing (dyspnea). Tracheal compression can arise from enlarged thyroid gland, enlarged lymph nodes or from aneurysm of arch of aorta
- Tracheostomy is a procedure to make an artificial opening just above the sternal notch in case of obstruction in upper airway.
- The trachea can be felt just above the sterna notch. The deviation of trachea in case of pnemothorax can be felt at this site. The aneurysm of the arch of the aorta can cause tracheal tug.

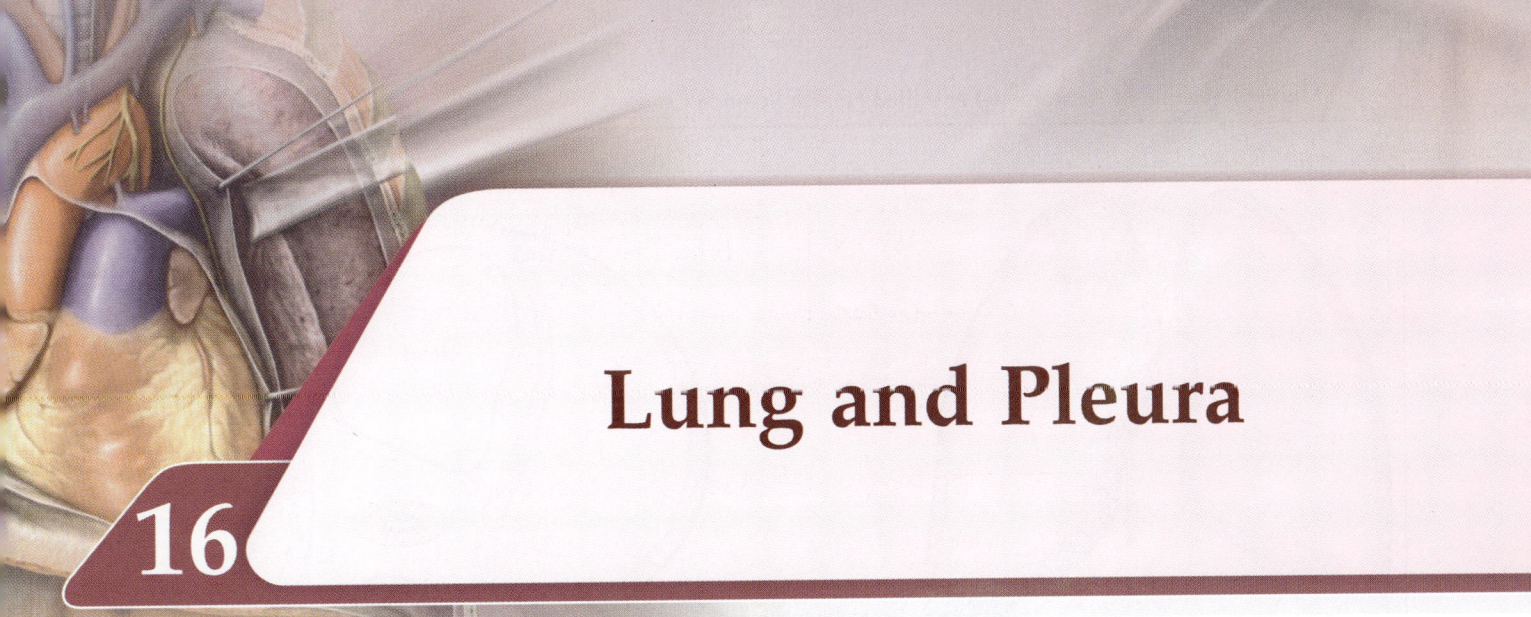

# Lung and Pleura

## 16

PLEURA

### PLEURA

It is a fibroserous membrane covering the lungs. Each pleural sac is invaginated by the lung from the medial side. The pleural sac consists of a visceral and a parietal layer.

1. Visceral (pulmonary) pleura: It closely invests the lungs, except at the hilum.
2. Parietal pleura: It is divided into different parts, according to the structures it lines. They are:

### Costal Pleura

Lines the inner surfaces of the sternum, ribs and their costal cartilages.

### Diaphragmatic Pleura

It covers the thoracic (upper) surface of the diaphragm.

### Cervical Pleura

It covers the apex of the lung at the root of the neck.

### Mediastinal Pleura

It covers the lateral aspect of the mediastinum.

### Pleural Cavity

The space between the visceral and parietal pleura forms the pleural cavity (or pleural space). Normally, it contains pleural fluid and is a narrow space. The fluid allows the lungs to glide freely without friction over thoracic wall during breathing movements. The pressure inside the pleural cavity is negative (about 2 mm Hg and during inspiration drops to 8 mmHg), which is necessary to retain the visceral pleura in contact with the parietal pleura. When the negative pressure collapse (entry of air or fluid), the lungs will collapse because of its elastic recoiling tendency.

### PLEURAL RECESSES

### Costomediastinal Recess

It is present in relation to the anterior border of the lungs. It is related to anterior border of the lungs. On the left side it is prominent because of cardiac notch (deviation in the anterior border of the left lung).

### Costodiaphragmatic Recess

It is prominent in the midaxillary line. It is a space between the lower limit of the pleural sac and the lower border of the lung (Figs 16.1 and 16.2).

- It makes a provision to allow expansion of the lung in full inspiration.
- It is the most dependent part of the pleural sac. If fluid appears in the pleural sac, it collects first in the costodiaphragmatic recess.
- The lower limit of the recess is 8th rib in the mid-clavicular line, 10th rib in the midaxillary line and 12th thoracic spine on the back.

### Nerve Supply to the Pleurae

The parietal pleura is innervated by the phrenic nerve and intercostal nerves. The visceral pleura is innervated by autonomic (sympathetic and parasympathetic) nerves. The visceral pleura is not sensitive to the pain, but when pleural infection or inflammation affects parietal pleura, it is very painful because it is sensitive to pain.

### Applied Aspects

1. *Pleurisy (pleuritis):* It is the inflammation of the pleura. It is characterized with sharp, stabbing pain, which gets aggravated with increased respiratory movements (exertion, such as climbing stairs). During normal respiratory

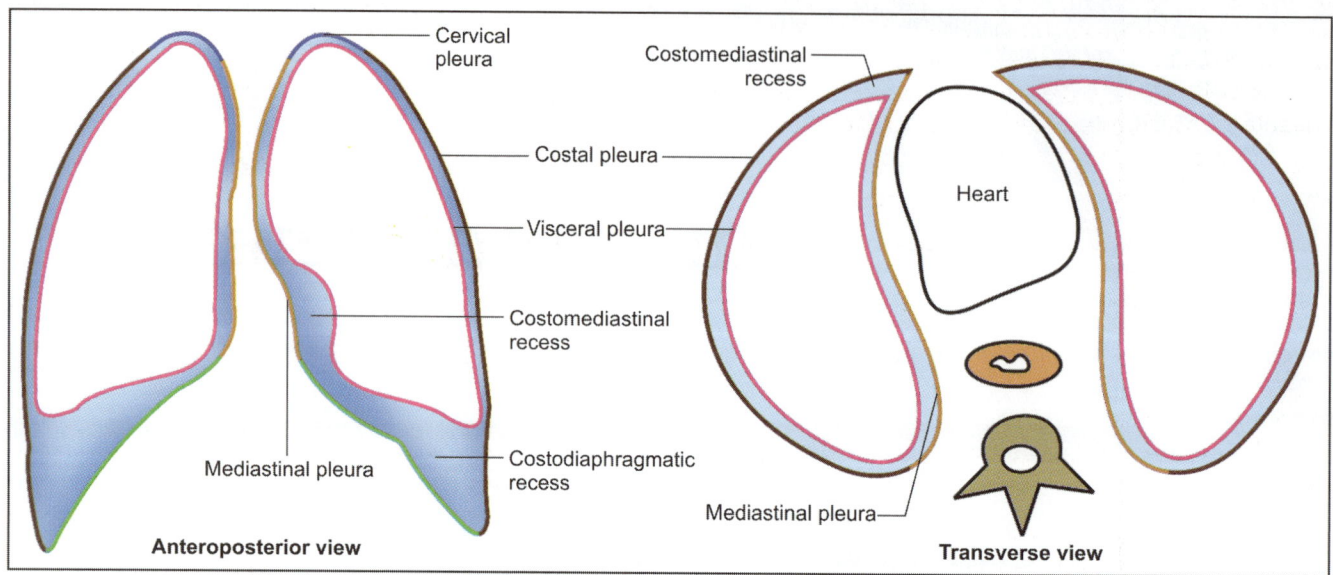

**Fig. 16.1:** Pleural recesses: Anteroposterior view and transverse view

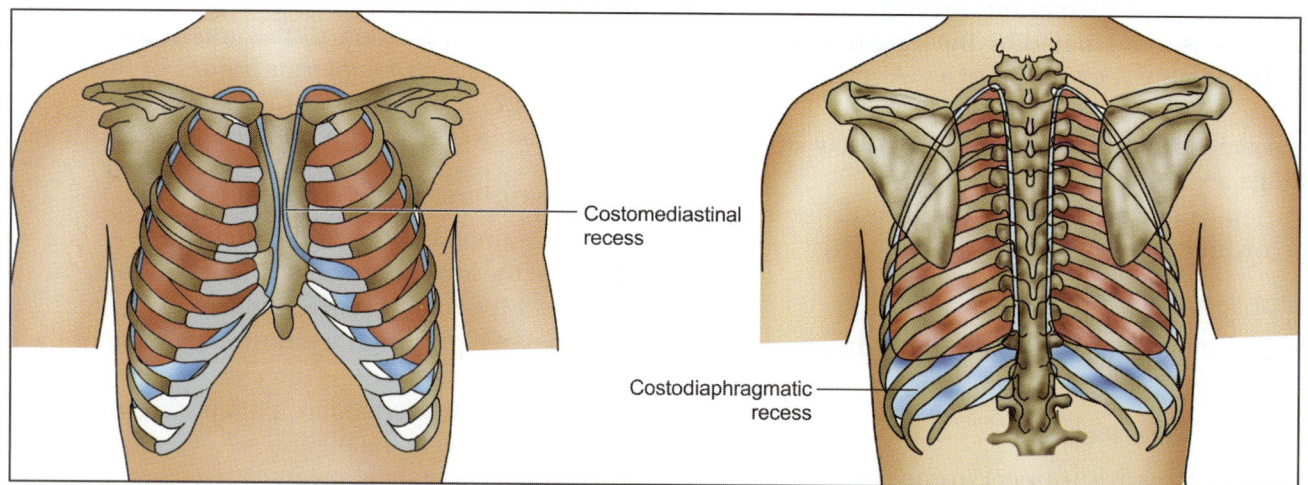

**Fig. 16.2:** Costomediastinal recess and costodiaphragmatic recess

movements, the sliding between parietal and visceral pleura is smooth, without any sounds during auscultation of the lungs, but in pleurisy, there will be a friction (pleural rub), which is detectable with a stethoscope. It sounds like a clump of hair being rolled between the fingers. The inflamed surfaces of the pleura may also cause the parietal and visceral layers of pleura to adhere.

2. *Pneumothorax (air in the pleural space):* The entry of the air into the pleural cavity can result from either penetrating wound of the parietal pleura (bullet entry or stab injury) or rupture of lung substance into the pleural cavity. The air in the pleural cavity leads to collapse of the lungs. Fractured ribs may also tear the visceral pleura and lung, thus producing the pneumothorax. The lowering of $O_2$ tension in blood gives rise to shortness of breath and cyanosis. The mediastinum shifts to the normal (opposite) side compressing the normal lung also. The mediastinal

shift can be confirmed by palpating the trachea just above the suprasternal notch.

3. *Pleural effusion (escape of fluid into the pleural cavity):* It is the accumulation of significant amount of fluid in the pleural cavity. It is associated with the disappearance of friction rub. This condition gives rise to dullness on percussion and reduction in the intensity of the breath sounds. Due to collapse of the lung on the affected side the mediastinum shifts to the normal (opposite) side, which can be confirmed by shift of the trachea. The Fluid level can be confirmed by radiographic examination.

Accumulation of significant amount of fluid in the pleural cavity is called **hydrothorax** and it may result from pleural effusion. The accumulation of blood in the pleural cavity is called **hemothorax**, accumulation of pus in the pleural cavity is referred as **pyothorax** and lymph fluid in the pleural cavity is called **chylothorax.**

4. *Thoracocentesis or pleural tap:* It is a procedure to remove excess fluid or blood or pus from the pleural cavity. This is performed with the patient in sitting posture. Usually the needle is inserted in the posterior axillary line or the midaxillary line through the lower part of **8th or 9th intercostal space.** The excess fluid accumulates in costodiaphragmatic recess. Performing thoracocentesis in either of these spaces **during expiration** will avoid the injury to the lung.

## LUNGS

Lungs are pair of respiratory organs. Lung is porous, highly elastic and spongy in texture. In the newborn, it is rosy pink in color. In adults, it is dark slaty grey due to the deposition of carbonaceous particles. Each lung is covered by pleura (or invaginates into pleural sac). Because of the negative intrapleural pressure, the parietal and visceral pleurae can slide over each other during respiration.

### EXTERNAL FEATURES OF THE LUNG

- Each lung presents an apex, a base, three surfaces (costal, medial and inferior/base) and three borders (anterior, posterior, and inferior).
- **Apex** of the lung extends into the root of the neck about 2.5 cm above the medial end of the clavicle. Apex is covered by cervical pleura and externally by suprapleural membrane. Subclavian vessels pass in front of the apex.
- **Base** is concave and rests on upper surface of the diaphragm. The diaphragm separates the base of the right lung from right lobe of the liver, and left lung from left lobe of the liver, fundus of stomach and spleen. The base is covered by diaphragmatic pleura.

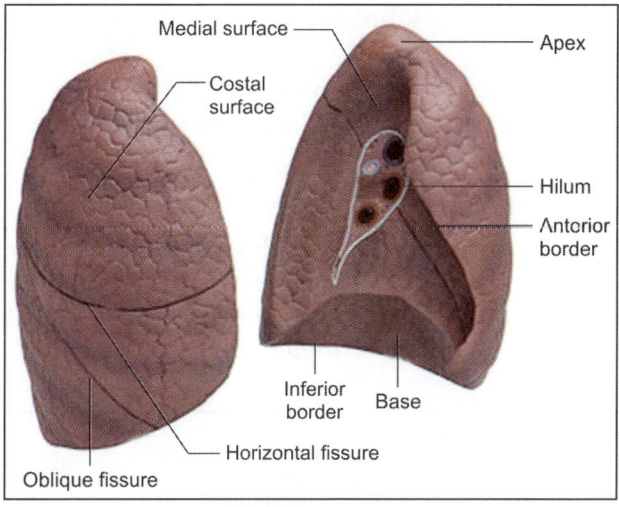

**Fig. 16.3:** Lung external features

- **Costal surface** is related to thoracic wall (ribs and intercostal spaces) and presents impressions of ribs and costal cartilages. It is covered by costal pleura and endothoracic fascia.
- **Medial surface** is divided into an anterior mediastinal part and posterior vertebral part (Figs 16.4 to 16.7)
- The vertebral part is related to bodies of the thoracic vertebrae and intervertebral discs between them. The mediastinal part is related to mediastinum. It presents hilum of the lung, cardiac impression.

### Lobes and Fissures of the Lung

Right lung presents three lobes upper, middle and lower separated by an oblique fissure and a horizontal fissure. Left lung presents two lobes—upper and lower, separated by an oblique fissure.

*Root of the lung:* It connects the hilum of the lung to the mediastinum. The root contains the principal bronchus,

| Table 16.1: Impression/relations of mediastinal surface of the lungs ||
|---|---|
| *Right lung* | *Left lung* |
| 1. Arch of azygos vein-above the hilum | 1. Arch of aorta—arching above the hilum |
| 2. Cardiac impression—right atrium, right auricle and right ventricle | 2. Descending thoracic aorta—behind the hilum and pulmonary ligament |
| 3. Groove for SVC and IVC | 3. Cardiac impression—left ventricle, left auricle and part of the right ventricle |
| 4. Trachea—in the upper part | 4. Esophagus—in the upper and lower part except at the level of hilum |
| 5. Esophages—at the level of hilum | 5. Left-subclavian artery—from the groove for arch of aorta to apex of the lung |
| 6. Brachiocephalic trunk—behind the right brachiocephalic vein | 6. Pulmonary trunk—in front of the hilum above the level of cardiac impression |
| 7. Nerves—right phenic nerve-descends in front of the root<br>Right vagus nerve-descends behind the root | 7. Nerves—left vagus, left phrenic and branches to superficial cardiac plexus and left recurrent laryngeal nerve winding around the arch of the aorta |

16

pulmonary vessels, bronchial vessels, lymphatics and nerves.

*Mediastinal surface:* The impressions and relations to the mediastinal surfaces of the lungs is listed in Table 16.1 and shown in Figs 16.4 and 16.5.

## Hilum of the Lung

Hilum is an area through which the structures enter or emerge from the lung. It consists of a pair of pulmonary veins, one pulmonary artery, two bronchi on the right side and one bronchus on the left side (Figs 16.6 and 16.7).

The arrangement of the structures at the hilum from above downwards (Fig. 16.8) are:

| | |
|---|---|
| Right lung | Eparterial bronchus |
| | Pulmonary artery |
| | Hyparterial bronchus |
| | Inferior pulmonary vein |
| Left lung | Pulmonary artery |
| | Left principal bronchus |
| | Inferior pumonary vein |

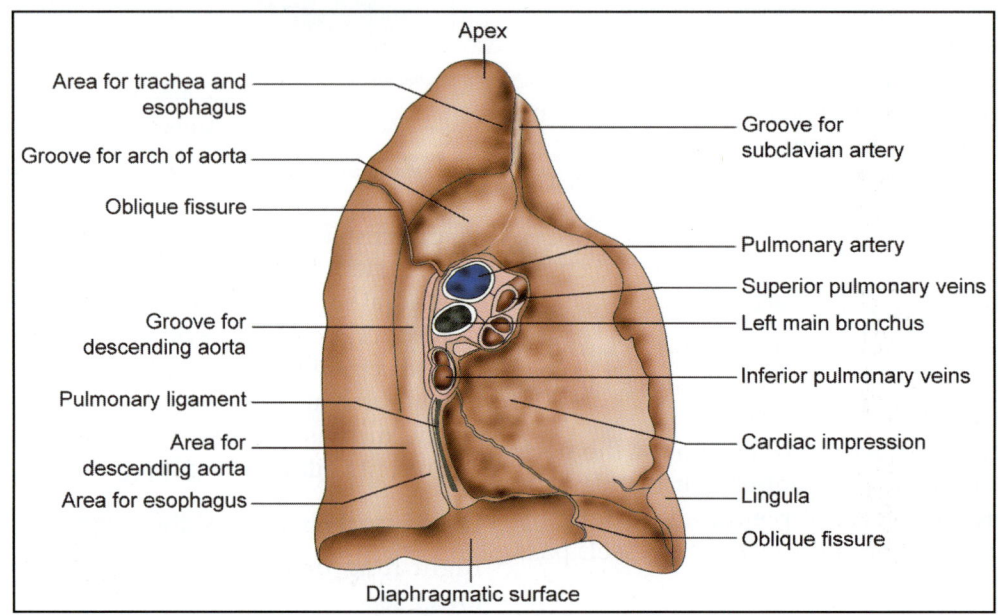

**Fig. 16.4:** Medial surface of the left lung

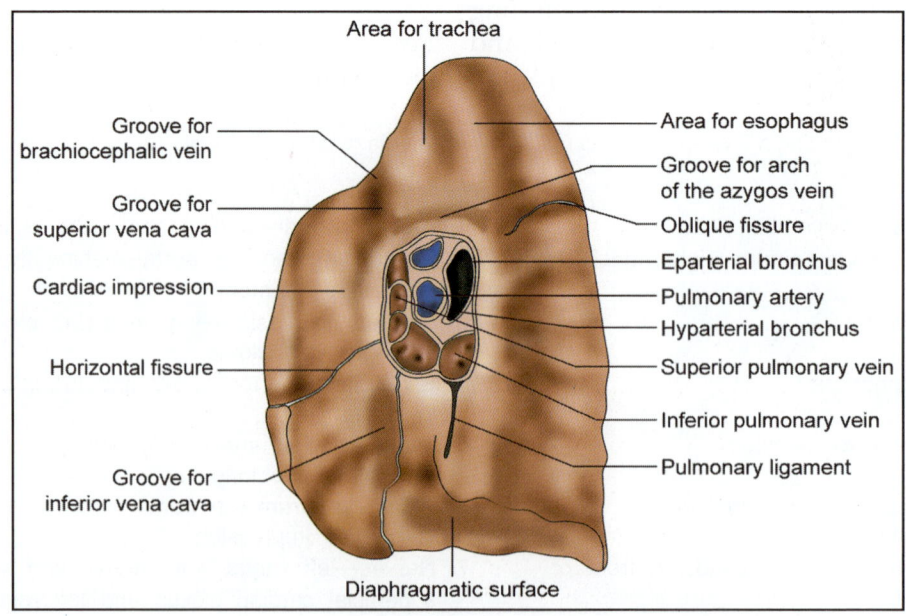

**Fig. 16.5:** Medial surface of the right lung

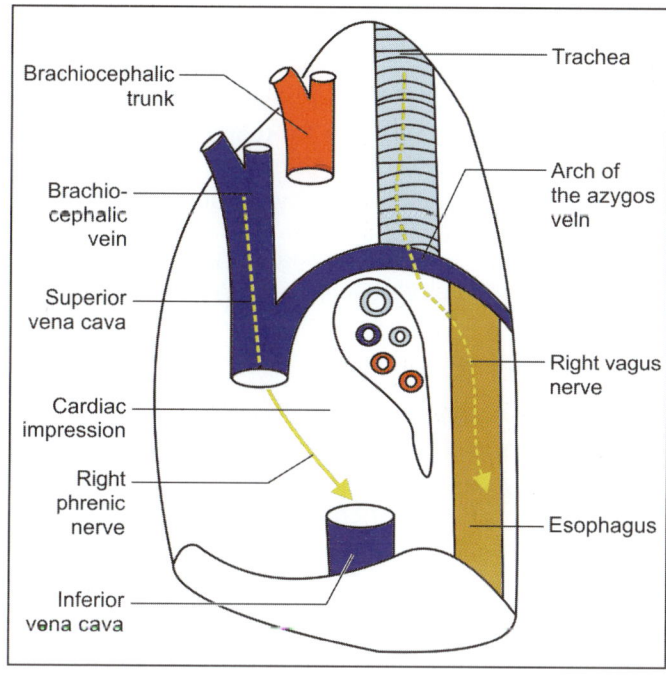

**Fig. 16.6:** Medial surface of the right lung

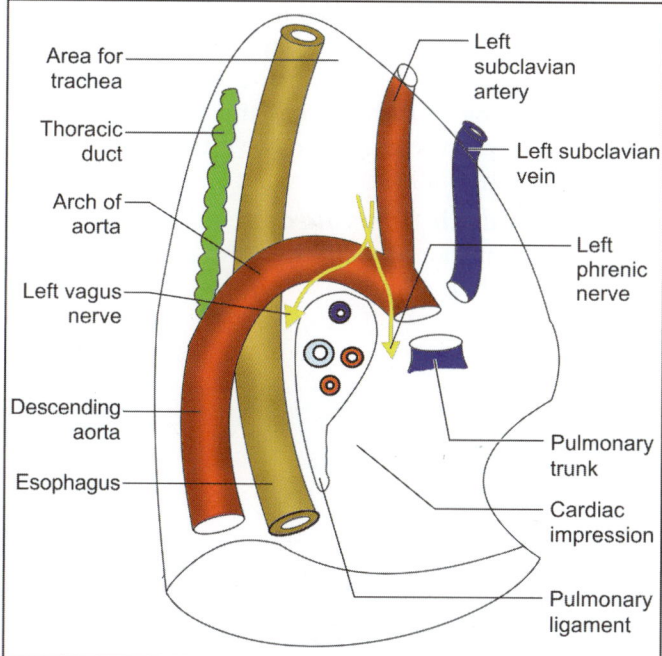

**Fig. 16.7:** Medial surface of the left lung

In a given cadaveric specimen of lung, identify the hilar structures of lung.

The bronchus is identified by the presence of rigid cartilage in its wall. The anteriormost structure is superior pulmonary vein and the inferior most is the inferior pulmonary vein.

- Anterior border separates costal and medial surfaces. It occupies costomediastinal recess of pleura. The anterior border of the left lung shows a cardiac notch. The tongue like extension of the lung below the cardiac notch is called 'lingula'.
- The posterior border is ill defined and separates vertebral part of the medial surface from costal surface
- The inferior border separates costal surface from the inferior surface or base.

## DIFFERENCES BETWEEN TWO LUNGS

| Right lung | Left lung |
|---|---|
| 1. Shorter, wider | Longer, narrower |
| 2. Weight - about 625 gm | About 565 gm |
| 3. Three lobes and fissure | Two lobes and one two fissures |
| 4. Absence of cardiac notch | Presence of cardiac notch |
| 5. Absence of lingula | Presence of lingula. |

## BRONCHIAL TREE

Trachea divides into right and left principal bronchi at the root of the lung. Each principal bronchus again divides into secondary (or lobuar) bronchi, one for each lobe (3 on right lung and 2 on left lung). Each secondary bronchus subdivides into tertiary or segmental bronchi. There are 10 such tertiary bronchi in each lung. The tertiary bronchi divide repeatedly to form 'terminal' and further 'respiratory bronchioles'. The wall of the

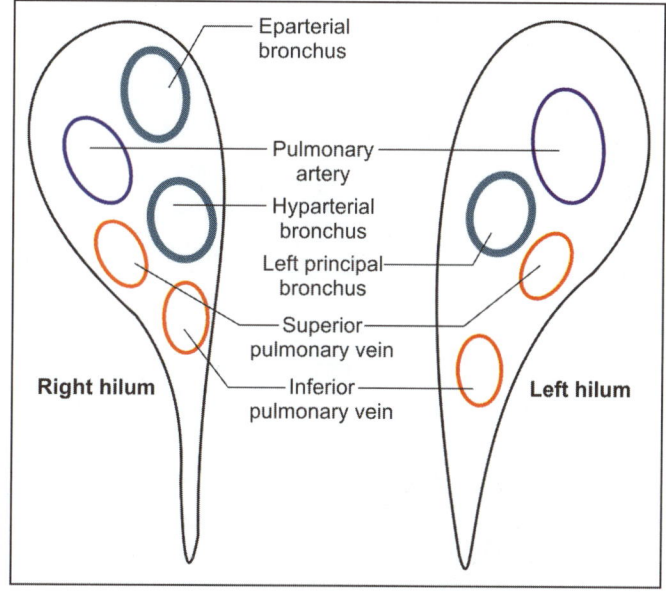

**Fig. 16.8:** Hilum of the lungs

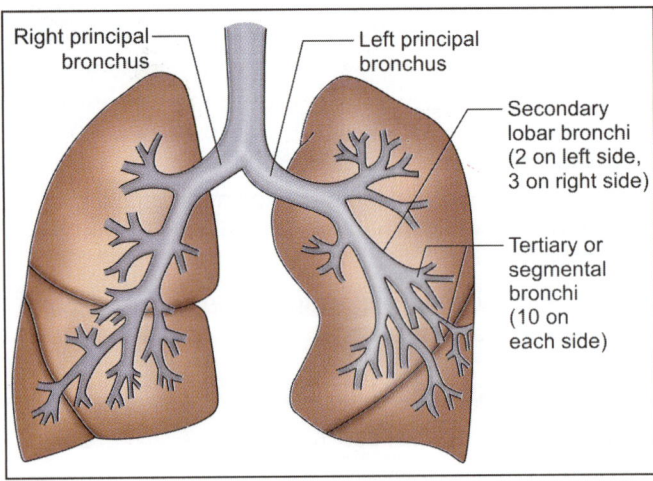

**Fig. 16.9:** Bronchial tree

bronchus is made up of cartilages however they are absent in bronchioles (Fig.16.9).

The respiratory bronchiole terminates in alveoli where oxygenation of blood takes place.

## BRONCHOPULMONARY SEGMENTS

These are well-defined pyramidal shaped independent units of the lung aerated by tertiary (segmental) bronchi with separate branch of pulmonary artery and drained by adjacent veins.

The apex of each segment is directed towards the hilum and base towards lung surface. Each segment is separated from the other by connective tissue. There are 10 bronchopulmonary segments in each lung, which are named in Table 16.2 and Figs 16.10 and 16.11.

## Clinical Significance

1. Spreading of infection from one segment to the other is prevented by connective tissue. However these connective tissues septa are no barriers for tuberculosis of the lung and tuberculosis can break this barrier.
2. The apical segment of the lower lobe and posterior segment of the upper lobe are common sites for lung abscess due to aspiration of infected material. These are the most dependent segments in supine position.

## BLOOD SUPPLY TO THE LUNG

1. *Pulmonary vessels:* The pulmonary trunk divides into right and left pulmonary artery for each lung. They carry deoxygenated blood to the lungs for oxygenation. The branches of the pulmonary artery and bronchi are paired in the lung.
2. *Bronchial vessels:* They carry oxygenated blood to the lungs and enter through the hilum. On right side there is one bronchial artery and on the left side there are two.

## NERVE SUPPLY TO THE LUNG

1. **Sympathetic fibers** are divided from upper thoracic segments ($T_1$ to $T_5$) of the spinal cord. They are bronchodilators (inhibitor to the smooth muscles in the wall of the bronchial tree) and vasomotor. They are inhibitor to the glands in the mucous membrane of the respiratory tract.
2. **Parasympathetic fibers** are derived from the vagus. They act as bronchoconstrictors and are secretomotor to the bronchial glands.

| | Table 16.2: Bronchopulmonary segments of the lung | |
|---|---|---|
| | *Right lung* | *Left lung* |
| Upper lobe | 1. Apical | 1. Apical (Apicoposterior) |
| | 2. Posterior | 2. Anterior |
| | 3. Anterior | 3. Posterior (may be separate) |
| Middle lobe | 4. Lateral | 4. Superior lingular |
| | 5. Medial | 5. Inferior lingular |
| Lower lobe | 6. Superior (apical basal) | 6. Superior (Apicobasal) |
| | 7. Medial basal | 7. Anterior basal |
| | 8. Anterior basal | 8. Lateral basal |
| | 9. Lateral basal | 9. Posterior basal |
| | 10. Posterior basal | 10. Medial basal (may be suppressed) |

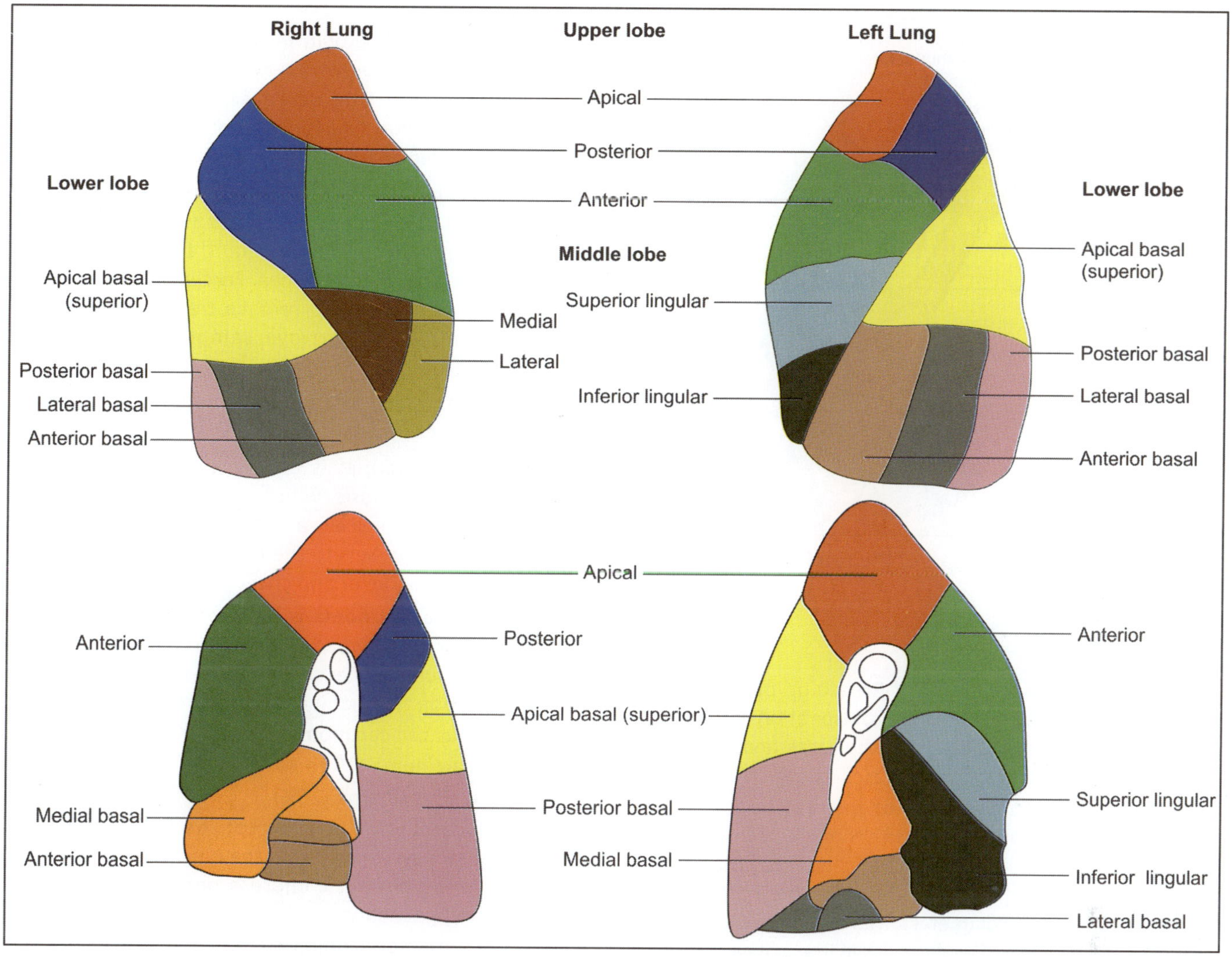

**Fig. 16.10:** Bronchopulmonary segments of the right lung and left lung

Right Lung — Upper lobe — Left Lung

Apical
Posterior
Anterior

Lower lobe

Lower lobe

Apical basal (superior)
Apical basal (superior)

Middle lobe

Superior lingular — Medial

Posterior basal

Posterior basal — Lateral

Lateral basal

Lateral basal — Inferior lingular

Anterior basal

Anterior basal

Apical

Anterior — Posterior — Anterior

Apical basal (superior)

Medial basal — Posterior basal

Superior lingular

Anterior basal — Medial basal

Inferior lingular

Lateral basal

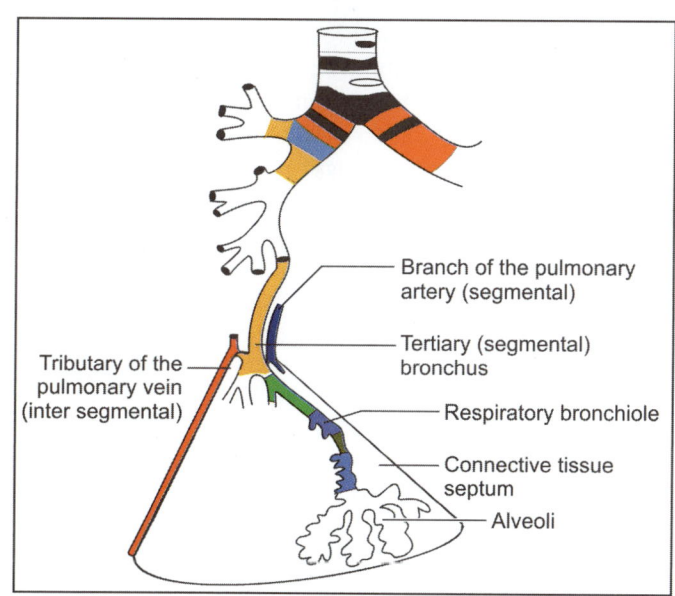

Tributary of the pulmonary vein (inter segmental)

Branch of the pulmonary artery (segmental)

Tertiary (segmental) bronchus

Respiratory bronchiole

Connective tissue septum

Alveoli

**Fig. 16.11:** Bronchopulmonary segment

## Microscopic Structure

The alveoli of the lung are lined by simple squamous cells. The alveoli are set close to the capillaries derived from the pulmonary artery (carrying deoxygenated blood). The structures intervening between air of lung alveoli and blood of pulmonary capillaries constitutes air-blood barrier. The structures include (Fig. 16.12):

a. Flattened epithelium of the alveoli
b. Its basement membrane
c. Basement membrane of the capillary
d. Endothelial cells lining the capillaries

The average thickness of this barrier is about 0.2 μm. The total surface area of alveoli is about 70–100 sq. meters (both lungs).

The alveoli also present some specialized cells (type II alveolar cells), which secrete fluid which acts as 'surfactant' by reducing the surface tension and thereby preventing the collapse of alveoli during expiration.

16

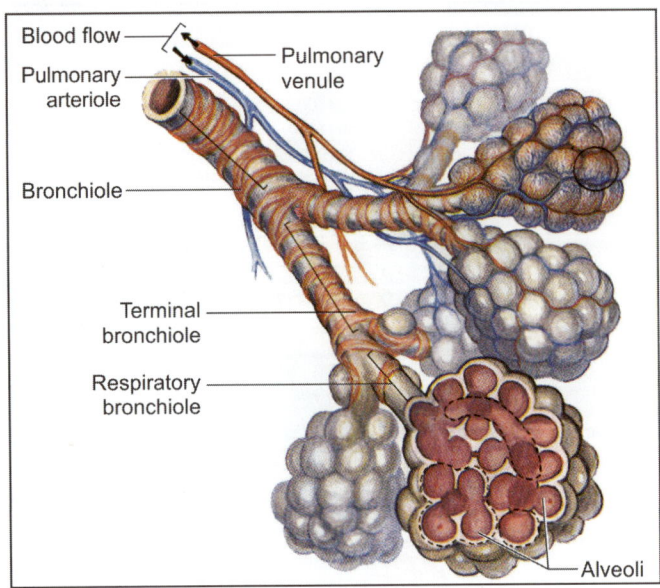

**Fig. 16.12:** Terminal part of the respiratory tract

## Applied Anatomy

1. **The anatomy of ventilation:** Breathing or pulmonary ventilation consists of two phases, inspiration (inhalation), the period when air flows into the lungs and expiration (exhalation), the period when gases exit the lungs.

   • **Inspiration:** The process of inspiration is easy to understand if you visualize the thoracic cavity as a box with single entrance at a top—the trachea. The volume of this box is changeable and can be increased by enlarging all of its diameters, thereby decreasing the gas pressure within it. The decrease in internal gas pressure in turn causes air to enter the box from atmosphere since air always flow along their pressure gradients. The inrushing air enters the lungs. The muscles involved in enlarging the volume of the thoracic cavity are diaphragm and external intercostal muscles.

   • **Expiration:** Quiet expiration in healthy individual is chiefly a passive process. As the inspiratory muscle relax the rib cage drops under the force of gravity and the relaxing diaphragm moves up. At the same time, the

many elastic fibres within the lungs recoil. Thus the volume of the thorax and the lung decrease simultaneously. The decrease in volume raises the pressure within the lungs and air moves along its pressure gradient, out of the lungs.

2. **Bronchoscopy:** Use of a viewing tube to examine the internal surface of the main bronchi in the lung. The tube is inserted through the nose or mouth and guided inferiorly through the larynx and trachea. Forceps may be attached to the tip of the tube to remove trapped objects, take biopsy samples or retrieve samples of mucous for examination.

3. **Pneumonia:** Infection and inflammation of the lungs in which fluid accumulates in the alveoli.

4. **Tuberculosis (TB):** It is caused by bacterium *Mycobacterium tuberculosis*, which primarily enters the body in inhaled air. TB typically affects the lungs but can spread through lymph vessels to the other organs. Symptoms of TB are coughing, fever and chest pain.

5. **Bronchogenic carcinoma** is the most common cancer in men. Cancer cells spread mostly by the lymphatics. Over 90% of the lung cancer patients are smokers. The three most common types of lung cancer are:

   • Squamous cell carcinoma (20 to 40% cases)
   • Adenocarcinoma (25 to 30%)
   • Small cell carcinoma (20%)

   In case of carcinoma, the lymph nodes at the hilum (bronchopulmonary) and root of the lung (tracheobronchial) may enlarge which mat compress phrenic, vagus or left recurrent laryngeal nerves.

6. Infections are more common on the right lung because of wide and vertically placed right principal bronchus. Inhaled particles tend to pass more frequently on right side.

7. The apical segment of the lower lobe and posterior segment of the upper lobe are common sites of lung absess by aspiration because these segments are most dependent parts of the lung.

8. Posterior segment of the right upper lobe is frequently the site of tuberculosis: anterior segment of the upper lobe for carcinoma.

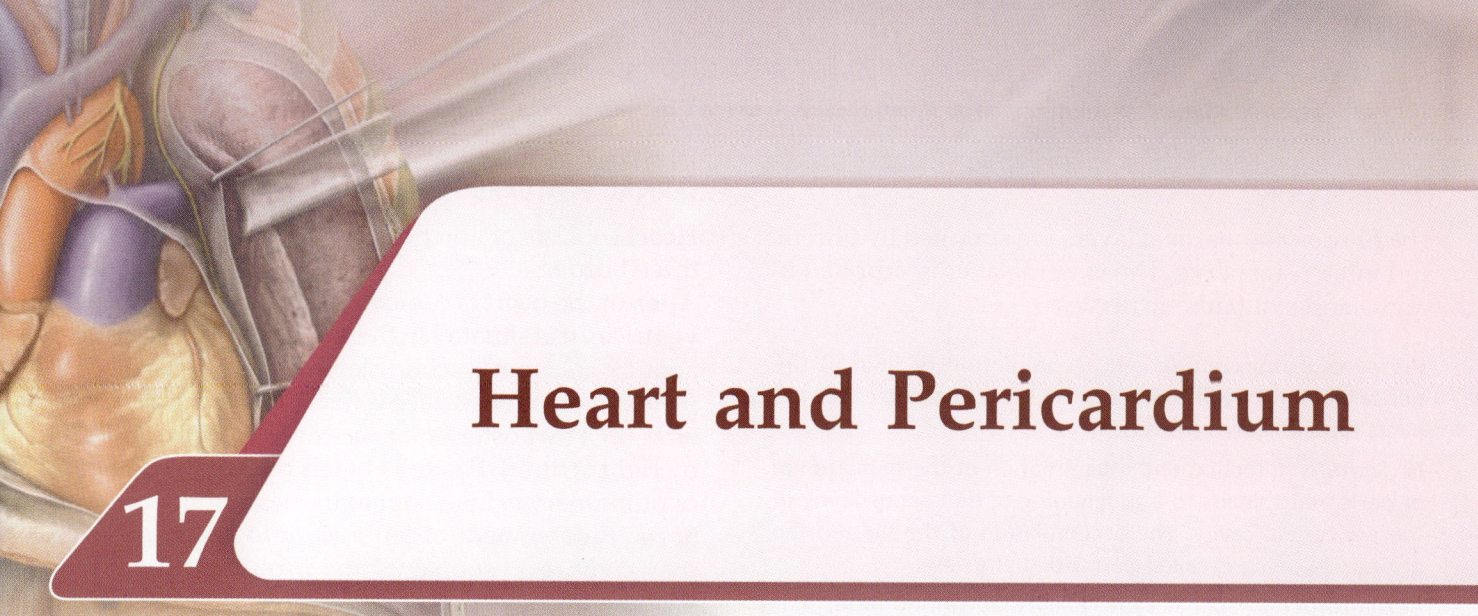

# Heart and Pericardium

## 17

### PERICARDIUM

Heart is covered by a fibro-serous membrane called 'pericardium'. Pericardium consists of outer fibrous layer and inner serous layer. The pericardium keeps the heart in position and prevents its over-distention. The pericardium is having following parts.

The inner serous pericardium is having an outer parietal layer, which is blended with fibrous pericardium. The visceral layer (epicardium) of the serous pericardium is closely applied to the heart.

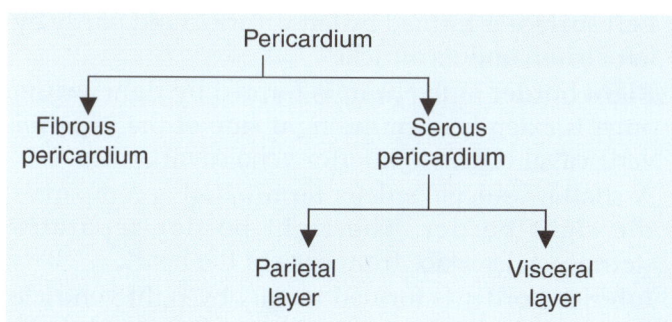

The space between the two layers of serous pericardium is called 'pericardial cavity', which contains thin layer of fluid, which allows the free movement of the heart within the fibrous pericardium (Fig. 17.1).

### PERICARDIAL SINUSES

These are parts of the pericardial cavity with special significance (Fig. 17.2).

a. *Transverse sinus:* It is a transverse gap behind the pulmonary trunk and ascending aorta and in front of superior vena cava.
b. *Oblique sinus:* It is part of the pericardial cavity behind the left atrium.

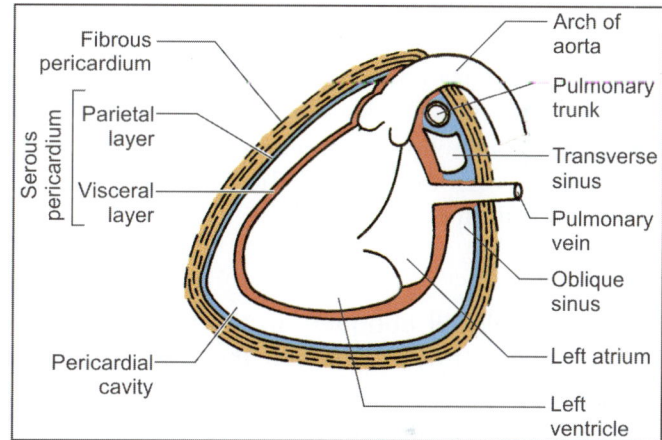

**Fig. 17.1:** Pericardium and its sinuses

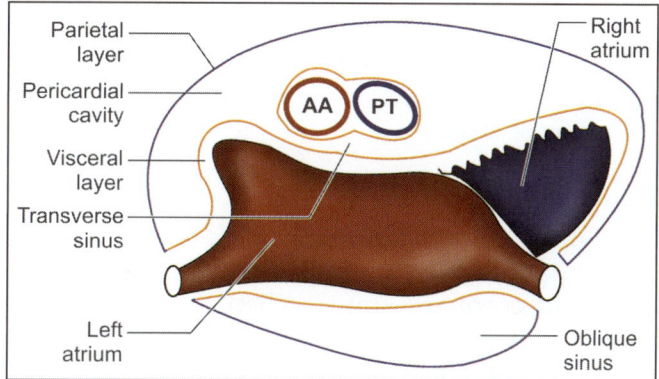

**Fig. 17.2:** Pericardial sinuses (transverse section)

### Arterial Supply

Fibrous and parietal layer are supplied by branches of internal thoracic artery and descending thoracic aorta. The visceral layer is supplied by coronary arteries.

## Nerve Supply

The fibrous and parietal layers are supplied by phrenic and intercostal nerve. The visceral layer is supplied by vagus and sympathetic nerves.

*Pericardial tamponade:* An accumulation of fluid in the pericardial cavity will compress the heart and decreases the heart rate. It causes chest pain.

*Pericarditis:* Infection and inflammation of the pericardium or pericarditis, leads to a roughening of the serous lining of the pericardial cavity. The accumulation of the fluid in the pericardial cavity is called pericardial effusion.

*Pericardiocentesis:* In case of cardiac tamponade, it is necessary to drain excess fluid from the pericardial cavity. The procedure by which the excessive fluid of the pericardial cavity is removed is called pericardiocentesis.

## HEART

Human heart is a hollow muscular organ, which pumps the blood to various parts of the body to meet the nutritive requirement.

## SITUATION

The heart is placed obliquely in the thoracic cavity (middle mediastinum) between the two lungs and behind the sternum.

*Measurement:* The normal adult heart measures about 12 cm vertically and about 6 cm anteroposteriorly. The average weight of the male heart is 300 g and female heart is 250 g. The size of the heart is about the clenched fist in normal individual.

The heart consists of four chambers. They are—right and left atria, right and left ventricles. Auricles are the extensions of atria.

## CIRCULATION OF BLOOD

Right atrium receives deoxygenated blood from the whole body through the superior and inferior vena cavae and coronary sinus. When it contracts, the blood passes to the right ventricle through the right atrioventricular orifice. When the right ventricle contracts, blood passes to the lungs through the pulmonary trunk and pulmonary arteries. In the lungs it gets purified, returns to the left atrium through the pulmonary veins and reaches the left ventricle through the left atrioventricular orifice. When the left ventricle contracts, the blood passes to the aorta and through its branches, to the different parts of the body.

## EXTERNAL FEATURES

- **Heart** consists of an apex, a base, three surfaces and three borders.
- **Apex** of the heart is conical and is formed by the left ventricle. It is situated in the left 5th intercostal space, about 9 cm from the middle line.
- **Base** or posterior surface is fixed. It is formed by two atria (2/3 by posterior surface of left atrium and 1/3 by right atrium). Posteriorly it is related to right pair of pulmonary veins, esophagus, descending thoracic aorta. Enlargement of left atrium in mitral stenosis may compress esophagus and produce difficulty in swallowing.
- **Sternocostal surface** is formed by right atrium with its auricle, right ventricle and left ventricle. This surface is related to posterior aspect of the sternum and adjoining costal cartilages (3rd to 6th costal cartilage) but separated by pericardium, anterior margins of lung with pleura. Due to the cardiac notch of left lung, lungs do not cover a portion of right ventricle on this surface. This area is called area of superficial cardiac dullness.
- **Diaphragmatic (inferior) surface** rests on the central portion of the diaphragm and separates the heart from liver and fundus of stomach. The diaphragmatic surface is formed by two ventricles, 2/3rd by left ventricle and 1/3rd by right ventricle.
- **Left surface** is formed by left ventricle and partly by left atrium and its auricle.
- **Right border** of the heart is formed by right atrium only. It extends from the right side of the superior vena caval orifice to inferior vena caval orifice.
- A shallow sulcus **'sulcus terminalis'** accompanies the right border. The right border separates sternocostal surface from base of the heart.
- **Inferior border** is formed mainly by right ventricle and partly by left ventricle. This border extends from inferior vena caval orifice to apex of the heart. Inferior border separates diaphragmatic surface from the sternocostal surface.
- **Left border** is ill defined and extends from apex of the heart to the left auricle. It is formed by left ventricle and partly by left auricle. Left border separates sternocostal surface from left surface.
- The atria are separated from ventricles externally by atrioventricular groove or **coronary sulcus**.
- The right anterior coronary sulcus extend downwards and is occupied by right coronary artery.
- The left anterior coronary sulcus intervenes between left auricle and left ventricle and is occupied by circumflex branch of left coronary artery and great cardiac vein.

- The posterior part of the coronary sulcus intervenes between base of the heart and its diaphragmatic surface. On the left side, it is occupied by coronary sinus and circumflex artery and on right side by right coronary artery.
- The right and left ventricles are separated externally by anterior interventricular sulcus (on sternocostal surface) and posterior interventricular sulcus (on diaphragmatic surface). They are occupied by anterior and posterior inteventricular arteries respectively (Figs 17.3 to 17.5).
- **Crux of the heart** is the meeting point of posterior interventricular, atrioventricular and posterior interatrial grooves.

## CHAMBERS OF THE HEART

### Right Atrium

#### External Features

- It forms the part of the sternocostal surface, entire right border and 1/3 of the base.

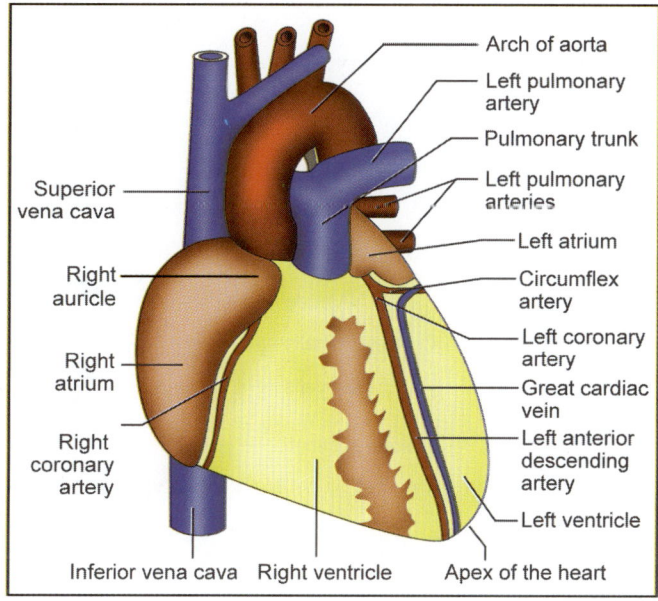

**Fig. 17.4:** Heart—sternocostal surface

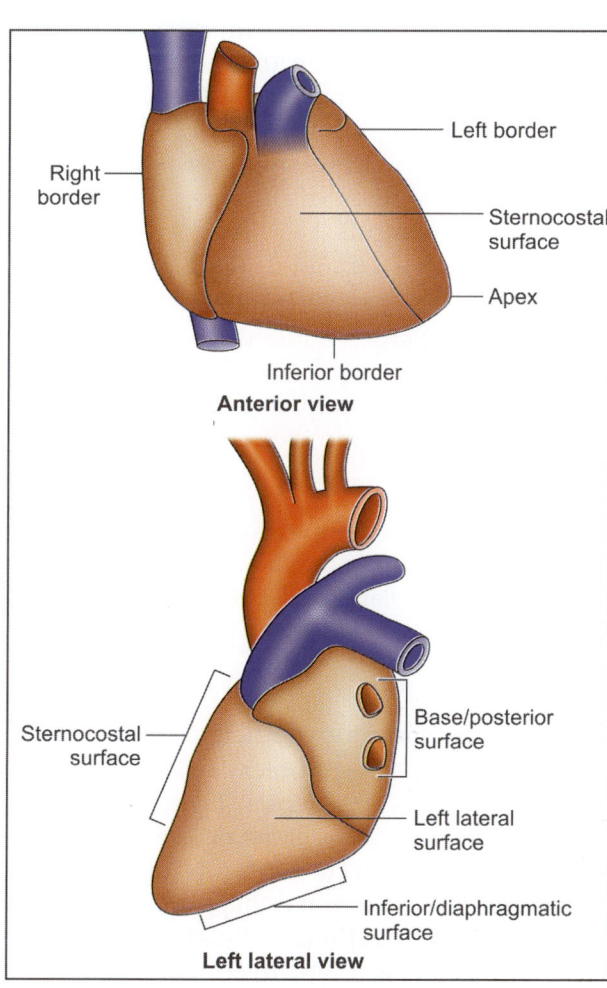

**Fig. 17.3:** Heart—borders and surfaces

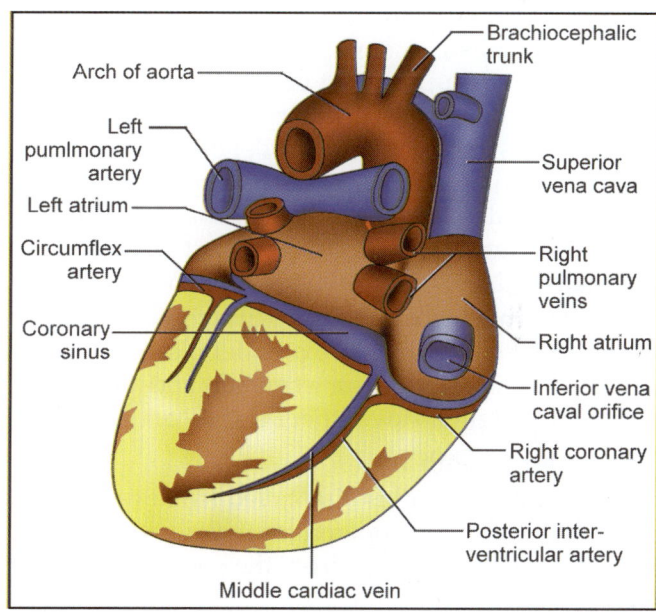

**Fig. 17.5:** Heart—diaphragmatic surface and base

- Right auricle is the conical projection of right atrium towards ascending aorta.
- Sulcus terminalis is a shallow groove, which extends from superior vena caval orifice to inferior vena caval orifice. It corresponds to a ridge inside the right atrium called 'crista terminalis'.

#### Interior of the Right Atrium

The cavity of the right atrium presents three walls (anterior, posterior and septal) (Fig. 17.6).

17

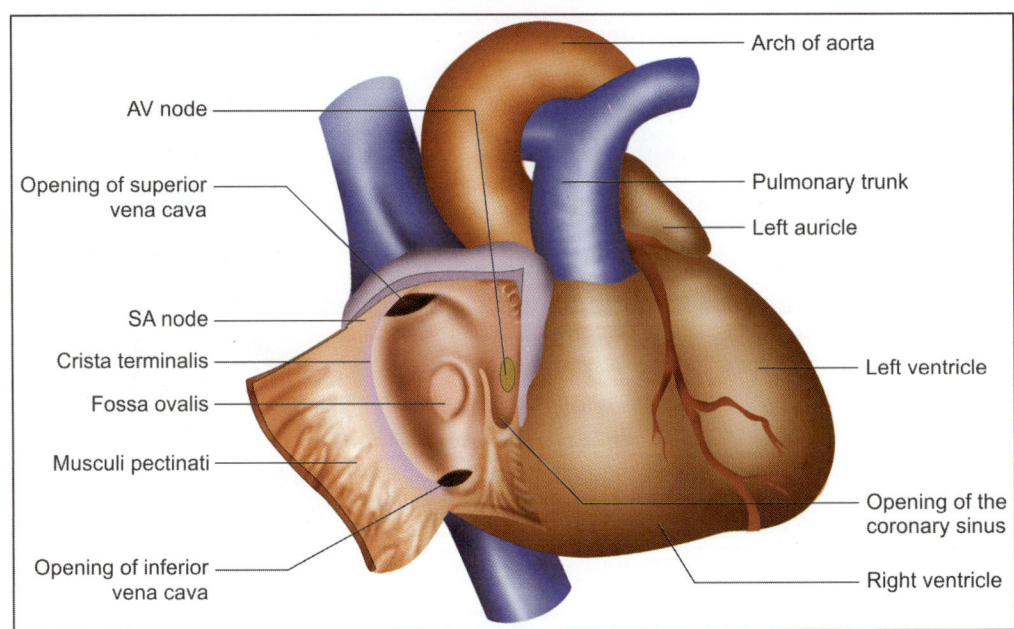

**Fig. 17.6:** Interior of the right atrium

### 1. Anterior rough wall

Crista terminalis is a smooth muscular ridge, which extends from the upper part of the interatrial septum. It passes in front of the superior vena caval orifice and then descends along the right border of the heart. Below it ends by joining with right horn of eustachian valve. Crista terminalis separates anterior rough wall from the posterior smooth wall. Upper part of the crista terminalis lodges sinuatrial node (SA node).

The roughness of anterior surface is because of **musculi pectinati** which are parallel placed muscular ridges extending from crista terminalis and are directed towards the right atrioventricular orifice.

### 2. Posterior smooth wall

Posterior smooth wall is also called sinus venarum. It presents the following openings for major veins, which bring deoxygenated blood from the body and the heart itself.

- Opening of the superior vena cava in the upper part
- Opening of the inferior vena cava in the lower part. This opening is guarded by a semilunar valve called 'eustachian valve' which presents right and left horns
- Opening of coronary sinus: The venous blood from musculature of the heart is drained into coronary sinus which opens into the right atrium between inferior vena caval orifice and right atrioventricular orifice.

### 3. Septal wall

Septal wall separates the right atrium from left atrium, which is placed posteriorly and to the left. It presents the following features.

- Fossa ovalis—an oval depression. In the fetal life the right and left atria are communicated through a foramen called 'foramen ovale'. This opening is closed immediately after the birth. The depression below this opening forms fossa ovalis.
- Limbus fossa ovalis—it is the sharp margin surrounding the fossa ovalis in its upper, anterior and posterior margins.
- Triangle of Koch is a triangular area behind the septal leaflet of the tricuspid valve and opening of coronary sinus. The atrioventricular node (AV node) is lodged in this area.
- Torus aorticus is a bulging produced by the right posterior aortic sinus in the septal wall.

### Right Atrioventricular Orifice

It is an oval opening communicating right atrium with right ventricle. The blood flows in posteroanterior direction since the plane of the orifice is vertical. This orifice is guarded by tricuspid valve.

### Right Atrioventricular/Tricuspid Valve

- It guards the right atrioventricular orifice
- It consists of three cusps or leaflets. They are named anterior, posterior and septal. They are attached to the corresponding sides of the orifice. The other end (free margin) of each cusp extends into the cavity of right ventricle. This free margin provides attachments to the 'chordae tendinae'. The chordae tendineae arise from the apical part of the papillary muscles present in the rough part of the right ventricle.

17

The papillary muscles contract when rest of the ventricle contracts (during ventricular systole), and they pull on the chordae tendineae to prevent the AV valve from everting. They do not act to open these valves.

## Right Ventricle

Right ventricle forms sternocostal surface, diaphragmatic surface and inferior border of the heart.

### Internal Features

The interior of the right ventricle is semilunar on cross-section due to bulging of interventricular septum towards the ritght ventricular cavity. The interior of the right ventricle consists of two parts:
- Rough inflowing part (ventricle proper)
- Smooth outflowing part (infundibulum)

**Rough inflowing part**

It receives blood from the right atrium. Roughness of this part is due to the presence of muscular ridges called 'trabeculae carneae'. Trabeculae carneae are of 3 types.

a. *Ridges:* These are muscular elevations, e.g. supraventricular crest which separates the smooth part from the rough part of the right ventricle.
b. *Bridges:* The two ends are connected to the wall of the ventricle with central free portion, e.g. septomarginal trabecula (moderator band) which extend from the interventricular septum to the base of the anterior papillary muscle. It conveys right branch of the atrioventricular bundle.
c. *Papillary muscles:* These are conical muscular projections usually three in number (anterior, posterior and septal). These anterior and posterior papillary muscles provide attachments to the chordae tendineae, which anchor the cusps of the tricuspid valve. The septal papillary muscles are divided into number of small ridges (Figs 17.7 and 17.8).

**Smooth outflowing part (infundibulum)**

The apex of the infundibulum presents pulmonary orifice, which is guarded by three semilunar cusps. The free margins of the cusps are directed into the pulmonary trunk.

## Left Atrium

It is situated posteriorly and to the left of right atrium. It forms the base and part of left surface and border. Left auricle is the projection of left atrium towards the root of pulmonary trunk (Fig. 17.8).

### Interior of the Left Atrium

The wall of the left atrium is smooth except at the auricle, which presents musculi pectinati. Posterior wall

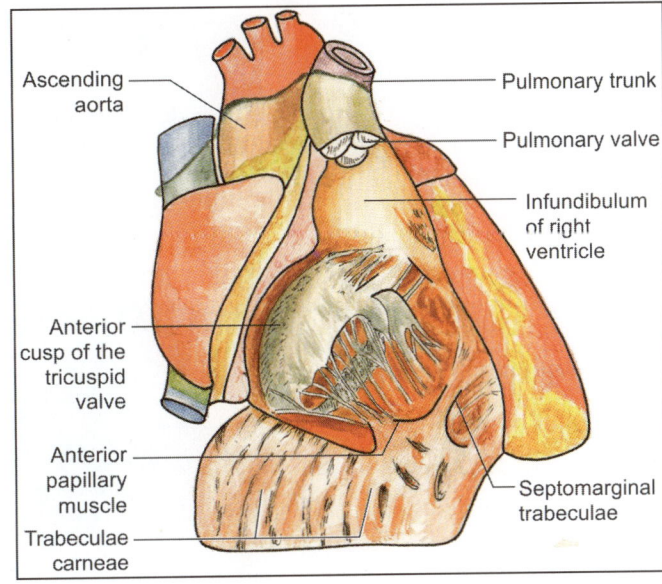

**Fig. 17.7:** Interior of the right ventricle—schematic

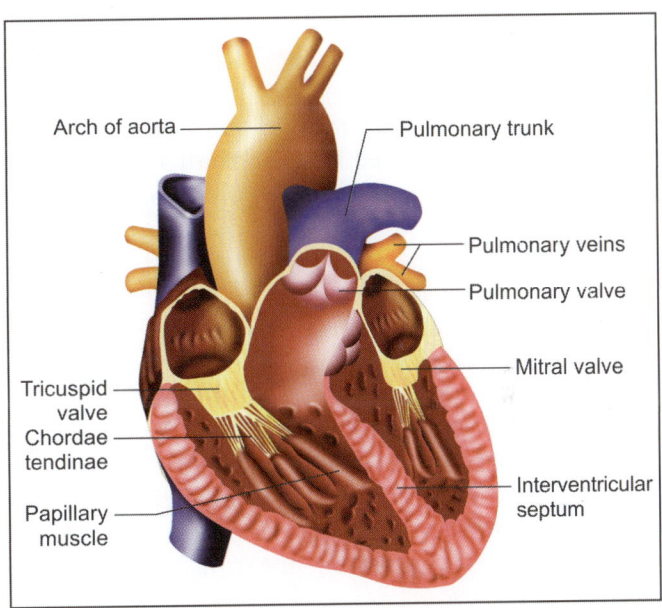

**Fig. 17.8:** Coronal section through the heart

of the left atrium receives the openings of four pulmonary veins.

Anteriorly, it communicates with left ventricle through left atrioventricular orifice, which is guarded by 'mitral valve'.

The septal wall separating it from the right atrium presents a 'lunate fossa' corresponding to the fossa ovalis.

## Left Ventricle

It forms the sternocostal, diaphragmatic and left surfaces and left border of the heart. The apex of the

17

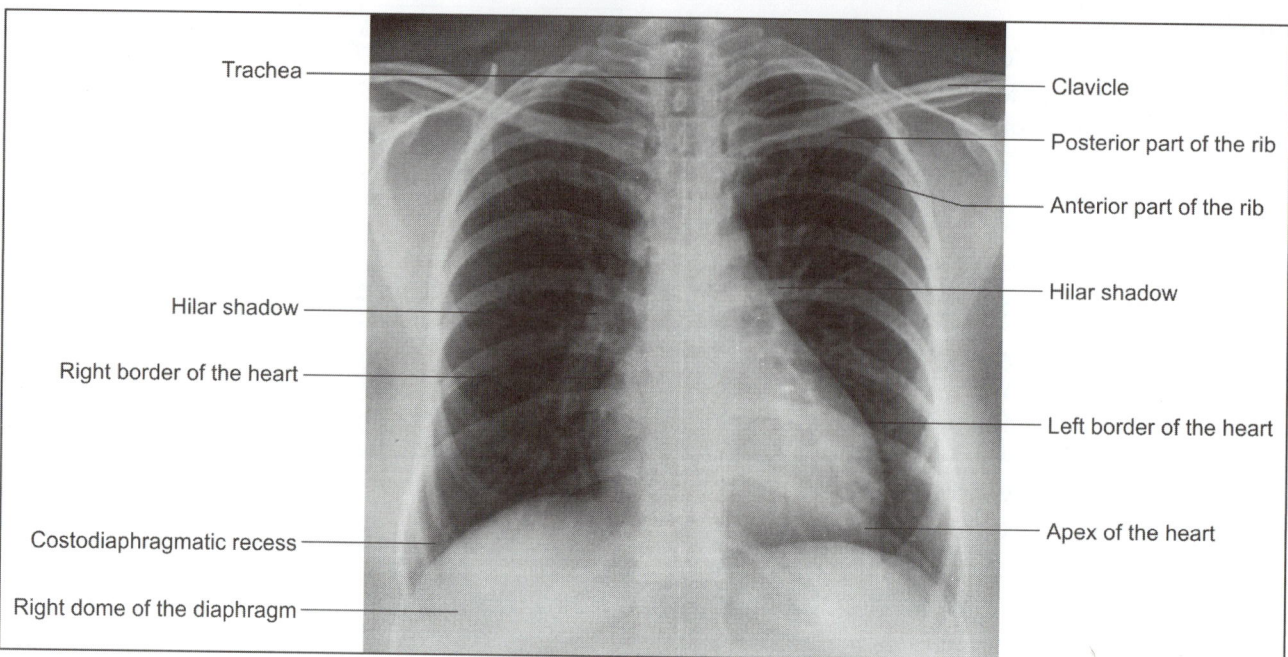

**Fig. 17.9:** Chest radiograph—PA view

heart is formed by left ventricle. The wall of the left ventricle is three times thicker than that of right ventricle to pump the oxygenated blood to all parts of the body.

### Interior of the Left Ventricle

The interior is circular in cross-section due to bulging of the interventricular septum towards the cavity of right ventricle.

The interior of the left ventricle also presents an inflowing rough part and a smooth out flowing part. The rough inflowing part presents left atrioventricular orifice with mitral valve and trabeculae carneae. The trabeculae carneae present anterior and posterior papillary muscles.

### Left Atrioventricular/Bicuspid/Mitral Valve

- It consists of two cusps anterior and posterior.
- These cusps are attached to the margin of left atrioventricular orifice. Their free ends provide attachment to the chordae tendineae. These chordae tendineae arise from papillary muscles present in the left ventricle.

The outflowing part of the left ventricle is called 'aortic vestibule'.

The summit of the vestibule presents three semilunar cusps (aortic valve). Above the cusps the wall of the ascending aorta presents three dilatations called 'aortic sinuses'.

The mitral valve is under the most strain because it must resist the powerful contraction of left ventricle. Therefore, it is often involved in valve disorders.

## BLOOD SUPPLY TO THE HEART
### Arterial Supply

The blood within the chambers of the heart will only supply the endocardium and subendocardial tissue. The thick musculature of the heart needs additional source of arterial supply. Heart is supplied by right and left coronary arteries (Fig. 17.10).

### 1. Right Coronary Artery
#### Origin

It arises from anterior aortic sinus of the ascending aorta.

#### Course

a. The artery appears between right auricle and pulmonary trunk and passes into right anterior coronary sulcus.
b. It descends obliquely downwards towards lower part of the right border and curves around this border to enter the right posterior coronary sulcus.
c. It reaches the crux and ends a little to the left of the crux by anostomosing with circumflex branch of the left coronary artery.

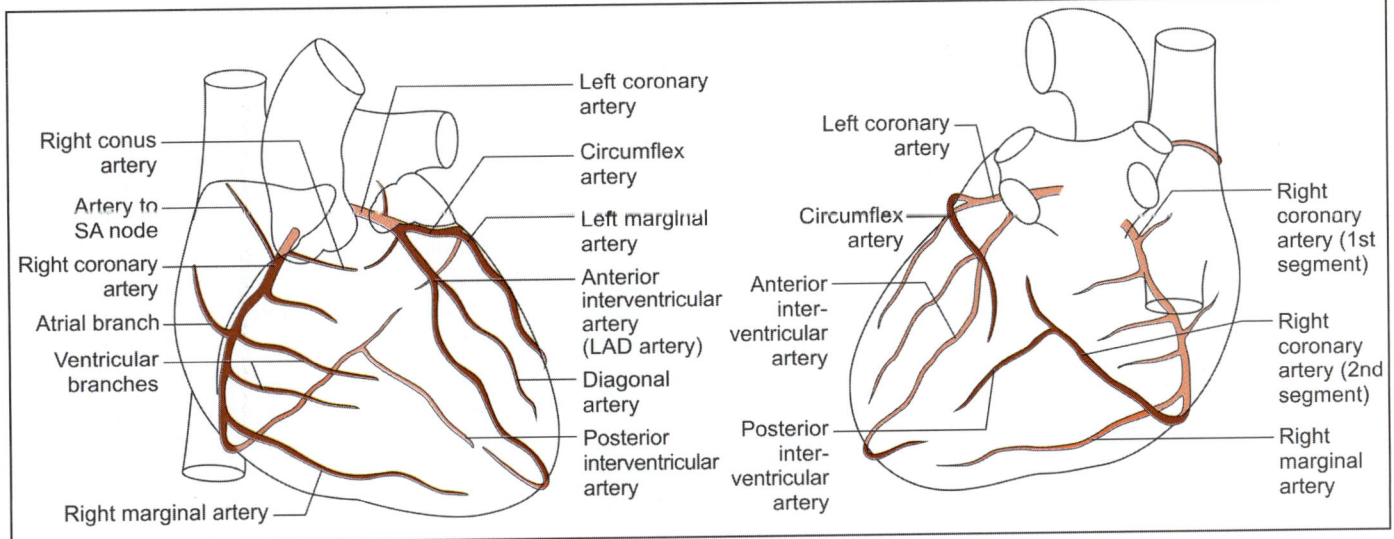

**Fig. 17.10:** Coronary arteries—anterior view and posterior view

## Branches

1. *Right conus artery:* It forms an arterial circle around the pulmonary trunk by anastomosing with similar branch from the left coronary artery. This arterial circle is called 'annulus of Vieussens'.

2. *Atrial branches:* They are classified into anterior, lateral and posterior groups. One of the anterior atrial branches is called 'artery to the sinuatrial node'. This nodal branch forms a loop at the base of the superior vena cava. From this loop, a prominent branch arises and it is called 'ramus cristae terminalis', which traverses the SA node.

3. *Ventricular branches:* These arteries are classified into anterior and posterior groups. The anterior group traverses the sternocostal surface and posterior group diaphragmatic surface.

4. *Right marginal artery:* This branch arises when right coronary artery crosses the right border of the heart. This marginal branch passes along the inferior border of the heart up to the apex.

5. *Posterior interventricular artery:* This branch arises close to the crux and proceeds in posterior interventricular groove. This artery is accompanied by middle cardiac vein. The posterior interventricular artery gives many septal branches and one of the septal branches supplies AV node.

### Areas of Distribution

a. Right atrium.
b. Greater part of the right ventricle except the right ventricle at the anterior interventricular groove.

c. Small portion of left ventricle adjoining posterior interventricular groove.
d. The entire conducting system of the heart except the left branch of the AV bundle.
e. Posterior part of the interventricular septum.

## 2. Left Coronary Artery

### Origin

It arises from the left posterior aortic sinus of the ascending aorta.

### Course

The artery passes between pulmonary trunk and left auricle and enters left anterior coronary sulcus. Soon it divides into two (or three) branches.

### Branches

1. *The anterior interventricular artery (the left anterior descending artery/LAD):* It descends in the anterior interventricular groove. It is accompanied by 'great cardiac vein'. The anterior interventricular artery gives following branches:

a. Right anterior ventricular branches
b. Left anterior ventricular branches: one of these branches is large and is called 'left diagonal artery'.
c. Left conus artery: It forms an arterial ring around the pulmonary trunk along with right conus artery.
d. Septal branches: Supply anterior part (anterior 2/3) of the interventricular septum.

17

2. *Circumflex artery:* This artery traverses the left anterior coronary sulcus and then curves around the left border of the heart. It partly runs in the left posterior coronary sulcus. It terminates (little to the left of the crux) with terminal branches of the right coronary artery. Circumflex artery gives following branches.

 a. Left marginal artery: It descends along the left border up to the apex of the heart.

 b. Anterior and posterior ventricular branches

 c. Atrial branches are classified into anterior, posterior and lateral groups

 d. Kugel's anastomotic artery traverses the anterior interatrial sulcus to establish direct or indirect anastomosis with right coronary artery.

### Areas of Distribution

a. Left ventricle.

b. Greater part of the left ventricle except at the posterior interventricular groove.

c. Small part of the right ventricle at the anterior interventricular groove.

d. A part of the left branch of the AV bundle.

### Special Features of the Coronary Arteries

- The diameter of the coronary artery varies from 1.5 to 5.5 mm
- Left coronary artery is larger in calibrae, supplying greater volume of the myocardium
- Coronary arteries are the only vessels where the blood flows in diastole
- Posterior interventricular artery normally arises from right coronary artery and is referred as 'right dominance'.
- Sympathetic stimulation constricts the epicardial arteries and dilates the intramuscular arteries.

### Applied Aspects

**Angina pectoris:** Angina pectoris is the term referring to pain originating from heart. It is a severe constricting pain as tightness in the thorax, deep to the sternum. The pain is the result of ischemia of the myocardium. This ischemia cause cellular necrosis (infarction) in myocardium, because of which the myocardium will not able to pump the blood. The common cause for angina is narrowing of the coronary artery. This results in reduced blood flow, reduced oxygen supply to the cardiac muscle cells. Strenuous exercise, sudden exposure to cold and stress are the added factors in a patient with narrowed coronary vessels to cause angina, because all these requires increased activity of the heart. After a heavy meal more blood flow into the digestive tract, for which some blood

may be diverted from heart also. This can also cause angina in patients with narrowed coronary vessels.

The stable angina is characterized by chest discomfort and pain precipitated by some activity (running, walking, etc.) with minimal or non-existent symptoms at rest. The unstable angina, the chest discomfort and pain occurs even at rest and it is severe and of new onset (i.e. within the prior 4–6 weeks). The pain resulting from myocardial infarction is more severe than angina pectoris and the pain does not subside after 1–2 minute of rest.

Sublingual nitroglycerin is placed under the tongue for rapid absorption, which dilates the coronary arteries. Such angina warns the patient about occlusion or narrowed coronary arteries indicating healthcare intervention. The cardiac referred pain (angina pectoris) is felt as radiating from the substernal and left pectoral regions to the left shoulder and the medial aspect of the left upper limb.

**Myocardial infarction (heart attack):** A sudden occlusion of the coronary artery or its major branch by an embolus cause infarction of the myocardium (and followed by its necrosis) in the area of the heart supplied by it. This is called 'myocardial infarction'. An area of the myocardium that has undergone necrosis constitutes a myocardial infarction. The most common cause for such sudden occlusion of the coronary artery is due to atherosclerotic changes changes in the coronary artery. Apart from severe chest pain (tightness in the chest), the victims of the heart attack may also have dyspnea, nausea, vomiting, sweating, pain in the left arm pit and medial side of the arm. Abnormalities in the electrical activity usually occur with heart attacks and ECG can identify the areas of heart muscle that are deprived of oxygen and/or areas of muscle that have died. Apart from ECG estimation of cardiac enzymes will also help in diagnosing the myocardial infarction. Cardiac enzymes are proteins that are released into the blood by dying heart muscles. These cardiac enzymes are creatine phosphokinase (CPK), special sub-fractions of CPK, and troponin, and their levels can be measured in blood. These cardiac enzymes typically are elevated in the blood several hours after the onset of a heart attack.

The left anterior descending (LAD)/anterior interventricular artery is most often involved artery in myocardial infarction. It supplies major part of the interventricular septum and wall of the ventricle especially on the left side.

**Coronary angiography:** This is a radiographic technique in which the coronary arteries are visualized. A catheter is introduced into the femoral artery or radial artery then guided into ascending aorta with the help of a monitor. Under the fluoroscopic control, the tip of the catheter is placed just inside the coronary artery. A radiopaque contrast material is injected and radiographs are taken. The radiograph shows the lumen of the coronary arteries and its branches and also stenotic area if any.

**Coronary angioplasty:** In certain people with coronary obstruction, the cardiologists use percutaneous transluminal coronary angioplasty. A catheter with inflatable balloon attached to its tip is introduced to the lumen of coronary artery at the site of obstruction. Then the balloon is inflated, flattening the atherosclerotic plaque against the arterial wall. The artery is stretched to increase the size of the lumen, thus improving the blood flow. Sometime 'thrombokinase'an enzyme dissolves the blood clot Is Injected through the catheter. It is also possible to introduce 'intravascular stent' to maintain the dilation. These intravascular stents are rigid or semirigid tubular meshes.

**Coronary bypass graft (CABG):** It is also called "the cabbage procedure", which is indicated in patients with coronary obstruction and severe angina. A segment of the vein or an artery from elsewhere in the patient's body are grafted into the coronary artery to improve the circulation. The one end of the arterial graft is connected to aorta or coronary artery proximal to the block and another end to the coronary artery distal to the site of block. A portion of the great saphenous vein is commonly used (in reverse direction) for coronary graft because its diameter is equal or greater than coronary arteries and can be easily dissected from the lower limb. Other alternatives include usage of radial artery and internal thoracic artery.

## VENOUS DRAINAGE OF THE HEART

The venous blood from the heart is drained into the right atrium through
A. Coronary sinus
B. Anterior cardiac veins
C. Venae cordis minimae (thebesian veins)

### Coronary Sinus

It is a venous sac about 2 to 3 cm long, situated in the left posterior coronary sulcus. It opens into the right atrium by an orifice, which is guarded by a valve. Following are the tributaries of the coronary sinus (Fig. 17.11).

1. *Great cardiac vein:* It begins near the apex, ascends in the anterior interventricular groove and then traverses the coronary sulcus. It receives left marginal vein.

2. *Small cardiac vein:* It passes along the right posterior coronary sulcus.

3. *Middle cardiac vein:* It begins near the apex and traverses the posterior interventricular groove.

4. *Posterior vein of the left ventricle:* It is present on the diaphragmatic surface of the left ventricle.

5. *Oblique vein of the left atrium (of Marshall):* It descends obliquely on the back of the left atrium to join the coronary sinus.

### Anterior Cardiac Veins

They drain anterior part of the right ventricle and are usually two or three in number. They ascend to open directly into right atrium.

### Venae Cordis Minimae

They are numerous in the right atrium and ventricle and open into all the chambers.

### NERVE SUPPLY TO THE HEART

Though the cardiac muscle contracts rhythmically and automatically, the nerves supplying the heart alter the cardiac rate. The sympathetic fibers are derived from upper 5 or 6 thoracic segment ($T_1$–$T_6$) of the spinal cord, while parasympathetic is derived from vagus nerve.

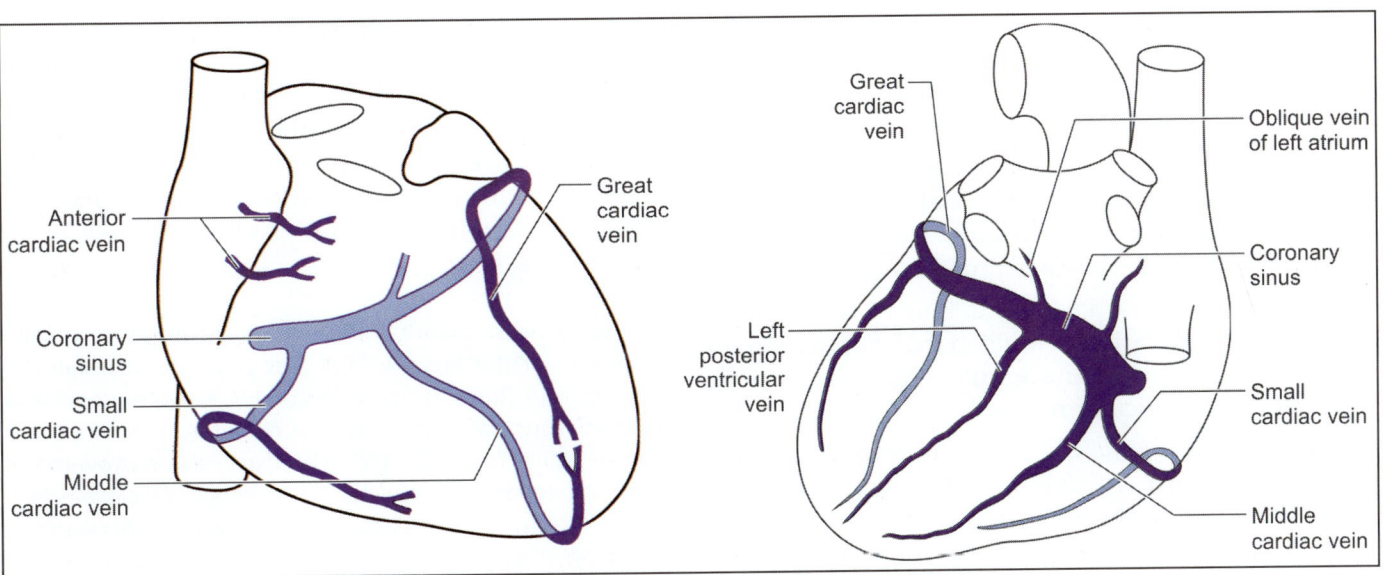

**Fig. 17.11:** Venous drainage of the heart —anterior view and posterior view

The sympathetic and parasympathetic fibers supplying the heart form two cardiac plexuses-superficial and deep.

### a. Superficial Cardiac Plexus

It is situated below the arch of aorta and in front of the right pulmonary artery. Fibers from the superficial cardiac plexus pass into deep cardiac plexus and pulmonary plexus.

*Formation*

1. A branch from the left superior cervical sympathetic ganglion.
2. Lower cervical cardiac branch of the left vagus nerve.

### b. Deep Cardiac Plexus

It is situated in front of the bifurcation of the trachea.

*Formation*

1. Cardiac branches of the both (right and left) cervical sympathetic ganglia (except from left superior)
2. Cardiac branches form the upper four or five thoracic sympathetic ganglia
3. Cardiac branches of the both vagus (except lower cervical cardiac branch of left vagus)

*Functions*

1. Sympathetic fibers increase the heart rate and cardiac output and parasympathetic fibers diminish it.
2. Sympathetic fibers produce vasodilatation in intramuscular branches and vasoconstriction of epicardial arteries.
3. Sympathetic fibers also carry pain sensation from the heart.
4. The parasympathetic fibers slows the heart rate, reduces the force of contraction and constricts the coronary arteries.

### CONDUCTING SYSTEM OF THE HEART

The conducting system consists of specialized cardiac muscle fibers. It includes pacemaker and Purkinje muscle fibers. These structures are capable of initiating and conducting the cardiac impulses (Fig.17.12).

1. *Sinuatrial node (SA node):* It is known as the 'pace maker' of the heart. It is situated in the upper part of the crista terminalis. The impulses from the SA node reach atrioventricular node.
2. *Atrioventricular node (AV node):* It is located in the triangle of Koch, which is placed in the lower part of the interatrial septum.
3. *Atrioventricular bundle (AV bundle or bundle of His):* It begins from the AV node traverses the membranus

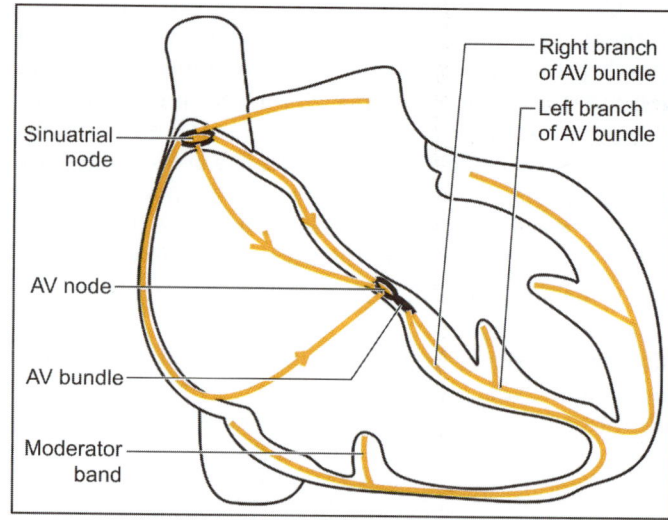

**Fig. 17.12:** Conducting system of heart

part of the interventricular septum and then divides into right and left branches.

a. The right branch passes to the right side of the interventricular septum. Majority of the fibers enters septomarginal trabecula (moderator band) to reach the base of the anterior papillary muscle.
b. The left branch is distributed in the wall of the left ventricle.

4. Purkinje fibers form a subendocardial plexus.

### STRUCTURE OF THE HEART

Heart consists of three coats from outside to inside-epicardium, myocardium and endocardium.

1. *Epicardium:* It is derived from the visceral layer of serous pericardium.
2. *Myocardium:* It is made up of cardiac muscles, which present striations with centrally placed nucleus. The muscle fibers branch and anastamose with adjacent fibers. Intercalated discs connect the adjacent muscle cells (myocytes). Some of the cardiac muscle fibers are specialized to form 'Purkinje fibers', which constitute the conducting system of the heart.
3. *Endocardium:* It is the lining endothelial cells of the chambers.

Abnormal heart sounds, called murmurs, often arise from disorders of the heart valves. For example, if a valve is incompetent (does not close properly), leakage produces a swishing sound after the valve has closed. A stenotic valve is one in which fused or stiffened cusps have narrowed the opening (stenosis = narrowing). Both stenotic and incompetent valves increase the workload on the heart and decrease its pumping efficiency. A faulty valve may be replaced with a synthetic valve.

The AV node is damaged by various forms of heart disease. The only route for impulse transmission from the atria to the ventricles is through the AV node. Therefore, damage to this node is called 'heart block', interferes with the ability of the ventricles to receive the impulses. Without these signals, the ventricles beat at an intrinsic rate that is slower than that of the atria and too slow to maintain adequate circulation. In such cases an artificial pacemaker set to discharge at the appropriate rate is usually implanted.

# Blood Vessels of the Thorax, Abdomen, Head and Neck

**18**

## ARTERIES OF THE THORAX

The thoracic cavity presents heart in middle mediastinum. The ascending aorta begins from the cavity of the left ventricle and carries oxygenated blood to all parts of the body. The ascending aorta itself gives two coronary arteries, which supply the musculature of the heart.

### 1. ARCH OF AORTA

- It is the continuation of the ascending aorta at the level of manubriosternal joint.
- Arch of aorta is situated behind the manubrium sterni. It passes upwards, backwards and to the left forming an arch.
- It terminates at the same level where it is formed (manubriosternal joint or lower border of fourth thoracic vertebra). It gives three branches (Fig. 18.1).
    a. Brachicephalic trunk (innominate artery) which further divides into right common carotid and right subclavian arteries.
    b. Left common carotid artery.
    c. Left subclavian artery.

*Relations*
- Anteriorly—medial surface of the left lung and left phrenic nerve.
- Posteriorly—tracheal, esophagus, body of $T_4$ vertebra.

A localized dilatation of the arch of aorta is called 'aortic aneurysm' which is due to the weakness in the wall of the aorta. The dilated aorta can compress the nearby structures mentioned above. It can be fatal if it ruptures.

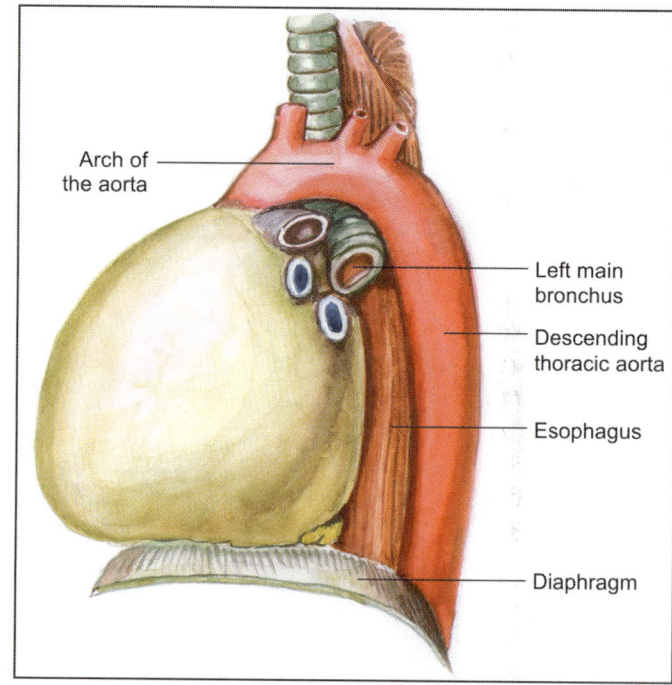

**Fig. 18.1:** Arch of aorta—lateral view

### 2. DESCENDING THORACIC AORTA

- It is the continuation of the arch of aorta.
- It descends in the posterior mediastinum of the thorax and closely related to esophagus.
- It enters the abdominal cavity by passing through the diaphragm at the level of twelfth thoracic vertebra.
- In the abdomen it continues as abdominal aorta.
- The descending thoracic aorta gives many branches.
- They include third to eleventh posterior intercostal arteries on each side. These arteries supply the thoracic wall.
- The other branches from the thoracic aorta are esophagel and mediastinal arteries (Figs18.2 and 18.3).

210

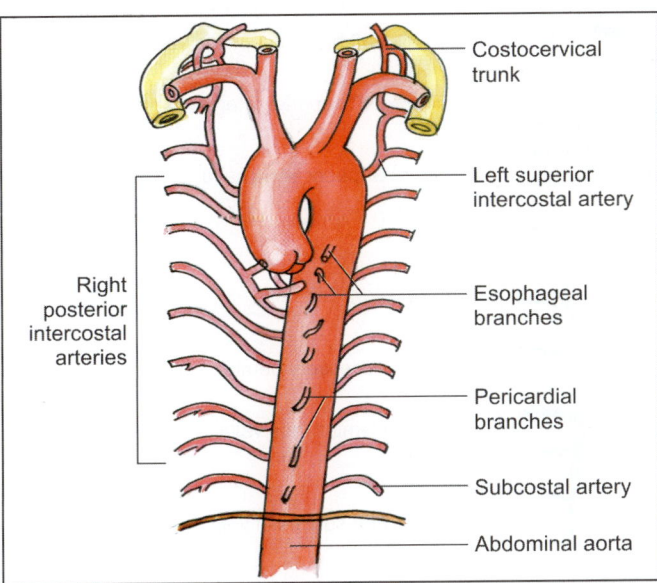

**Fig. 18.2:** Descending thoracic aorta

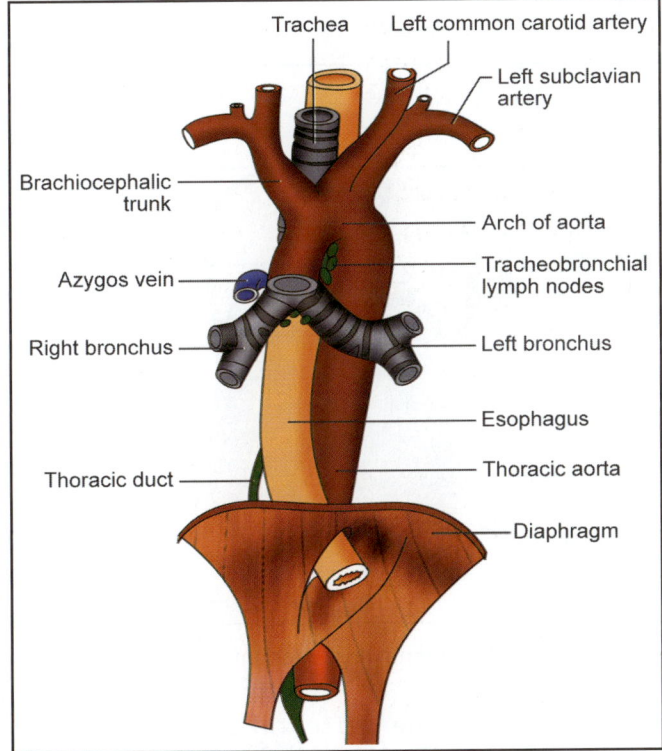

**Fig. 18.3:** Thoracic aorta and esophagus

## 3. INTERNAL THORACIC ARTERY (INTERNAL MAMMARY ARTERY)

- It is a branch from the first part of the subclavian artery.
- On each side it descends in the anterior thoracic wall behind the costal cartilages.

- At the sixth intercostal space it terminates by dividing into superior epigastic artery and musculophrenic artery.
- The internal thoracic artery gives two anterior intercostal arteries in each intercostal space (upper six intercostal spaces). It is the chief artery supplying mammary gland in females.
- The superior epigastric artery enters the rectus abdominus muscle of the abdomen by passing through the gap present between the sternal and costal origin of the diaphragm (foramen of Morgagani). It anastomoses with inferior epigastric artery arising from the external iliac artery within the rectus abdominis muscle.
- The musculophrenic artery descends obliquely along the costal margin supplying lower intercostal spaces and diaphragm.

The internal thoracic artery can be used as the bypass vessel for coronary bypass surgery. The use of this artery has some advantages over the traditional use of great saphenous vein. Internal thoracic artery is a thick walled artery and less likely to be damaged by the pressure of heartbeat and therefore less likely to develop atherosclerosis. The internal thoracic artery remains attached to the subclavian artery (the origin of the artery is not cut) and its distal end is sutured onto the obstructed coronary artery in the wall of the heart.

## VEINS OF THE THORAX

The inercostal spaces of thorax are drained by anterior and posterior intercostal veins. The anterior intercostal veins terminate in internal thoracic vein. However, the mode of termination of posterior intercostal veins differ on two sides. They drain into azygos (azygos = unpaired) system of veins (Fig. 18.4).

### 1. AZYGOS VEIN

It is an important vein draining the venous blood from the posterior abdominal wall and major portion of the thoracic wall.

### Formation

It is formed within the abdominal cavity by many combinations. Usually, it is formed by the union of right ascending lumbar vein (which is formed by the union of four lumbar veins) and right subcostal vein. Sometimes a lumbar azygos vein (a vein arising from the inferior vena cava) can also contribute to the formation of azygos vein. It ascends through aortic opening of the diaphragm. It ascends in the posterior mediastinum on the right side.

18

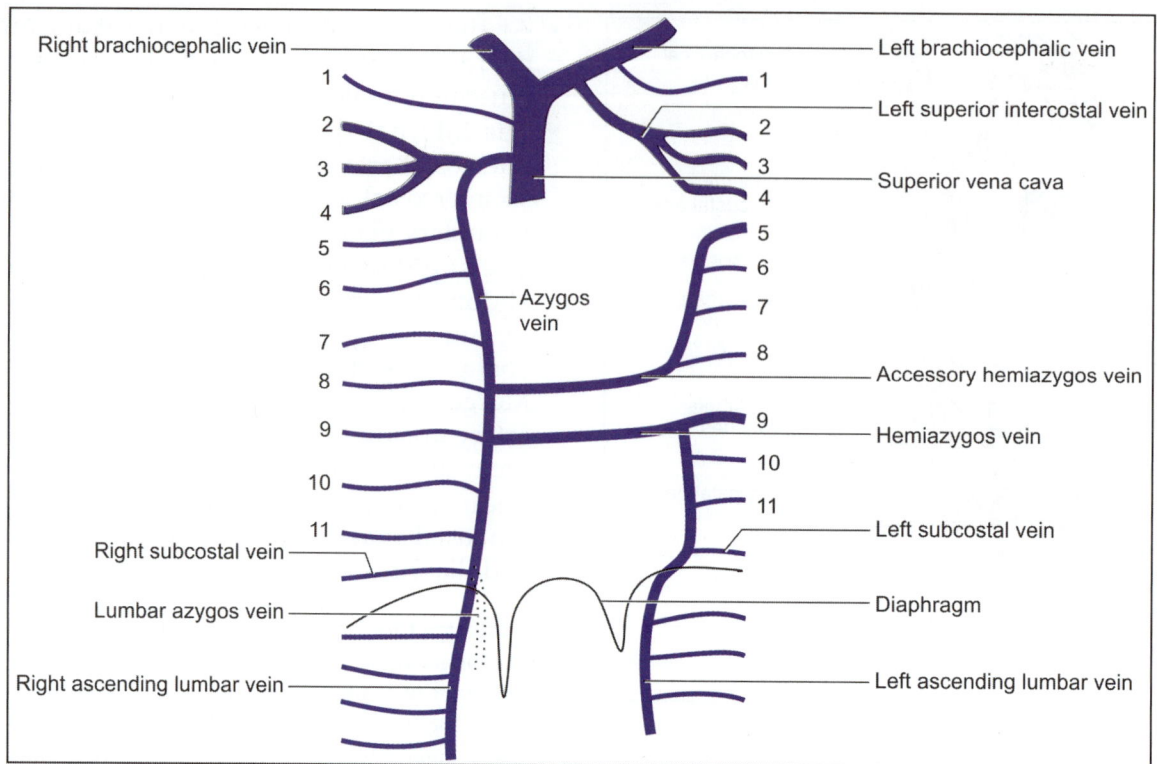

**Fig. 18.4:** Azygos system of veins

## Termination

It arches over the root of right lung and opens into the superior vena cava.

## Tributaries

i. All the posterior intercostal veins on the right side open directly or indirectly except the right first posterior intercostal vein.

ii. Posterior intercostal veins of the left side terminate in to the azygos vein by forming accessory hemiazygos (which is formed by the union of fifth to eighth left posterior intercostal veins) and hemiazygos vein (which is formed by the union of left ascending lumbar vein and left subcostal vein. In the posterior mediastinum the hemiazygos vein receives lower three posterior intercostal veins (Fig. 18.4).

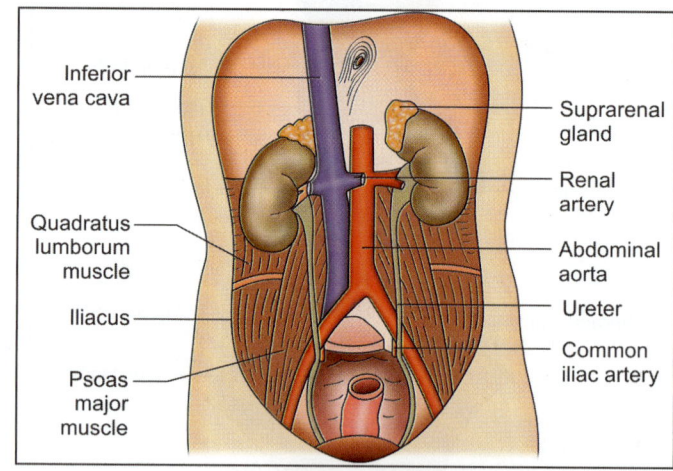

**Fig. 18.5:** Abdominal aorta and inferior vena cava

### ARTERIES OF ABDOMEN AND PELVIS

## ARTERIES

### The Abdominal Aorta

It is the main artery supplying abdominal wall and organs. It is the continuation of the thoracic aorta at the level of $T_{12}$ vertebra (where it appears through the diaphragm). It descends on the posterior abdominal wall in front of the vertebral bodies and their intervertebral discs. Anteriorly, it is covered by peritoneum and it is placed to the left of the inferior vena cava. It terminates at the level of lower border of fourth lumbar vertebra by dividing into right and left common iliac arteries (Fig. 18.5).

The branches of the abdominal aorta can be classified into anterior/ventral (those supplying gastrointestinal tract and related organs) and lateral (supplying kidney and suprarenal glands).

18

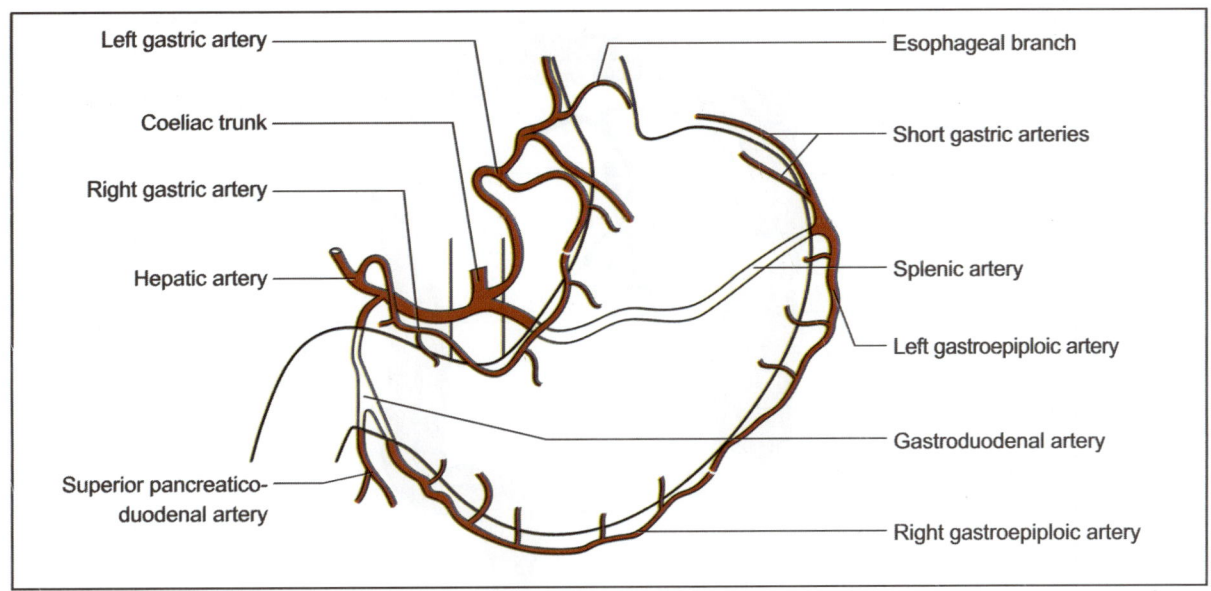

**Fig. 18.6:** Coeliac trunk and its branches

The three ventral branches are:

### 1. Coeliac Trunk

It is an arterial trunk, which arises from ventral aspect of the abdominal aorta and soon divides into three terminal branches. The branches include (Fig. 18.6).

i. *Left gastric artery:* It ascends towards the lower end of the esophagus and then descends along the lesser curvature of the stomach within the lesser omentum. In addition to supplying the stomach it gives a branch to the lower end of the esophagus.

ii. *Common hepatic artery:* It passes horizontally towards right side along the upper border of the pancreas. It gives a right gastric artery, which runs along the lesser curvature of the stomach within the lesser omentum to anastomose with left gastric arery. After giving another branch called gastoduodenal artery the common hepatic artery ascends in the right free margin of the lesser omentum as hepatic artery proper and terminates in the porta hepatis of the liver by dividing into right and left terminal branches.

The gastroduodenal artery divides into superior pancreaticoduodenal artery and right gastoepiploic artery (which passes along the greater curvature of the stomach) (Fig. 18.6).

iii. *Splenic artery:* This tortuous artery passes horizontally to the left along the upper border of the body of the pancreas behind the stomach. Its terminal part enters the peritoneal ligament called lienorenal ligamnet along with the tail of the pancreas and near the hilum of the spleen it divides into many branches for the spleen. It gives the following branches.

a. Many pancreatic branches supplying the pancreas.

b. Left gastroepiploic artery, which passes along the greater curvature of the stomach and anastamoses with right gastoepiploic artery.

c. Short gastric arteries: They enter the gastrosplenic ligament to supply the fundic portion of the stomach.

To summarize, the coeliac trunk supplies stomach, part of the duodenum, liver, gallbladder, pancreas and spleen.

In gastric ulcers, acidic contents can erode the posterior wall of the stomach and erode splenic artery which cause internal bleeding.
Ulcers affecting first part of the duodenum can perforate posteriorly to involve gastroduodenal artery causing severe bleeding.

### 2. Superior Mesenteric Artery

It arises from the ventral aspect of the abdominal aorta behind the body of the pancreas just below the origin of the coeliac trunk. It supplies mainly the small intestine. It gives following branches (Fig. 18.7).

i. *Inferior pancreaticoduodenal artery:* It ascends in the groove between duodenum and pancreas and anastomoses with superior pancreaticoduodenal artery.

18

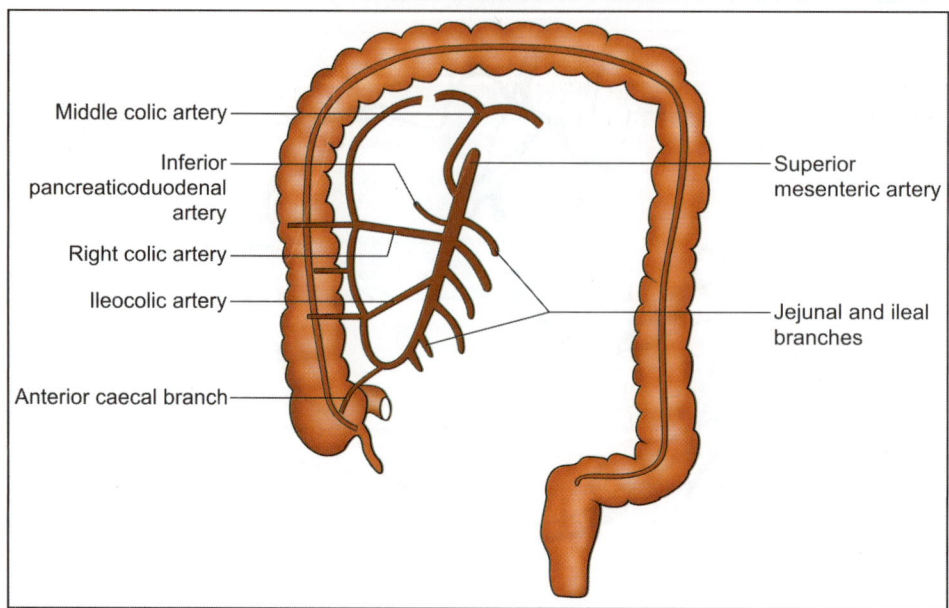

**Fig. 18.7:** Superior mesenteric artery and its branches

ii. *Many jejunal and ileal branches* arising from the left convex margin of the parent artery enter the mesentery (peritoneal fold suspending the jejunum and ileum) and supply jejunum and ileum.

iii. *Ileocolic artery:* It passes behind the peritoneum towards the caecum. Where it gives many branches (anterior and posterior caecal arteries, appendicular artery, ascending branch and ileal branch). It supplies terminal part of the ileum, caecum, appendix and lower part of the ascending colon.

iv. *The right colic artery:* It passes towards the ascending colon and divides into ascending and descending branches. The descending branch anastomose with ascending branch of the ileocolic artery and ascending branch with right terminal branch of the middle colic artery.

v. *The middle colic artery:* It passes towards transverse colon within the transverse mesocolon and divides into right and left branches. The right terminal branch anastomoses with ascending branch of the right colic artery and left branch with ascending branch of the left colic artery.

### 3. Inferior Mesenteric Artery

It arise from the ventral aspect of the abdominal aorta just above its termination. It supplies the large intestine. It gives the following branches (Fig.18.8).

   i. *The left colic artery:* It passes towards the descending colon where it divides into ascending and descending branches. The ascending branch

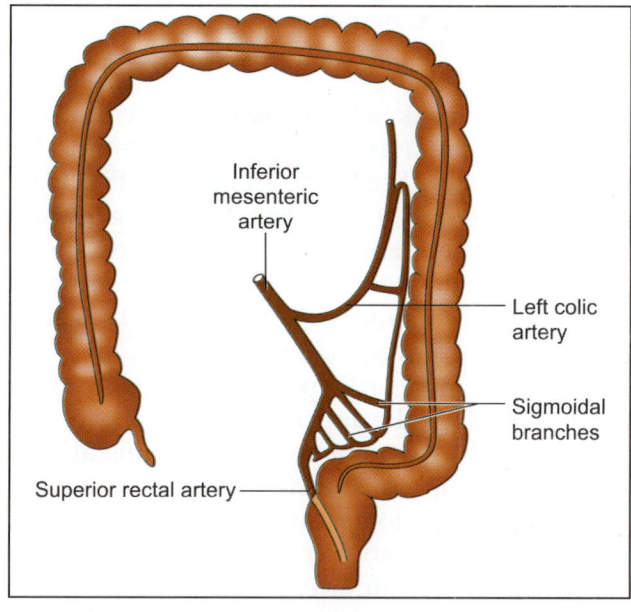

**Fig. 18.8:** Inferior mesenteric artery and its branches

anastomoses with left terminal branch of the middle colic artery and descending branch with highest sigmoidal artery.

   ii. *Sigmoidal branches:* They supply the sigmoid colon.

iii. *The superior rectal artery:* It is the continuation of inferior mesenteric artery. It descends along the posterior aspect of the rectum. It pierces the outer musculature of the rectum and its final radicals appear in the anal columns.

The lateral branches of abdominal aorta include.

## 4. Renal Arteries

The right renal artery is longer than left and it passes behind the inferior vena cava. Each renal artery divides into branches before entering the hilum of the kidney. Each renal artery gives inferior suprarenal artery(s).

## 5. Gonadal Arteries (Testicular or Ovarian Artery)

They arise from the lateral aspect of the abdominal aorta and descend on the posterior abdominal wall deep to the peritoneum. In males, the testicular artery enters the inguinal canal as the content of the spermatic cord and passes along the posterior border of the testis.

In females, the ovarian artery after descending on the posterior abdominal wall deep to the peritoneum enters the suspensory ligament of the ovary (which extend from the lateral pelvic wall) and finally reaches the ovary through mesovarium (peritoneal fold connecting the posterior layer of the broad ligament of the uterus to ovary). The ovarian artery apart from ovary also supplies uterine tube, part of the uterus and ureter.

## 6. Middle Suprarenal Arteries

They supply suprarenal glands.

## 7. Inferior Phrenic Arteries

They are the first branches from the abdominal aorta arising just below the diaphragm and supply the under surface of the diaphgram. They give superior suprarenal arteries.

## 8. Lumbar Arteries

On each side, usually they are four in number and supply posterior abdominal wall.

## Common Iliac Arteries

One on each side they arise as the terminal branches of the abdominal aorta. Each artery passes downwards and laterally and terminates by dividing into external iliac and internal iliac arteries (Fig. 18.9).

## External Iliac Artery

It extends downwards to the anterior aspect of the thigh. It passes deep to the inguinal ligament. At the midinguinal point it enters the thigh as femoral artery. The external iliac artery gives two named branches.

## Inferior Epigastric Artery

It enters the rectus abdominis muscle to anastomose with superior epigastric artery.

## Deep Circumflex Iliac Artery

It passes towards anterior superior iliac spine.

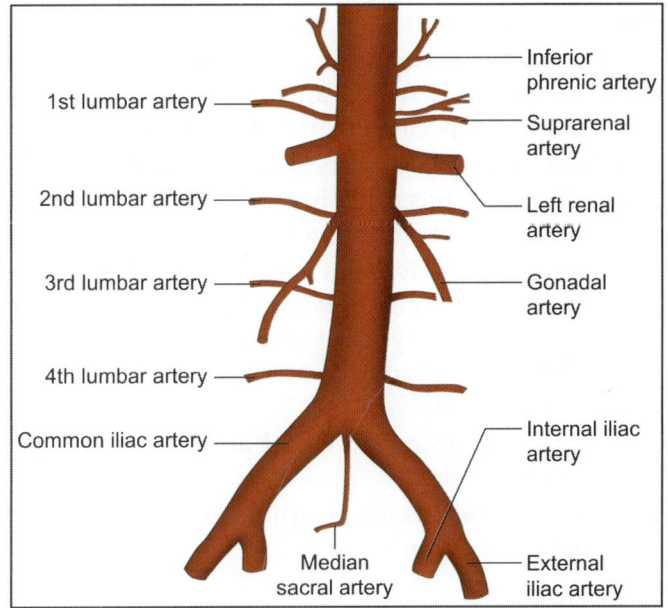

**Fig. 18.9:** Abdominal aorta and its lateral branches

## Internal Iliac Arteries

The internal iliac artery, with its following branches supplies the pelvic organs (anal canal, prostate, perineum, urethra, urinary bladder, uterus, etc.) and also gluteal region.

 i. *Superior and inferior gluteal arteries:* These branches passes into the gluteal region through greater sciatic foramen.

 ii. *Internal pudendal artery:* It also passes into the gluteal region by passing through greater sciatic foramen and then it curves around the ischial spine. It enters

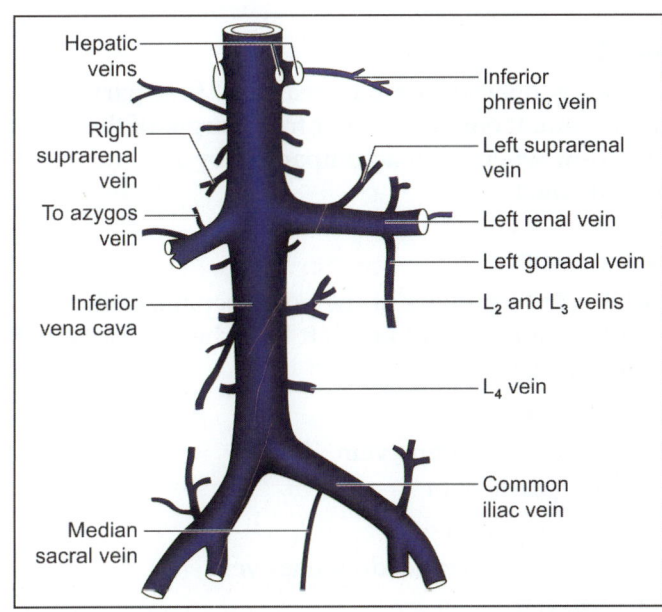

**Fig. 18.10:** Inferior vena cava and its tributaries

the lesser sciatic foramen along with pudendal nerve to travese the pudendal canal (in the lateral wall of the ischiorectal fossa) and supplies structures present in the perineum and external genitalia.

iii. *Obturator artery:* It descends into the medial side of the thigh by passing through obturator canal accompanying the obturator nerve.

iv. *Uterine artery:* In females it is an important artery which ascends along the lateral border of the uterus within the two layers of the broad ligament. In addition to the uterus it also supplies ovary, uterine tube and vagina.

v. Superior and inferior vesical arteries supply the urinary bladder.

vi. Middle rectal artery supplies seminal vesicle, prostate and rectum.

## PORTAL VEIN

Portal vessels begin from capillaries and terminate in capillaries (Fig. 18.11).

Portal vein brings venous blood from abdominal part of the gastrointestinal tract (which contains absorbed materials of digestion) liver, pancreas and spleen to the liver for further metabolism.

It is about 8 cm long.

The normal portal pressure is about 5–15 mmHg.

### Formation

Portal vein is formed behind the neck of the pancreas by the union of superior mesenteric and splenic veins.

### Course

It ascends deep to the pancreas and first part of the duodenum. It enters the right free margin of the lesser omentum where it is accompanied by hepatic artery and bile duct.

### Termination

Portal vein terminates at the porta hepatis of the liver by dividing into right and left branches. *Tributaries of the portal vein:*

1. Splenic vein
2. Superior mesenteric vein
3. Right gastric vein
4. Left gastric vein
5. Superior pancreaticoduodenal vein
6. Cystic vein
7. Paraumbilical vein

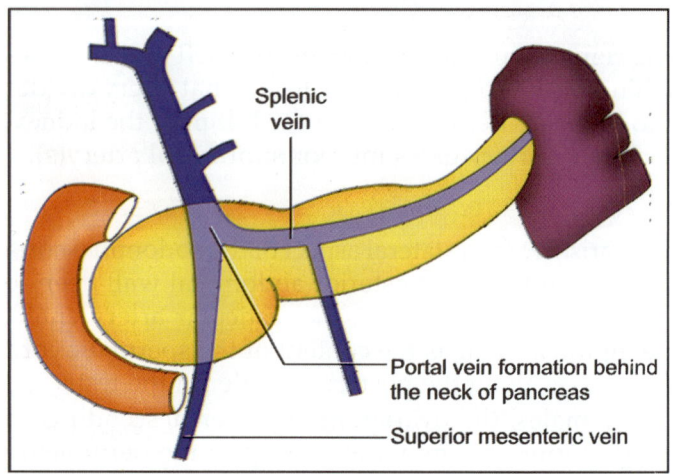

**Fig. 18.11:** Portal vein, formation

### Portocaval Anastomosis

These are the communications between the tributaries of portal vein (ending in liver) and systemic veins (ending in right atrium of the heart through vena cava).

These anastamoses are important in case of portal obstruction, where these vessels dilate and form an alternate route of venous drainage.

Such portocaval anastomoses are present at the following places (Fig. 18.12).

1. *At the umbilicus:* Para umbilical veins (portal) anastamosing with veins of the anterior abdominal wall (systemic)
2. *At the lower end of the oesophagus:* Tributaries of the left gastric vein (portal) anastomosing with tributaries of hemiazygos vein (systemic)
3. *At the anal canal:* The superior rectal vein (portal) anastamosing with middle and inferior rectal veins (systemic)
4. *In the posterior abdominal wall:* Veins of duodenum, ascending and descending colon (portal) anastamosing with renal and azygos veins (systemic)
5. *At the Bare area of the liver:* Hepatic venules arising from the liver (portal) anastamosing with inferior phrenic vein (systemic).

### Applied Aspects

In increased portal pressure (portal hypertension) as in cirrhosis of the liver, the portocaval anastamoses enlarge and can cause:

- *Caput medusae:* Superficial veins of the anterior abdominal wall dilate and radiate from the umbilicus
- *Esophageal varices:* Dilated venous sacs at the lower end of the esophagus and it may rupture causing severe hematemesis
- *Piles in the anal canal:* Dilated venous sacs in the anal canal.

18

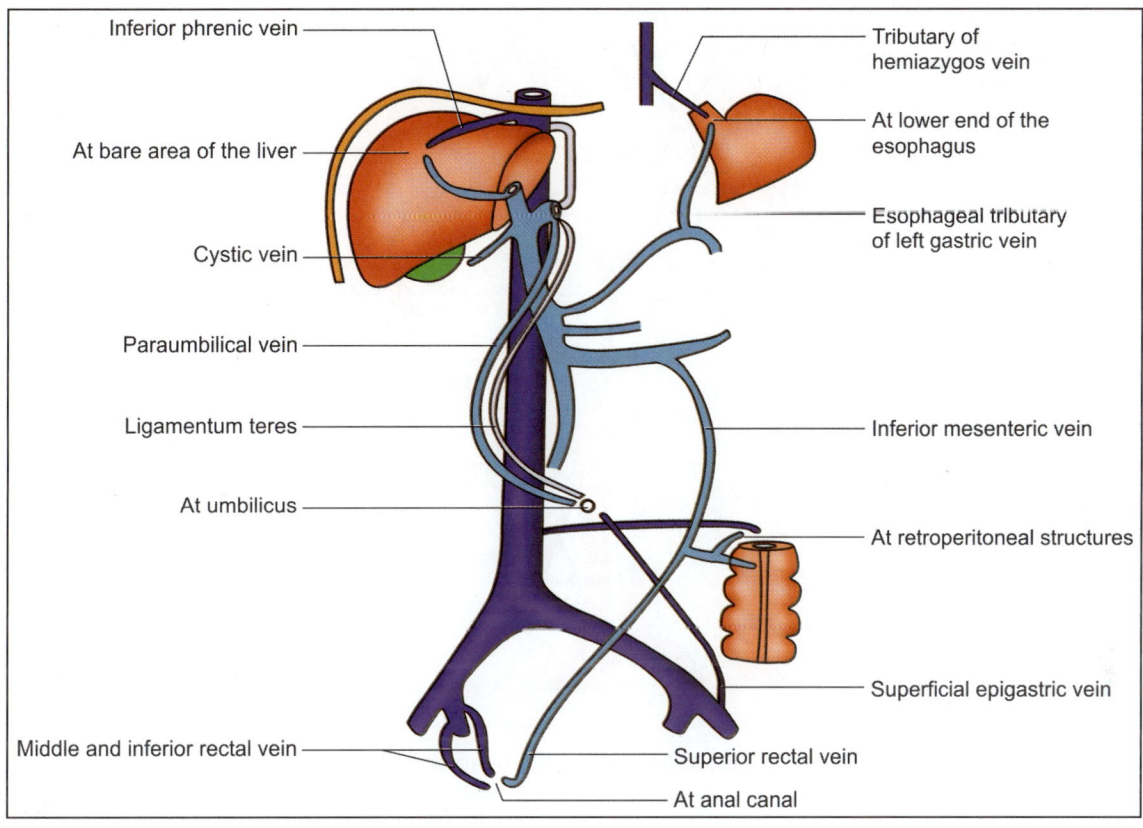

**Fig. 18.12:** Sites of portocaval anastomosis

## INFERIOR VENA CAVA

It is the main vein carrying venous blood from lower limb, pelvis and the abdominal cavity. It drains into the right atrium of heart (Fig. 18.10).

It is formed by the union of right and left common iliac veins at the level of lower border of fifth lumbar vertebra. It ascends infront of the lumbar vertebral bodies to the right of abdominal aorta. Then it grooves the posterior surface of the liver and finally passes through the central tendon of diaphgram to open into the right atrium.

It receives renal veins and right gonadal vein, right suprarenal vein and hepatic veins.

### ARTERIES OF HEAD AND NECK

## ARTERIES

The main artery supplying the neck and greater part of the head is external carotid and subclavian arteries (Fig. 18.13).

### External Carotid Artery

It is one of the terminal branches of the common carotid artery given at the level of upper border of the lamina of the thyroid cartilage (Fig. 18.14).

It ascends through the neck and enters the parotid salivary gland. It terminates within the parotid gland at the level of neck of the mandible.

It gives the following branches:

1. *Ascending pharyngeal artery:* It ascends along the wall of the pharynx supplying pharynx and palatine tonsil.

2. *Superior thyroid artery:* It passes along with external laryngeal nerve and supplies thyroid gland. It also gives superior laryngeal artery.

3. *Lingual artery:* It passes towards tongue deep to the hyoglossus muscle. This muscle divides the artery into three parts. The proximal part of the artery is crossed by hypoglossal nerve.

4. *Facial artery*
   - It ascends deep to the posterior belly of the digastric muscle, then winds around the superficial part of the submandibular salivary gland.
   - It enters the face at the anteroinferior angle of the Masseter muscle.
   - In the face the artery is tortuous and reaches the point little lateral to the angle of the mouth.
   - Then it ascends along the lateral side of the nose.

18

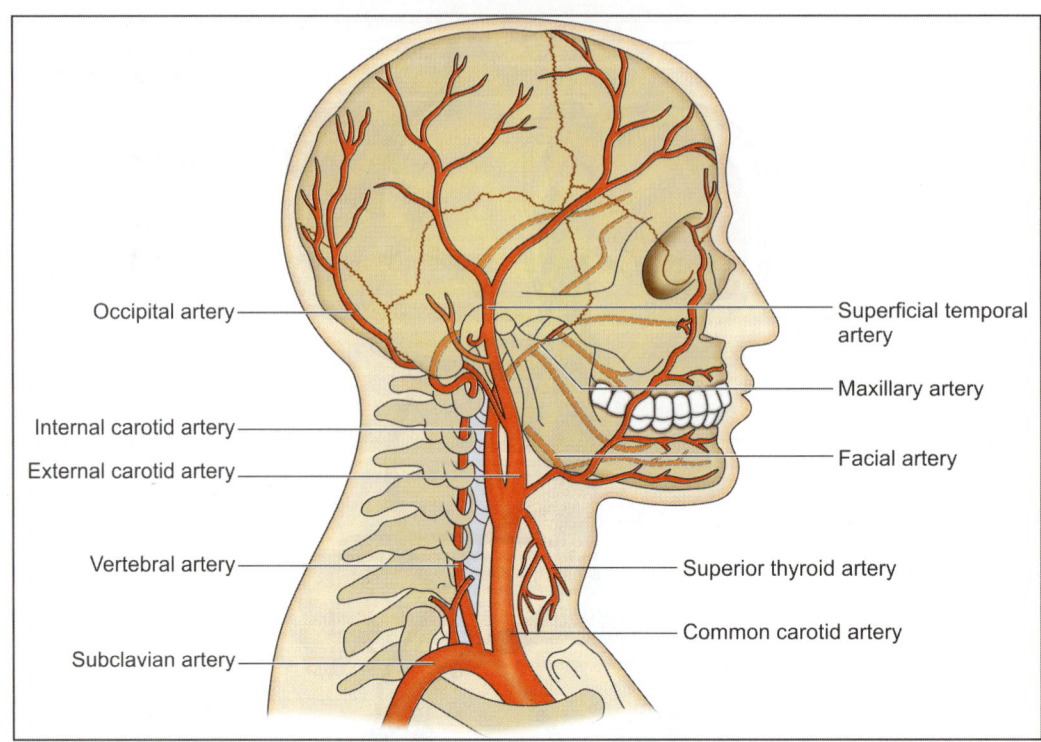

**Fig. 18.13:** Arteries of the head and neck

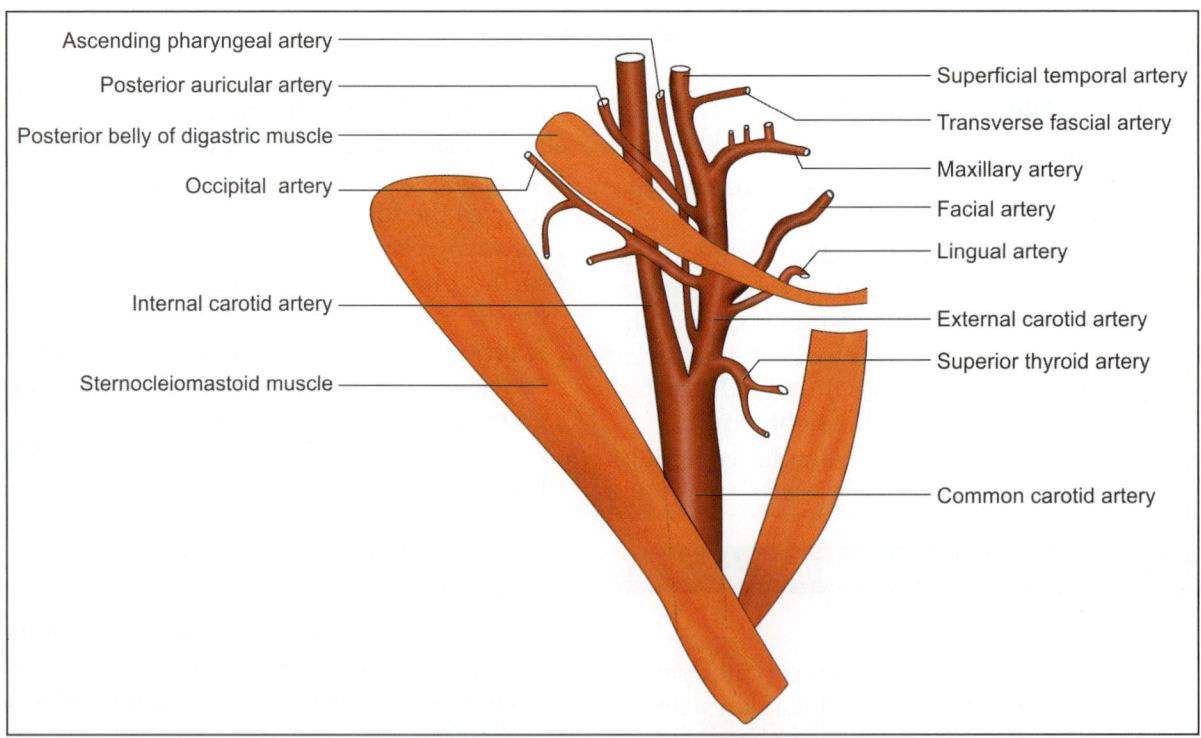

**Fig. 18.14:** External carotid artery and its branches

- It terminates at the medial angle of the eye by anastomosing with dorsal nasal branch of the ophthalmic artery.

*Branches of facial artery in the neck*

a. Ascending palatine artery

b. Tonsillar artery

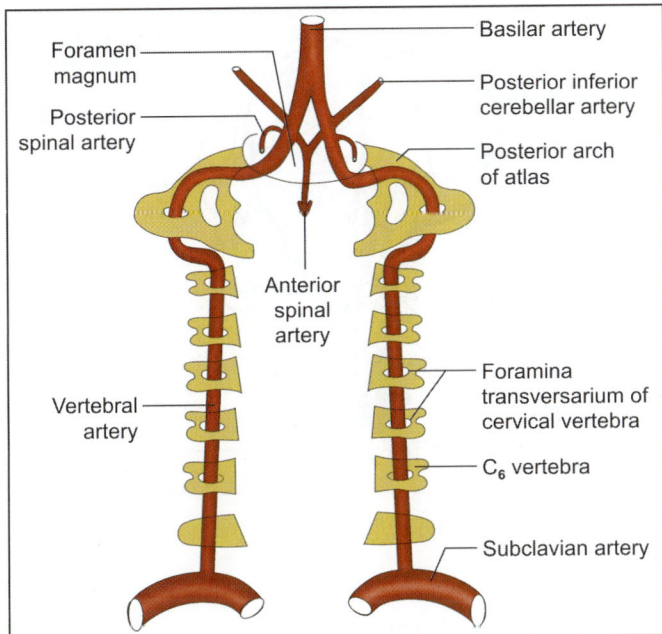

**Fig. 18.15:** Vertebral arteries

c. Submental artery

d. Glandular branches to submandibular gland.

*Branches of the facial artery in the face*

a. *Inferior labial artery:* To lower lip

b. *Superior labial artery:* It gives alar and septal branches to the nose

c. Lateral nasal branch.

5. *Posterior auricular artery:* It passes posteriorly along the upper border of posterior belly of the digastric muscle. It supplies external ear and posterior quadrant of the scalp.

6. *Occipital artery:* It also passes posteriorly along the lower border of the posterior belly of the digastric muscle. It supplies posterior quadrant of the scalp.

7. *Superficial temporal artery:* It is one of the terminal branches of the external carotid artery. It ascends in front of the ear along with auriculo-temporal nerve. It gives transverse facial artery, which appears on the face. The superficial temporal artery supplies temporal region and anterior quadrant of the scalp.

8. *Maxillary artery*

- It is the other terminal branch of the external carotid artery.
- It passes anteriorly in the infratemporal fossa.
- The artery is divided into three parts by lateral pterygoid muscle.
- The first part extends from its origin to the lower border of the lateral pterygoid muscle (Mandibular part). This part gives following branches

a. *Deep auricular artery:* It supplies external ear.

b. *Anterior tympanic artery:* It enters the middle ear

c. *Middle meningeal artery:* It enters the cranial cavity and supplies meninges

d. *Accessory meningeal artery:* It also enters the cranial cavity and supplies meninges

e. *Inferior alveolar artery:* It supplies all the lower teeth and mandible.

The second part lies either superficial or deep to the lower head of the lateral pterygoid muscle (pterygoid part). It gives many muscular branches like deep temporal arteries, buccal artery, pterygoid arteries and masseteric artery.

The third part extends between the two heads of lateral pterygoid muscle to the pterygopalatine fossa (pterygomaxillary part). It enters the fossa through the pterygomaxillary fissure. It gives the following branches; some of which arise even before the maxillary artery enters the pteygopalatine fossa.

a. *Posterior superior alveolar artery:* It enters the maxillary air sinus and supplies upper molar and premolar teeth.

b. *Infra orbital artery:* It terminates on the face.

c. *Greater palatine artery:* It descends in the greater palatine canal. It gives lesser palatine branch. It supplies palate and nasal cavity.

d. *Pharyngeal artery:* It enters the nasopharynx and supplies nasopharynx and auditory tube.

e. *Artery of the pterygoid canal:* It traverses the pterygoid canal. It supplies nasopharynx, auditory tube and middle ear cavity.

f. *Spheno-palatine artery:* It supplies posterior part of the lateral wall of the nasal cavity and nasal septum.

Middle meningeal artery is clinically important. It enters the skull through foramen spinosum and supplies inner surfaces of the skull bone and underlying dura mater. Blows to the sides of the head often tear this artery producing an increased hematoma that can compress the cerebrum and disrupt brain function.

## SUBCLAVIAN ARTERY

### Origin

On the right side it arises from the brachiocephalic trunk and on the left side it arises as a direct branch from the arch of aorta.

### Course

Each artery arches laterally in the root of the neck, in front of the apex of the lungs and cervical pleura. It passes over the superior surface of the first rib. At the

18

outer border of the first rib the artery continues as axillary artery.

### Parts

The subclavian artery is divided into three parts by Scalenus anterior muscle.

The first part, medial to the muscle gives the following branches.

a. *Vertebral artery:* It is explained in 'blood vessels of the brain'.

b. *Internal thoracic artery:* It is explained in 'blood vessels of the thorax'.

c. *Thyrocervical trunk:* This arterial trunk soon divides into three branches—the inferior thyroid artery, supra scapular artery and transverse cervical artery (superficial cervical artery).

The second part is deep to the scalenus anterior muscle. It gives costocervical trunk (this arterial trunk gives superior intercostal and deep cervical arteries).

The third part distal (lateral) to the scalenus anterior muscle is in the posterior triangle. It gives dorsal scapular artery.

### VEINS OF THE HEAD AND NECK

#### INTERNAL JUGULAR VEIN (Fig. 18.16)

It is the continuation of sigmoid sinus. It descends in the neck along with internal carotid and common carotid artery and vagus nerve inside the carotid sheath.

It terminates by joining with subclavian vein to form brachiocephalic vein.

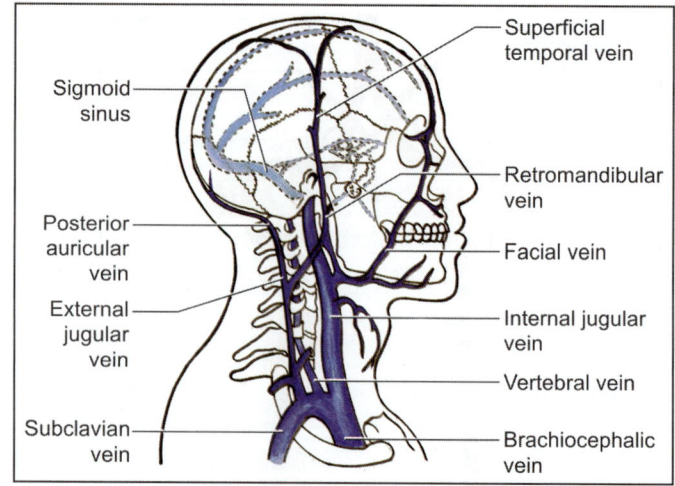

**Fig. 18.16:** Major veins of the head and neck

The internal jugular vein has the following tributaries.
- Inferior petrosal sinus
- Pharyngeal veins
- Common facial vein
- Superior thyroid vein
- Middle thyroid vein
- Deep lingual vein

Lymph from the lower limb, pelvis abdomen and part of the thorax is drained into thoracic duct, which opens at the junction of left internal jugular vein and left subclavian vein.

#### EXTERNAL JUGULAR VEIN

It is formed by the union of posterior division of retro-mandibular vein and posterior auricular vein (Fig. 18.17).

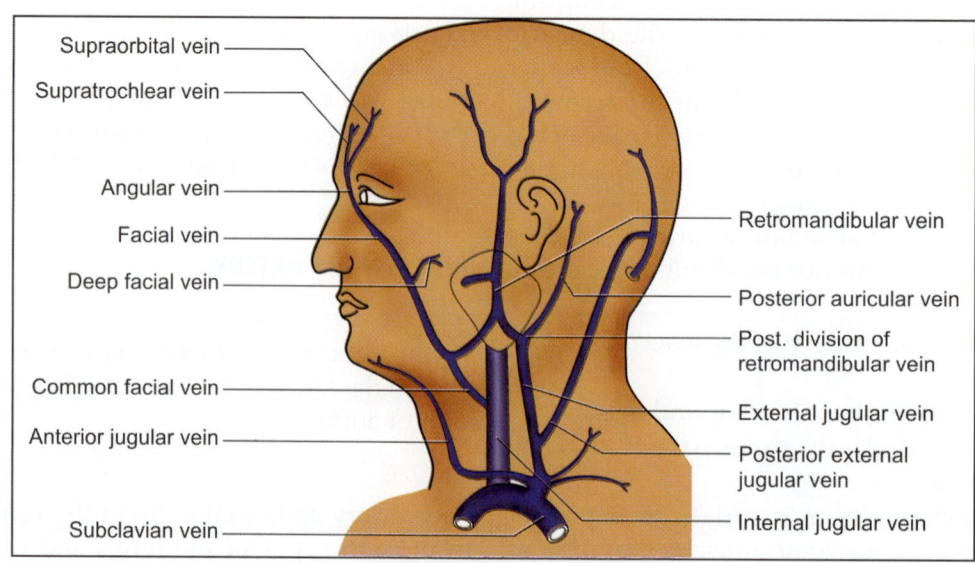

**Fig. 18.17:** Facial vein and deep facial vein

It descends superficially over the sternocleidomastoid muscle and then on the roof of the posterior triangle of the neck. It pierces the deep facia and terminates into subclavian vein.

## RETROMANDIBULAR VEIN

This is formed inside the parotid salivary gland by the union of maxillary and superficial temporal veins. It terminates at the apex of the gland by dividing into anterior and posterior divisions. The anterior division joins with facial vein to form common facial vein. The posterior division joins the posterior auricular vein to form the external jugular vein.

*Deep facial vein:* This vein connects the facial vein with pterygoid plexus of veins present around the lateral pterygoid muscle. These pterygoid plexus of veins are connected with cavernous sinus through emissary veins. Squeezing pimples on the nose or upper lip can spread infection through deep facial vein into the cavernous sinus. For this reason, the nose and upper lip is called 'dangerous area of the face'.

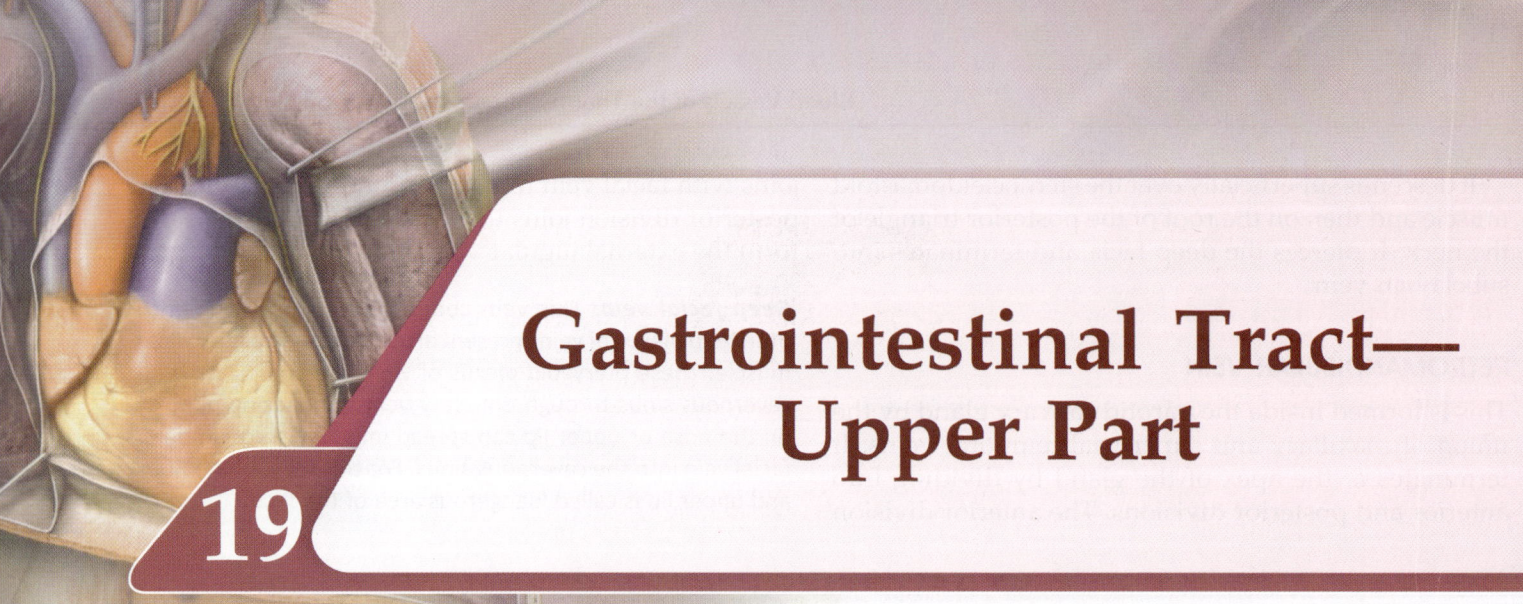

# Gastrointestinal Tract— Upper Part

## 19

Digestive system consists of gastrointestinal tract (GIT) and many glands associated with digestion.

The gastrointestinal tract extends from the mouth to the anus. It includes, oral cavity, pharynx, esophagus, stomach, small intestine (duodenum, jejunum, ileum), and large intestine (cecum with appendix, ascending, transverse, descending, sigmoid colon, rectum and anal canal).

Structurally, it is designed for deglutition, digestion, absorption of food substances, and expelling the waste products.

### GIT Consists of Following Parts

Oral cavity, pharynx, esophagus, stomach, small intestine and large intestine (Fig. 19.1).

### ORAL CAVITY

The oral cavity is divided into an outer smaller portion called vestibule and inner larger part called oral cavity proper.

### VESTIBULE

It is a narrow space bounded externally by lips and cheeks and internally by gums and teeth. The parotid duct opens into it opposite the crown of the upper 2nd molar tooth. Except the teeth, the entire vestibule is lined by mucous membrane.

### ORAL CAVITY PROPER

It is bounded anterolaterally by the teeth, gums and alveolar arches of the jaws. The roof is formed by hard palate, which separate it from the nasal cavity. Floor is formed posteriorly by the dorsum of the tongue, and anteriorly by the sublingual region (*see* Fig. 19.2).

*Gums* (gingivae) are soft tissues, which envelop the alveolar processes of the upper and lower jaws.

### TEETH

They form a part of the masticatory apparatus and are fixed to the jaws. In man, the teeth are replaced only once. The teeth of the first set (dentition) are known as milk or deciduous teeth and the second set as permanent teeth.

The milk teeth fall out between the ages of 6 and 12 years.

Deciduous teeth are 20 in number. Permanent teeth are 32 in number (8 incisors, 4 canines, 8 premolars, 12 molars) (*see* Fig. 19.2).

Generally all permanent teeth except the third molars have erupted by the end of adolescence. The third molars, also called 'wisdom teeth' emerge between the ages of 17 and 25 years. The wisdom teeth often fail to erupt and in some people they are completely absent.

Each tooth has three parts (Fig. 19.3):

1. A crown (projecting beyond the gum)
2. Root (embedded in the jaw)
3. Neck (between the crown and the root)

The crown is covered with a layer of enamel. Enamel is the hardest substance in the body. Calcium salts make 99% of its mass and it contains no cells or vessels.

Dentine underlies the enamel cap and forms the bulk of the tooth. Dentine is harder than bone and is made up of 'dentine tubules' filled with cellular processes of an odontoblast. The pulp cavity in the center of the tooth is filled with pulp, a loose connective tissue containing the tooth's vessels and nerves. The part of the pulp cavity in the root is root canal.

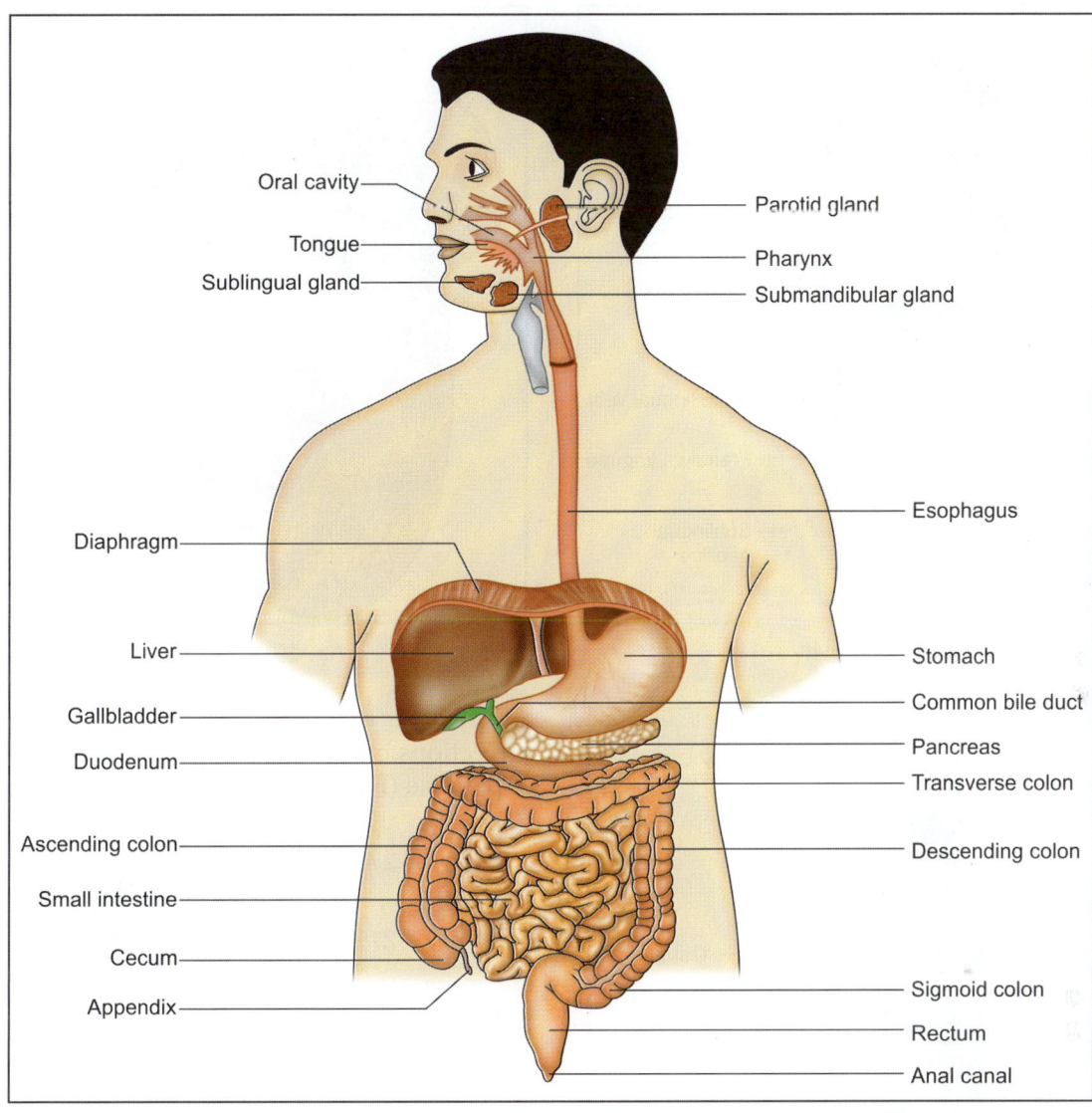

**Fig. 19.1:** Parts of the gastrointestinal tract

*Cementum:* The external surface of the tooth root is covered by a calcified connective tissue is called cementum.

The dental formula is a shorthand way of indicating the numbers and relative positions of the different classes of teeth in the mouth. This formula is written as a ratio, uppers over lowers for just half of the mouth.

For permanent dentition (Fig. 19.2):

$$\frac{2I, 1C, 2P, 3M}{2I, 1C, 2P, 3M} \times 2 = 32$$

For deciduous teeth:

$$\frac{2I, 1C, 2M}{2I, 1C, 2M} \times 2 = 20$$

When the tooth is damaged by a blow or by a deep cavity, the pulp becomes infected. In such cases root canal treatment (RCT) is performed. In this procedure, all of the pulp is drilled out and the pulp cavity is sterilised and filled with an artificial inert material. The tooth is then capped.

Dental cavities or caries result from a gradual demineralisation of the enamel and dentine by bacterial action. The decay process begins with the accumulation of dental plaque, a film of sugar, bacteria and other debris that adhere to the inflammation of the gums (gingivitis).

Upper teeth are supplied by maxillary and lower teeth are supplied by mandibular nerves.

## TONGUE

Tongue is a muscular organ situated in the floor of the oral cavity and oropharynx. It has a free tip at the

19

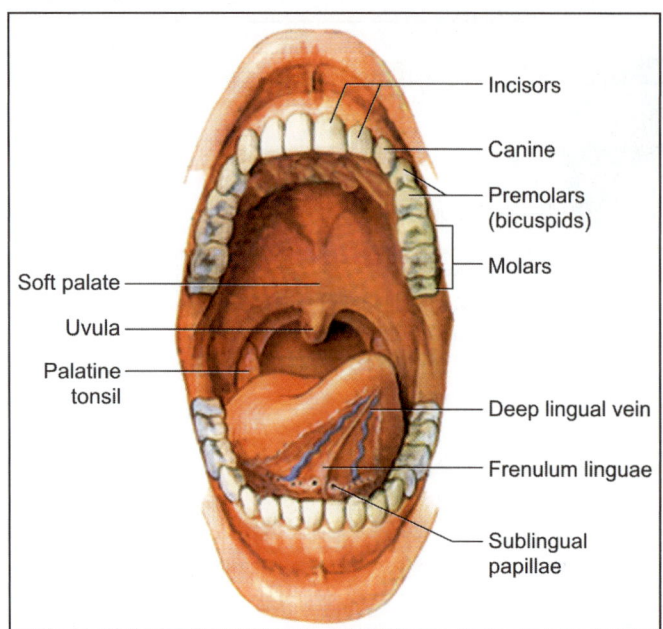

**Fig. 19.2:** Oral cavity

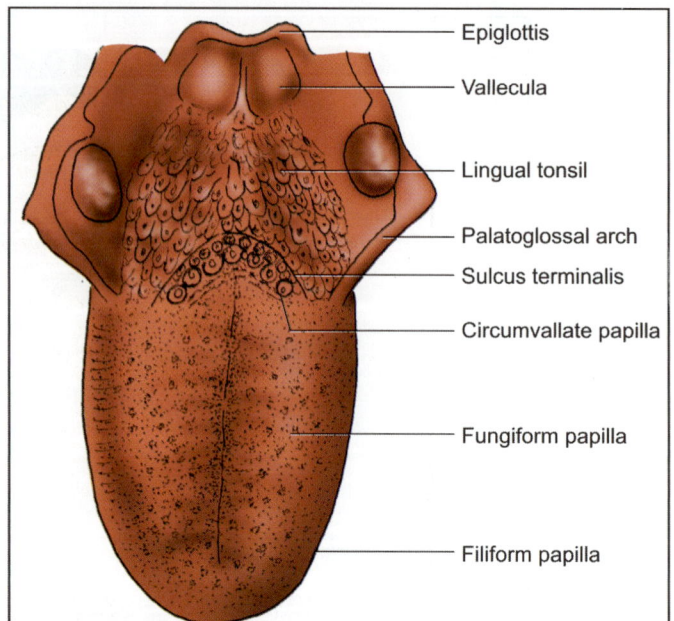

**Fig. 19.4:** Tongue—dorsum

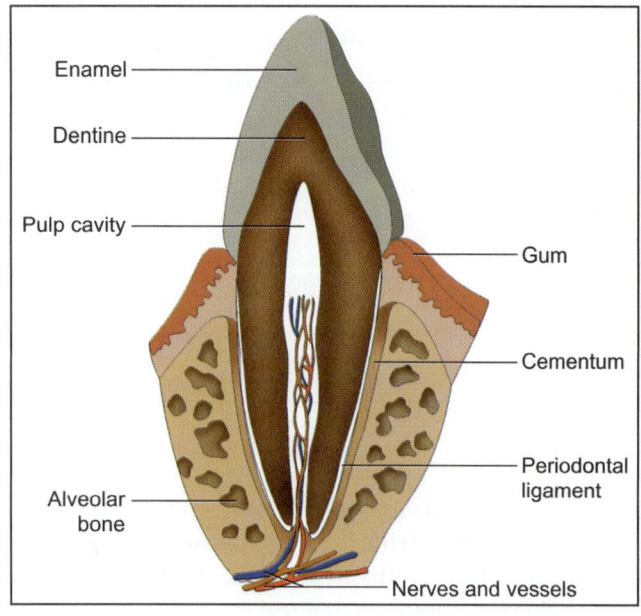

**Fig. 19.3:** Tooth

membrane of the anterior 2/3 presents conical projections called papillae. There are three main types of papillae (Fig. 19.4).

a. *Filiform papillae:* They are numerous all over the anterior 2/3 of the dorsum.

b. *Fungiform papillae:* They are scattered over the anterior 2/3 of the dorsum

c. *Circum-vallate papillae:* They are located in front of the sulcus terminalis. They present a number of taste buds.

The mucous membrane of the posterior 1/3 of the tongue presents lymphatic tissue, hence called lingual tonsil.

### Nerve Supply

The mucous membrane of the anterior 2/3 is supplied by lingual nerve (general sensation) and taste sensation is carried by chorda tympani branch of the facial nerve.

The mucous membrane of the posterior 1/3 is supplied by glossopharyngeal nerve, which carry both general sensation and taste sensation.

The posterior most part (vallecula) of the tongue is supplied by internal laryngeal branch of the vagus nerve.

### Muscles of the Tongue

Muscles of the tongue are classified into intrinsic and extrinsic groups. The intrinsic muscles alter the shape of tongue (Fig. 19.5).

anterior end and a root attached posteriorly to mandible. It has dorsal and ventral surfaces. The ventral surface is confined to the oral cavity and is connected to the floor of the mouth by a frenulum (Fig. 19.2).

### Dorsum of the Tongue

The dorsal surface (dorsum) is divided into anterior 2/3 or oral part and posterior 1/3 or pharyngeal part by a 'V' shaped sulcus terminalis. The mucous

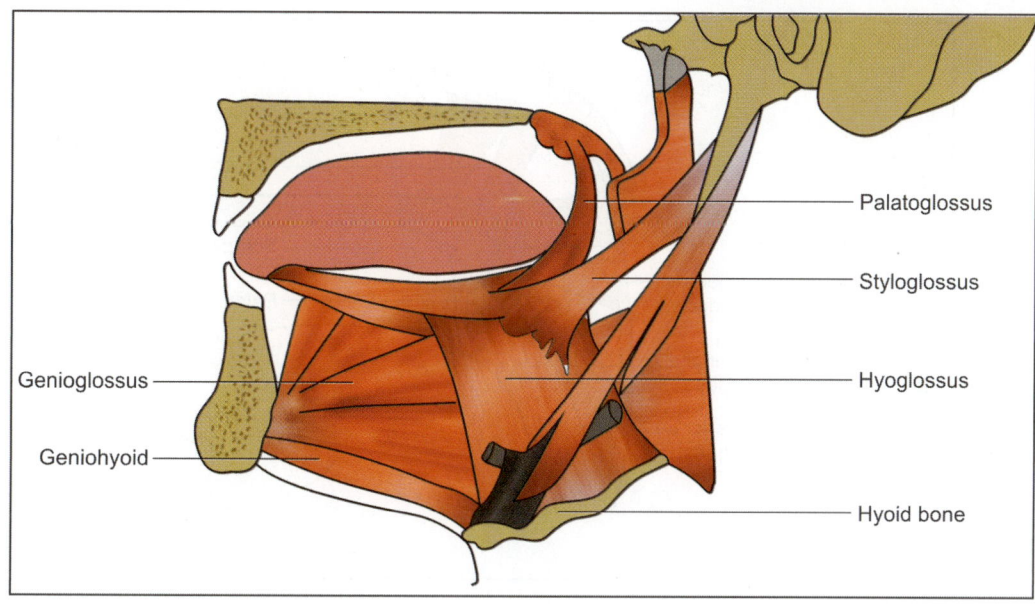

**Fig. 19.5:** Tongue muscles—lateral view

Extrinsic muscles bring about the movements of the tongue. They include genioglossus, hyoglossus, styloglossus and palatoglossus.

All the muscles of the tongue are supplied by the hypoglossal nerve except the palatoglossus, which is supplied by the cranial part of the accesory nerve, through the vagus.

### PALATE

It consists of anterior bony part (hard palate) and a posterior muscular part (soft palate).

### Hard Palate

It is a partition between the oral cavity below and nasal cavity above. It is formed by two bones—palatine processes of maxillae and horizontal plates of palatine bones. Its posterior margin is continuous with the soft palate. Its upper surface is lined by respiratory mucosa and lower surface by oral mucosa.

### Soft Palate

It is a movable muscular fold, suspended from the posterior border of the hard palate (Fig. 19.6). It separates the nasopharynx from the oropharynx. Structurally, it is made up of muscles, and is enclosed by mucous membrane. The muscles are attached to palatine aponeurosis.

The mucous membrane of the soft palate is supplied by lesser palatine and glossopharyngeal nerve.

*Muscles:* The muscles of the soft palate (Fig. 9.6) are:
1. *Tensor palati (tensor veli palatini)*

*Origin:* Scaphoid fossa at the base of the medial pterygoid plate, spine of the sphenoid and lateral membranous wall of the auditory tube.

*Insertion:* Its tendon winds around the pterygoid-hamulus. It spreads out in the soft palate to become the palatine aponeurosis, which is attached to the posterior border of the hard palate.

*Actions*: It tenses (stretches) the soft palate. The muscle fibers attached to the auditory tube helps in opening the auditory tube during deglutition and yawning.

2. *Levator palati (levator veli palatini)*
*Origin:* Apex of the petrous temporal bone, medial (cartilaginous) wall of the auditory tube.

*Insertion:* The muscle along with the auditory tube passes along the upper margin of the superior constrictor muscle (sinus of Morgagni), piercing the pharyngobasilar fascia. It is inserted into upper surface of the palatine aponeurosis.

*Action:* Bilateral action of the muscles elevates the soft palate towards the posterior wall of the pharynx, thus closing the communication between nasopharynx and oropharynx during swallowing.

3. *Musculus uvulae*
*Origin:* Each muscle takes origin from the posterior nasal spine of the hard palate.

*Insertion:* Each muscle proceeds backwards within the palatine aponeurosis. It is inserted into mucosa of the uvula.

*Action:* It shortens the uvula by pulling forward to its own side.

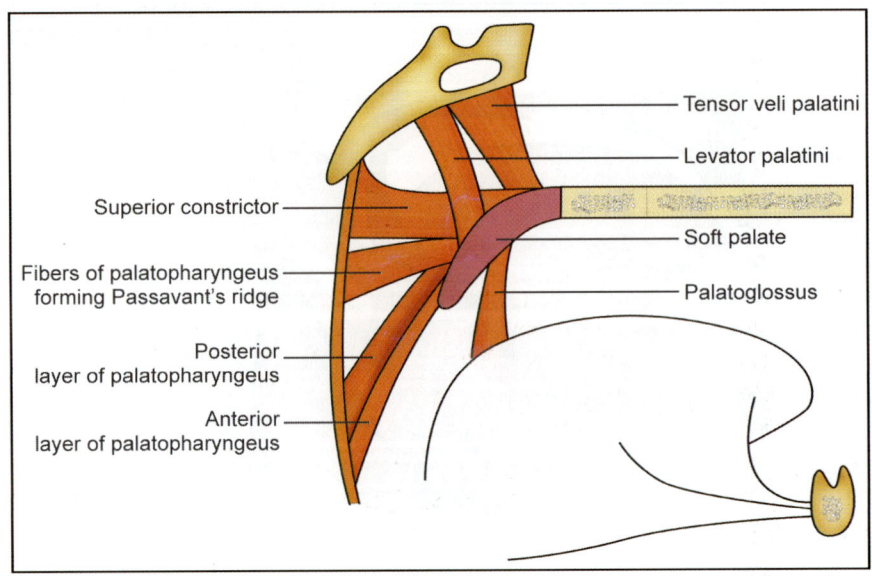

**Fig. 19.6:** Muscles of the soft palate

4. *Palatoglossus*

   *Origin:* From the under surface of the palatine aponeurosis

   *Insertion:* The muscle passes downward and forward and inserted into side of the tongue at the junction of oral (anterior 2/3rd) and posterior 1/3rd (pharyngeal part). The muscle is covered by mucous membrane and is called palatoglossal arch, which forms the anterior boundary of the palatine tonsil in the lateral wall of the oropharynx.

   *Action:* Muscles of the two sides acting together elevates the base of the tongue to close the oropharyngeal isthmus (communication between oral cavity and oropharynx).

5. *Palatopharyngeus*

   *Origin:* It takes origin by two slips. The anterior slip takes origin from the posterior border of the hard palate and the posterior slip from the upper surface of the palatine aponeurosis. The two slips are separated by insertion of levator palati muscle.

   *Insertion:* Both slips join to form a single muscle which passes downwards and backwards in the lateral wall of the oropharynx. The mucous membrane covering the muscle forms palatopharyngeal arch which forms the posterior boundary of the palatine tonsil. The palatopharyngeus join with salphingopharyngeus and the stylopharyngeus muscles in the wall of the pharynx and with them it is inserted into posterior border of the lamina of the thyroid cartilage. Some of its fibers spreads along the pharyngeal wall and are inserted into pharyngeal raphe.

*Passavant's ridge:* A few fibers of the palatopharyngeus sweep backwards and join with the similar muscle of the opposite side in the wall of the pharynx at the level of superior constrictor muscle. When the soft palate is elevated, this muscle band appears as a ridge known as 'Passavant's ridge' at the junction of nasopharynx and oropharynx and act as a sphincter. During swallowing the Passavant's ridge and soft is approximated by the contraction of this sphincter, closing the nasopharyngeal isthmus. It prevents regurgitation of food into the nasopharynx.

## Nerve Supply

These muscles are supplied by cranial part of the accessory nerve through the vagus, except tensor palati, which is supplied by mandibular nerve.

**Paralysis of muscles of soft palate:** There are many causes for paralysis of muscles of soft palate like tumors in posterior cranial fossa compressing the vagus nerve or vascular lesion affecting nucleus ambiguous in the medulla oblongata. A unilateral lesion of nucleus ambiguous or vagus nerve will result in atrophy and paralysis of all palatine muscles ipsilateral to the lesion, except the tensor veli palatini. Because of the palate paralysis, the patient's speech may be nasal. Due to the hemiplegic palate the patient may complain of nasal regurgitation of liquids since he/she is unable to shut off completely the nasopharynx from the oropharynx. Moreover, during phonation (say ahhh!) the soft palate is elevated on the normal side and the uvula deviates towards the opposite (normal) side (contralateral to the lesion;

contrast this with lesions of the hypoglossal nucleus). Paralysis of the soft palate produces nasal regurgitation of liquids, disturbance in the voice and flattening of the palatal arch.

**Cleft palate:** Cleft palate is a result of non-fusion of the right and left halves of the embryonic palate. This leaves an opening between the mouth and the nasal cavities that interfere with baby's sucking ability. Cleft palate can lead to aspiration (inhalation) of food into the nasal cavity and lungs, resulting in pneumonia. Cleft palate is repaired surgically.

## PHARYNX

It is a wide muscular tube, situated behind the nose, the mouth and the larynx. It is about 12 cm in length and subdivided into three parts.

### 1. NASOPHARYNX

It is the upper part of the pharynx situated behind the nasal cavity and above the soft palate. Its wall is rigid and non-collapsible. It is respiratory in function (lined by ciliated columnar epithelium) and no food ever enters it. Infections are common in this part. Hence it presents many lymphatic aggregations in its wall.

The roof and posterior wall is formed by body of the sphenoid, basilar part of the occipital bone and anterior arch of the atlas. The roof presents the following features (Figs 19.7 to 19.9).

a. *Nasopharyngeal tonsil:* It is formed by aggregation of lymphoid tissue deep to the mucous membrane. It projects from the roof like a conical mass. It is more

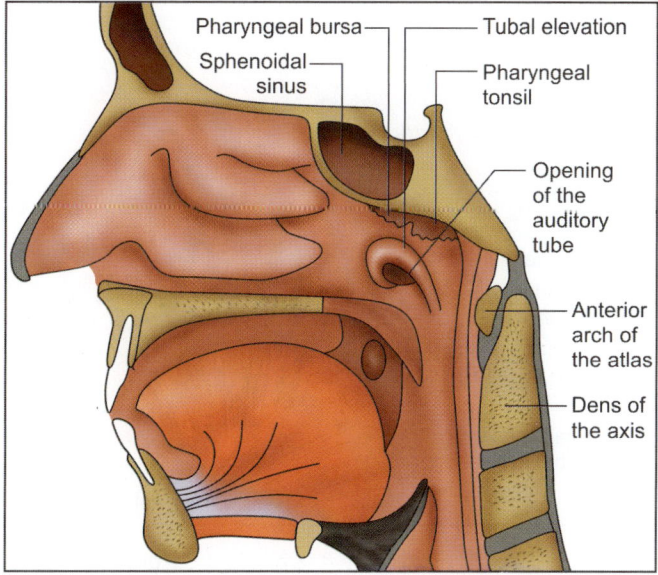

**Fig. 19.8:** Lateral view of the nasopharynx and oropharynx

prominent in children and its enlargement due to infection is known as 'adenoids'.

b. *Pharyngeal bursa (pouch of Luschka):* It is a mucous diverticulum extending into the nasopharyngeal tonsil.

The lateral wall of the nasopharynx presents the following features:

a. *Opening of the auditory tube:* The other end of the tube opens into the middle ear.

b. *Tubal elevation:* The upper and posterior part of the opening of the auditory tube shows this elevation. It is produced by cartilaginous part of the auditory tube.

c. *Tubal tonsil:* Aggregation of lymphoid tissue over the tubal elevation, deep to the mucous membrane.

d. *Two mucous folds* extend downwards from the tubal elevation. They are called salpingopharyngeal fold and salpingopalatine fold.

e. *Pharyngeal recess* (fossa of Rosenmüller): It is a mucous diverticulum behind the tubal elevation.

### 2. OROPHARYNX

It is situated behind the oral cavity. Posteriorly, it is bounded by $C_2$ and $C_3$ vertebrae. Below it continues with laryngopharynx.

The communication between nasopharynx and oropharynx is called 'pharyngeal isthmus', which is bounded above by soft palate and posteriorly by Passavant's ridge and on each side by the palato-pharyngeal arch. During swallowing this isthmus (communication) is closed and prevents the entry of food into nasopharynx.

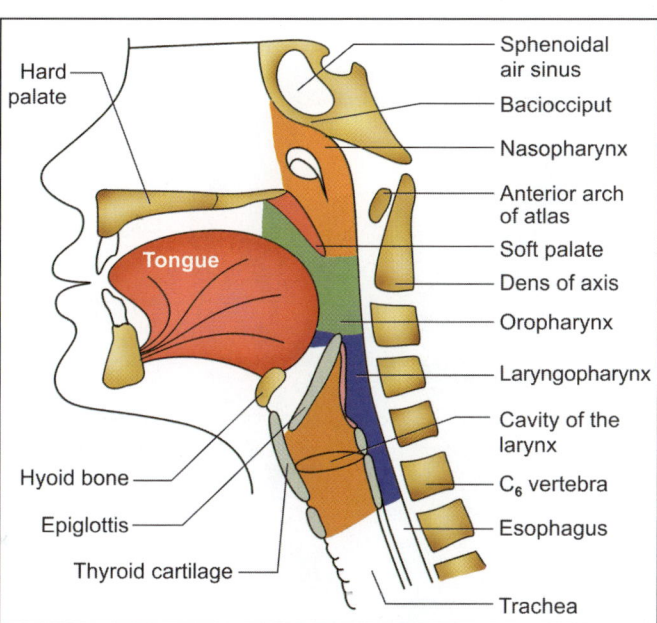

**Fig. 19.7:** Sagittal section of the pharynx showing its parts

19

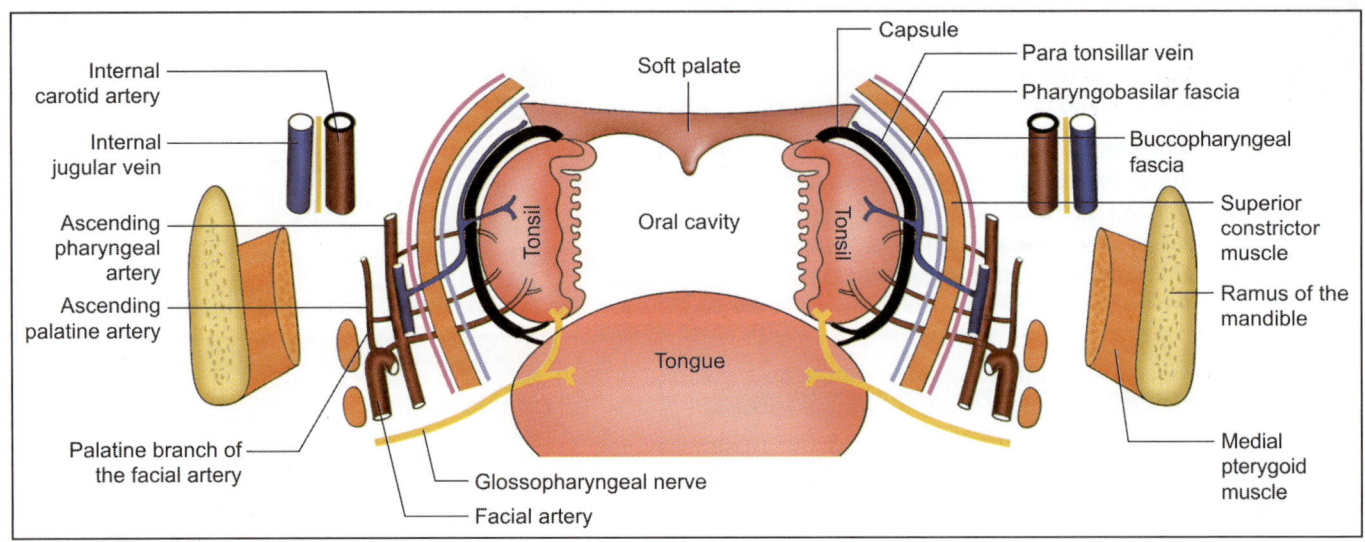

**Fig. 19.9:** Coronal section showing lateral relations of tonsil

The lateral wall of the oropharynx presents on each side the palatine tonsil.

### Palatine Tonsil

It is a lymphatic organ situated in the lateral wall of the oropharynx.

#### Relations

*Anteriorly:* Palatoglossal mucous arch with underlying palatoglossus muscle.

*Posteriorly:* Palatopharyngeal mucous arch with underlying palatopharyngeus muscle.

*Above:* Soft palate.

*Below:* Posterior part of the dorsum of the tongue.

*Medial surface:* It is covered by mucous membrane (stratified squamous non-keratinized epithelium). This surface shows many small openings called 'tonsillar pits'. One of the pits is deep and is called 'intratonsillar cleft'.

The lateral surface (tonsillar bed) is related to pharyngobasilar fascia, superior constrictor muscle of the pharynx and buccopharyngeal fascia.

#### Arterial Supply

The palatine tonsil is supplied mainly by branches of facial artery. The other arteries supplying palatine tonsil are branches of lingual artery, ascending palatine artery, ascending pharyngeal artery and greater palatine artery (Fig. 19.10).

**Fig. 19.10:** Arterial supply to the tonsil

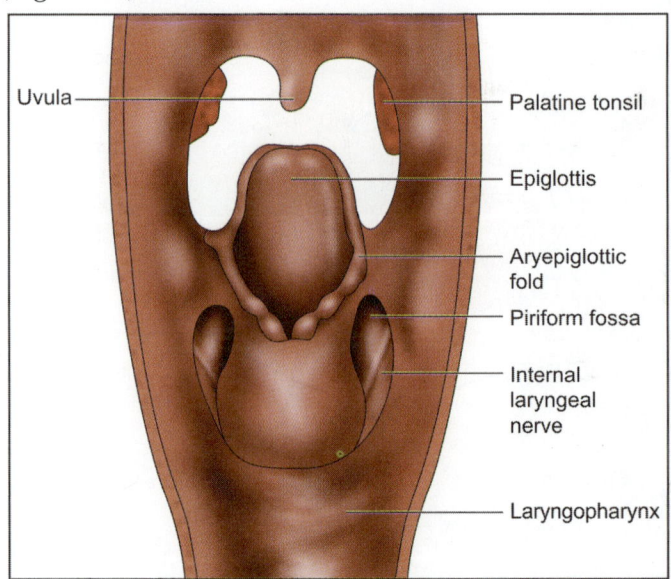

**Fig. 19.11:** Piriform recess (pharynx seen from behind)

19

## Nerve Supply

The mucous membrane of the tonsil is supplied by glossopharyngeal and lesser palatine nerves.

### Applied Aspects

- Tonsil being a lymphatic organ prevents infections. But sometimes tonsils themselves get infected which leads to their enlargement. It is common in children. Removal of tonsil is called 'tonsillectomy'. There is a possibility of severe bleeding due to high vascularity during removal of palatine tonsil. Glossopharyngeal nerve is also likely to be damaged during the surgery.
- The capsule covering the lateral surface of the tonsil is separated from superior constrictor muscle by a space filled with loose areolar tissue called peritonsillar space.
- Peritonsillar abscess (quinsy): Quinsy is a peritonsillar abscess in the loose connective tissue outside the capsule of the tonsil (peritonsillar space).

The aggregations of lymphoid tissue (palatine tonsil, tubal tonsil, pharyngeal tonsil and lingual tonsil) around the oropharyngeal isthmus is called **Waldeyer's lymphatic ring**.

## 3. LARYNGOPHARYNX

It is situated behind the larynx. It extends from the upper border of the epiglottis to the lower border of the cricoid cartilage. The lateral wall presents a depression called the **piriform fossa**, on each side of the inlet of the larynx (Fig. 19.11). Foreign bodies tend to be lodged in this fossa. Removal of such foreign bodies from the fossa can damage the internal laryngeal nerve, which lies deep to it.

The internal laryngeal nerve carries sensory fibers from the upper part of the larynx, vallecula of the tongue and laryngopharynx. Damage to this nerve can cause anesthetization of upper larynx. Accidental entry of food and water in to the laryngeal cavity cannot be sensed in such case.

### Structure of the Pharynx

The pharynx is composed of following 5 layers from within outwards.
1. Mucosa
2. Submucosa
3. Pharyngobasilar fascia
4. Muscular coat
5. Buccopharyngeal fascia

### Muscles of the Pharynx (Fig. 19.12)

- *Stylopharyngeus:* It extends from the styloid process and enter the wall of the pharynx between superior and middle constrictors.

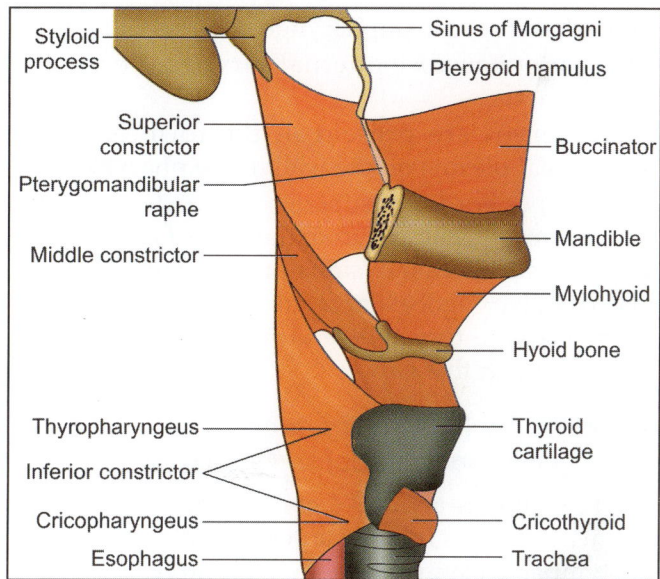

**Fig. 19.12:** Muscles of the pharynx

- *Palatopharyngeus:* It arises from palatine aponeurosis of soft palate
- *Salpingopharyngeus:* It arises from cartilaginous part of the auditory tube.

All these muscles join with each other in the wall of the pharynx and then it is inserted into posterior border of the lamina of the thyroid cartilage. They are responsible for elevating the pharynx, larynx during deglutition.

The circular muscles are:
- Superior constrictor
- Middle constrictor
- Inferior constrictor

All the constrictor muscles take origin anteriorly from bones and ligaments. The muscles of the two sides inserted into a fibrous raphe in the posterior midline of the pharynx. The lower part of the superior constrictor is overlapped by middle constrictor and the lower part of the middle constrictor by inferior constrictor. The lower part of the inferior constrictor is the weak part of the pharyngeal wall, without such overlapping of muscle to strengthen the wall.

### Nerve Supply to the Pharynx

*Motor:* All these muscles are supplied by the cranial part of the accessory nerve through the vagus except stylopharyngeus. The stylopharyngeus is supplied by glosspharyngeal nerve.

*Sensory:* The mucous membrane of the pharynx is supplied by:
- Nasopharynx—pharyngeal branch of pterygo-palatine ganglion (maxillary nerve)

- Oropharynx—glossopharyngeal nerve
- Laryngopharynx—internal laryngeal branch of vagus nerve.

The nerves are present in the form of plexus (pharyngeal plexus) on the wall of the pharynx.

The upper border of superior constrictor muscle of the pharynx is separated from the base of the skull by a gap. This gap is called 'sinus of Morgagni', which is closed by pharyngobasilar fascia and buccopharyngeal fascia. The auditory tube and levator palati muscle passes through this gap.

### Auditory Tube (Eustachian tube/ Pharyngotympanic tube)

Auditory tube is about 3.6 cm. It has a lateral bony part, which opens into the anterior wall of the middle ear (tympanic cavity). The medial fibro-cartilagenous part which opens at the lateral wall of the nasopharynx. It maintains an equal air pressure on either side of the tympanic membrane.

Infections from the nasopharynx can spread into middle ear through auditory tube. It is common in children due to wide and horizontally placed auditory tube.

Inflammation of the tubal tonsil can block the auditory tube. This can retract the tympanic membrane.

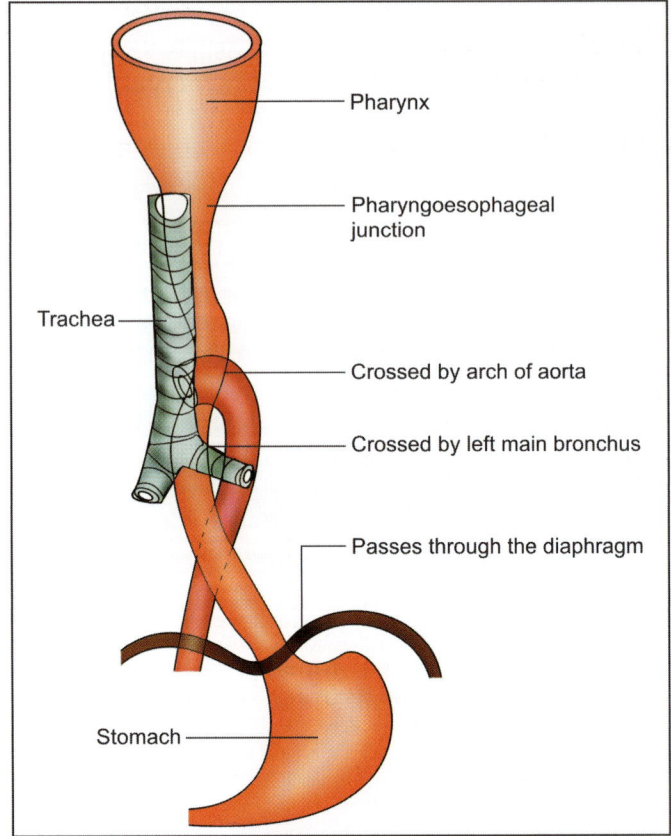

Fig. 19.13: Normal esophageal constriction

### ESOPHAGUS

- It is a muscular tube of about 25 cm in length.
- It extends from the laryngopharynx (at the level of C6 vertebra or lower border of cricoid cartilage) to the cardiac end of the stomach (at the level of $T_{11}$ vertebra) (Fig. 19.13).
- The esophagus has 3 parts:
  - Cervical (4 cm)
  - Thoracic (20 cm)
  - Abdominal (1.25 cm).
- The esophagus is related posterior to the trachea in the upper part and thoracic aorta to the left and posterior in the lower part.
- Esophagus passes through the oesophageal orifice of the diaphragm (at the level of 10th thoracic vertebra) and enters the abdominal cavity. It presents 4 normal constrictions, which are important during instrumentation through it.
  - a. *First constriction:* At the pharyngoesophageal junction ($C_6$ vertebra) It is about 6 inches from the incisor teeth.
  - b. *Second constriction* is where it is crossed by arch of aorta ($T_4$ vertebra) It is about 9 inches from the incisor teeth.
  - c. *Third constriction* is where it is crossed by left bronchus ($T_6$ vertebra) It is about 11 inches from incisor teeth.
  - d. *Fourth constriction* is where the esophagus passes through the diaphragm ($T_{10}$ vertebra) It is about 15 or 16 inches from the incisor teeth.

### Arterial Supply

Esophagus is supplied by the branches of the following arteries—inferior thyroid artery, descending thoracic aorta, bronchial arteries and left gastric artery.

### Microscopic Structure of the Esophagus

The wall of the esophagus is made up of four layers from inside to outside.

1. *Mucosa (mucous membrane):* It has three parts.
   - a. Lining epithelium—stratified squamous non-keratinized epithelium.
   - b. Lamina propria—made up of connective tissue fibres.
   - c. Muscularis mucosa—layer of smooth muscle fibres.
2. *Submucosa:* It presents plenty of mucous secreting esophageal glands.

3. *Muscularis externa (muscle coat):* It consists of outer longitudinal and inner circular layers. The upper part of esophagus presents striated, middle part mixed variety and lower part smooth muscle fibers.

4. Outer fibrous coat is made up of areolar tissue.

## Applied Anatomy

**Dysphagia**: It means difficulty in swallowing. Any structure related to esophagus can compress it, causing dysphagia. Such compression can be due to aneurysm of the arch of aorta, enlarged lymph nodes, enlarged left atrium (mitral stenosis), retrosternal goiter aberrant right subclavian artery

**The gastroesophageal reflux:** The lower end of the esophagus is guarded by a physiological sphincter which prevents gastro-esophageal reflux. However, it can become compromised, usually by a loss of muscle tone or sliding hiatal hernia (explained in the Chapter on-diaphragm). The acidic peptic chyme burns and inflames the esophageal mucosa (esophagitis). It causes uncomfortable sensation or heart burn, and dysphagia.

**Carcinoma of the esophagus:** The squamous cell carcinoma arises from the epithelium lining the esophagus (association with tobacco and alcohol consumption) and the adenocarcinoma arises from glandular cells that are present at the junction of the esophagus and stomach (associated with a history of gastroesophageal reflux).

**Esophagealvarices:** It occurs in portal hypertension. The anastamoses between the tributaries of systemic and portal vessels at the lower end of the esophagus dilate. The varices (dilated veins) lie immediately beneath the mucosa, where they are subjected to mechanical trauma during deglutition, or the passage of diagnostic instruments. They produce no symptoms until they rupture, causing massive hematemesis (vomiting of blood).

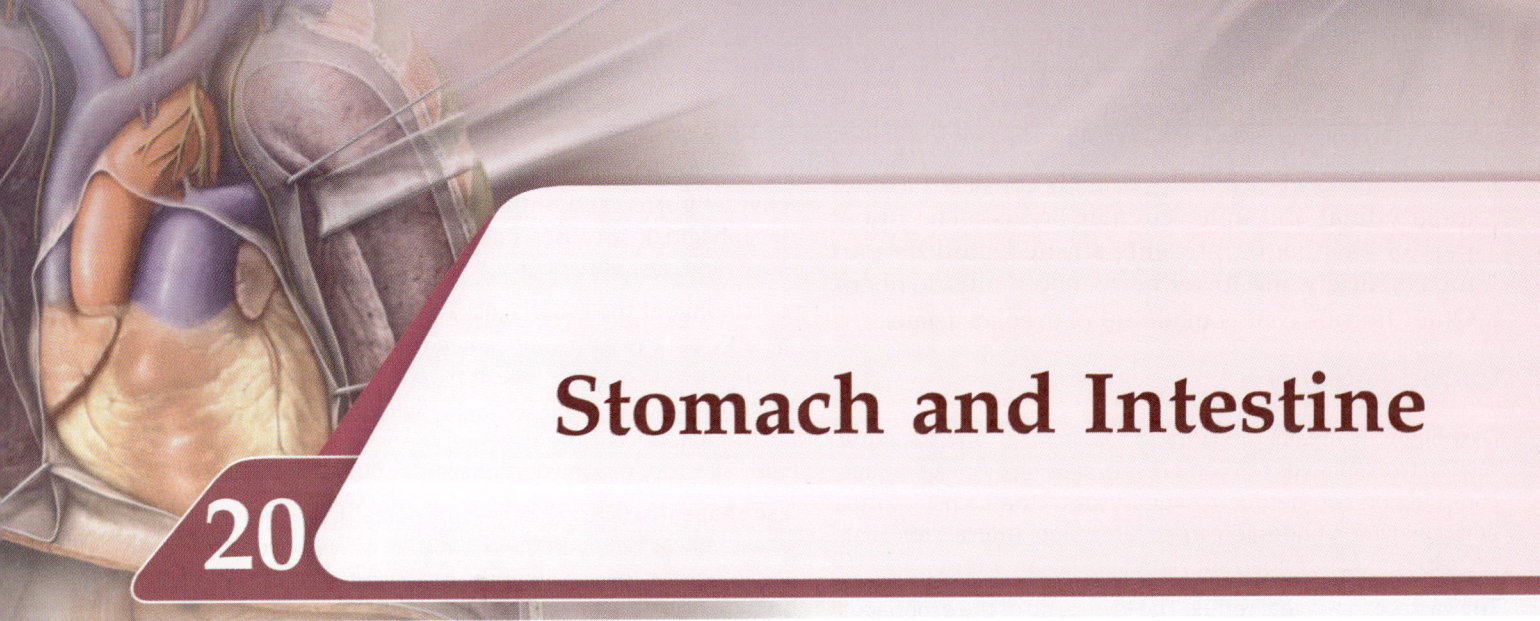

# Stomach and Intestine

## 20

Before studying the abdominal organs one should have some idea about the peritoneum and its cavity.

### THE PERITONEAL CAVITY AND PERITONEUM

Peritoneum is a fibroserous membrane lining the abdominopelvic cavity. The mesothelial cells lining the inner surface of the peritoneum secrete, thin film of fluid into the peritoneal cavity. It provides slippery surface for the free movements of the viscera.

The peritoneum consists of visceral and parietal layers. The visceral peritoneum covers the external surface of many digestive organs and is continuos with the parietal peritoneum, which lines the walls of the abdominal cavity. Between the visceral and parietal peritoneum is the peritoneal cavity, containing serous fluid.

Some of the abdominal organs are fixed to the abdominal wall by peritoneum and others are suspended by peritoneal folds. Such peritoneal folds allow the free movements of those organs.

*Omenta* are the peritoneal folds of the stomach.

*Mesentery* is the peritoneal fold of the intestine.

The general peritoneal cavity is divided into greater and lesser sacs.

In male pelvis, the peritoneal pouch between the urinary bladder and the rectum is called 'rectovesical pouch'. In females the peritoneum lining of the pelvic organs forms two pouches. 'Rectouterine pouch' (pouch of Douglas) between rectum and uterus and 'utero-vesical pouch' between uterus and urinary bladder.

The visceral peritoneum is supplied by nerves and vessels supplying the viscera. The parietal peritoneum is supplied by nerve supplying the body wall (somatic nerve). Hence infections affecting parietal peritoneum are painful and are referred in the body wall.

## STOMACH (GASTER/VENTER)

The stomach is a muscular bag, forming the widest and most distensible part of the digestive tube. It connects the lower end of the esophagus to the duodenum. The stomach acts as a reservoir of food and helps in the digestion of protiens, milk and fats. The stomach lies obliquely in the upper and left part of the abdomen (Fig. 20.1).

### Shape

The shape of the stomach varies according to the distention of the stomach and the surrounding viscera. When empty it is somewhat 'J' shape. When distended it becomes pear shaped or pyriform. In obese persons, it is placed horizontally.

### Features

#### Two Orifices

Cardiac orifice is joined by lower end of esophagus. Pyloric orifice is where it opens into the duodenum.

#### Two Curvatures

Lesser curvature gives attachment to the lesser omentum. Greater curvature gives attachment to the greater omentum and gastrosplenic ligament.

#### Two Parts (Fig. 20.1)

1. Cardiac part, divided into fundus (upper convex dome above the level of cardiac orifice) and body.
2. Pyloric part divided into pyloric antrum and pyloric canal.

#### Two Surface

1. Anterosuperior suface
2. Posteroinferior surface

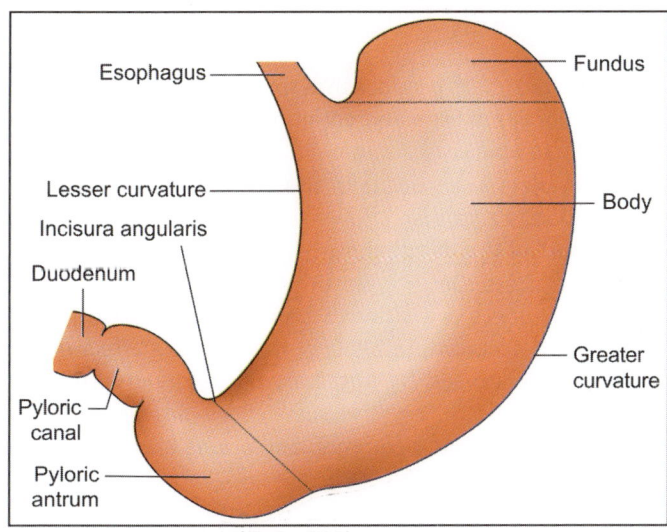

Fig. 20.1: Parts of the stomach

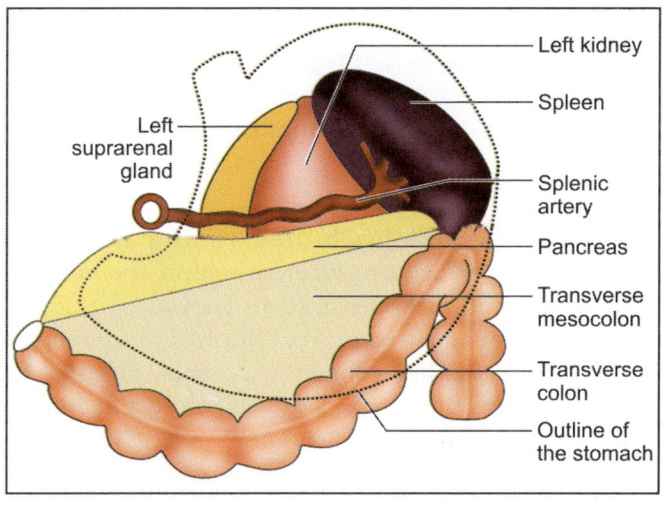

Fig. 20.2: Posterior relation of the stomach—schematic

## Relations

*Anteriorly*: It is related to the anterior abdominal wall, liver and diaphragm. In case of complete esophageal obstruction, a feeding tube can be introduced through the anterior surface of the stomach where it is in direct contact with anterior abdominal wall.

*Posteriorly*: It is related to the lesser sac, left kidney, left suprarenal gland, splenic artery, pancreas, splenic flexure of the colon, transverse mesocolon and the spleen. A posterior perforation of the stomach due to gastric ulcers can cause damage to all these structures especially splenic artery. This may lead to bleeding in the peritoneal cavity (Fig. 20.2).

## Blood Supply

1. Right and left gastric arteries along the lesser curvature
2. Right and left gastroepiploic arteries along the greater curvature
3. A few short gastric arteries supplying stomach

Corresponding veins drain into the superior mesenteric, splenic and the portal vein (Fig. 20.4).

## Nerve Supply

Stomach is supplied by the both sympathetic and parasympathetic nerves. Sympathetic is from $T_5$–$T_9$ spinal segments and parasympathetic by vagus nerve.

The parasympathetic fibers stimulate the gastric musculature, inhibit the pyloric sphincter and

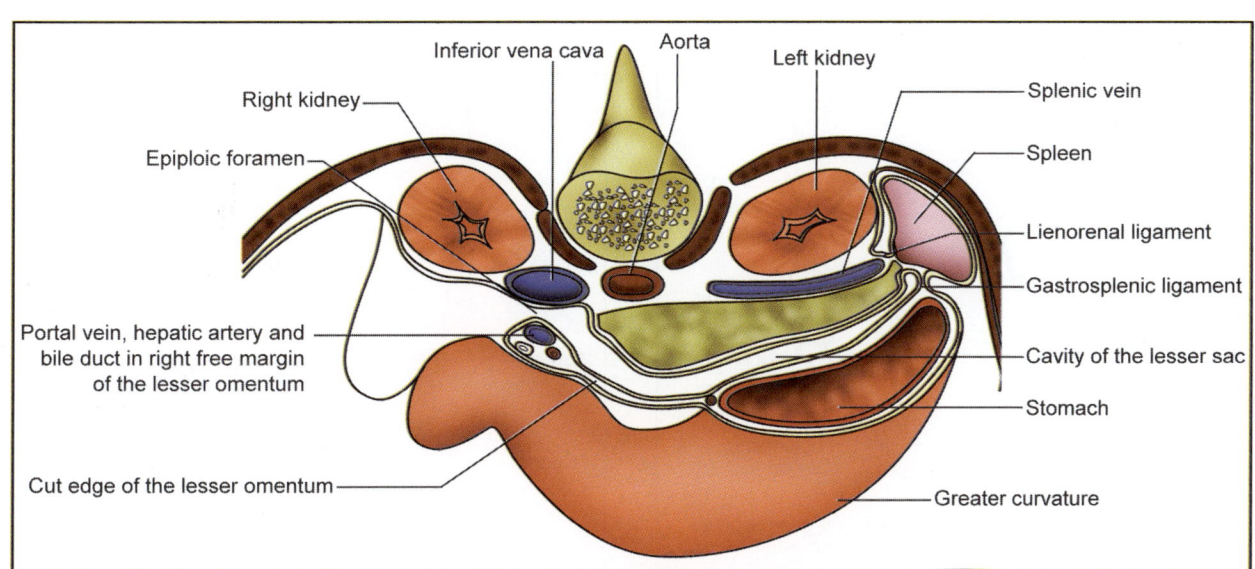

Fig. 20.3: Posterior relations of the stomach

secretomotor (stimulates) to the gastric glands. They also carry sensation of hunger and nausea.

Sympathetic fibres are motor to the pyloric sphincter and inhibit the gastric musculature.

### Lymphatic Drainage

The lymph from stomach drains into pancreatico-splenic nodes which are located behind the stomach along the splenic artery (Fig. 20.4). They also drain into left gastric, right gastroepiploic lymph nodes which are located close to the respective vessels. Finally, the lymph from all these nodes drians into coeliac group of lymph nodes.

### Structure

The wall of the stomach is made up of 4 layers—mucosa, submucosa, muscularis externa and serosa.

The mucous membrane is lined by simple columnar cells.

The mucous folds are called rugae. The mucosa presents gastric glands and pyloric glands. The outer muscular coat consists of smooth muscle fibers. The gastric glands of stomach present following types of cells.

a. *Chief/peptic cells (zymogenic):* They secrete pepsinogen and gastric lipase.

b. *Parietal/oxyntic cells:* They secrete HCl.

c. *Neck mucous cells:* They secrete mucous and protects the lining of the stomach from acids and enzymes.

d. *Argentaffin cell:* They secrete gastrin and they also contain 5-HT (seratonin).

### Applied Aspects

1. Gastric disorders produces "dyspepsia". It is characterized by anorexia, nausea and vomiting. There is a discomfort or pain in epigastric region.
2. Peptic ulcers can occur in the sites of pepsin and HCl secretion, viz stomach, lower part of the esophagus and first part of the duodenum.
3. Gastric ulcers: Occur typically along the lesser curvature. Gastric ulcers are slow to heal and persist for years together. To promote healing, the irritating effect of HCl can be minimised by antacids, partial gastrectomy or vagotomy.
4. Gastric carcinoma is common and occurs along the lesser curvature.

The muscularis externa consists of smooth muscle fibers. At the pylorus, these muscles are thickely set to form pyloric sphincter. In a given cadaveric specimen you will able to distinguish the cardiac end from the pyloric end by feeling the thick pyloric sphincter.

### SMALL INTESTINE

### GENERAL FEATURES OF SMALL INTESTINE

- Small intestine is about 6.5 meters in length. It extends from pylorus of the stomach to cecum (Fig. 20.5).
- It has following parts—Duodenum (proximal fixed part-about 25 cm in length), jejunum (about 8 feet in length) and Ileum (about 12 feet in length).
- The jejunum and ileum are suspended by a peritoneal fold called the mesentery.

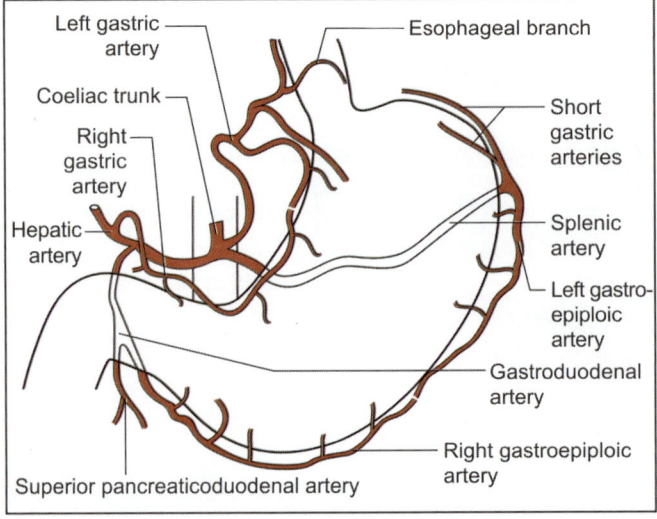

**Fig. 20.4:** Arterial supply to the stomach

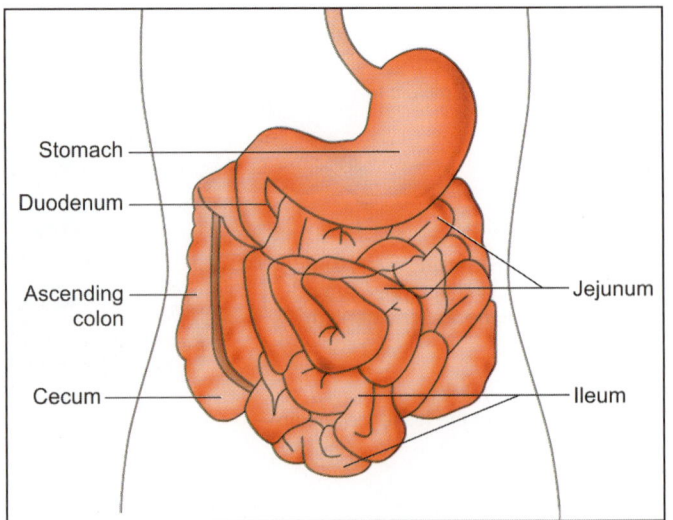

**Fig. 20.5:** Parts of the small intestine

- The arterial supply to the small intestine is mainly from superior mesenteric artery. The venous blood drains into portal vein.
- Structurally, the small intestine is designed for digestion and absorption
- A large surface area for absorption of food substances is provided by means of plenty of circular mucous folds (plicae circularis) and intestinal villi
- Small intestine is supplied by sympathetic ($T_9$–$T_{11}$) and parasympathetic fibres by vagus nerve. Sympathetic fibres inhibit the peristaltic movement and parasympathetic stimulates.

## 1. Duodenum

- It is the proximal fixed part of the small intestine (Fig. 20.6).
- It is about 10 inches in length with 4 parts (first, second, third and fourth parts).
- It is a retroperitoneal structure and fixed to the posterior abdominal wall except for small portion at its beginning (Fig. 21.6).
- It lies opposite to the $L_1$, $L_2$ and $L_3$ vertebrae and it almost surrounds the head of the pancreas.
- The interior of the 2nd part of the duodenum shows an opening at major duodenal papilla. It is about 8–10 cm distal to the pylorus. The bile secreted in the liver is poured into the second part of the duodenum. The bile duct (from liver) and pancreatic duct (from pancreas) join to form hepatopancreatic ampulla, which opens into the major duodenal papilla.
- Minor duodenal papilla is occasionally present. It lies 6–8 cm distal to the pylorus.

- Duodenum is supplied by superior and inferior pancreaticoduodenal arteries.
- The third part of the duodenum is crossed in front by superior mesenteric vessels and behind by abdominal aorta. This compress the third part of the duodenum.

## 2. Jejunum

- The width is about 4 cm, its wall is thicker and more vascular.
- Circular mucous folds are more and closely set.
- Its villi are long and leaf like.
- It is supplied by the jejunal branches of the superior mesenteric artery.

## 3. ILEUM

- The width is about 3.5 cm and its wall is thinner and less vascular.
- The circular mucous folds are smaller and sparse.
- Its villi are shorter.
- Payer's patches are present, which are the aggregations of lymphatic follicles.
- Both jejunum and ileum are suspended in theabdominal cavity by a fold of peritoneum called the mesentery. The blood vessels, nerve fibers and lymphatic reach them through this fold.

The jejunum and ileum are supplied by jejunal and ileal branches of the superior mesenteric artery.

There are about 12 to 15 branches arising from the left convex margin of the superior mesenteric artery. They reach the intestinal border between the two layers of the mesentery and form arterial arches (or **arcades**),

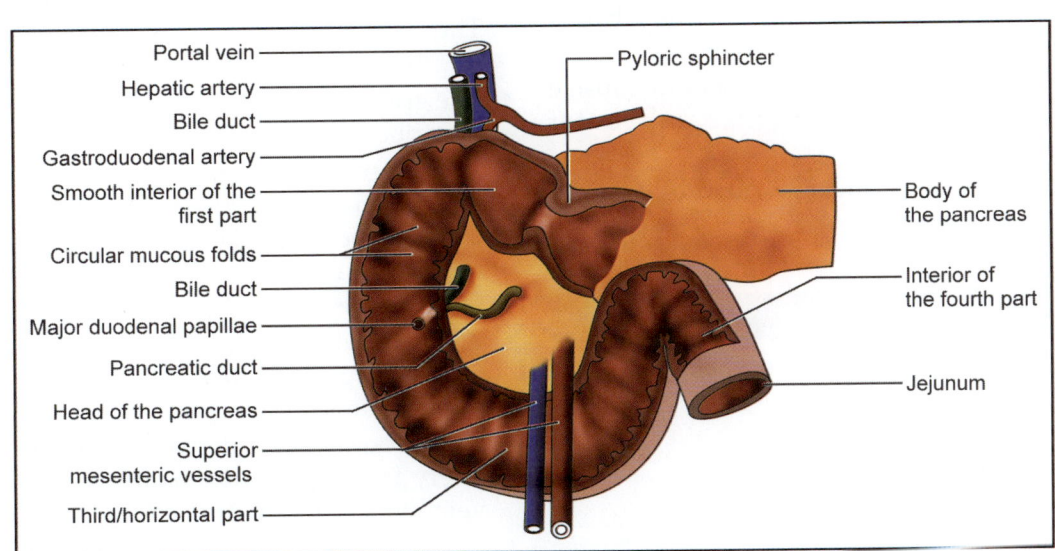

**Fig. 20.6:** Interior of the duodenum

20

which are interconnections between the adjacent branches. These arterial arcades are important in providing the collateral circulation in case of obstruction in one or other jejunal or ileal branches. The branches arising from the terminal arches are called **vasa recta** which enters the wall of intestine. These branches enter alternatively between the mesenteric and free borders of the intestine. The vasa recta are end arteries. In jejunum, the arterial arcades are few and the vasa recta are longer, while in ileum the arcades are more, hence vasa recta are shorter.

Occlusion of the vasa recta by emboli (blood clot) results in ischemia of the part of the intestine affected. It can leads to necrosis and obstruction of the intestine. It causes severe colicky pain along with the abdominal distension, vomiting and fever. It needs to be diagnosed and treated early.

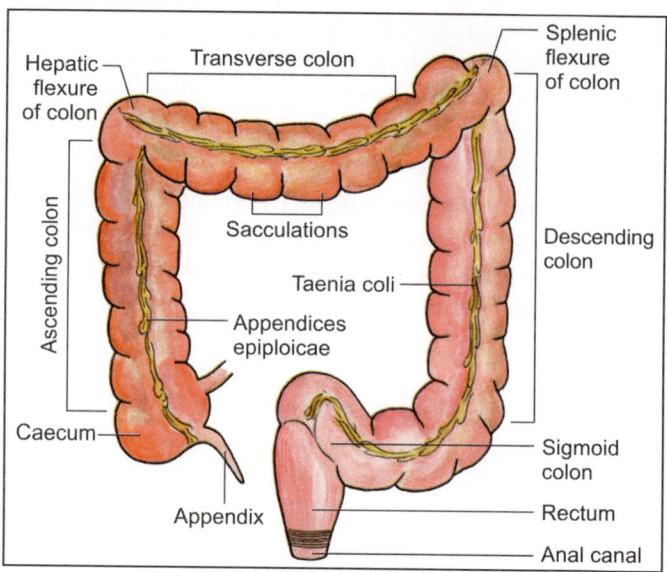

**Fig. 20.7:** Parts of the large intestine

### Microscopic Structure of Small Intestine

The wall of the intestine is made up of 4 layers from inside to outside.

1. *Mucosa:* The mucous membrane presents many villi. The villi are tall in duodenum and jejunum but short and stout in ileum. The lining epithelium is simple columnar with microvilli on their luminal surface. The number of goblet cells (mucous secreting) will increase towards the distal part of the gut. The lamina propria of mucosa presents plenty of intestinal glands (crypts of Lieberkühn). The muscularis mucosa is responsible for local contraction of the mucous membrane.

2. *Submucosa:* The submucosa of the ileum shows aggregation of lymphocytes in the form of follicles. They are called 'Peyer's patches'. They are actually present in the lamina propria and they break muscularis mucosa to enter the submucosa.

3. *The muscularis externa* is made of smooth muscle fibers arranged in inner circular and outer longitudinal layers.

4. *Serosa* is the outer layer and is formed by visceral layer of the peritoneum.

### LARGE INTESTINE

It extends from ileocecal junction to anal canal. It is about 1.5 meters long.

### Subdivisions (Fig. 20.7)

1. *Cecum and appendix:*
   - Cecum—6 cm long
   - Appendix—9 cm long

2. *Colon*
   - Ascending—15 cm
   - Transverse—50 cm
   - Descending—25 cm
   - Sigmoid—40 cm

3. Rectum—12 cm

4. Anal canal—3.8 cm

### CHARACTERISTIC FEATURES OF THE LARGE INTESTINE

- Structurally, it is adapted for storage of the fecal matterand for absorption of the fluid and solutes from it.

- The villi are absent, and the mucous membrane presents plenty of mucous secreting goblet cells.

- The large intestine is wider in caliber than the small intestine.

- The greater part of the large intestine is fixed, except the appendix, transverse colon and sigmoid colon.

- **Taeniae coli** are aggregations of the outer longitudinal muscle coat. They are 3 in number (taenia libera, taenia mesocolica and taenia omentalis). Because of these taeniae, the major part of colon presents sacculations.

- **Appendices epiploicae** are peritoneal pouches containing fat. They are absent in the cecum, appendix and the rectum.

- The blood supply is derived from inferior mesenteric artery and the veins drain into the inferior mesenteric vein, which finally drains into the splenic vein.

- The specific arteries include ileocolic, right colic, middle colic, left colic and sigmoidal branches. The terminal ends of these arteries are connected to each other close to the wall of the gut to form 'marginal artery'. Marginal artery provides collateral circulation in case of obstruction in one of the main artery feeding the colon.

Taeniae coli, appendices epiploicae and sacculations are the 3 cardinal features of the large intestine.

## Applied Aspects

1. *Colitis:* Irritation of the colon, leading to abnormal bowel function.
2. *Gastroenteritis:* Vomiting and diarrhea caused by an extremely powerful irritating stimulus.
3. *Enteritis:* Irritation of small intestine by toxins or other irritants.

## 1. Cecum

Cecum is the commencement of the large intestine. It is about 6 cm in length and 7.5 cm in breadth. It lies in the right iliac fossa. Shape of the cecum varies and is of following types:

1. *Fetal type:* 2% (where the appendix arises from the apex of cecum)
2. *Infantile type:* 3% (appendix arises from the depressed bottom of the cecum)
3. *Normal type:* 90% (appendix arises from posteromedial wall of the cecum)
4. *Exaggerated type:* 4 to 5% (apendix arises very close to the ileal attachment)

Interior of the cecum is continuos above with the ascending colon. The ileum opens into the cecum at the ileocecal orifice, which is guarded by an ileocaecal valve. It prevents the reflux from the cecum to the ileum. It regulates the passage of ileal contents into cecum. Appendicular orifice is 2 cm below the ileocecal orifice on the posteromedial wall of the cecum. It is supplied by the ileocolic branch of the superior mesenteric artery (Fig. 20.8).

## 2. Vermiform Appendix

It is a worm like diverticulum of the cecum, arising from the posteromedial wall of the cecum. The length varies from 2 to 20 cm with an average of 9 cm. The base of the appendix is fixed into the cecum but the tip can point in any direction (Fig. 20.9).

Accordingly following positions are explained:

a. 11 o'clock position (paracolic)
b. 12 o'clock position (retrocolic)
c. 2 o'clock position (splenic)
d. 3 o'clock position (promontoric)

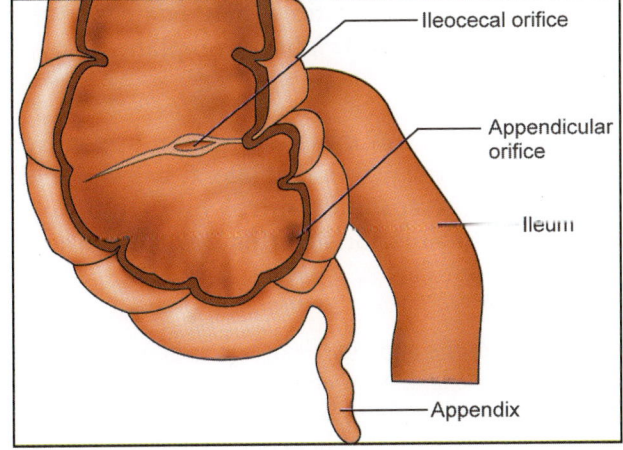

**Fig. 20.8:** Interior of the cecum

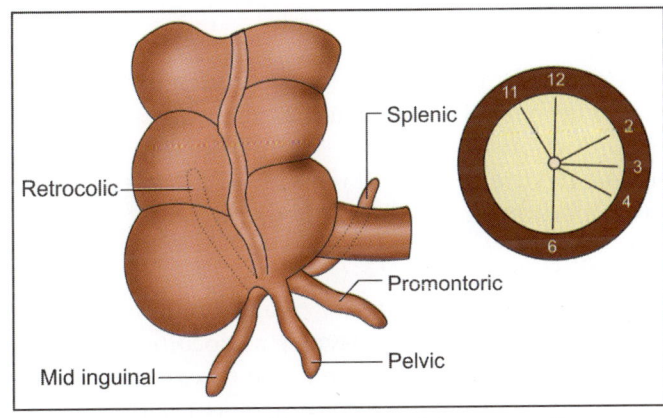

**Fig. 20.9:** Possible position of the appendix

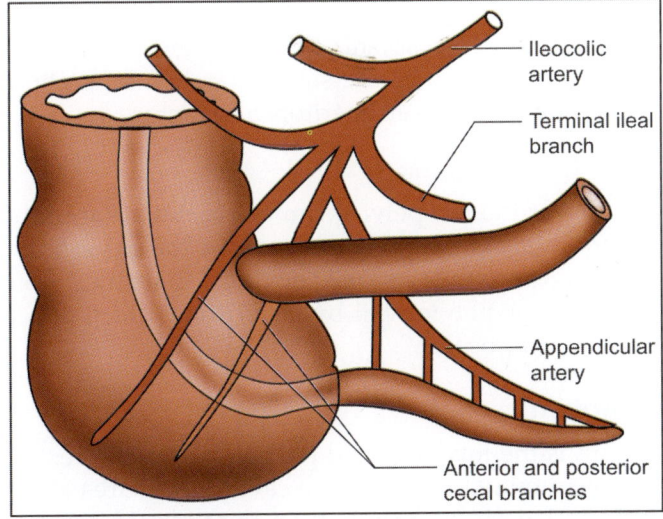

**Fig. 20.10:** Arterial supply to the cecum and appendix

e. 4 o'clock position (pelvic)
f. 6 o'clock position (mid inguinal)

Appendicular orifice is situated about 2 cm below the ileocecal orifice. It is occasionally guarded by a

20

"valve of Gerlach". The orifice is marked on the surface by a transtubercular and right lateral planes.

### McBurney's Point

It is the site of maximum tenderness in appendicitis. The point lies at the junction of lateral 1/3 and medial 2/3 of the right spinoumbilical line (line joining umbilicus to the anterior superior iliac spine).

## Appendicitis

Inflammation of the appendix is known as appendicitis. Pain is felt around the umbilicus, and then at the right iliac fossa. Pain is followed by vomiting and fever (Murphy's symptom). If the removal of appendix is not done immediately, a tender and fixed lump develops in the right iliac fossa.

### Ascending Colon

It extends from the cecum to the undersurface of the liver where it turns to the left as the transverse colon. This junction is called the right flexure of colon or hepatic flexure of colon. It is about 15 cm in length. It is a retroperitoneal structure (fixed).

### Transverse Colon

It is suspended in the cavity of abdomen by a fold of peritoneum called the transverse mesocolon. It extends from hepatic flexure of colon to left flexure of colon (or splenic flexure) where it continues as the descending colon. It is about 50 cm in length.

### Descending Colon

It extends from the splenic flexure to left pelvic brim where it continues as the sigmoid colon. It is about 25 cm long and is a retroperitoneal structure.

### Sigmoid Colon (pelvic colon)

It begins at the left pelvic brim as continuation of the descending colon and ends in front of the $S_3$ vertebra. Its average length is about 40 cm. It is suspended from the posterior pelvic wall by a peritoneal fold called "sigmoid mesocolon".

## 3. Rectum

Rectum is the lower dilated part of the large intestine and is contained in the pelvic cavity, measures about 12 cm in length. It extends from the sigmoid colon to the anal canal at the anorectal junction. The lower end of the rectum dilates to form the rectal ampulla. The peritoneum covers in front and sides of the upper 1/3rd of the rectum and in front in the middle 1/3rd of the rectum. Then the peritoneum passes into upper part of the base of the urinary bladder in males forming a

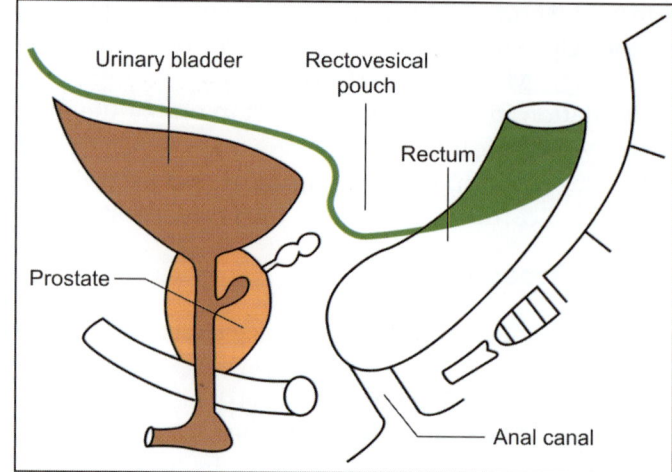

**Fig. 20.11:** Peritoneal relation of rectum in males

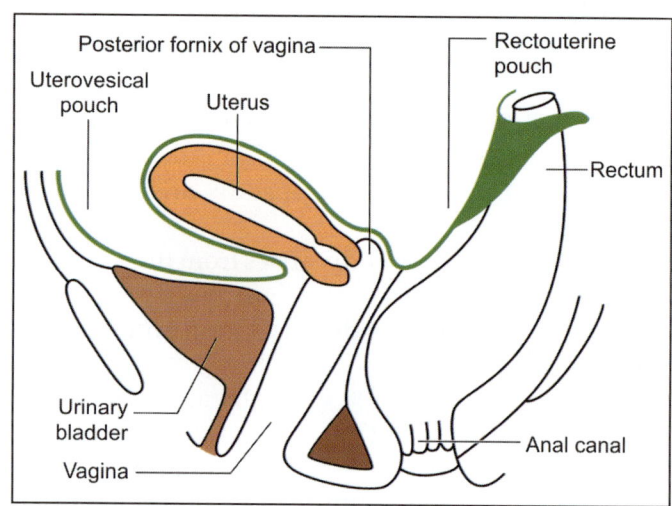

**Fig. 20.12:** Peritoneal relation of rectum in females

shallow **rectovesical pouch** (Fig. 20.11). In females the peritoneum passes into posterior fornix of the vagina and then into posterior surface of the cervix of the uterus. The peritoneal pouch between rectum and uterus is called **rectouterine pouch** or Douglas pouch (Fig. 20.12). This is the most dependent part of the female pelvic cavity and fluid tends to accumulate in this pouch.

The lower part of the anterior wall of the rectum is related to seminal vesicle and prostate gland. Enlargement of these structures can be felt through digital rectal examination.

The interior of the rectum shows 4 mucous folds called Houston's valves. In the male, the rectum is related anteriorly to the urinary bladder (Fig. 20.11), but separated by the rectovesical pouch. In females, the rectum is separated from the uterus by a rectouterine pouch.

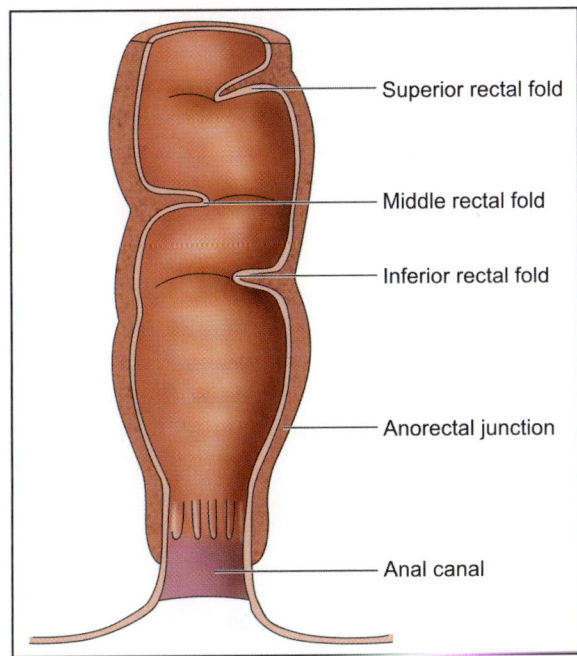

**Fig. 20.13:** Interior of the rectum (coronal section)

## 4. Anal Canal

It is the terminal part of the alimentary tract. It extends from anorectal junction to the anal office, passing through the pelvic diaphragm. It is about 3.8 cm in length. Externally, the anal canal is surrounded by internal and external anal sphincters. Internal anal sphincter surrounds the upper part of the anal canal.

It is made up of smooth muscle fibers (involuntary). It is supplied by sympathetic nerves.

External anal sphincter surrounds the entire length of the anal canal. It is made up of striated (voluntary) muscles. It is supplied by pudendal nerve.

The external anal sphinctra has 3 parts: Subcutaneous part, superficial part and deep part (Figs 20.13 to 20.15).

Interior of the anal canal: Interior is subdivided into 3 parts:

a. *Upper part (mucous):* It is about 1.5 cm in length, below lined by pectinate line. The mucosa is reddish in color. The mucosa shows about the mucosa shows about 6–10 vertical folds called **anal columns** (columns of Morgagni). The mucous membrane deep to the anal column presents terminal radicles of inferior mesenteric vessels. In case of portal obstruction these vessels enlarge to form internal piles (hemorrhoids). Rupture of these vessels leads to bleeding. The lower ends of the anal columns are connected by crescentic mucous folds, called the **anal valves**. The recesses (spaces) above the anal valves are called **anal sinuses**. The mucous membrane is lined by simple columnar epithelium.

b. *Intermediate area (pecten part):* It is a transitional zone and about 1.5 cm in length. It extends from the pectinate line to the Hilton's line. It is lined by stratified squamous non-keratinized epithelium. With internal rectal venous plexus deep to it, it is bluish in color.

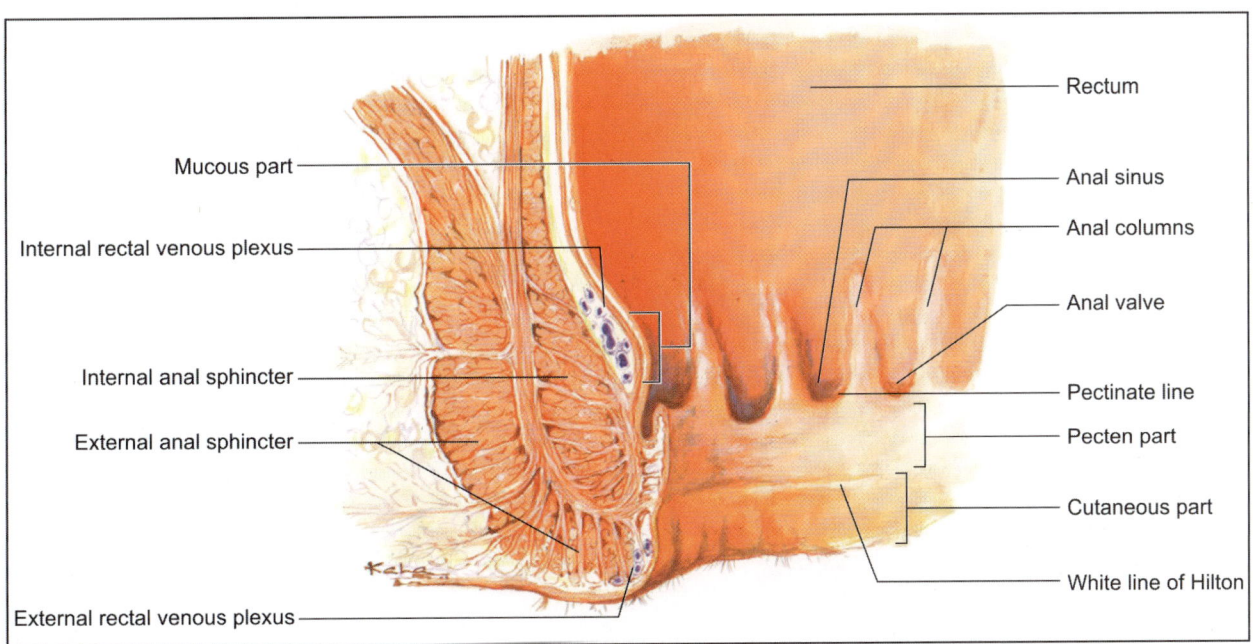

**Fig. 20.14:** Interior of the anal canal (coronal section)

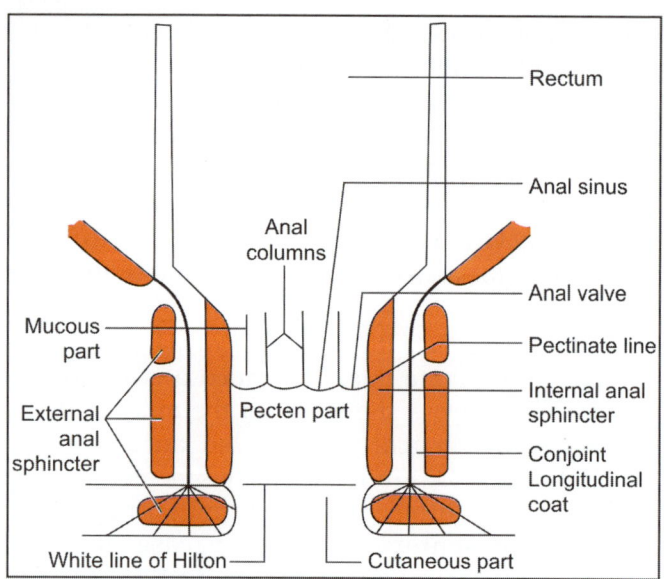

**Fig. 20.15:** Interior of the anal canal—schematic

c. *Lower area (anal verge):* It is about 8 mm in length and lined by skin. Associated with skin there are sweat and sebaceous glands.

## Blood Supply

The area above the pectinate line by superior rectal artery and below by inferior rectal artery. The venous blood drains into 2 sets of plexus. The internal rectal venous plexus present deep to the mucosa of the anal canal mainly drain into superior rectal vein and finally into portal vein. The external rectal venous plexus situated around the subcutaneous part of the external anal sphincter drain mainly into internal pudendal vein, finally into systemic vein. The two venous plexus communicate each other, hence anal canal is one of the site of portacaval anastomose.

## Nerve Supply

Above the pectinate line by sympathetic ($L_1$ & $L_2$) and parasympathetic (pelvic splanchnic/S2, 3, 4) nerves. They are insensitive to pain. Below the pectinate line, it is by inferior rectal nerve (somatic nerve), hence this area is sensitive to pain.

## Applied Anatomy

**1. Piles (Hemorrhoids)**

Piles are dilatation of veins and they project into the lumen of the anal canal as mucous bulging. The internal piles occur above the pectinate line. It occurs in 3,7 and 11 o'clock positions of the anal wall when viewed in lithotomy position. The piles can rupture and bleed during straining to pass stool. The external piles occur below the pectinate line. It is very painful and does not bleed on straining while passing stool.

**2. Anal fissure**

It is due to the rupture of anal valves during passage of dry hard stool. The condition is very painful.

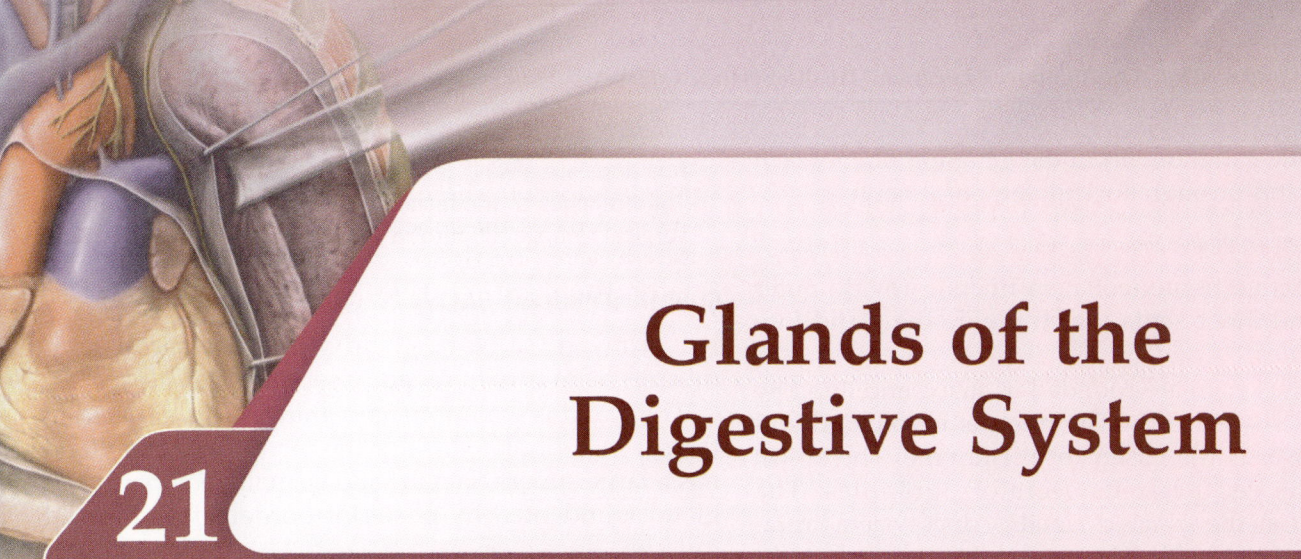

# Glands of the Digestive System

**21**

## SALIVARY GLANDS

There are three pairs of large salivary glands, namely parotid, submandibular and sublingual glands (Fig. 21.1). The secretions of these glands are carried by their ducts into the oral cavity. Salivary glands are not essential for life. Salivary amylase present in the saliva is a carbohydraye splitting enzyme acts only on cooked starch. In addition to this, saliva has cleansing, solvent and lubricating actions.

### PAROTID SALIVARY GLAND

It is the largest salivary gland situated in front and below the external acoustic meatus.

Each gland is inverted pyramid in shape. It presents apex, base, 3 surfaces (superficial, anteromedial and posteromedial) and 3 borders (anterior, posterior and medial).

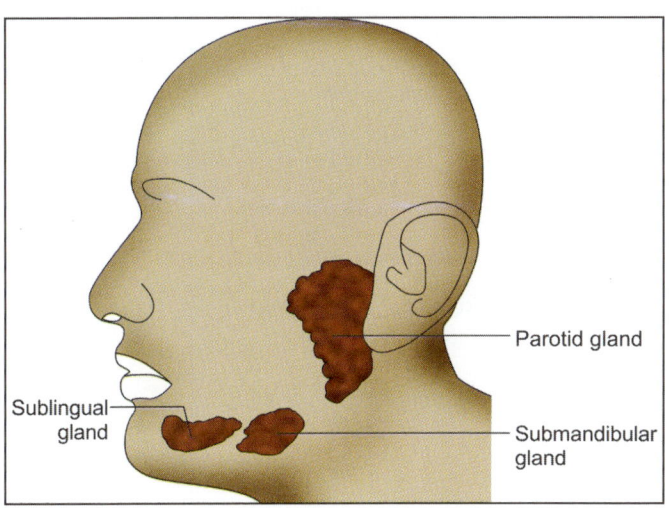

**Fig. 21.1:** Salivary glands

- **Apex** is directed downwards towards the neck. The retromandibular vein and cervical branch of the facial nerve emerge from the apex.
- **Base** is related to external acoustic meatus. The auriculotemporal nerve and superficial temporal vessels emerge from the base.
- The **superficial (or lateral) surface** is related to skin, platysma and parotid fascia.
- The **anteromedial surface** is related to posterior border of the ramus of the mandible with masseter muscle outside and medial pterygoid muscle inside.
- The **posteromedial surface** is related to mastoid and styloid processes with muscles attached to them.
- The terminal branches of the facial nerve, parotid duct and transverse facial artery emerge from under cover of the anterior border (Fig. 21.2).

### Structures Inside the Parotid Gland (Outside to Inside)

1. Facial nerve and its branches
2. Retromandibular vein
3. External carotid artery and its branches

### Parotid Duct (Stensen's Duct)

It is about 5 cm in length. It emerges from the anterior border of the gland and proceeds forward then turns medially. It pierces buccal pad of fat, buccopharyngeal fascia and buccinator muscle successively. The duct opens in the vestibule of the mouth opposite the crown of upper second molar tooth.

### *Nerve Supply*

The secretomotor parasympathetic fibers are derived from glossopharyngeal nerve. A branch of glosso-pharyngeal nerve called lesser petrosal nerve relay the fibers in otic ganglion. From the ganglion fibers reach parotid gland through auriculotemporal nerve.

### Structure of Parotid Salivary Gland

The connective tissue (collagen fibers) provide outer capsule and inner septa which divide the gland into many lobules.

The serous acini are rounded in shape and lined by pyramidal shaped cells. The nucleus is rounded and placed towards the basement membrane. The apical part of the cell presents secretory granules. The secretion from the acini is drained by duct system (intralobular duct = found in between acini. Interlobular duct = found in the connective tissue septum between the lobules).

### Applied Ananomy

- A bad oral hygiene can cause bacterial parotitis (infection spread through parotid duct) resulting in slight swelling of the gland.
- A bacterial infection localized in the parotid gland usually produces an abscess. It is extremely painful due to unyielding nature of the parotid fascia covering it.
- **Mumps**—a viral infection that most often affects the parotid salivary glands. The mumps virus may also cause inflammation of the parotid duct, causing redness in the area of opening of the duct. The pain produced by the mumps is mistaken for toothache.
- A rapidly growing carcinoma of the gland can show the involvement of facial nerve. Hence, the facial muscle

functions are always tested in case of any parotid tumors. The branches of the facial nerve may be damaged during surgical removal of parotid tumors

## SUBMANDIBULAR SALIVARY GLAND

It is a mixed salivary gland with both serous and mucous acini (predominantly serous type).

The gland is walnut in appearance. It is situated in the submandibular fossa of the mandible. The gland has a large superficial part and a small deep part. The gland is indented by posterior border of mylohyoid muscle.

The superficial part of the gland is looped by facial artery. The submandibular duct opens in the floor of mouth on a sublingual papilla on each side of frenulum linguae (see Fig. 19.2).

Structurally it is a mixed salivary gland having both serous and mucous acini.

### Nerve Supply

The secretomotor parasympathetic fibers to both submandibular and sublingual glands are derived from facial nerve and its branch chorda tympani. The fibers from chorda tympani join the lingual nerve. Before reaching the gland fibers are relayed in submandibular ganglion.

### Structure of Mucous Salivary Gland

The mucous acini are larger when compared to serous acini. On cut section they are oval or elongated and

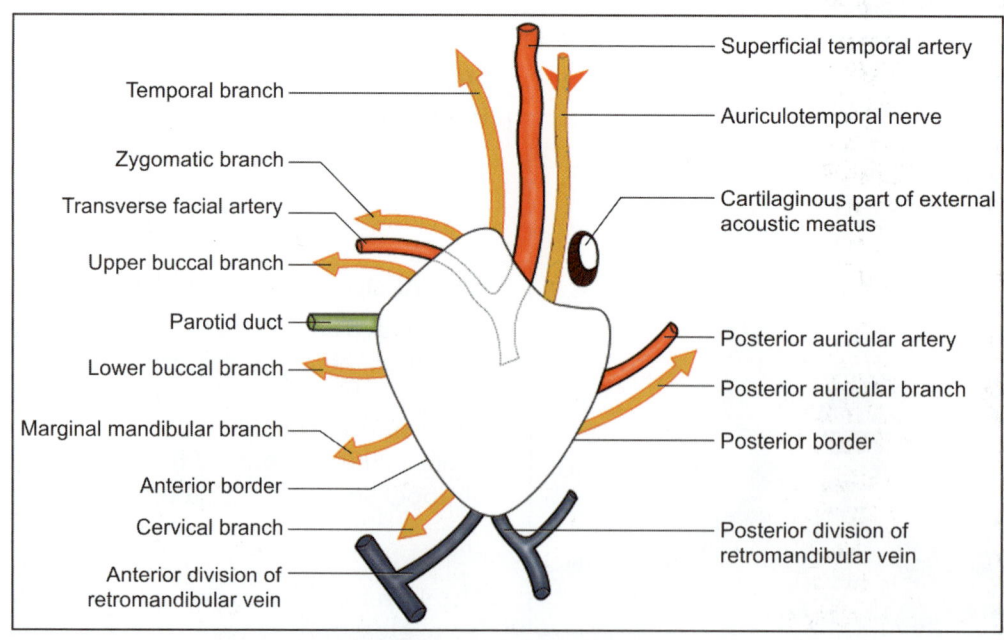

**Fig. 21.2:** Lateral view of parotid with structures emerging from its anterior border (left side)

Labels:
- Temporal branch
- Zygomatic branch
- Transverse facial artery
- Upper buccal branch
- Parotid duct
- Lower buccal branch
- Marginal mandibular branch
- Anterior border
- Cervical branch
- Anterior division of retromandibular vein
- Superficial temporal artery
- Auriculotemporal nerve
- Cartilaginous part of external acoustic meatus
- Posterior auricular artery
- Posterior auricular branch
- Posterior border
- Posterior division of retromandibular vein

lined by columnar cells. The nuclei are flat and placed at the basement membrane. The lumen is prominent.

## SUBLINGUAL SALIVARY GLAND

It is situated in the floor of the mouth between the mucous membrane and mylohyoid muscle. Many ducts arising from the gland opens at the summit of the sublingual fold. Structurally it is made up of mucous acini.

---

## EXTRAHEPATIC BILIARY APPARATUS

It consists of structures, which store and transmit bile into the duodenum. Following are the parts (Fig. 21.3):
1. *The right and left hepatic ducts*—which emerge at the porta hepatis (hilum of liver) from right and left lobes of the liver.
2. *Common hepatic duct*—it is formed by the union of right and left hepatic ducts.
3. *Gallbladder*
4. *Bile duct*

## GALLBLADDER

*Function:* Gallbladder stores (30–50 ml) and concentrates the bile, which is secreted by the liver.

*Location:* Gallbladder is located at the inferior surface of the liver.

*Parts:* It has fundus, body and neck. The neck continues to form the cystic duct, which joins with the common hepatic duct to form the bile duct.

*Major relations:* Its upper surface is in contact with undersurface of the liver. Its under surface is related to

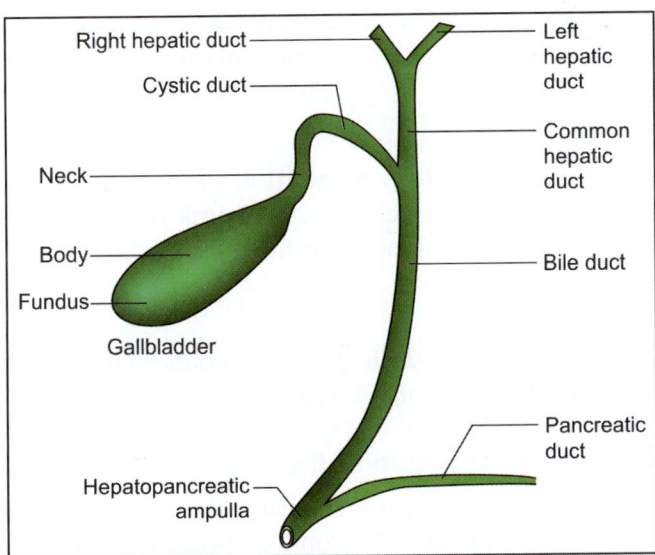

**Fig. 21.3:** Parts of the extrahepatic biliary apparatus

first and second parts of the duodenum, hepatic flexure of colon. The funds can be marked at surface of the body at the tip of the right 9th costal cartilage.

*Blood supply:* Cystic artery is a branch from right terminal branch of the hepatic artery.

*Nerve supply:* The sympathetic fibers supplying the gall-bladder are derived from $T_7$ to $T_9$ segments of the spinal cord.

### Structure

The wall of the gallbladder shows 3 layers:
a. The inner mucous membrane is thrown into small folds and lined by simple columnar epithelium with microvilli (brush border) on the luminal surface. Deep to the mucous membrane is the lamina propria. The muscularis mucosa and submucosa are absent.
b. The fibromuscular coat consists of fibroelastic fibers and smooth muscle fibers
c. The outer serous coat is derived from peritoneum (only on under surface of gallbladder).

### BILE DUCT

- It is formed by the union of cystic duct and common hepatic duct.
- It is about 8 to 9 cm in length.
- It descends in the right free margin of the lesser omentum along with portal vein and hepatic artery.
- It passes deep to the first part of the duodenum and head of the pancreas.
- It joins with pancreatic duct and opens into the second part of the duodenum on the summit of the major duodenal papilla.
- The terminal part of the bile duct is surrounded by **sphincter of Boyden**, while hepatopancreatic ampulla is surrounded by **sphincter of Oddi.**
- When the gastric contents appears in the duodenum, cholecystokinin (CCK) hormone released from the intestine to the blood causes contraction of gallbladder and relaxation of the sphincters, allowing the bile to enter the duodenum (Fig. 21.3).

*Gallstones and cholecystitis:* A common clinical problem of the gallbladder is the development of the gallstones. Bile is composed of various salts, pigments and cholesterol. Normally cholesterols remain in solution, but under certain conditions they precipitate to form solid crystals called gallstones. It may block the bile flow at neck of the gallbladder or in the bile duct. This may cause inflammation of the gallbladder which is called 'cholecystitis'. The gallstones are common in females and incidence increases with the age. At time gallbladder can rupture and erode the wall of the

21

duodenum or colon, so that gallstones can enter these structures. Pain from the gallbladder develops in epigastric region and later shifts to right hypochondriac region at the tip of the right 9th costal cartilage.

## LIVER

Liver is the largest gland of the body. It has metabolic (carbohydrate, protein and fat), synthetic (bile and prothrombin), excretory, protective and storage functions. It is a wedge shaped structure, situated in the right upper quadrant of the abdomen.

### Weight

- In adult male 1.4 to 1.8 kg
- In adult female 1.2 to 1.4 kg

### External Features

- *Liver presents 5 surfaces:* Superior, inferior, anterior, right and posterior (Fig. 21.5).
- The superior surface is separated from the heart and lungs by the diaphragm (Fig. 21.4).
- Its anterior surface is related to the anterior abdominal wall.
- The right surface related to diaphragm throughout, pleura in the upper and middle third and right lung in the upper third.
- The posterior and inferior surfaces are related to many abdominal viscera.
  - The left lobe is related to esophagus and stomach.
  - The right lobe is related to second part of the duodenum, right kidney, right suprarenal gland and right flexure of the colon (Fig. 21.6).
  - The bare area of the liver is not covered by peritoneum and it is in direct contact with diaphragm.
- It also presents fissure for ligamentum teres (at inferior surface) and fissure for ligamentum venosum (at posterior surface).
- Following peritoneal ligaments are attached to liver—falciform ligament, right and left triangular ligaments and coronary ligaments.
- Liver also presents caudate and quadrate lobes.
- Porta hepatis is the hilum of the liver in which right and left hepatic ducts, right and left branches of portal vein and hepatic artery are present.
- A gallbladder fossa is present, which lodges the gallbladder (Fig. 21.6).

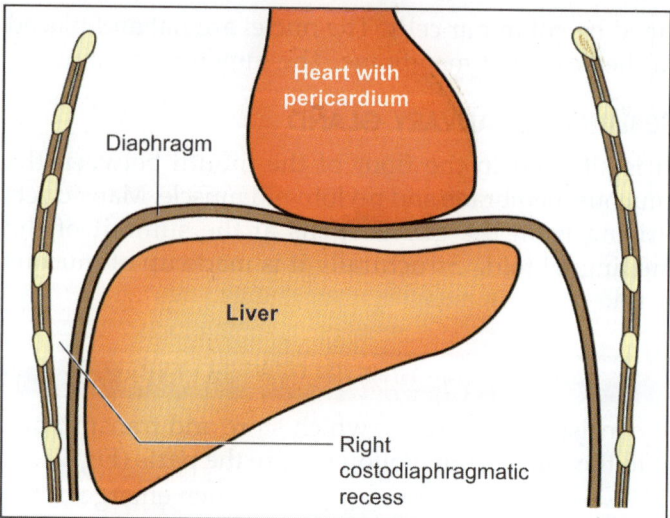

**Fig. 21.4:** Relations of the superior surface of the liver

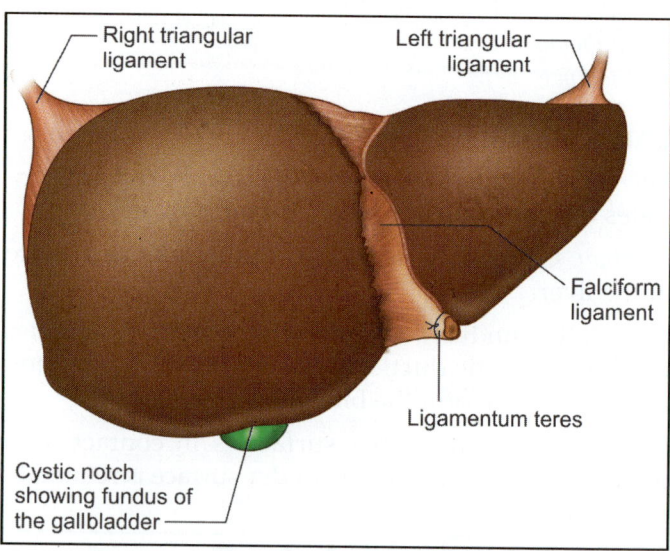

**Fig. 21.5:** Anterior surfaces of the liver

### Arterial Supply

20% of the blood (oxygenated) is received from the hepatic artery (branch of coeliac trunk of abdominal aorta). 80% of the blood from the portal vein.

### Venous Drainage

The venous blood is drained by the hepatic veins, which drain into the inferior vena cava.

### Microscopic Structure of the Liver

- The connective tissue covering the liver is called 'Glisson's capsule'. This connective tissue divides the liver substance into a number of lobules.

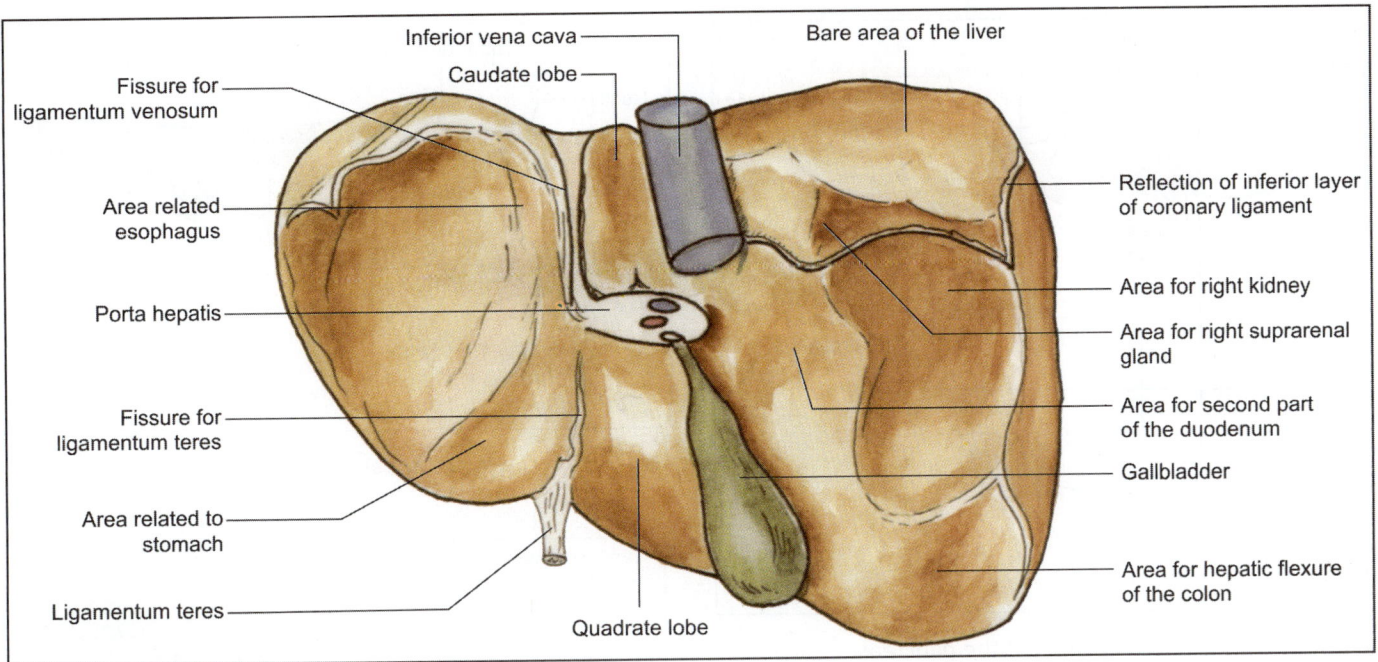

**Fig. 21.6:** Posterior and inferior surface of the liver

- Liver presents plenty of hepatic lobules, which are hexagonal in shape. The center of the lobule is traversed by a vein (central vein).
- Liver cells (hepatocytes) are polygonal in shape arranged in laminae, which radiate from the central vein. These hepatic laminae consist of two rows of cells with bile canaliculi intervening between them. The space between the adjacent hepatic laminae is occupied by sinusoids.
- The periphery of the hepatic lobules presents portal canals (portal triads). Each portal canal consists of three structures:
  a. A radical of portal vein
  b. A branch of hepatic artery
  c. Interlobular bile ductule
- The sinusoids between the hepatic laminae receive blood from both portal vein and hepatic artery. After providing nutrition to the hepatocytes, the blood of the sinusoids drains into the central vein. Central veins join successively to form hepatic veins, which open into inferior vena cava.
- The bile canaliculi present between the rows of hepatocytes receive 'bile' which opens into interlobular bile ductule of portal triad.
- Space of Disse is present between the walls of the sinusoids and hepatic laminae. These space contain blood plasma which opens into space of Mall which is present at the portal canal. The lymphatics of the liver begin at this space.

- Kupffer cells are reticuloendothelial cells present in the walls of the sinusoids.
- Portal lobule of the liver is a triangular area supplied by structures in the portal canal. Hence, it consists of centrally placed portal canal and central veins at three corners.

## Applied Aspects

1. Clinically the hepatocellular damage is manifested by jaundice.
2. Cirrhosis of the liver is a condition in which the liver hardens and shrinks due to fibrosis, often in a chronic alcoholic. It leads to portal hypertension. After suffering for several years, the patients die in hepatic failure.

## PANCREAS

- Pancreas is a partly exocrine and a partly endocrine gland (Fig. 21.7).
- The exocrine part secretes pancreatic juice and endocrine part secretes insulin and glucagon.
- Pancreas is transversely placed in the posterior abdominal wall (retroperitoneally) at the level of $L_1$ and $L_2$ vertebrae.
- It is a J-shaped structure about 6–8 inch longs and weighs about 90 gm.

## Parts

1. Head with uncinate process
2. Neck

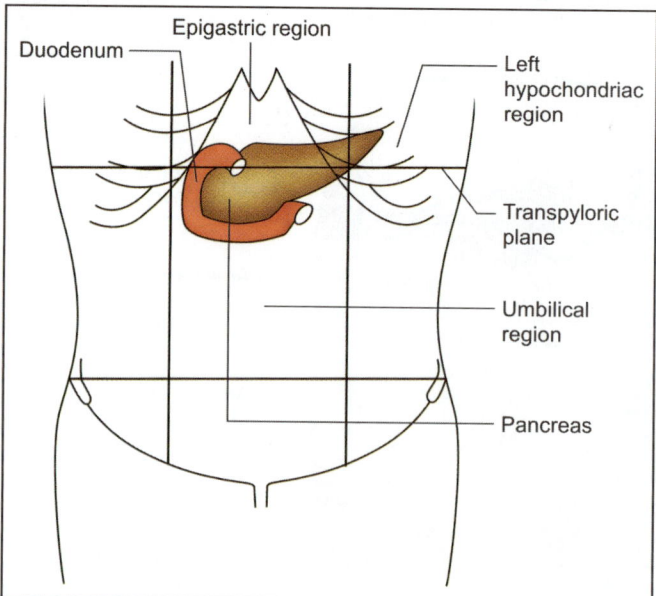

Fig. 21.7: Position of the pancreas

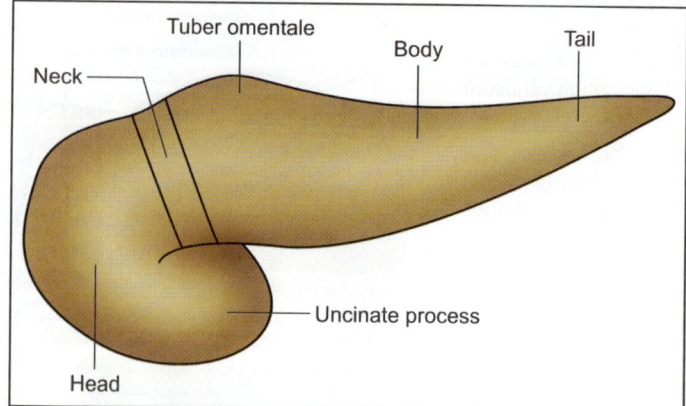

Fig. 21.8: Parts of the pancreas

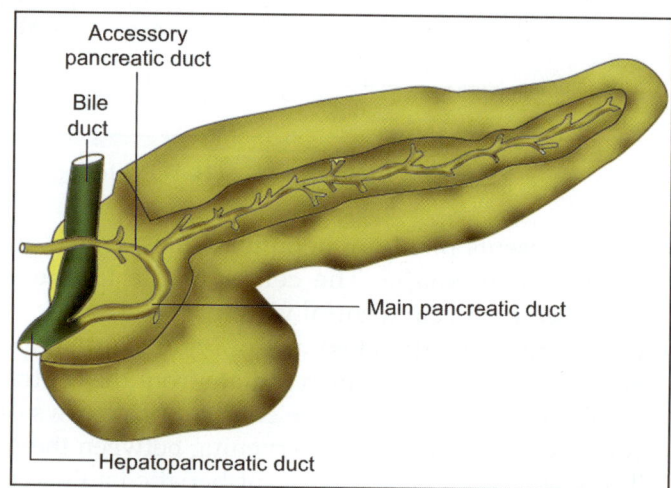

Fig. 21.9: Duct system of the pancreas

3. Body with tuber omentale
4. Tail

- The head of the pancreas is situated within the concavity of the duodenum.
- Posteriorly it is related to inferior vena cava and bile duct.
- Neck is the constricted part between the head and body. The portal vein is formed behind the neck.
- The body of the pancreas is anteriorly overlapped by stomach. Posteriorly it is related to abdominal aorta, left kidney and left suprarenal gland.
- Tail extends into hilum of spleen in a peritoneal fold called lienorenal ligament and is accompanied with splenic artery (Fig. 21.8).

Structurally pancreas presents pancreatic acinus, which secretes pancreatic juice. The acini are lined by pyramidal shaped cells with round nucleus placed towards basement membrane. The islets of Langerhans are small isolated masses throughout the pancreas but more towards the tail. They secrete hormones like insulin and glucagon.

*Pancreatic duct:* The pancreatic juice is drained by pancreatic duct which joins with bile duct (from liver) to form hepatopancreatic ampulla. It opens into the second part of the duodenum on the summit of major duodenal papilla. An accessory pancreatic duct may be present, which opens on the minor duodenal papilla.

Pancreas is supplied by splenic artery, superior and inferior pancreaticoduodenal arteries. The venous blood is drained into the portal vein (Fig. 21.9).

## Applied Aspects

1. Diabetes mellitus: Deficiency of insulin, which is characterized by polyuria, polydipsia, polyphagia, glycosuria and hyperglycemia. The patients are susceptible to infections, which are quite resistant to treatment.
2. Acute pancreatitis is a grave disease. It begins with acute agonising pain over the epigastrium, piercing deep to the back-associated with vomiting, and the collapse of the person.
3. Carcinoma is common in the head of the pancreas. Which may compress the bile duct to cause obstructive jaundice. Pancreatic cancer has the worst prognosis of all types of cancers due to spongy, vascular nature of this organ.

## SPLEEN

Spleen is situated in the abdominal cavity along the long axis of the left tenth rib (Fig. 21.10).

21

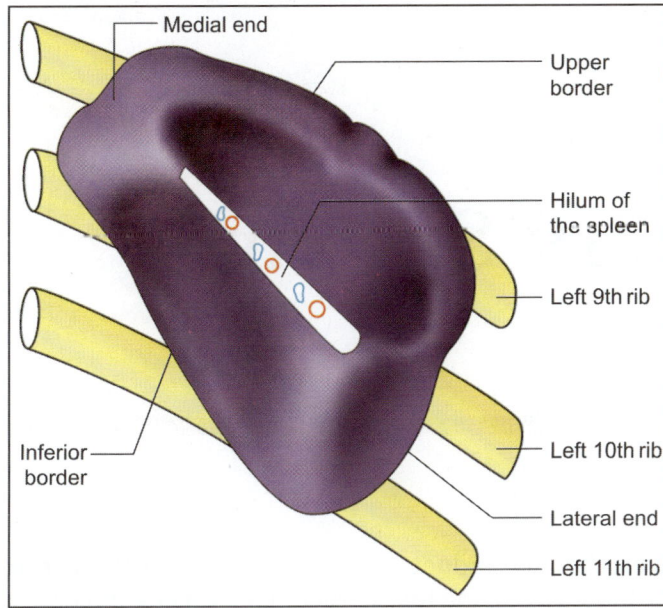

**Fig. 21.10:** Position of the spleen

## External Features

- Spleen presents an expanded anterior end and a pointed posterior end.
- It has convex diaphragmatic surface which is related to the diaphragm at the level of left ninth, tenth and eleventh ribs.
- Its visceral surface presents hilum through which the splenic vessels enter the spleen through a peritoneal ligament (lienorenal ligament). The visceral surface shows following impressions (Fig. 21.11).

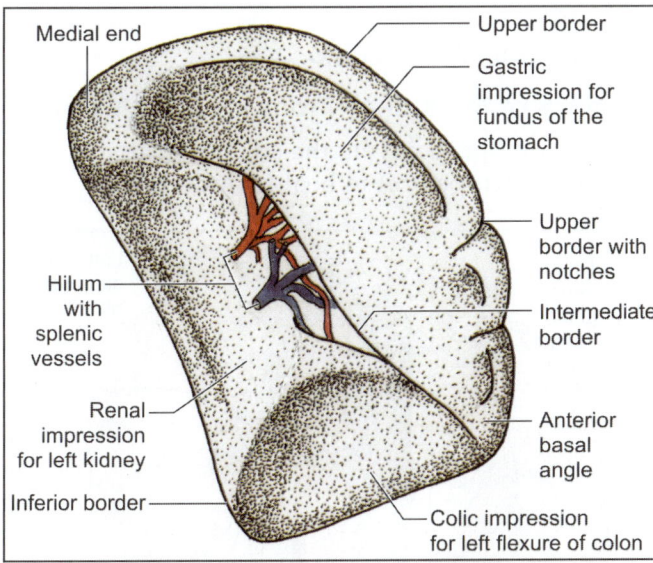

**Fig. 21.11:** Visceral surface of the spleen

- The gastric impression for the fundus of the stomach
- The renal impression for the left kidney
- The colic impression for the left flexure of the colon.
- The tail of the pancreas extends into the lower part of the hilum.

## Blood Supply

The splenic artery is a branch from the coeliac trunk. The splenic vein forms the portal vein after joining with superior mesenteric vein.

## Structure

The interior of the spleen shows white pulp and red pulp. The white pulp is the aggregation of the lymphocytes around an arteriole. The remaining area of the spleen shows cut sections of blood vessels with red pulp, which is made up of RBCs, lymphocytes, macrophages and platelets. All these cells rest on reticular variety of connective tissue fibers.

## Functions

- It filters the blood, phagocytose bacteria (spleen has largest aggregation of macrophages), degenerated blood cells and platelets.
- It provides immunity by producing lymphocytes and plasma cells.
- It is a reservoir of RBC.
- It extracts iron from hemoglobin and also bilirubin from hemoglobin.
- In fetal life, it produces all blood cells.

## Applied Anatomy

- The enlargement of the spleen is called **splenomegaly**. It occurs in infections, such as malaria and typhoid and also in portal hypertension and leukemia.
- Spleen is protected by 9th to 12 ribs, but their fracture can injure it (sharp bone fragment may lacerate the spleen). Even blunt trauma in this region of the abdomen (e.g. impact of handlebars of motor cycle) can tear the thin capsule of the spleen leading to profuse bleeding. Repair of ruptured spleen is difficult, hence a splenectomy (removal of spleen) is often performed to prevent bleeding.
- Normal spleen is not palpable, but when it enlarges to the double of its size, it is palpable under the left costal margin.

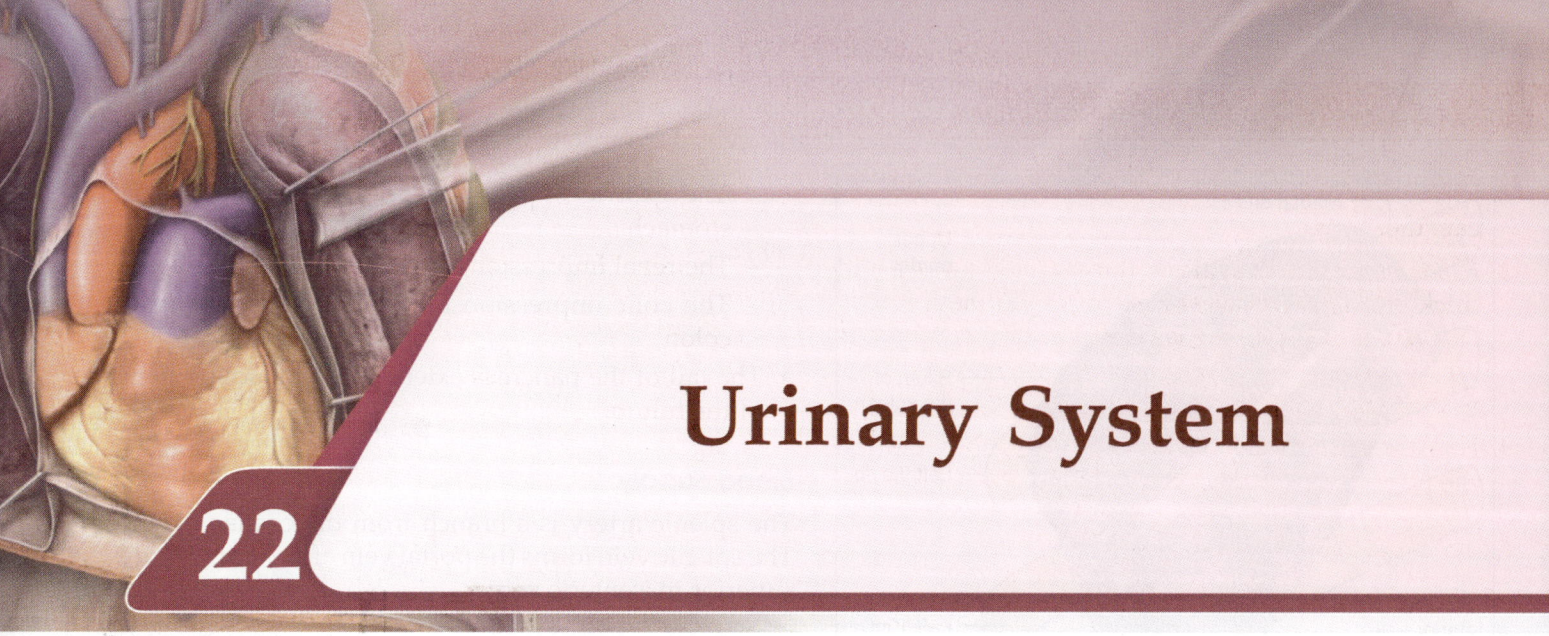

# Urinary System

## 22

The urinary system consists of those organs, which excrete urine and eliminate it from the body. They are kidneys (paired), ureters (paired), urinary bladder and urethra (Fig. 22.1).

The production of urine and its elimination from the body are vital functions since together they constitute one of the most important mechanisms for maintaining homeostasis.

### KIDNEY

Kidneys are a pair of excretory organs, which eliminate the waste products of metabolism in the form of urine and maintain electrolyte and water balance of the body.

Everyday, the kidneys filter many liters of fluid from the blood, allowing toxins, metabolic wastes and excess ions to leave the body in urine and returning needed substances from the filtrate to the blood.

### Situation

Kidneys are placed retroperitoneally on the posterior abdominal wall on either side of vertebral column, at the level of $T_{12}$–$L_3$ vertebrae. Right kidney is slightly lower than left (due to the liver) and left kidney is narrower and longer (Fig. 22.2).

### Measurements

Average measurements of each kidney are:
- Length—11 cm
- Breadth— 6 cm
- Anteroposterior thickness—3 cm

### Coverings of the Kidney (from within outwards)

1. *Fibrous capsule:* It covers the entire organ and it can be easily stripped off in healthy individuals.

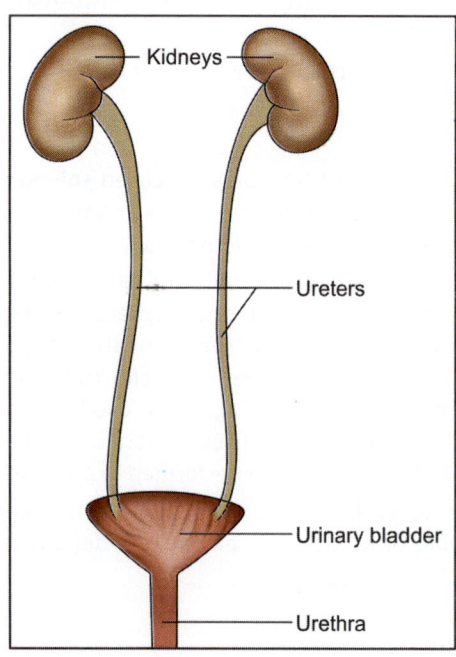

Fig. 22.1: Parts of the urinary system

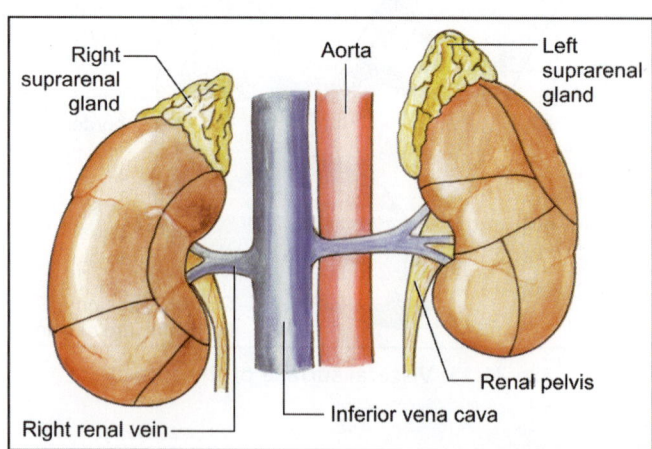

Fig. 22.2: Kidney in *situ*—anterior view

2. *Perinephric fat:* Thin layer of fat outside the fibrous capsule.

3. *Renal fascia:* It is thin along the anterior surface and thick on the posterior surface of the kidney. Above it encloses the suprarenal gland and is continuous with the fascia of the diaphragm. Hence kidney moves with respiration.

4. *Pararenal pad of fat:* This layer of fat is abundant on the posterior surface of the kidney.

## External Features

Each kidney has
- Two poles—superior and inferior (upper and lower)
- Two surfaces—anterior and posterior
- Two borders—medial and lateral.

*Superior (upper pole)* is broad and is in close contact with the corresponding suprarenal glands. The lateral border is convex.

The *medial border* is convex above and below and concave in the middle. The middle part shows a depression, the hilum through which structures enter or leave the kidney. They are renal vein, renal artery and renal pelvis (from anterior to posterior).

## Relations of the Kidney (Figs 22.3 and 22.4)

The relations to kidney on its anterior and posterior aspects is listed in Table 22.1.

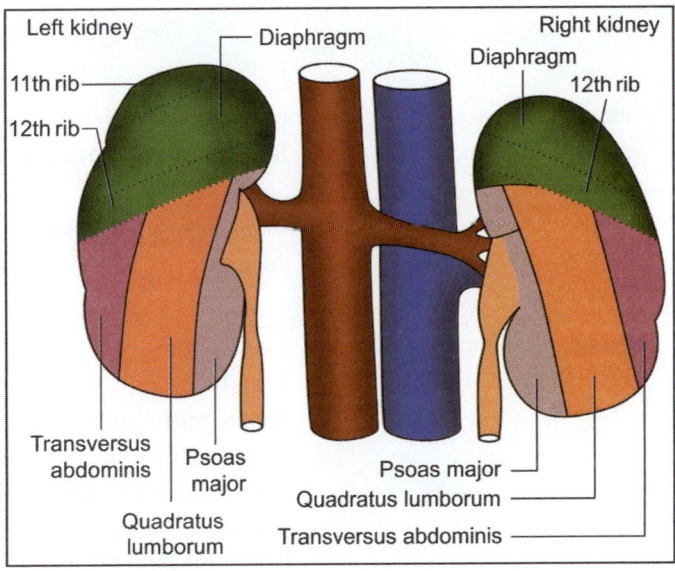

**Fig. 22.4:** Posterior relations of the kidney

## Macroscopic Structure (Fig. 22.5)

In the naked eye examination the coronal section of kidney shows:

a. An outer reddish brown cortex.

b. An inner pale medulla—consisting of renal pyramids and in between the adjacent pyramids the renal columns.

c. A space—renal sinus.

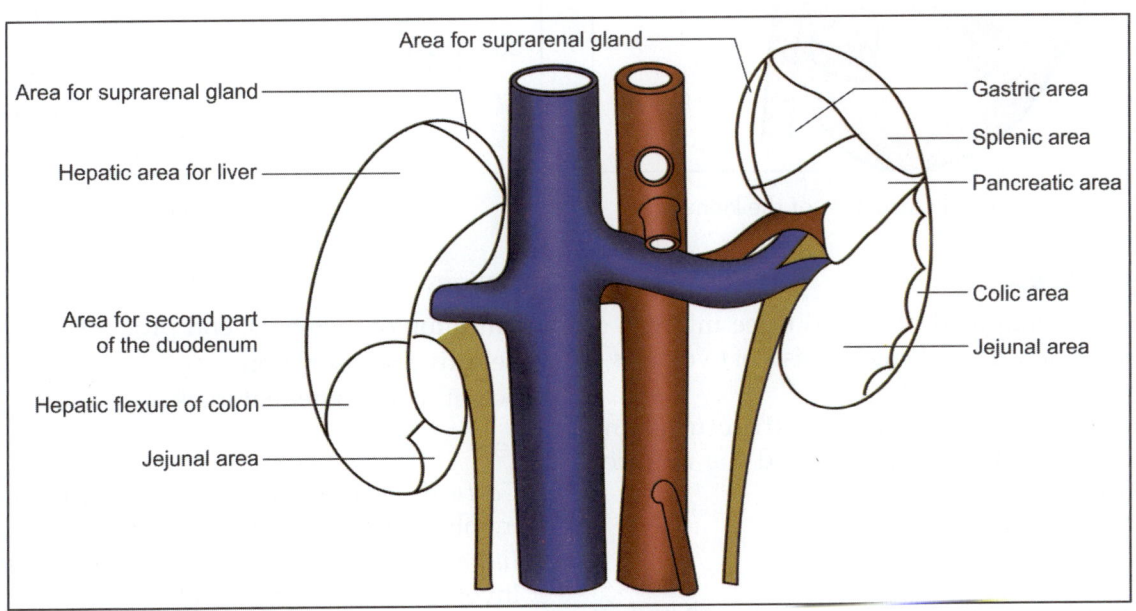

**Fig. 22.3:** Anterior relations of the kidney

22

**Table 22.1:** Relations of the kidney

| | Right kidney | Left kidney |
| --- | --- | --- |
| Anterior surface | Right suprarenal gland | Left suprarenal gland |
| | Second part of duodenum | Spleen |
| | Liver | Stomach |
| | Right flexure of colon | Pancreas |
| | Jejunum | Left flexure of colon |
| | | Jejunum |
| Posterior surface | Diaphragm | Diaphragm |
| | 12th rib | 11th and 12th rib |
| | Psoas major muscle | Psoas major muscle |
| | Quadratus lumborum muscle | Quadratus lumborum muscle |
| | Transverse abdominis | Transverse abdominis |
| | Subcostal vessels and nerves | Subcostal vessels and nerves |
| | Iliohypogastric nerve | Iliohypogastric nerve |
| | Ilioinguinal nerve | Ilioinguinal nerve |

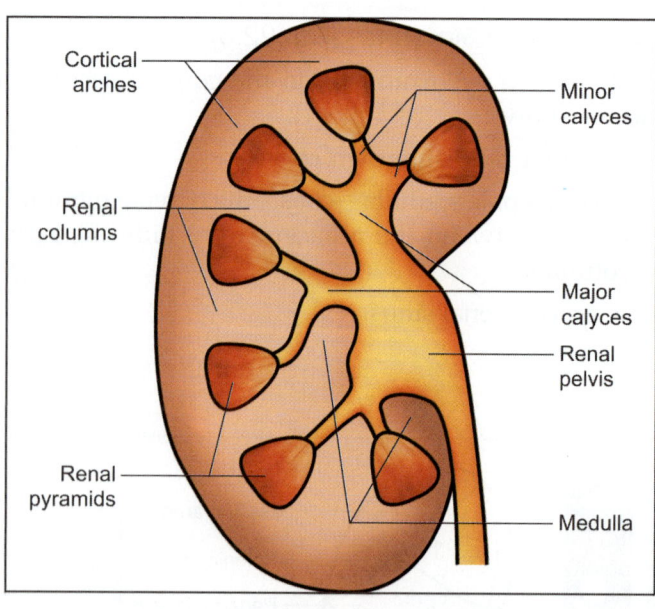

**Fig. 22.5:** Macroscopic structure of the kidney

**Fig. 22.6:** Nephron and collecting duct

## Microscopic Structure

Each kidney is composed of one to three millions of uriniferous tubules. Each tubule consists of two parts—secretory and collecting parts.

a. Secretory part consists of the structural and functional unit of the kidney called the nephron (Fig. 22.6).

## Nephrons

There are about one million of nephrons in each kidney. Its length varies from 50 to 55 mm.

## Functions

- Filtration of metabolic end products
- Selective reabsorption
- Secretion of some materials

## Types

- *Cortical nephrons (about 85%),* which are mainly involved in reabsorption of Na$^+$.
- *Juxtamedullary nephrons (15%),* which are mainly involved in reabsorption of water.

*Nephron* presents the following parts (Fig. 22.6)

1. *Bowman's capsule:* It is a bilaminar structure covering the tuft of capillaries called glomerulus. These glomeruli are derived from the terminal branches of renal artery (afferent arteriole). The filtration of the blood occurs at this site. The filtrate is collected by Bowman's capsule.

   *Structures intervening* between the blood of the glomerular capillaries and the Bowman's capsular space are the following from within outwards:

   • Flattened endothelium of the capillaries (which are fenestrated)
   • Basement membrane of the capillary endothelium
   • Foot plates of the podocyte cells (part of the Bowman's capsule).

   The total filtration surface of the glomeruli of both kidney are 1.5 m$^2$

2. *Proximal convoluted tubule:* The Bowman's capsule is continuous with the proximal convoluted tubule. Columnar cells with microvilli on their luminal surface line proximal convoluted tubule. Each tubule is about 60 μm in diameter.

4. *Loop of Henle:* The proximal convoluted tubule continues as loop of Henle, which has a descending limb, loop and ascending limb. It is lined by flattened cells.

5. *Distal convoluted tubule:* The loop of Henle continues as distal convoluted tubule which later joins the collecting tubule. Distal convoluted tubule is lined by cuboidal or low columnar cells with or without microvilli on their luminal surface. The distal tubule is 30 to 40 μm in diameter.

## Collecting Tubules

Collect the urine formed in the nephron. Many collecting tubules unite to form the ducts of Bellini, which open into the minor calyx.

The filtrate (urine) collected in the ducts of Bellini pass into the minor calyx (7 to 13 in number). The minor calices unite to form major calyces (2 or 3 in number) which open into renal pelvis. The urine collected in the renal pelvis passes through the ureter to be collected in the urinary bladder.

• 1700 liters of blood circulates/24 h
• 170 liters of filtrate is collected/24 h
• 1.5 liters of urine is excreted/24 h

## Blood Supply to the Kidney

### Arterial Supply (branching pattern of renal artery inside the kidney)

Under normal resting conditions, the large renal arteries deliver about one-fourth of the heart's systemic output to the kidneys. The renal arteries arise from the abdominal aorta. The right renal artery is longer than the left. Normally each renal artery divides into five segmental arteries that enter the hilus. Within the renal sinus, each segmental artery branches into several lobar artries, which lie in the renal columns between the medullary pyramids. They further divides into arcuate and interlobular arteries. Afferent arterioles from these interlobular arteries form 'glomerulus' (tufts of capillary plexus within the Bowman's capsule). From the other end of the glomerulus 'efferent arteriole' (note, it is not a venule) leaves the Bowman's capsule.

Because of the high blood pressure in the glomerulus the filtrate is forced out of the blood into Bowman's capsule.

The kidneys generate 1 liter of this filtrate every 8 minutes, but of which 1% ends up in urine, the other 99% is reabsorbed by the uriniferous tubules and returned to the blood. The efferent arterioles arising from the glomerulus form two types of capillaries.

a. *Vasae rectae:* These capillary loops extend into the medulla, running along side the loops of Henle. The vasae rectae are part of the kidney's urine-concentrating mechanism. The vasae rectae finally join interlobular veins.

b. *Peritubular capillary plexuses:* They are low-pressure, porous capillaries that readily absorb solutes and water from the tubules (PCT and DCT), and these peritubular capillary plexuses join the interlobular vein.

### Venous Drainage

Interlobular veins join to form arcuate veins, which further form interlobar and finally renal vein. Each renal vein drains into inferior vena cava.

### Juxtaglomerular Apparatus

Group of cells which are involved in increasing the glomerular filtration rate and thereby bringing back the normal volume of blood in the body. The cells are:

1. *Macula densa:* These are the specialized cells lining the distal convoluted tubule where it is in contact with afferent arteriole.

2. *Cells of Polkissen (lacis cells):* These are clusters of cells between the vascular pole of nephrons and the distal convoluted tubules.

3. *Juxtaglomerular cells:* These are the cells in the tunica media of the afferent arteriole and situated very close to the macula densa.

### Functions

When the afferent arteriolar pressure tends to fall, the macula densa releases 'renin'. The renin-angiotensin

22

mechanism results in secretion of angiotensin II, which directly acts on the smooth muscles of the arterioles producing vasoconstriction; therefore the blood pressure is raised. It also acts on the zona glomerulosa of the suprarenal cortex and stimulates the secretion of aldosterone. The latter increases the blood volume by retaining sodium and water.

### Applied Aspects

1. The renal fascia and fat around the kidneys hold them in their normal position. A loss of this fat (as with rapid weight loss) can drop the kidneys to a lower position. The kinking of the ureter and blood vessels can damage the kidney.
2. Surgery is performed on the kidneys for a variety of reasons (tumor removal or kidney transplant). Surgeons usually approach the kidney by cutting through the posterolateral abdominal wall, where the kidney lies closest to the body surface. However, the incision must be made inferior to the level of 12th rib to avoid puncturing the pleural cavity, which lies posterior to the superior third of each kidney. When 12th rib is absent or is too short to be felt, the 11th rib may be mistaken for the 12th and chances of opening the pleura are maximum. Puncturing the pleural cavity leads to pneumothorax and collapse of the lungs.
3. *Pyelitis:* Infection of the renal pelvis and calyces. When the infection involves the rest of the kidney as well, it produces pyelonephritis.
4. The three main waste products, excreted in urine are urea, uric acid and creatinine. Kidney functions are estimated by calculating their levels in blood.
5. *Multiple kidneys:* More than one kidney may be present on one or both sides. Kidney may be absent on one side
6. *Abnormal position:* Kidney may be placed in the pelvic cavity
7. A kidney with stenosis of renal artery produces systemic hypertension.

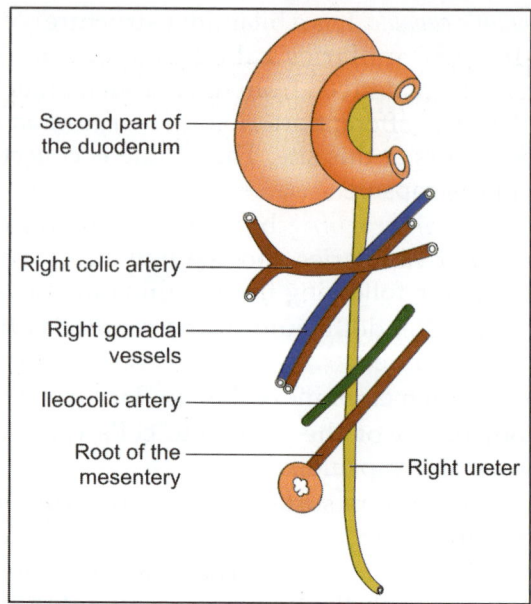

**Fig. 22.7:** Relations of the abdominal part of the right ureter

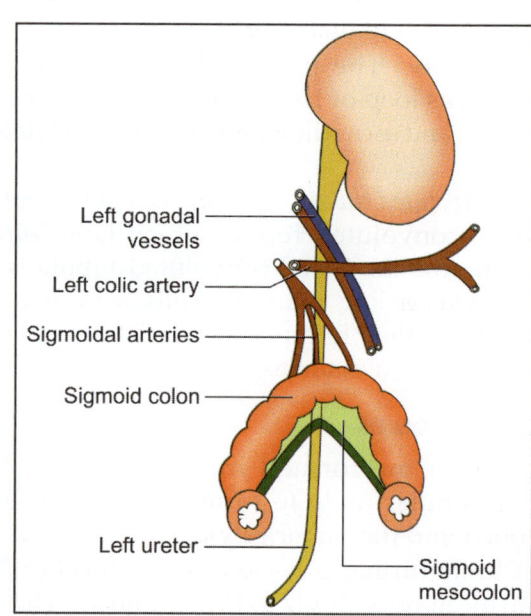

**Fig. 22.8:** Relations of the abdominal part of the left ureter

---

## URETERS

The ureters are a pair of narrow thick muscular tubes, which convey urine from the kidneys to the urinary bladder. They lie deep to the peritoneum, on the posterior abdominal wall in the upper part and on the lateral pelvic wall in the lower part (Figs 22.7 and 22.8).

### Measurements

Length is about 25 cm (12.5 cm in the abdomen and 12.5 cm in the pelvis). It measures about 3 mm in diameter.

### Normal Constrictions

The ureter is slightly constricted at three places
a. At the pelvi-ureteric junction
b. At the brim of lesser pelvis
c. At the entry of the urinary bladder
   A ureteric stone may lodge in one of these constrictions.

### Structure of Ureter

It has an outer fibrous coat, middle muscular coat and inner mucous coat. The smooth muscles of the muscular coat are arranged in outer circular and inner longitudinal layers. The mucous membrane is lined by transitional epithelium.

The lumen of the ureter is star shaped, when empty.

## Arterial Supply

Ureter is supplied by branches of following arteries - Renal artery, gonadal artery, lumbar artery, internal iliac artery and inferior vesical artery.

## URINARY BLADDER

The urinary bladder is a muscular reservoir of urine, which lies in the anterior part of the pelvic cavity (Figs 22.9 and 22.10).

## Capacity of the Bladder

The mean capacity of the urinary bladder is 220 ml. and the average capacity is between 120 and 320 ml.

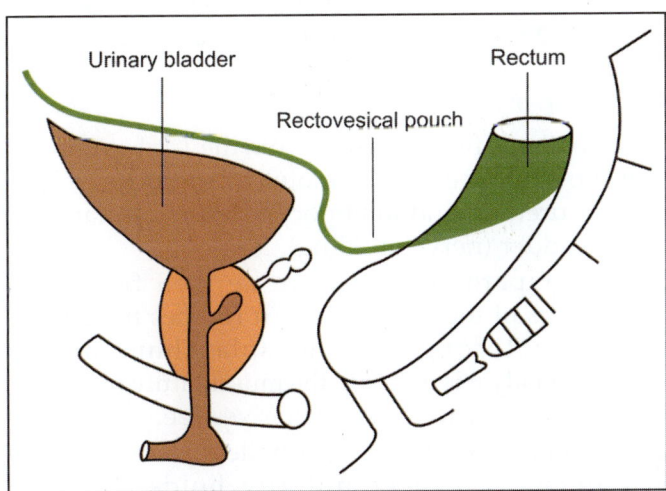

**Fig. 22.9:** Urinary bladder in male

## External Features

An empty bladder is tetrahedral in shape when it is distended it becomes ovoid. An empty bladder has (Fig. 22.11):

a. Apex
b. Base
c. Neck
d. Three surfaces—superior, inferolateral (right and left)
e. Four borders—anterior, posterior and two lateral borders.

- **Apex** is directed towards upper part of pubic symphysis. It is connected with umbilicus by median umbilical ligament.
- **Base (posterior surface/fundus)** is directed backwards. In males, it is related to a pair of seminal vesicles and terminal parts of the vasa deferentia and rectum from which it is separated by a peritoneal pouch called rectovesical pouch (Fig. 22.9). In females it is related to anterior wall of the vagina.
- **Neck** is the lowest part of the urinary bladder where urethra begins. It is situated about 3 to 4 cm behind the lower border of pubic symphysis. It is pierced by internal urethral orifice. In males the neck rests on the prostate gland. In females it is related to pelvic fascia that surrounds the upper part of the urethra.
- **Superior surface** is covered by peritoneum and related to coils of ileum. In females it is related to supravaginal part of the cervix and body of the uterus. It is separated from the uterus by a peritoneal pouch called 'uterovesical pouch' (Fig. 22.10).

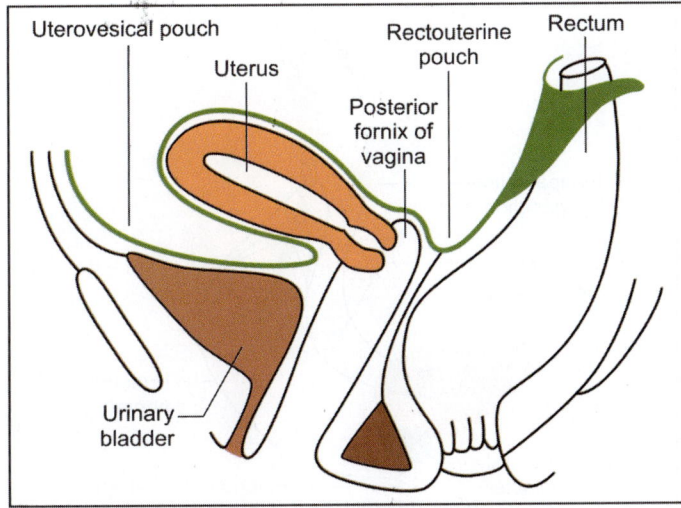

**Fig. 22.10:** Urinary bladder in female

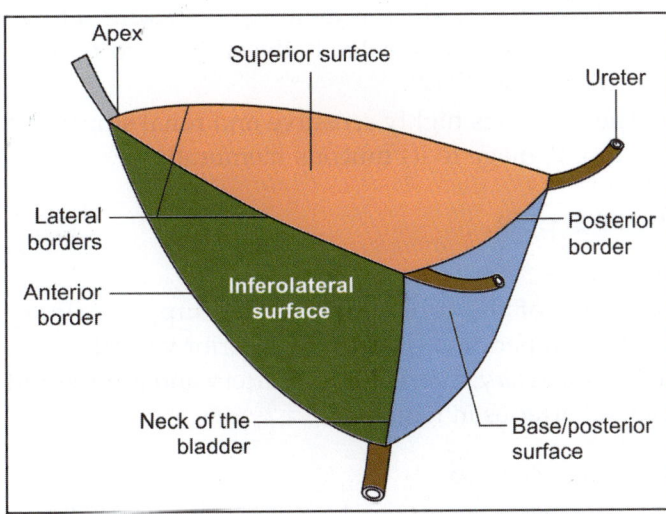

**Fig. 22.11:** External features of empty urinary bladder

- **Inferolateral surfaces:** On each side, it is related to obturator internus and levator ani muscles. It is separated from the body of the pubis by 'retropubic space'. This space is filled with fat and vesical plexus of veins. Surgical approach to the bladder is performed through this surface when bladder is distended.
- **Anterior border** extends from apex to the neck of the bladder. It separates the two inferolateral surfaces.
- **Posterior border** separates superior surface from the base. The two ureter opens at the lateral ends of the posterior border.
- **Lateral borders** separate superior surface from the inferolateral surfaces.

### Structure of Urinary Bladder

The wall of the urinary bladder consists of an outer serous layer, a thick coat of smooth muscle and a mucous membrane (from outside to inside).

### Trigone of the Bladder

- It is a small triangular area inside the urinary bladder, over the lower part of the base. Its inferior angle is formed by internal urethral orifice.
- The posterolateral angles are formed by openings of ureters.
- In an empty bladder the greater part of the mucous membrane forms irregular folds. In the region of the trigone, mucous membrane of the bladder is firmly attached to the underlying muscular coat.
- **Uvula vesicae** is an elavation in the interior of the urinary bladder produced by the median lobe of the prostate gland. Mucous membrane presents a ridge called interureteric ridge between the two ureteric orifices (Fig. 22.12).
- The trigone is highly sensitive and renal stones can cause damage to its mucous membrane.

### Blood Supply

#### Arterial Supply

Branches of the following arteries supply urinary bladder, superior vesical artery, inferior vesical artery, obturator artery, inferior gluteal artery and uterine and vaginal arteries in females.

#### Venous Drainage

The veins from the urinary bladder form vesical plexus, which drains into the internal iliac veins.

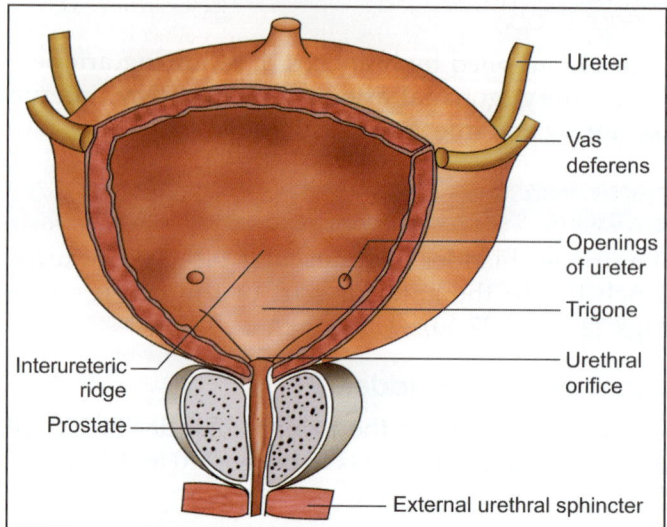

**Fig. 22.12:** Interior of the male urinary bladder

### Nerve Supply

1. Sympathetic fibers derived from the $T_{11}$–$L_2$ segments of the spinal cord. It is motor to sphincter vesicae (refer urethra) and inhibitory to the musculature of the bladder (nerve of filling).
2. Parasympathetic fibers are derived from $S_2$–$S_4$ segments of the spinal cord. It reaches the urinary bladder through pelvic splanchnic nerves. Functionally it is motor to the musculature of bladder and inhibitory to the sphincter vesicae.
3. Pudendal nerve ($S_2$, $S_3$, $S_4$) supplies external urethral sphincter which voluntarily holds the urine (Fig. 22.13).

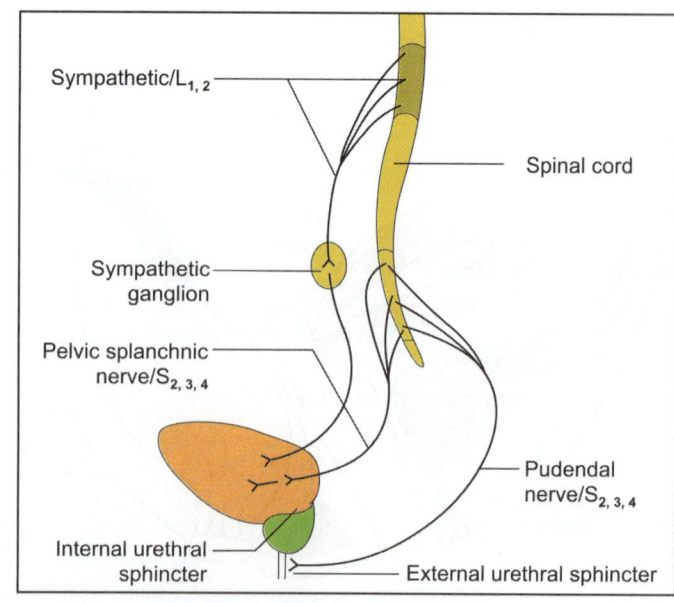

**Fig. 22.13:** Nerve supply to the bladder

4. Both sympathetic and parasympathetic nerves carry pain sensation from the urinary bladder (by distention or spasm of the urinary bladder).

## Applied Anatomy

1. Obstruction to the out flow of urine causes hypertrophy of the bladder, hydroureter and hydronephrosis (fluid accumulation inside the kidney).
2. Cystoscopy: Examination of the interior of urinary bladder.
3. Pyelography: The radiographic procedure for examining the ureters and renal calyces is called 'pyelography'. The contrast medium can be injected into the ureter through a catheter in the bladder (retrograde pyelography). The contrast medium can also be injected into a vein so that it reaches the ureters when excreted by the kidney (intravenous pyelography—IVP).
4. Renal calculi (Renal stones): On occasion, calcium, magnesium or uric acid salts in urine may crystallize and precipitate in the renal pelvis, forming kidney stones or renal calculi. Most calculi pass through the urinary tract without causing serious problems. Larger calculi however can block the drainage of urine, which raises the pressure inside the kidney. Calculi tend to lodge in the three normal constrictions of the ureter. The clinician identifies these constrictions of ureter in X-ray films at
   a. Tip of the transverse process of the $L_2$ vertebra (pelvi ureteral junction)
   b. The sacroiliac joint (brim of the lesser pelvis)
   c. Medial to the ischial spine (where the ureter enters the bladder).
5. Pain due to kidney stones radiates to the posterior abdominal wall on the same side of the body (loin to groin). The kidney stone causes the spasm of the ureteric musculature. When urine is dilute, the salts it contains cannot precipitate out of solution to form calculi. Hence patients with kidney stones are encouraged to drink large quantity of water.
6. Incontinence—the inability to control micturition is normal in babies who have not learned to use their external urethral sphincter.
7. Injuries to the spinal cord affect the function of urinary bladder. Transection of the spinal cord above the level of $S_{2,3,4}$ segments of the spinal cord, the patient loses voluntary control over bladder function. Bladder fills and empties reflexly. If injury involves $S_{2,3,4}$ segments of the spinal cord, the patient loses voluntary control and bladder fails to act reflexly. It overfills and overflows.

## URETHRA

Urethra is the passage through which urine is expelled out from the urinary bladder.

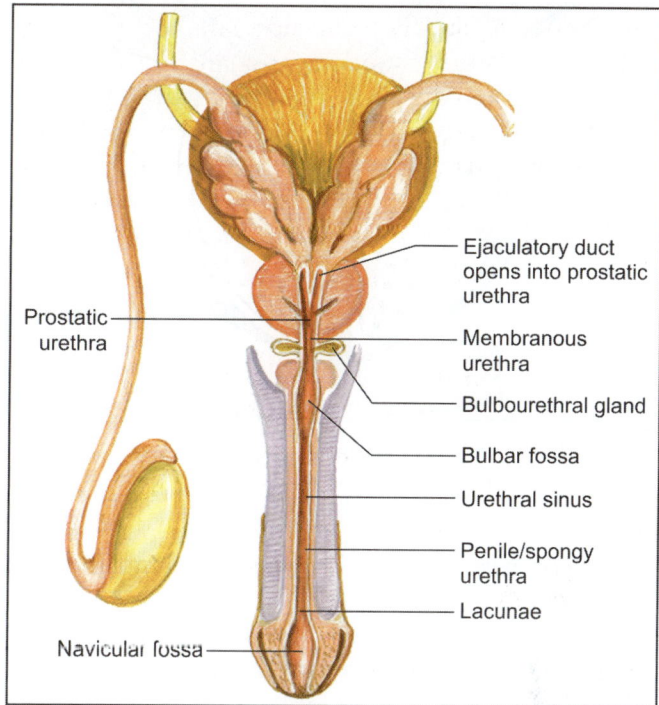

**Fig. 22.14:** Parts of the male urethra with male genital organs

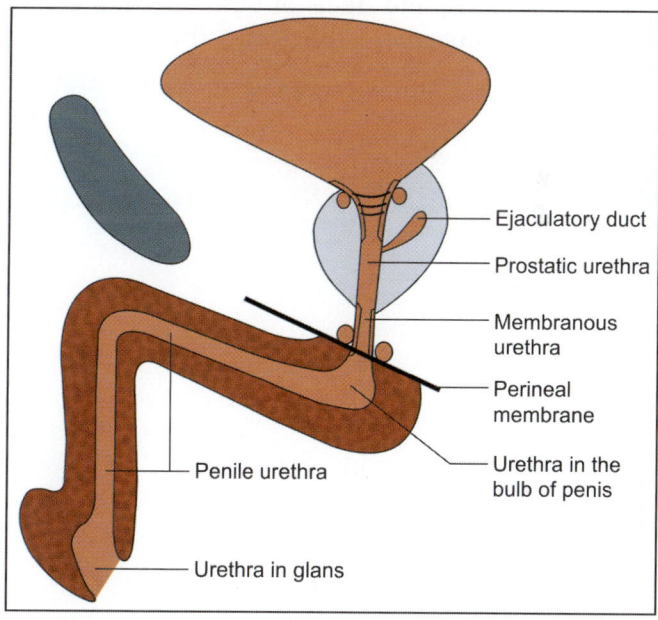

**Fig. 22.15:** Male urethra—lateral view

## THE MALE URETHRA

The male urethra is 18–20 cm long. It extends from internal urethral orifice at the neck of the urinary bladder to the external urethral orifice at the tip of the penis (Figs 22.14 and 22.15).

22

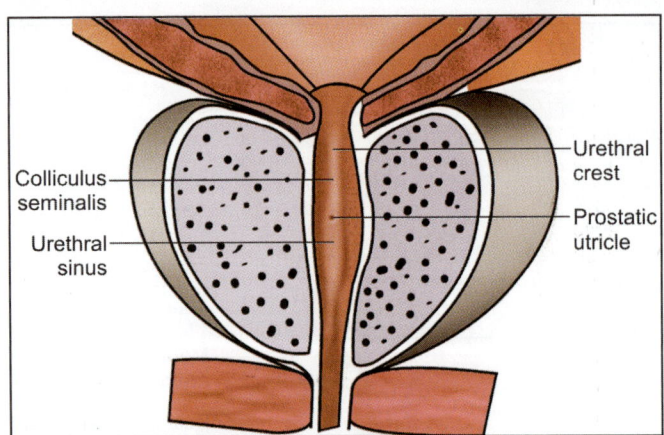

**Fig. 22.16:** Prostatic urethra

### Parts

1. *Prostatic part:* Within the prostate gland (3 cm in length) (Fig. 22.16).
2. *Membranous part:* Within the deep perineal pouch surrounded by sphincter urethrae muscle (2 cm in length).
3. *Spongy part:* Within the bulb and corpus spongiosum of the penis (15 cm in length). It receives the opening of many urethral glands. Mucous secreted by urethral glands, and ducts of bulbourethral glands at its commencement lubricates the urethra and

retards the entry of pathogens into the urinary bladder.

### SPHINCTERS OF THE URETHRA

1. *Internal urethral sphincter or sphincter vesicae:* It consists of smooth muscle fibers surrounding the internal urethral orifice in the form of U-shaped loop, and is involuntary in nature. It is absent in females.
2. *External urethral sphincter or sphincter urethrae:* It is made up of striated muscle fibers surrounding the membranous urethra and is voluntary in nature.

### FEMALE URETHRA

The female urethra is only 4 cm long and 6 mm in diameter. It corresponds to the upper part of the prostatic part of male urethra. It begins at the internal urethral orifice and traverses the urogenital diaphragm, and ends in the external urethral orifice in the vestibule of the vagina.

Sometimes a catheter is introduced through urethra (in case of retention of urine in the bladder). In such procedures one should know about the presence of lacunae (small pit-like recesses in spongy part) which may intercept the tip of the catheter. The membranous part of the urethra is the least dilatable part of male urethra.

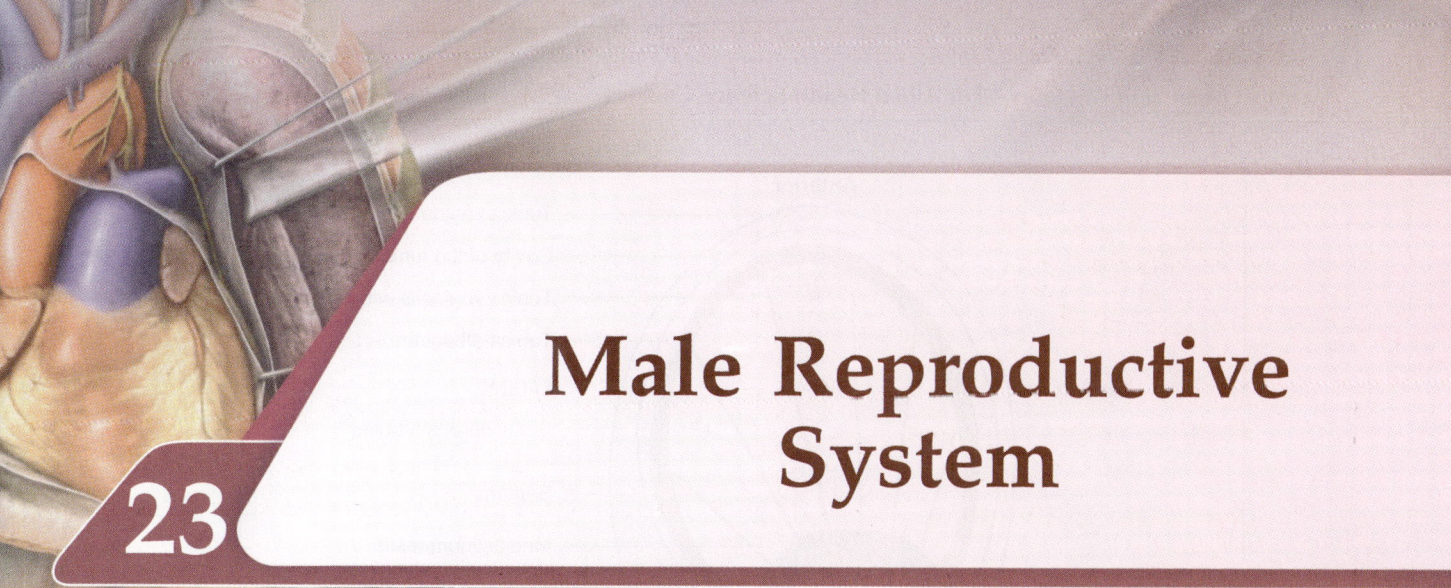

# Male Reproductive System

**23**

The male genital organs include the testis, epididymis, ductus deferens, ejaculatory ducts and penis. It also includes the accessory glandular structures like seminal vesicles, prostate and bulbourethral glands.

The testes are the primary reproductive organs or gonads. Epididymis, ductus deferens and ejaculatory ducts are tubular structures, which link the epididymis and prostatic part of the urethra. Penis is the male copulatory organ (Fig. 23.1).

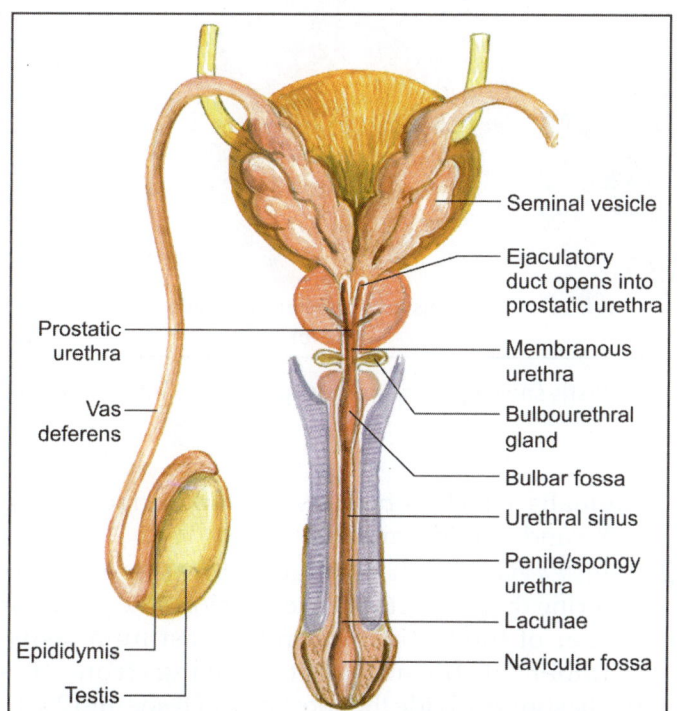

Fig. 23.1: Parts of the male reproductive system

*(Figure labels:)*
- Seminal vesicle
- Ejaculatory duct opens into prostatic urethra
- Prostatic urethra
- Membranous urethra
- Vas deferens
- Bulbourethral gland
- Bulbar fossa
- Urethral sinus
- Penile/spongy urethra
- Lacunae
- Epididymis
- Navicular fossa
- Testis

### Situation

Testis is suspended in the scrotal sac (scrotum) by the spermatic cord and covered by scrotal layers. The scrotal layers include dartos muscle (smooth muscles) and cremaster muscle. Sperms cannot be produced at body temperature (37 °C) thus the testes are situated in the scrotum which provides a temperature about 3° cooler. Furthermore, the scrotum responds to changes in the external temperature.

### Shape and Dimensions

Testis is oval in shape and is compressed from side to side.

Left testis lies about 1 cm lower than the right testis.

### Measurements

Length—5 cm
Breadth—2.5 cm
Thickness—3 cm
Weight 10 to 14 gm.

### External Features

The testis has:
Two poles—upper and lower
Two borders—anterior and posterior
Two surfaces—medial and lateral

Upper end is overlapped by the head of the epididymis and connected to it by efferent ductules. The posterior border is related to body of the epididymis on posterolateral aspect and vas deferens on posteromedial aspect (Figs 23.2 and 23.3).

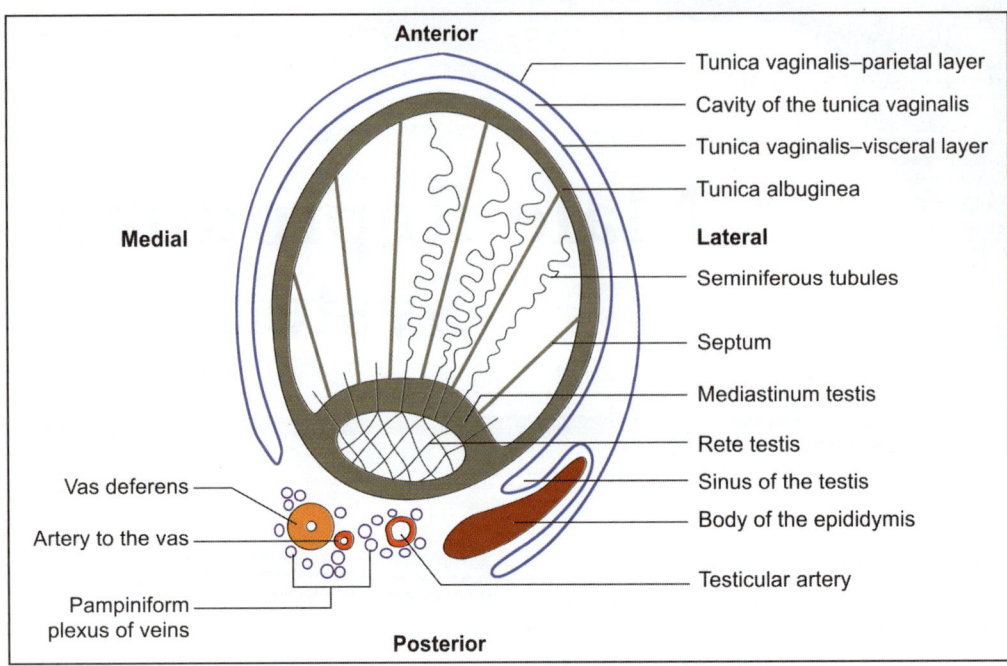

**Fig. 23.2:** Transverse section through right testis

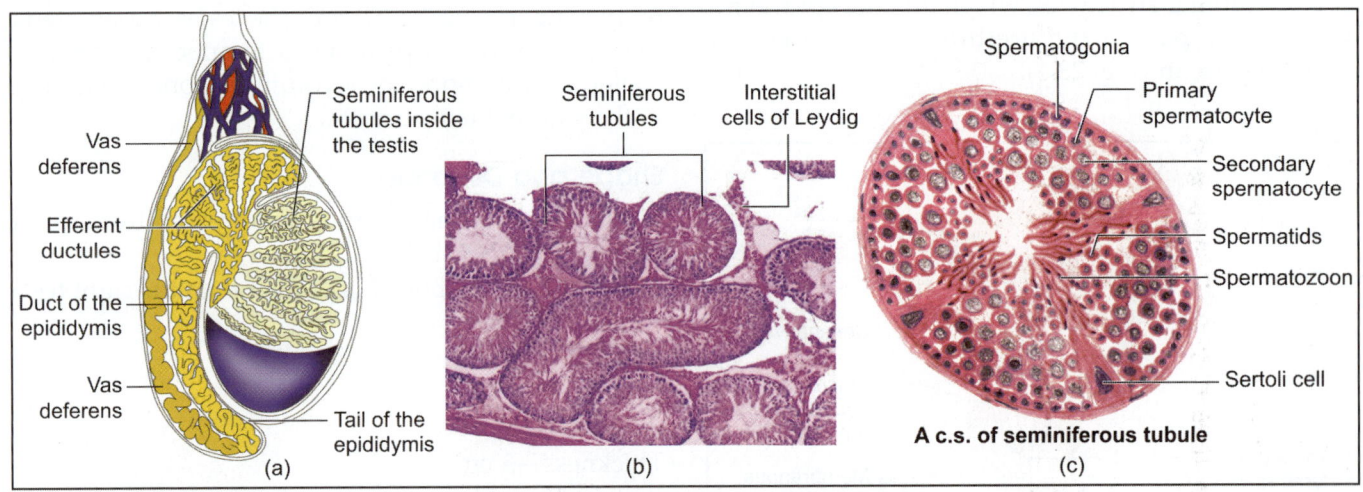

**Fig. 23.3:** (a) Duct system of the testis; (b) microscopic structure of the testis showing seminiferous tubules and interstitial cells of Leydig (H&E staining); (c) enlarged seminiferous tubule

The lateral surface of the testis is separated from epididymis by a recess called 'sinus of the epididymis' (Fig. 23.2) (part of the cavity of the tunica vaginalis).

### Coverings of the Testis (from outside inwards)

1. *Tunica vaginalis:* It is a peritoneal extension, covering the testis except at the posterior border. It is having two layers (outer parietal and inner visceral) with a cavity between them. Sinus of the epididymis is the part of the cavity of the tunica vaginalis which is between lateral surface of the testis and epididymis.

2. *Tunica albuginea:* It is a thick fibrous membrane covering the testis. It is thickened along the posterior border of the testis to form mediastinum testis. Number of fibrous septa arising from this mediastinum divide the substance of testis into 200 to 300 lobules. Each lobule is occupied by seminiferous tubules and interstitial cells of Leydig. (Fig. 23.3)

3. *Tunica vasculosa* is a vascular membrane.

## Microscopic Structure of the Testis

The testis is divided into 200–300 lobules by numerous septa that arise from the mediastinum testis. Within each lobule there are 2–3 seminiferous tubule.

**The interstitial cells (of Leydig)** are large polyhedral cells lying in the connective tissue that intervenes between the coils of the seminiferous tubules. These cells secrete male sex hormone, **testosterone**.

## Seminiferous Tubule

An uncoiled seminiferous tubule is about 70–80 cm in length and about 0.2 mm in diameter.

Each seminiferous tubule is covered by basement membrane. There are two varieties of cells inside the seminiferous tubule (Fig. 23.3).

a. *Spermatogenic cells:* These cells represent different stages in the formation of a spermatozoon. It includes spermatogonia, primary spermatocytes, secondary spermatocytes, spermatids and spermatozoa in lumen.

b. *Sertoli cells:* These cells support and nourish the spermatogenic cells.

The seminiferous tubules at the apices of the lobules become straight to form straight tubules, which enter the mediastinum. Here they form a network called rete testis. The rete testis gives rise to 12–20 efferent ductules, which emerge near the upper pole of the testis and enter the epididymis. The tubules end in a single duct, which is coiled on itself to form the body and tail of the epididymis. Tail continues as ductus deferens.

### Arterial Supply

Testicular artery, a direct branch of abdominal aorta.

### Venous Drainage

Drained by pampiniform plexus of veins, which later unite to form the testicular vein, which drains into the inferior vena cava on the right side and renal vein on the left side.

### Lymphatic Drainage

Testis drains into pre- and para-aortic group of lymph nodes while scrotum drains into superficial inguinal lymph nodes.

## Applied Aspects

Cryptorchidism: It is a congenital condition in which one or both testes fail to descend into the scrotum. The testis may be in the inguinal canal or in the pelvis. A testis that remains undescended is sterile, however the interstitial cells secrete 'testosterone' in normal quantities.

Varicocele: Varicose veins in the pampiniform plexus of the spermatic cord, which can lead to low sperm count or sterility. Such vericocele is common on left side, may be because of the load of the sigmoid colon on the left vein and the left testicular vein opens into left renal vein at acute angle.

Hydrocele: A swelling in the scrotum, caused by an excessive accumulation of fluid in the cavity of the tunica vaginalis. Hydrocele may result from an infection or injury to the testis that causes the layers of the tunica vaginalis to secrete excess serous fluid.

## Epididymis

It is a tortuous canal and the first part of the efferent route from the testis. It is much folded and tightly packed to form a mass, which is attached to the testis. Epididymis stores sperms in their last stage of maturation. Sperms are also stored in the ductus deferens.

### Parts

Head, body and tail.

Head is the enlarged upper end, and is connected to the upper pole of the testis by efferent ductules. Body is the middle part. The lower part is the tail. The head is made up of highly coiled efferent ductules. The body and tail are made up of single duct of epididymis (about 6 meters in length if uncoiled), which is highly coiled, on itself. At the lower end of the tail this duct becomes continuous with the ductus deferens.

## Ductus Deferens (vas deferens)

It is the distal continuation of the duct of the epididymis. It is about 45 cm in length.

It ascends along the posterior border of the testis. From the superior pole of the testis, it ascends in the posterior part of the spermatic cord. It passes through the inguinal canal, lateral pelvic wall and the floor of the pelvis to reach the base of the urinary bladder. It then descends to the base of the prostate where it joins with the duct of the seminal vesicle to form the ejaculatory duct, which opens into the prostatic urethra (Fig. 23.4).

### Structure (from outside inwards)

1. Outer fibrous coat
2. Middle muscular coat—smooth muscles are arranged in outer longitudinal and inner circular layers.
3. Mucous membrane is lined by simple columnar epithelium.

23

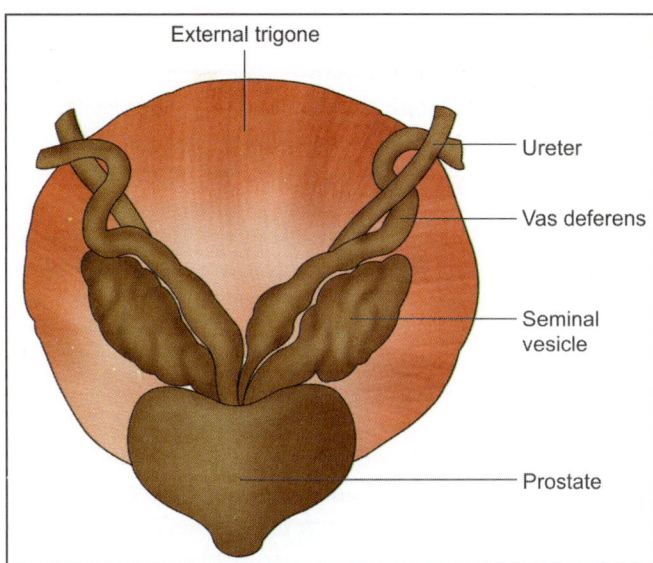

**Fig. 23.4:** Prostate—posterior view

**Vasectomy**
Bilateral ligation of the vas deferens is applied as one of the methods of family planning.

## PROSTATE GLAND

The prostate is an accessory gland of the male reproductive system. Secretion of this gland is added to the seminal fluid.

### Position, Shape and Measurements

Prostate lies in the lesser pelvis below the neck of urinary bladder. It resembles an inverted cone measuring about 4 cm transversely at the base, 3 cm vertically and 2 cm anteroposteriorly. It weighs about 8 grams.

### Coverings

Prostate is covered by an inner true capsule and outer false capsule. The space between the true and false capsule is occupied by the venous plexus.

### Parts

1. *Apex:* Directed downwards.
2. *Base:* Continuous with the neck of the urinary bladder.
3. *Four surfaces:* Anterior, posterior and two inferolateral.

### Lobes of the Prostate (Fig. 23.5)

Prostate is divided into 5 lobes by prostatic urethra and ejaculatory duct.

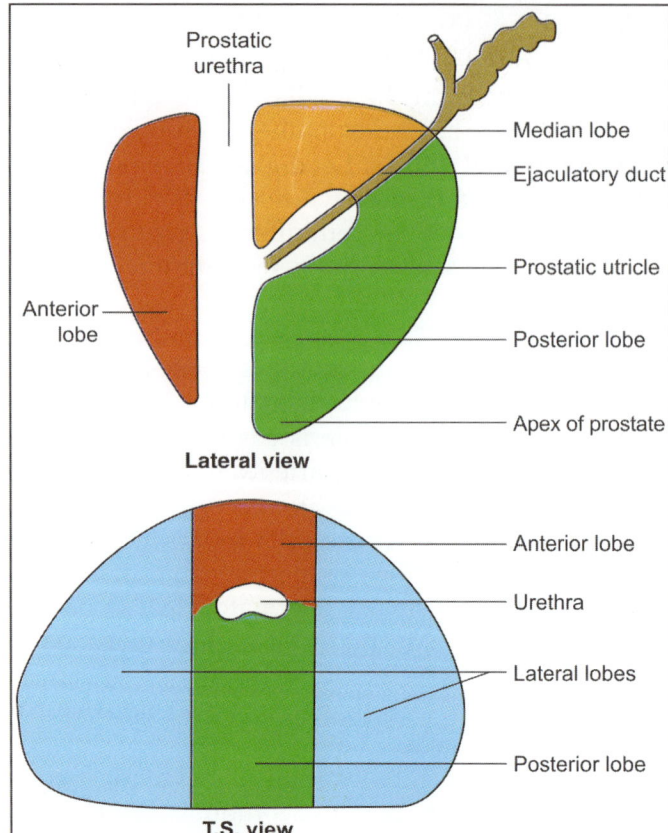

**Fig. 23.5:** Lobes of the prostate gland

*Anterior lobe:* Small portion in front of the prostatic urethra.

*Posterior lobe:* It lies behind the prostatic urethra and below the ejaculatory ducts.

*Lateral lobes:* They lie one on each side of the prostatic urethra.

*Median lobe:* It is the portion of prostate above and in front of the ejaculatory ducts. It projects into the trigone of the urinary bladder and this projection is called 'uvula vesicae' when this median lobe is enlarged (in old age), can obstruct the outlet of the bladder, causing difficulty in urination.

### Zonal Anatomy of the Prostate Gland

Recently the instead of surgical or anatomical lobes, zonal anatomy of the prostate is gaining clinical importance. According to which there are 3 zones:

1. *Outer peripheral zone (about 70% of prostate tissue)*—which is prone for carcinoma.
2. *Central zone (about 25% of prostate tissue)*—which surrouns the ejaculatory duct and occupies posterior to upper prostatic urethra.
3. *Transitional zone (about 5% of prostate tissue)*—which occupies around the distal part of the preprostatic

urethra, just proximal to the central zone. The BPH is more common in this zone.

## Blood Supply

1. The arteries supplying the prostate gland are inferior vesical, middle rectal and internal pudendal.
2. The veins form a 'prostatic plexus' between its true and false capsule and drains into internal iliac vein.

## Structure

Structurally, the gland has a fibromuscular stroma, within which lies the glandular tissue in the form of numerous follicles. These are tubuloalveolar glands. Each follicle is lined by columnar epithelium. The follicles drain into 12–20 excretory ducts, which open into the prostatic urethra (Fig. 23.6).

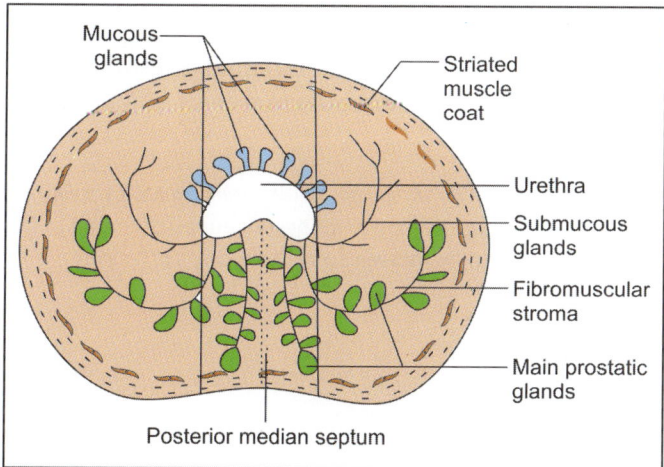

**Fig. 23.6:** Transverse section through the prostate showing passage of urethra and glandular arrangements

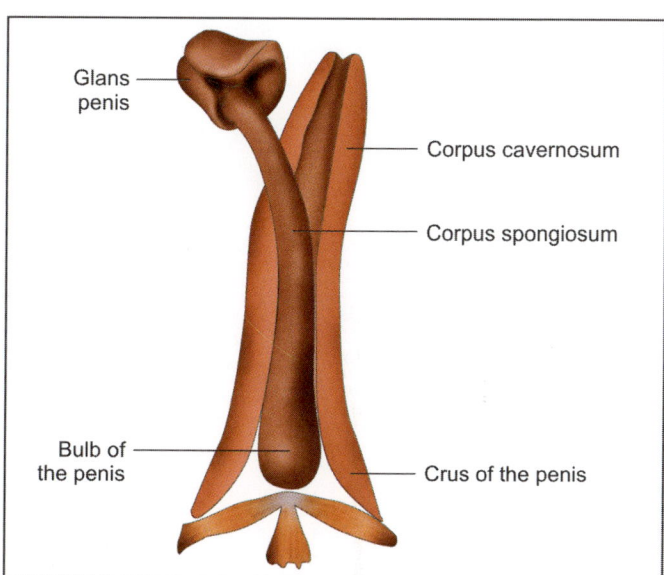

**Fig. 23.7:** Parts of the penis

The prostate produces a secretion, which forms a considerable part of the semen. The secretion is rich in enzymes (acid phosphate, amylase and protease) and citric acid. The prostate also produces substances called prostaglandins.

## Applied Aspects

*Benign prostatic hypertrophy (BPH):* It involves proliferation of fibromuscular stroma and epithelial cells of the prostate causing its enlargement. The enlarged prostate compresses the urethra and obstructs the urinary outflow. The median lobe is more frequently affected, which obstruct the internal urethral orifice. The more the person strains, the more the valve-like prostatic mass occlude the urethra. BPH can cause nocturia (need to void during the night), dysuria (difficulty and or pain during urination), and urgency (sudden desire to void). Obstruction to urethra can result in bladder infections as well as kidney damage. Most prostatic tumors are detected when men seek medical treatment for this problem.

Prostate enlargement is confirmed by rectal examination, since prostate lies just anterior to the rectum, a finger in the anal canal can easily feel this gland through the anterior rectal wall provided the bladder is full. A full bladder offers resistance, holding the prostate gland in place and making it more readily palpable. The posterior lobe of the prostate is felt through this rectal examination.

The prostatic venous plexus communicate with internal vertebral venous plexus. Through this anatomical rote the carcinoma of the prostate spreads into vertebral column and rib cage.

## EJACULATORY DUCTS

These are formed on each side by union of duct of a seminal vesicle with the ductus deferens. Each is 2 cm in length. Each of them passes through the prostate to open into the prostatic part of urethra.

## SEMINAL VESICLES

These are sacculated contorted tubes placed between the bladder and rectum (Fig. 23.1). Each vesicle is about 5 cm long. The lower narrow end forms the duct of the seminal vesicle, which joins the ductus deferens, to form the ejaculatory duct. The secretion of this forms a large part of the seminal fluid.

## PENIS

The penis is the male organ of copulation. It is made up of (a) root and (b) body (Fig. 22.8).

a. *Root of the penis:* Root of the penis is situated in the superficial perineal pouch. It is composed of 3 masses of erectile tissue.

23

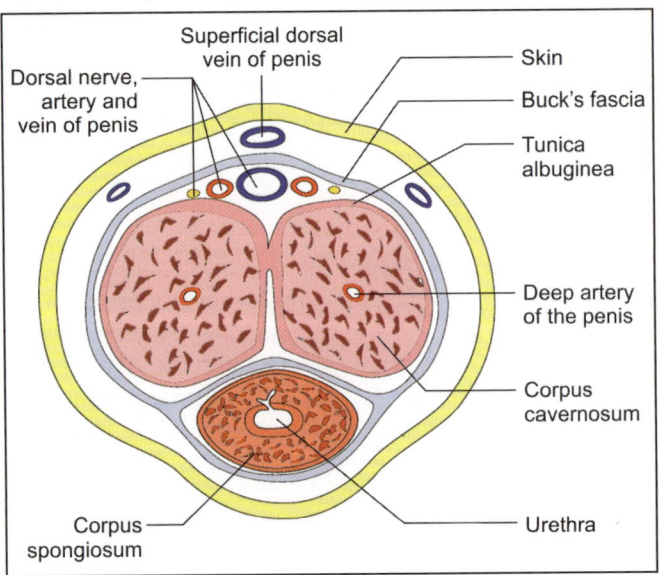

Labels on figure:
- Superficial dorsal vein of penis
- Dorsal nerve, artery and vein of penis
- Skin
- Buck's fascia
- Tunica albuginea
- Deep artery of the penis
- Corpus cavernosum
- Corpus spongiosum
- Urethra

**Fig. 23.8:** Cross-section through the body of the penis

Two crura and one bulb: Each crus is firmly attached to the margins of the pubic arch and covered by the muscle—ischiocavernosus. The bulb is attached to the perineal membrane and is covered by the bulbospongiosus muscle. Its deep surface is pierced by the urethra, which traverses its substance, to reach the corpus spongiosum in the body of the penis. Intrabulbar part of urethra shows a dilatation called the intrabulbar fossa.

b. *Body of penis:* It is the free portion of the penis. It is completely enveloped by skin. It is composed of three elongated masses of erectile tissue—right and left corpora cavernosa, and median corpus spongiosum, which is traversed by the urethra. During erection of the penis, these masses become engorged with blood, leading to considerable enlargement.

The terminal part of corpus spongiosum is expanded to form a conical enlargement called glans penis. The base of the glans penis has a projecting margin—the corona glandis, which overhangs an obliquely grooved constriction known as the neck of the penis. Within the glans, the urethra shows a dilatation called the navicular fossa. On the corona glandis and on the neck of the penis, there are numerous small preputial glands which secrete a sebaceous material is called the smegma.

**Circumcision:** In children or adults, circumcision may be required for a tightly constricting prepuce (phimosis). The prepuce (foreskin) is incised to release any adhesions.

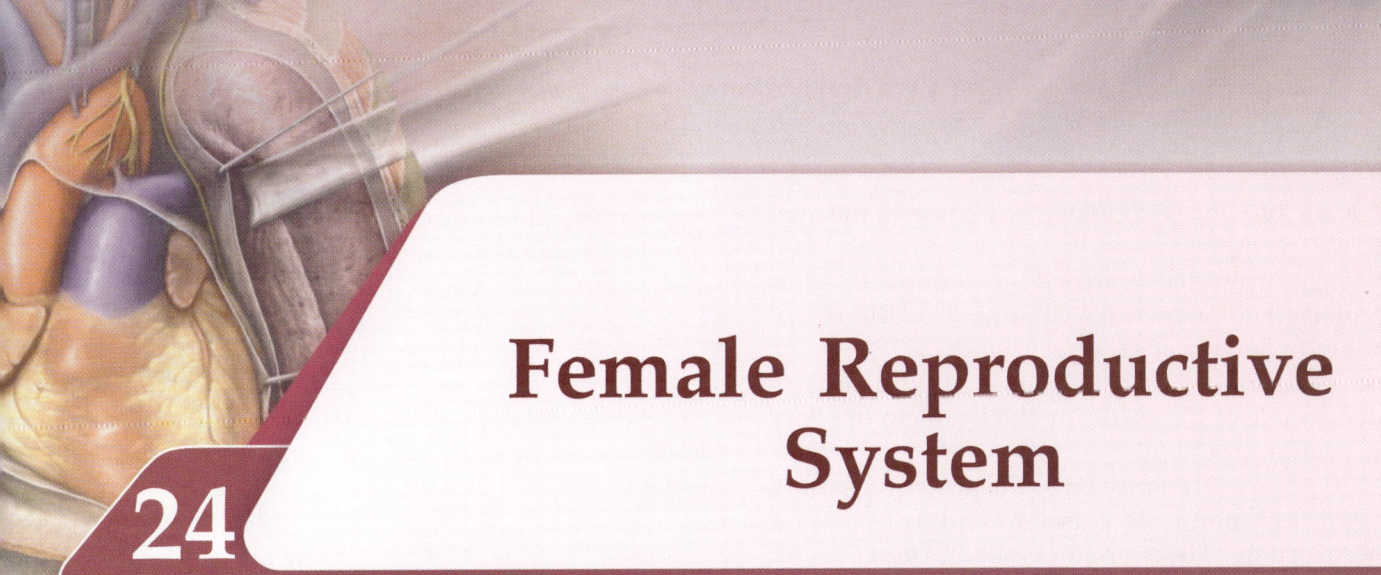

# Female Reproductive System

## 24

The female reproductive system consists of internal organs, namely ovaries, uterine tubes, uterus, vagina and external genital organs, namely mons pubis, labia majora and minora, clitoris, vestibular bulb, greater vestibular glands and vestibule.

### OVARY

The ovaries are the female gonads, which produce the ova.

### Situation

The ovary is situated in the ovarian fossa on the lateral pelvic wall, but the position of the ovary is variable. In nulliparus women, its long axis is nearly vertical and hence presents upper and lower poles (Fig. 24.1).

The ovarian fossa is bounded:
- Anteriorly by obliterated umbilical artery
- Posteriorly by ureter and internal iliac artery
- In young girls, before the onset of ovulation the ovaries have a smooth surface. After puberty the surface becomes uneven due to repeated ovulation. During pregnancy, the ovary rises to the abdominal cavity and after parturition it returns to the pelvic cavity and can occupy rectouterine pouch.

Though the normal ovaries are not palpable, enlarged ovaries and ovaries in rectouterine pouch are palpable by vaginal examination.

### Size and Shape

Each ovary is almond shaped, about 3 cm long, 1.5 cm wide and 1 cm thick.

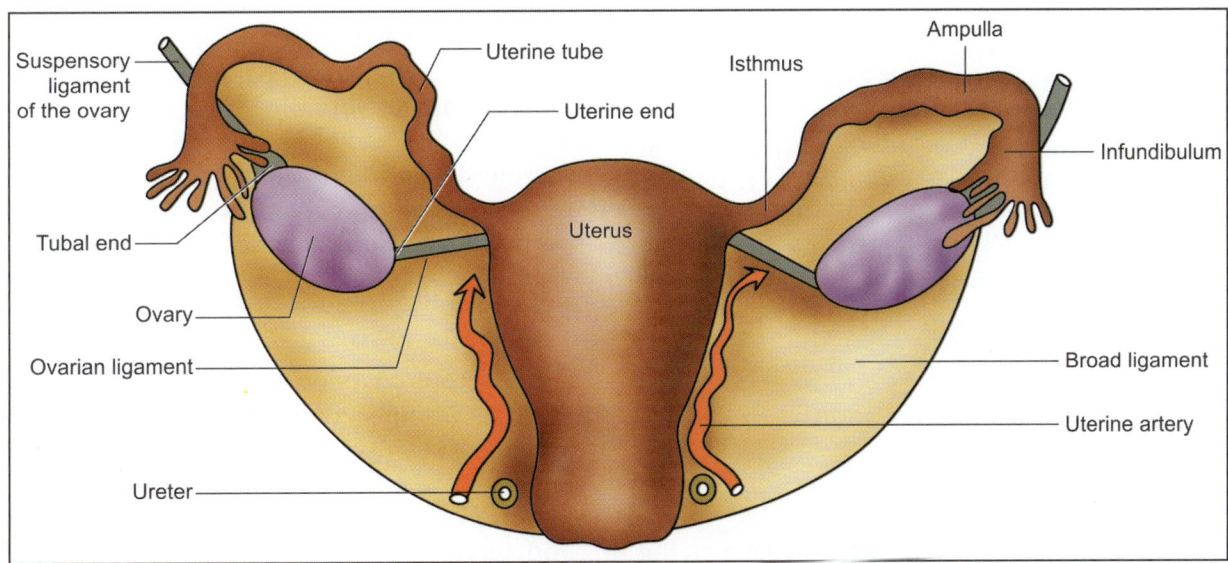

**Fig. 24.1:** Ovaries placed posterior to the broad ligament

## External Features

Each ovary presents two ends, two borders and two surfaces

i. *Upper end (tubal end)* is arched by uterine tube—it is connected to suspensory ligament of the ovary through which ovarian vessels enters.

ii. *Lower end (uterine end)* is connected with supero-lateral angle of the uterus by the ligament of ovary (or ovarian ligament)

iii. *Anterior border* is connected to the posterior layer of broad ligament by a peritoneal fold called 'mesovarium'. The ovarian vessels and nerves enter the ovary through it.

iv. *Posterior border* is convex and free

v. *Medial surface* is related to uterine tube

vi. *Lateral surface* rests in ovarian fossa

## Microscopic Structure

The ovary has an outer thick cortex containing ovarian follicles and corpora lutea and an inner vascular medulla.

At birth, the ovarian cortex contains many primary ovarian follicles. Each has a large central oogonium surrounded by a single layer of small cuboidal follicular cells. Many of these primary ovarian follicles degenerate during childhood. After puberty, some developing each month as vesicular ovarian follicles (graafian follicles) one usually maturing and rupturing. During the child bearing period (until menopause) the cortex contains ovarian follicles, corpora lutea and atretic follicles.

The graafian follicles consist of an outer layer of cells called tunica interna, which secrete 'Estrogen'. Estrogen stimulates the proliferative phase of the endometrium in menstrual cycle.

After ovulation the graafian follicle is converted into a mass called 'corpus luteum' which secretes 'progesterone'. If pregnancy occurs the corpus luteum persists for about three months, otherwise it will be converted into a mass called 'corpus albicans'. Progesterone maintains the integrity of the uterine endometrium and hence is required for maintenance of the pregnancy (Fig. 24.2).

## Arterial Supply

1. Ovarian artery from abdominal aorta
2. Branches from uterine artery

## Venous Drainage

Ovarian veins drains into the inferior vena cava on the right side, and renal vein on the left side.

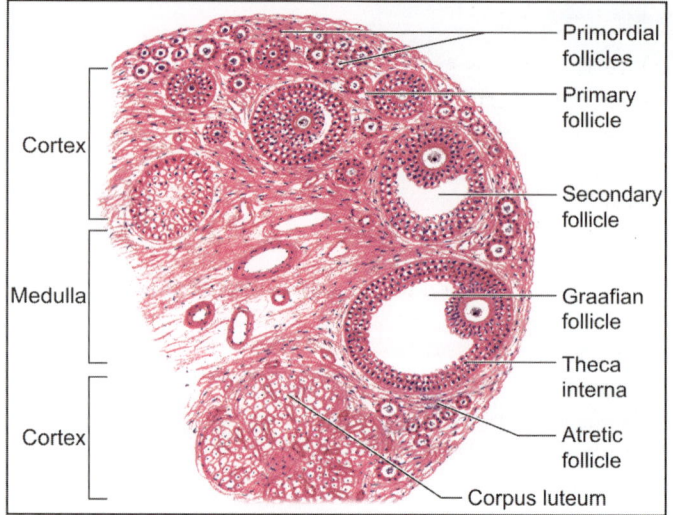

**Fig. 24.2:** Microscopic structure of ovary

## UTERINE TUBES (FALLOPIAN TUBES)

These are tortuous ducts, which convey ova from the ovary to the uterus. Each uterine tube is about 10 cm in length. At the lateral end, the uterine tube opens into the peritoneal cavity through its abdominal osteum. Medially it opens into uterus through uterine osteum (Fig. 24.1).

## Parts

a. *Infundibulum:* It is the lateral part of the uterine tube, which opens into the pelvic peritoneal cavity. Infundibulum shows many mucous folds called fimbriae, which collect the ovum, that is shed into the peritoneal cavity.

b. *Ampulla:* Infundibulum is followed medially by a dilated portion of the uterine tube called ampulla. Normally fertilization occurs here.

c. *Isthmus:* It is the medial part of the uterine tube. The musculature surrounding its wall is thick and acts as a sphincter and allows the fertilized ovum to the uterine cavity when it is in the morula stage.

d. *Uterine/intramural part:* This is the small medial portion of the uterine tube within the wall of the uterus.

## Structure of the Uterine Tube (from outside inwards)

1. Outer serous coat derived from the peritoneum.
2. Middle muscular coat: It consists of smooth muscles arranged in outer longitudinal and inner circular layers.
3. The mucous membrane shows primary, secondary and tertiary folds. It is lined by simple ciliated columnar cells.

## Blood Supply

1. Uterine tube is supplied by branches of uterine and ovarian arteries.
2. The venous blood is drained into uterine and ovarian veins.

## Applied Aspects

1. *Tubectomy:* It is one of the methods of family planning. A small segment of the tube is excised and cut ends are ligated.
2. *Salpingitis:* Inflammation of the uterine tube
3. *Tubal pregnancy (ectopic pregnancy):* Fertilized ovum fails to reach the uterine cavity and undergoes development within the uterine tube. This may cause rupture of the tube. This requires immediate surgical interference.

## UTERUS (WOMB)

It is the organ, which protects and provides nutrition to a fertilized ovum, enabling it to grow into a fully formed foetus. At the time of childbirth, contraction of muscles in the wall of the uterus results in expulsion of the fetus from the uterus.

## Situation and Position

It is situated in the lesser pelvis between the urinary bladder and rectum.

## Measurements

It is about 7.5 cm in length, 5 cm in breadth and nearly 2.5 cm in thickness and weighs about 30–40 g.

## PARTS OF THE UTERUS

Uterus is divisible into three parts (Fig. 24.3).
1. *Fundus:* It is the upper portion present above the level of openings of the uterine tubes.
2. *Body:* It is between the fundus and cervix.
3. *Cervix:* It is the lower cylindrical part, which enter the vagina, hence divisible into supravaginal and vaginal parts.

## Normal Axes of the Uterus

Uterus is not placed vertically in the true pelvis. It shows two forward angulations when urinary bladder and rectum are empty. These angles are important as they provide stability to uterus (Fig. 24.4).

1. *Angle of anteversion:* It is the forward angulation of uterus between the long axis of cervix and vagina. It is about 90°. Any backward tilt in this angle is called retroversion (retroverted uterus). A retroverted

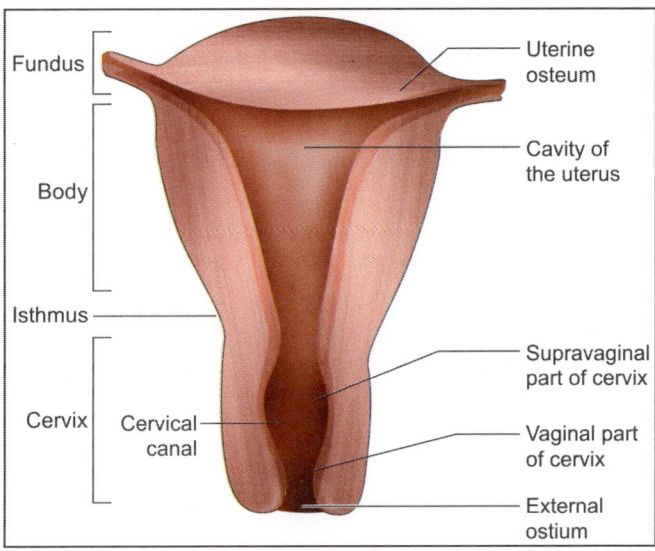

**Fig. 24.3:** Parts of the uterus (coronal section)

uterus comes in line with the axis of the vagina and may lead to prolapse of uterus.

2. *Angle of anteflexion:* It is the forward angulation between the body and cervix of the uterus. It is about 125°.

Because of these axes, the fundus and body presents upper and lower surfaces rather than anterior and posterior. The fundus and body almost rests on upper surface of the bladder. Externally the body is separated from the cervix by a constriction called 'isthmus'.

## Relations

### Fundus and Body

1. *The lower (anterior) surface* is flat and faces downwards and forwards. It is covered by peritoneum up to the isthmus. It is separated from the urinary bladder by uterovesical peritoneal pouch that may contain coils of ileum.

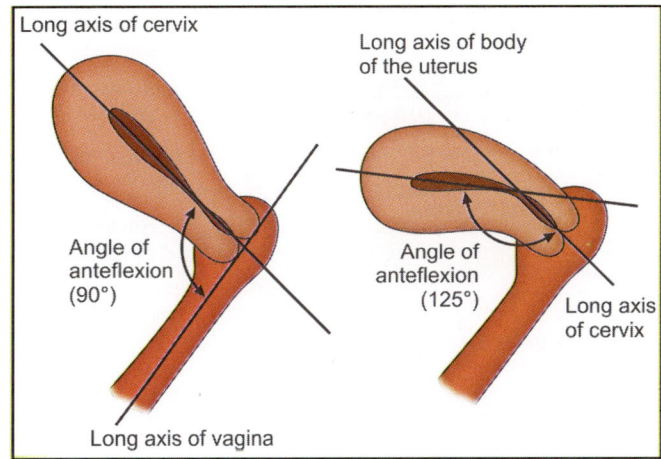

**Fig. 24.4:** Axis of the uterus

24

2. *The upper (posterior) surface* is convex and directed upwards and backward. It is covered by peritoneum up to the posterior fornix of the vagina (Fig. 24.5). It is separated from the rectum by rectouterine peritoneal pouch (pouch of Douglas). This pouch is occupied by coils of intestine and sigmoid colon.

3. *The lateral border* provides attachment to the broad ligament of the uterus. The uterine tube opens at the superolateral angle through uterine osteum. This superolateral angle (on lateral border of uterus) provides attachment to round ligament of uterus and ovarian ligament. The uterine artery ascends between the two layers of broad ligament along the lateral border.

### Cervix

It has two parts. The lower part projecting into the vagina is called the vaginal part and the part above the vagina is called the supravaginal part. The cavity of the cervix is called the cervical canal, which opens into vagina at the external osteum. Cervical canal communicates with the body above, through internal osteum and with vagina below through external osteum.

1. Anterior surface of the cervix is non-peritoneal and separated from the base of the urinary bladder by loose connective tissue.

2. Posterior surface is related to pouch of Douglas (rectouterine pouch).

3. On each side, the cervix is related to ureter, uterine vessels crosses the ureter from lateral to medial side.

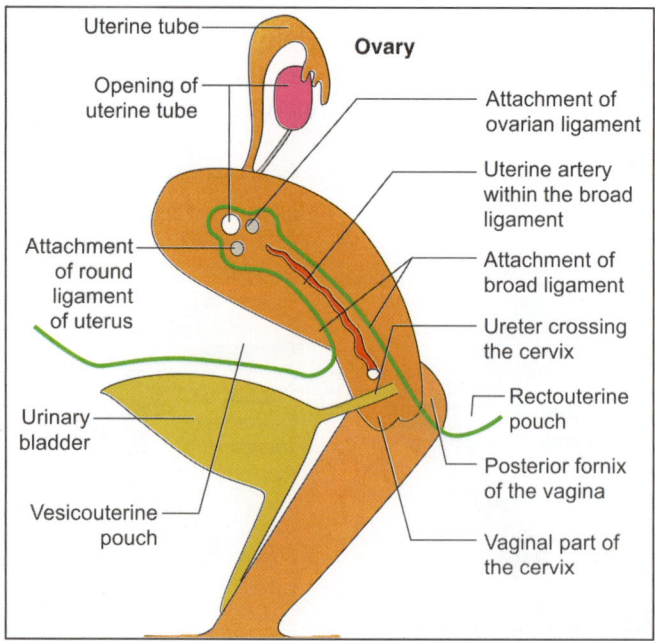

Uterine tube
Ovary
Opening of uterine tube
Attachment of ovarian ligament
Uterine artery within the broad ligament
Attachment of round ligament of uterus
Attachment of broad ligament
Ureter crossing the cervix
Urinary bladder
Rectouterine pouch
Posterior fornix of the vagina
Vesicouterine pouch
Vaginal part of the cervix

**Fig. 24.5:** Sagittal section of uterus

Transverse cervical ligament and paracervical lymph node close to the ureter.

The mucous membrane of the supravaginal part is lined by simple columnar epithelium and the vaginal part by stratified squamous epithelium.

### Microscopic Structure

Structurally uterus has three coats (from within outwards).

1. *Endometrium:* It is the mucous membrane of the uterus which consists of surface epithelium (simple columnar) and lamina propria. The lamina propria contains numerous tubular uterine glands and blood vessels. The cyclical changes that occur regularly every month, during the reproductive life of a female in the endometrium is called uterine or menstrual cycle. These changes are under the influence of estrogen and progesterone hormones secreted by ovary.

2. *Myometrium:* It is a muscular layer consisting of smooth muscle fibers. It is arranged in 3 ill-defined layers, outer longitudinal, middle circular and inner reticular.

3. *Perimetrium* is derived from peritoneum.

### SUPPORTS OF UTERUS

Uterus is a mobile organ, which undergoes extensive changes in size and shape during reproductive period of life.

It is supported or stabilized by a number of factors, which prevent its sagging down.

1. **Pelvic diaphragm:** It is a muscular structure forming the floor of the pelvis. It supports all the pelvic organs.

2. **Perineal body:** It is a fibromuscular node which acts as an anchor and maintains the integrity of the pelvic floor. It receives attachment of many perineal muscles.

3. **The external urethral sphincter** supports the vagina and thus indirectly supports the uterus.

4. **The axis of uterus** is an important mechanical factor stabilizing the uterus. The round ligaments of the uterus tend to pull the fundus forward and uterosacral ligaments tend to pull the cervix backwards. These ligaments maintain the normal axis of the uterus.

5. **The condensation of the pelvic fascia** in the form of the following ligament supports the uterus.
   a. *Pubocervical ligament:* It extends from the back of the body of the pubis to anterior aspect of the cervix.
   b. *Transverse cervical ligament:* It extends from the lateral wall of the pelvis (fascia covering the obturatorinternus) to lateral aspect of the cervix.

The uterine artery passes medially in this ligament.

c. *Uterosacral ligament:* It extends from sacrum to posterior aspect of the cervix.

### Arterial Supply (Fig. 24.6)

a. *Uterine artery:* It is a branch of internal iliac artery. It reaches the lateral aspect of the cervix through transverse cervical ligament in the floor of the pelvis. It ascends along the lateral border of the uterus crossing the ureter superficially from lateral to medial side. It ascends between the two layers of broad ligament.

b. *Ovarian artery:* It is a branch from the abdominal aorta. It passes through suspensory ligament of the ovary. Apart from ovary and uterine tube it also supplies uterus.

### Venous Drainage

Uterine, ovarian and vaginal veins which drain into internal iliac vein.

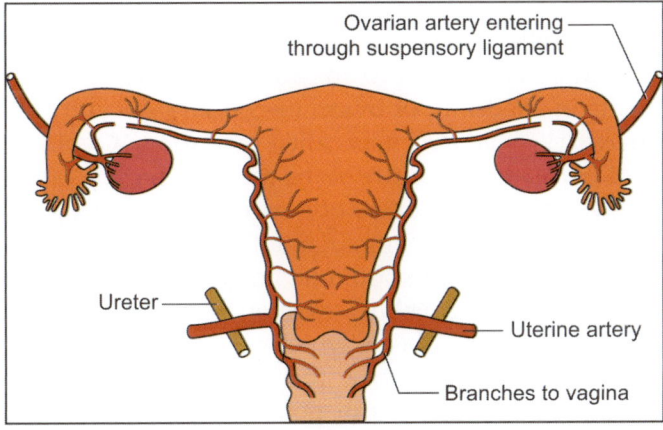

**Fig. 24.6:** Blood supply to uterus

### Applied Aspects

1. Among all the structures stabilizing the uterus the muscles of pelvic diaphragm and urogenital diaphragm is important. Most of the perineal muscles get attached to 'perineal body' which maintains the integrity of the pelvic floor. This perineal body is sometimes torn during childbirth. Subsequently the unsupported uterus may sink inferiorly. This condition is called prolapse of the uterus.
2. Hysterectomy—removal of uterus. It is very common operation, performed most often to treat tumors and cancers of the uterus.
3. Cesarean section—abdominal delivery of the baby by laparotomy and section of uterus.
4. Prolapse of uterus usually occurs in old age.
5. Retroverted uterus (backward tilt from the normal axis) causes dysmenorrhea (painful menstruation).

## VAGINA

The vagina is a fibromuscular canal forming the female copulatory organ. It extends from the vulva to the uterus. It is situated behind the bladder and urethra in front of the rectum and anal canal.

The diameter of the vagina gradually increases from below upwards. It is quite distensible and allows the passage of the head of fetus during delivery.

In the virgin the lower end of the vagina is partially closed by a thin annular fold of mucous membrane called the hymen.

The upper circular part of the vaginal cavity is protruded by lower part of the cervix. The portion of the vaginal cavity around the cervix of the uterus is called 'fornices'. They are anterior, posterior and two lateral. The posterior fornix is closely related to rectouterine pouch (pouch of Douglas). The rectouterine pouch is the most dependent part of the female peritoneal cavity and hence pus or blood tends to accumulate here. To drain the fluid the physician inserts a syringe needle superiorly through vagina at posterior fornix into the rectouterine pouch.

*Mons pubis:* It is a fat-filled subcutaneous area in front of the pubic symphysis. It is covered with pubic hair.

*Labia majora:* These are two thick folds of skin with subcutaneous fat forming lateral boundaries of pudendal cleft (or vulva). Its outer surface is covered with hair. The right and left labia majora join to form posterior commissure in front of the anus.

*Labia minora:* These are two thin folds of skin without fat.

*Clitoris:* It is an erectile organ homologous with the penis but not traversed by urethra. It is located in the anterior part of the pudendal cleft.

*Greater vestibular gland (Bartholin's gland):* It is located in the superficial perineal pouch. It corresponds to bulbourethral glands of males. It is partly overlapped by bulbospongiosus muscle. It has 2 cm long duct which opens into the vestibule deep to the labium minus, below the hymen. The glands secrete mucus into the vestibule during sexual arousal. The gland drains into superficial inguinal lymph nodes. The greater vestibular glands are usually not palpable, but when infected they are palpable. The gland is the site or origin of most vulvar cancers. Infection of this gland can result from number of pathogenic organisms. Infected gland can enlarge to a diameter 4–5 cm. These glands get infected in gonorrhea.

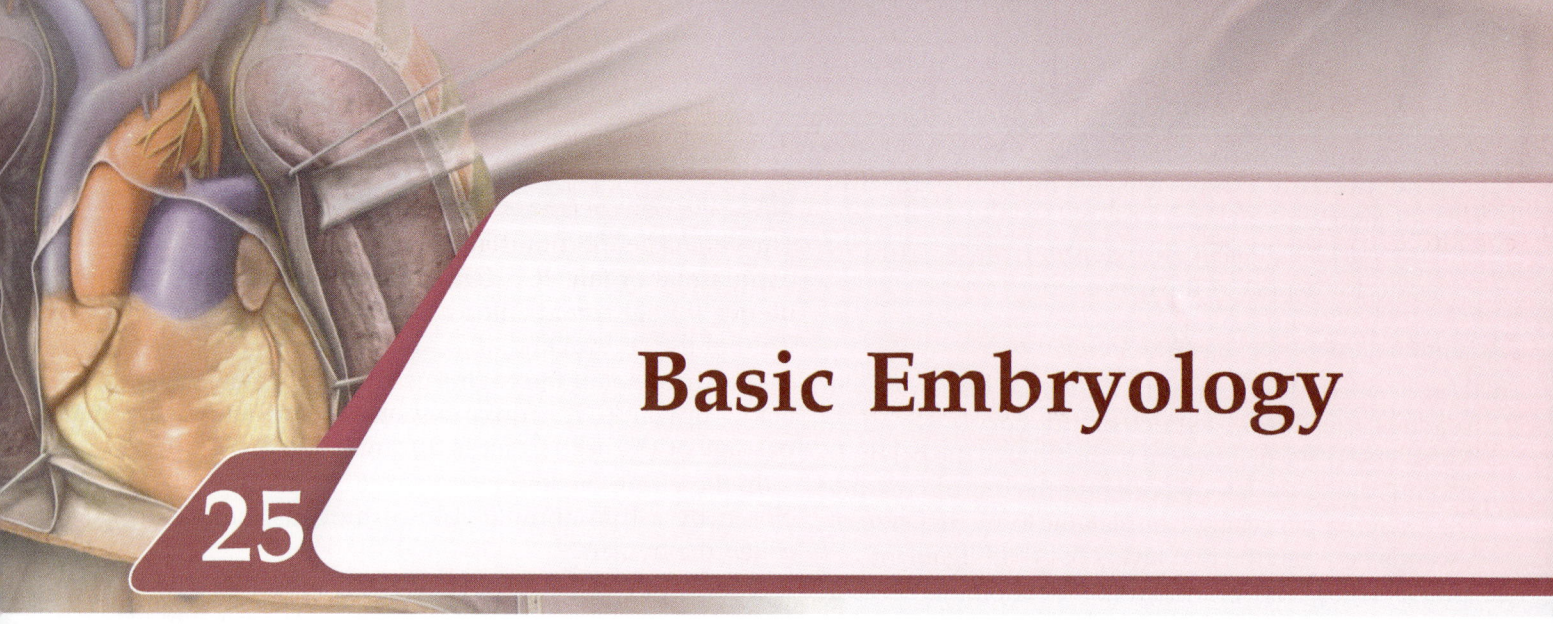

# Basic Embryology

## 25

Embryology is a branch of anatomy, which deals with human conception, intrauterine growth and development. This forms the basis for the understanding of an adult human body structure, function and provides anatomical basis for congenital anomalies.

### FEMALE ORGANS OF REPRODUCTION

Ovaries are a pair of female gonads. Every month they produce one ovum (female germ cell) and this process is called ovulation. This occurs from puberty to menopause.

Uterine tubes extend laterally from the uterus. The lateral end of the uterine tube opens into peritoneal cavity close to the ovary. The ovum released from the ovary is taken by the lateral end of the uterine tube. The spermatozoa (male germ cells) traverse vagina, uterus and then uterine tube. Fertilization occurs at the ampulla of the uterine tube (*see* Fig. 24.1).

Uterus is a childbearing organ where fertilized ovum is implanted within its endometrium. It provides nutrition and protection to the fetus till parturition (delivery of the baby).

Vagina is the female copulatory organ and forms lower part of the birth canal.

### OVARIAN CYCLE

During maturation of female germ cells (primary oocyte to ova) the stromal cells of the ovary provide a protective coat outside them.

The primary oocyte with single layer of follicular cells constitutes 'primary ovarian follicle'. These follicular cells multiply to form several layers. At this stage, it is called 'secondary follicle'. Later a cavity appears in follicular cells (which contains liquor

folliculi) and at this stage it is called tertiary follicle (Fig. 25.1).

This matured follicle is called 'Graafian follicle', which has secondary oocyte inside. The outer follicular cells differentiate into two layers—theca externa and interna. Cells of the theca interna secrete 'estrogen'. The stromal cells break and the follicle ruptures, which results in shedding of ovum (secondary oocyte) from the ovary. This process is called ovulation. Ovulation takes place at the middle of the menstrual cycle (about 14 days prior to the onset of next menstrual bleeding).

After ovulation, the graafian follicle is converted into a mass called 'corpus luteum', consisting of a mass of cells containing a yellow carotenoid pigment called lutein in their cytoplasm, which secrete 'progesterone' hormone. If the ovum is fertilized and pregnancy occurs, the corpus luteum persists for 3 to 4 months and is called corpus luteum of pregnancy.

In the absence of pregnancy, the corpus luteum (of menstruation) persists for only 12–14 days and then regresses and is converted into corpus albicans.

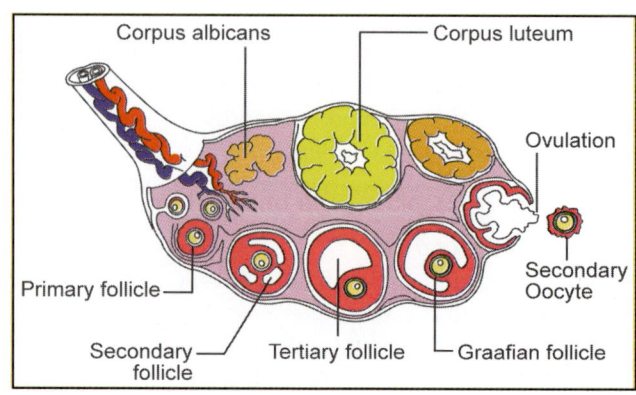

**Fig. 25.1:** Ovarian cycle

These cyclical changes inside the ovary comprising primary ovarian follicle to formation of corpus luteum constitute 'ovarian cycle'.

## OOGENESIS

The primary oocyte undergoes first meiotic division (reduction of chromosome number to half) to give secondary oocyte which has 22X chromosomes and first polar body. This division is unequal so that greater volume of cytoplasum passes into secondary oocyte (Fig. 25.2a).

This secondary oocyte further undergoes second meiotic division to give rise to 'mature ovum' which is having 22X chromosomes and second polar body. During ovulation the secondary oocyte is shed from the ovary. The second meiotic division occures only if fertilization takes place.

## MENSTRUAL CYCLE (UTERINE CYCLE)

The periodic structural changes of the endometrium of the uterus constitute 'menstrual cycle'. It occurs during the reproductive life of the female, from puberty to menopause. The cycle is counted from the first day of one menstrual bleeding to the first day of next menstrual bleeding (normally of 28 days). Hormones (estrogen and progesterone) liberated from the ovary during ovarian cycle are responsible for cyclical changes in the endometrium of the uterus.

If pregnancy fails to occur, the corpus luteum inside the ovary degenerates (12 to 14 days after ovulation). This results in sudden withdrawal of 'progesterone' from the circulating blood. This is followed by shedding of the endometrium (menstrual bleeding). This is due to rupture of the blood vessels in uterine endometrium.

If pregnancy occurs, the corpus luteum persists up to the end of 4th month of pregnancy and secretes 'progesterone' which maintains the integrity of the uterine endometrium where embryo is growing. Later its function is taken over by placenta.

## MALE ORGANS OF REPRODUCTION

Testes are male gonads suspended in the scrotum by spermatic cords. Semeniferous tubules present inside the testis produce 'spermatozoa' (male germ cells) (Fig. 25.2b).

Epididymis is a coiled single tube attached to the posterior aspect of the testis. The spermatozoa formed inside the seminiferous tubules pass out from the testis through 'efferent ductules'. These ducts join to form

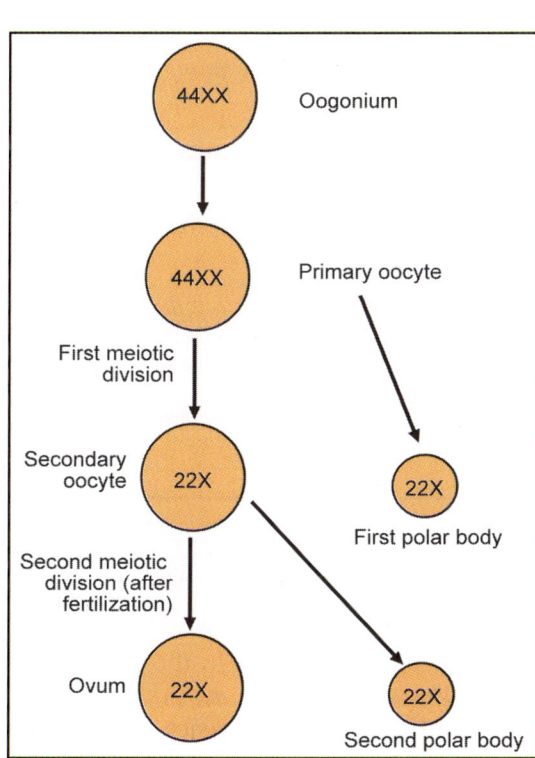

**Fig. 25.2a:** Oogenesis

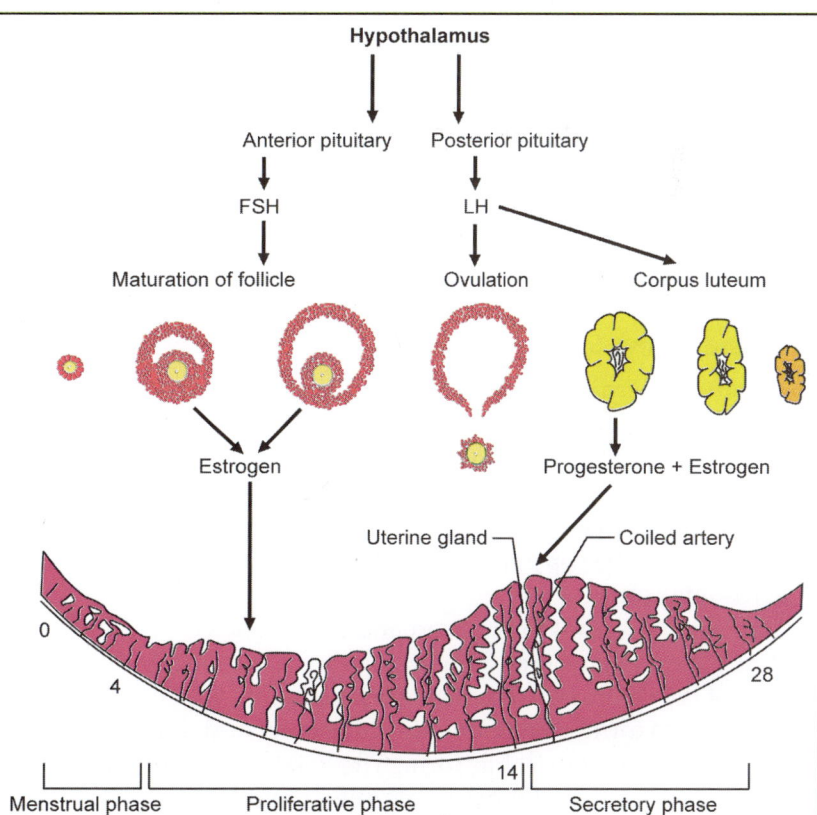

**Fig. 25.2b:** Endometrial changes with respect to ovarian cycle

25

single duct inside the epididymis. This duct of the epididymis continues as vas deferens (ductus deferens).

Vas deferens is a muscular tube transmitting spermatozoa from epididymis to prostatic urethra.

Seminal vesicles are two accessory glands of reproduction. Their secretion forms a large part of the seminal fluid. The duct of the seminal vesicle joins with terminal part of the vas deferens to form 'ejaculatory duct' which opens into prostatic urethra. Semen with spermatozoa passes through spongy part of the urethra (inside the penis) and then ejaculated.

Prostate gland is an accessory gland of male reproductive system and its secretion adds to the bulk of the seminal fluid.

Penis is the male organ of copulation.

### SPERMATOGENESIS

It is a process by which spermatozoa are formed in the seminiferous tubules of the testes. A single germ cell gives rise to many spermatozoa.

The spermatogonia undergo mitotic division to give rise to primary spermatocytes, each of which has 44XY chromosomes. The primary spermatocyte undergoes first meiotic division to give rise to secondary spermatocytes, each of them has 22X or 22Y chromosome. The secondary spermatocyte completes second meiotic division to give rise to spermatids. The spermatid is transformed into a spermatozoon/sperm and this process is called spermiogenesis (Fig. 25.3).

In a single ejaculation of the normal male, about 200 to 300 million sperms are emitted, and the amount of semen is about 2–5 ml. If the concentration of the spermatozoa in the semen is only 20 million or less per ml, the individual is usually sterile.

### Structure of the Spermatozoon

- A mature spermatozoon consists of head, neck, body (middle piece) and tail (principal piece).
- It measures about 50 microns of which the tail measures about 40 microns.
- The head consists of nucleus covered by a cell membrane. Its upper part is enveloped by an acrosomal cap.
- The neck lies distal to the head and is constricted. It consists of a centriole, with 2 cylinders. The distal part of the centriole presents 9 thick filaments which continue to form axial filaments of the body and tail.
- The body is cylindrical in form. The axial filaments are covered externally by many mitochondria. The tail consists of axial filaments surrounded by a thin cell membrane (Fig. 25.4).

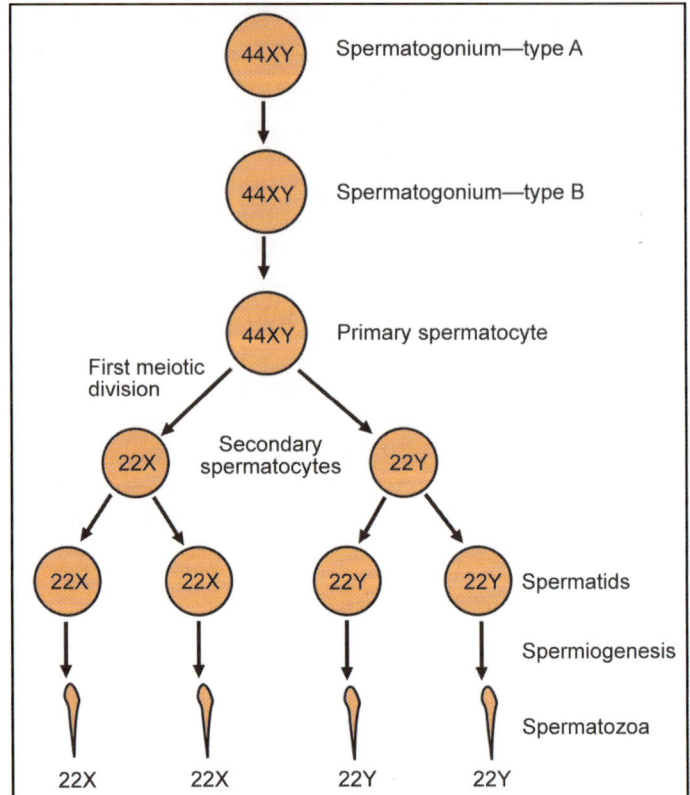

**Fig. 25.3:** Spermatogenesis

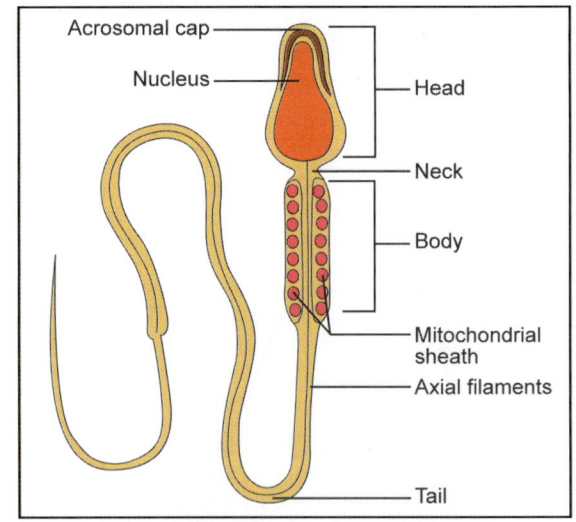

**Fig. 25.4:** Structure of a spermatozoon

### FERTILIZATION AND IMPLANTATION

The fertilization takes place usually in the ampulla of the uterine tube. The spermatozoa introduced inside the vaginal cavity during copulation, reach uterine tube by successive contraction of uterine musculature and also due to the motility of the sperms.

The ovum released from the ovary is taken inside the uterine tube by rhythmical contractions of the musculature of the uterine tube and also movements of cilia of the epithelium (Fig. 25.5).

During fertilization (head and neck of spermatozoon is taken inside the ovum) the normal chromosome number (44XX or 44XY) is restored. The fertilized product 'zygote' undergoes division and this process is called 'cleavage'. When the zygote is in 16-cell stage, it is called 'morula' (Fig. 25.6a).

The cells of the morula further differentiate into an inner cell mass and outer layer of cells (trophoblast) with the appearance of a cavity. The embryo at this stage of development is called 'blastocyst'. The blastocyst is formed about 5 days after fertilization (Fig. 25.6b).

On reaching the uterine cavity the blastocyst is implanted in the uterine endometrium 6 or 7 days after fertilization. The thickened endometrium of the uterus after fertilization is called 'decidua'.

The time of prenatal development or the time of pregnancy is called 'gestation' period. The human gestation period is usually 266 days or 280 days from the beginning of the last menstrual period to parturition or childbirth.

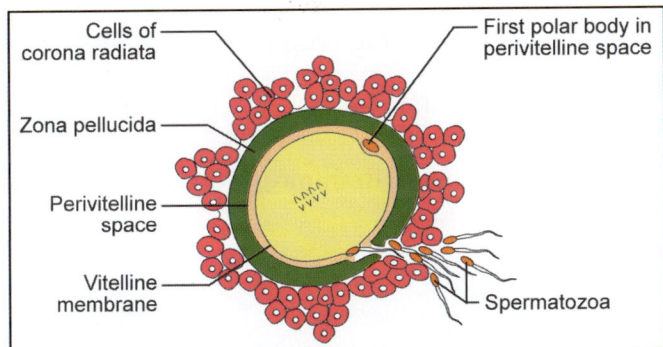

Fig. 25.5: Barriers for sperm around the secondary oocyte

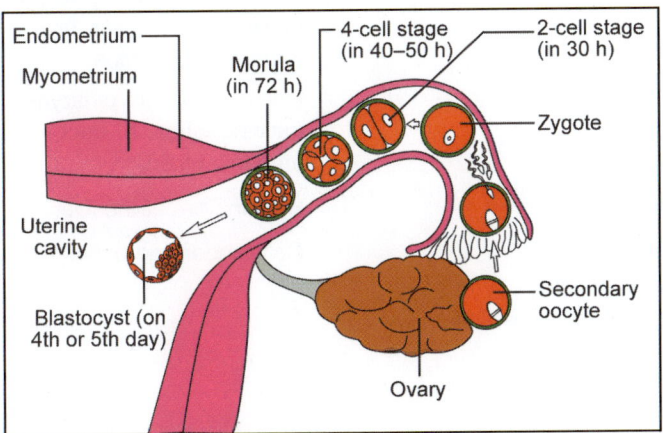

Fig. 25.6a: Transport of zygote

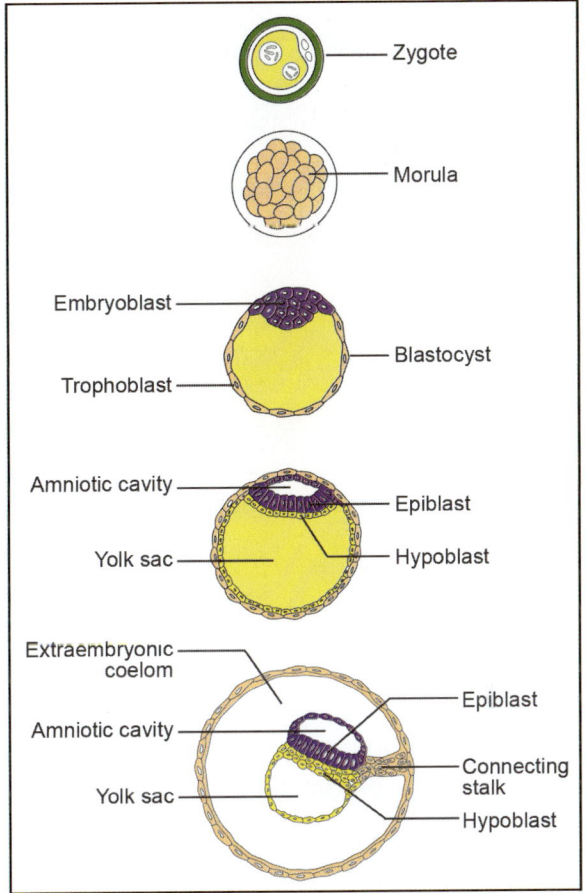

Fig. 25.6b: Cleavage and formation of bilaminar germ disc

## STAGES OF EMBRYOLOGY

The gestation period is subdivided into three stages.
1. *Germinal period:* 1st to 3rd week of development.
2. *Embryonic period:* Extends from 4th to 8th weeks.
3. *Fetal period:* Extends from 3rd month up to termination of pregnancy.

### Germinal Period

During this period following important events occur.
1. The outer cell mass (trophoblast) differentiates to give rise to extraembryonic mesoderm, which later involved in the formation of fetal membranes, placenta and umbilical cord.
2. The inner cell mass (embryoblast) differentiates into three germ layers (trilaminar germ disc). By a complicated further growth of the blastula, three embryonic germ layers are formed. These germ layers are (Fig. 25.7):
   1. Ectoderm
   2. Mesoderm
   3. Endoderm

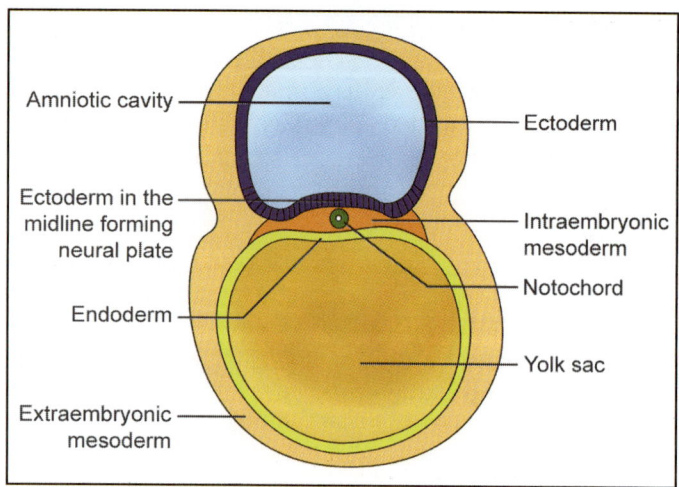

**Fig. 25.7:** Epiblast and hypoblast formation

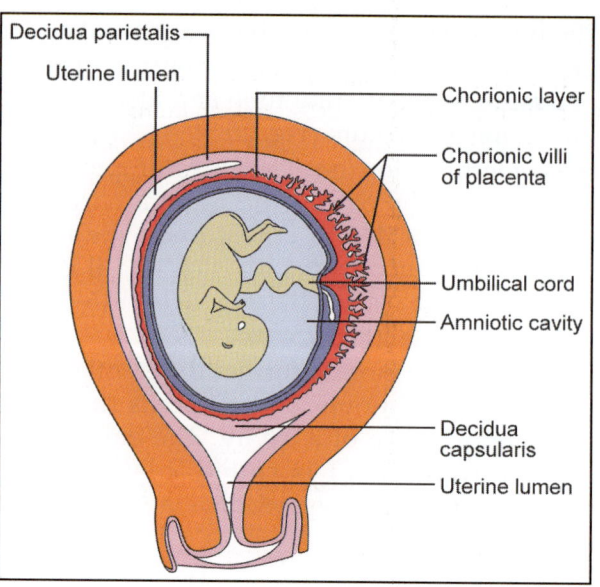

**Fig. 25.8:** Fate of amniotic cavity and fetal membranes

These layers later give rise to various structures of the body, which are listed in Table 25.1.

## Embryonic Period

During the embryonic period, all the body organs are formed along with placenta, umbilical cord and fetal membranes. During this period, the vascular connection between the uterus of the mother and the embryo is established through placenta.

## Amnion

It is a thin membrane, which loosely envelops the embryo, forming an amniotic sac that is filled with amniotic fluid (Fig. 25.8).

## Amniotic Fluid

It is a clear watery fluid which acts as a protective cushion for the embryo. The embryo is suspended by the umbilical cord and laterally swims in the fluid. The fluid maintains the uniform pressure for the symmetrical growth of the embryo. It cushions and protects the embryo. It allows the fetus to develop freely.

- At full term, the average volume of amniotic fluid is 1000 ml.
- Hydramnios (polyhydramnios)—increased volume of amniotic fluid.
- Oligamnios (oligohydramnios)—decreased volume of amniotic fluid.

| **Table 25.1:** Derivitives of the germ layers | | |
|---|---|---|
| *Ectoderm* | *Mesoderm* | *Endoderm* |
| Epidermis of skin | Muscles: | Epithelium of the pharynx, auditory tube, tonsils, thyroid, parathyroid, thymus |
| Epidermal derivatives: Hair, nails, glands of the skin | Arrector pilorum of the skin | |
| | Ciliaris muscle of the eye | |
| Lining epithelium of the oral, nasal, lower part of the anal and vaginal cavities | Muscles: Smooth, cardiac and skeletal | Lining epithelium of larynx, trachea, lungs, GI tract, urogenital tract |
| | Connective tissue, cartilages, bones | |
| Lens of the eye | Blood cells | |
| Enamel of the teeth | Dermis of the skin | Hepatocytes of the liver |
| Suprarenal medulla (neural crest cells) | Dentin of the teeth | Gallbladder and pancreas |
| Sphincter pupillae and dilator pupillae of the eye | Epithelium of the blood vessels, lymphatic vessels, bodies cavities and joint cavities | |
| Neural tube formed from ectoderm gives rise to spinal cord and brain | Internal reproductive organs | |
| | Kidney and ureter | |
| | Suprarenal cortex | |

## Amniocentesis

The aspiration of amniotic fluid is known as amniocentesis. This is done to investigate the nuclear sexing of the fetus in some sex-linked diseases. The enzyme estimation of the fluid and other chemical tests may be helpful to diagnose the gross fetal malformations.

## Chorion

The chorion is a highly specialized membrane that participates in the formation of the placenta. It is the outermost membrane and originates from trophoblast of the blastocyst. Numerous small finger-like extensions called chorionic villi form from the chorion and penetrate deeply into the uterine tissues. Initially, the entire surface of the chorion is covered with villi. But those villi on the surface towards the uterine cavity degenerate. Those, which penetrate the endometrium, form the placenta (Fig. 25.8).

### Chorionic Villus Biopsy

It is a technique used to detect the genetic disorders much earlier than amniocentesis permits. In chorionic villus biopsy, a catheter is inserted through the cervix to the chorion and a sample of chorionic villus is obtained by suction or cutting. Genetic tests can be performed directly on the villus samples since this sample contains much larger number of fetal cells than a sample of amniotic fluid.

## PLACENTA

Placenta is a structure, which connects the fetus with the uterine wall of the mother. It is a structure, where maternal and fetal tissues come in direct contact without rejection. Structurally, it contains the bulk of the chorionic villi.

At full term the placenta is a 'disc' shaped structure, 15 to 20 cm in diameter and 3 cm thickness in the central part. It weighs about 500 gm.

The placenta presents fetal and maternal surfaces and peripheral margin.

The fetal surface is smooth, covered by amnion and presents the attachment of the umbilical cord close to its center. The maternal surface is rough and irregular. It shows 15–30 cotyledons, which are limited by fissures. The peripheral margin is continuous with the fetal membranes.

## Structure

The placenta consists of chorionic plate on fetal side and basal plate on maternal side. These two plates are connected by stem villi, which present primary, secondary and tertiary chorionic villi. The space between the stem villi are called intervillous spaces, which are filled with maternal blood.

A tertiary chorionic villus contains fetal blood vessels in the center, surrounded successively by extra embryonic mesoderm, cytotrophoblast and syncytiotrophoblast.

## Placental Barrier

It consists of tissues, which intervene between fetal blood in the chorionic villi and maternal blood in the intervillous space. Through this barrier exchange of gases and metabolic products takes place between the fetus and the mother.

## Functions of Placenta

1. Exchange of gaseous and metabolic products between the maternal and fetal blood.
2. Placenta prevents the entry of pathogenic organisms from mother to fetus.
3. Transfer of maternal antibodies to fetus.
4. Secretion of hormones:
   - *Progesterone*: Which maintains the integrity of the uterine endometrium.
   - *Estrogen:* Which causes enlargement of the uterus and breasts.
   - *Human chorionic gonadotropin (HCG):* The presence of this hormone in urine is applied as an indicator of the pregnancy test.

## Placenta Previa

The attachment of the placenta may extend partially or completely into the lower uterine segment (cervix of the uterus). This condition is called placenta previa. It causes difficulty during childbirth, and may cause severe bleeding.

## UMBILICAL CORD

- It extends from the center of the anterior abdominal wall of fetus to the placenta.
- At full term pregnancy, the length of the umbilical cord is about 50 cm.
- The cord contains two umbilical arteries, which carry deoxygenated blood towards the placenta and one umbilical vein, which carries oxygenated blood from the placenta to the embryo.
- These vessels are surrounded by a mucoid connective tissue called 'Wharton's jelly'.
- The umbilical cord is externally covered by amnion.

## Twinning

Women's ovaries release two eggs at once that are fertilized by two different sperm. The result is nonidentical or fraternal twins, who resemble one another no more closely than typical brothers and sisters. Fraternal twins are also called dizygotic twins.

In some pregnancies, the inner cell mass of a single blastocyst splits into two at the end of first week of development. This produces identical twins (mono-zygotic = from one zygote).

## Some Important Terminologies used in Developmental Anatomy

*Abortion:* Premature removal of the embryo or fetus from the uterus. Abortion can be spontaneous (resulting from fetal death) or induced.

*Ectopic pregnancy:* A pregnancy in which the embryo implants in any site other than uterus. Ectopic pregnancy usually occurs in one of the uterine tubes, a condition known as tubal pregnancy. Such pregnancy will rupture the uterine tube resulting in severe bleeding which may threaten the woman's life.

*Teratology:* The scientific study of birth defects and fetuses with congenital deformities.

*Ultrasonography:* Non-invasive technique that uses ultrasound echoes to visualize the position and size of the fetus and placenta.

*Neonatal period:* It extends from birth to the end of four weeks of development.

*Infancy:* The period of infancy extends from the end of the neonatal period at 4 weeks to 2 years of age.

*Childhood:* Childhood is the period of growth and development extending from infancy to adolescence, at which time puberty begins.

*In vitro fertilization:*

It is the external fertilization of human ova.

In some cases when the female has normal ovaries, but congenital atresia of both uterine tubes, *in vitro* fertilization of the ovum is done with the husband's sperms. Thereafter, the embryo transfer is made to the uterine cavity of female after pretreatment.

## Developmental Anomalies

A deviation from the normal pattern of development is called developmental or congenital anomaly. In medical science, we come across numerous congenital anomalies.

Some of the significant and most common congenital anomalies of development are listed below. However, the cause and related complications are not discussed. Students of the allied health science courses are expected to be familiar with the names of these anomalies.

1. *Albinism:* Absence of pigment in skin, hair and eyes.
2. *Spina bifida:* The posterior parts (laminae) of the vertebrae (lumbosacral region) fail to fuse and hence present bifid spines. The spinal cord can protrude through this gap (meningocele).

3. *Congenital hydrocephalus:* It occurs due to blockage in the CSF circulation. The ventricular system of the brain is distended; cranial vault is expanded (huge head).
4. *Polydactyly:* Presence of additional digit (finger or toe).
5. *Harelip:* Presence of a cleft in the lip (normally in the upper lip).
6. *Oblique facial cleft:* A cleft arising from the medial angle of the eye to the mouth. The nasolacrimal duct is not formed.
7. *Cleft palate:* Presence of a cleft in the palate, which results in communications between the mouth and the nose.
8. *Situs inversus:* All the abdominal and thoracic viscera are transposed to the opposite side (e.g. appendix, ascending colon on left side, sigmoid colon on right side).
9. *Congenital diaphragmatic hernia:* Some part of the diaphragm fails to develop. There is a free communication between the pleural and peritoneal cavities. It may cause death of the infants due to respiratory distress caused by abdominal organs entering the chest cavity. Stomach can roll upwards until it becomes upside down.
10. *Interatrial septal defect:* Persistent foramen ovale (communication between right and left atria). This condition persists in about 25% of the normal subjects without mixing of blood.
11. *Fallot's tetralogy:* It is a combination of 4 cardiac anomalies
    - Pulmonary stenosis
    - Hypertrophy of the right ventricle
    - Interventricular septal defect
    - Aortic orifice (beginning of ascending aorta) is shifted over the upper free edge of interventricular septum (over riding of aorta).
12. *Patent ductus arteriosus (PDA):* The communication between arch of aorta and left pulmonary artery persists even after birth. The blood from aorta enters the pulmonary artery through ductus arteriosus. Normally this ductus arteriosus is converted into a ligament (ligamentum arteriosum) after birth.
13. *Anomalies of kidney:*
    - Instead of lumbar region, kidney may be placed in abnormal position (in pelvis)
    - Kidney's with different shapes are reported (horseshoe kidney, pan cake kidney, etc.)
    - Polycystic kidney: Plenty of cysts in the kidney.
14. *Cryptorchidism:* The testes fail to descend into the scrotum and will be placed at abnormal position. Spermatogenesis often fails to occur and are prone for a malignant tumor.
15. *Meningocele:* Meninges of the brain with CSF bulge outwards through a gap present in the back of the skull (at occipital bone).
16. *Coloboma of iris:* A slit in the inferomedial part of the iris. Such slit (gap) can also affect ciliary body, choroid.
17. *Anencephaly:* Brain substance is exposed to the surface as a mass, through a gap in the cranial vault (skull cap).

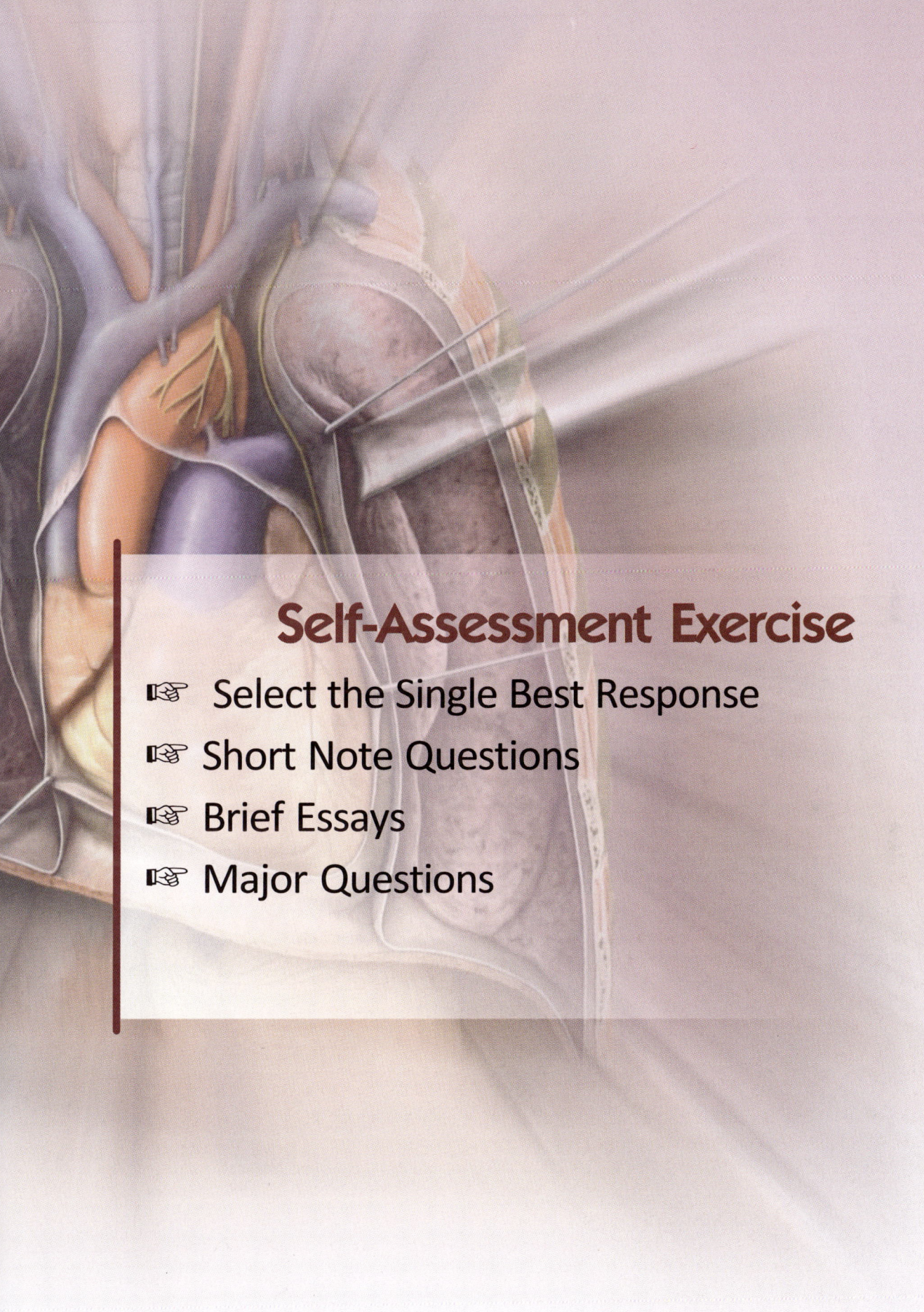

# Self-Assessment Exercise

☞ Select the Single Best Response

☞ Short Note Questions

☞ Brief Essays

☞ Major Questions

## Select the Single Best Response

1. **Which of these bones contributes to the nasal septum?**
   A. Labyrinth of ethmoid
   B. Perpendicular plate of palatine bone
   C. Perpendicular plate of ethmoid bone
   D. Lacrimal bone

2. **Ethmoidal bulla is produced by underlying:**
   A. Anterior ethmoidal air sinus
   B. Middle ethmoidal air sinus
   C. Posterior ethmoidal air sinus
   D. Maxillary air sinus

3. **Maxillary air sinus opens into:**
   A. Inferior nasal meatus
   B. Sphenoethmoidal recess
   C. Nasopharynx
   D. Hiatus semilunaris

4. **The length of the adult trachea is about:**
   A. 5 cm
   B. 10 cm
   C. 20 cm
   D. 25 cm

5. **Little's area of epistaxis is located at the:**
   A. Nasal septum
   B. Lateral wall of the nasal cavity
   C. Roof of the nasal cavity
   D. None of the above

6. **Which of these cartilages of larynx is not unpaired?**
   A. Arytenoid cartilage
   B. Epiglottis
   C. Thyroid cartilage
   D. Cricoid cartilage

7. **Vocal ligament is a thickened part of:**
   A. Thyrohyoid membrane
   B. Cricovocal membrane
   C. Quadrate membrane
   D. Mucous membrane

8. **The vocal cord is abducted by:**
   A. Posterior cricoarytenoid muscle
   B. Lateral cricoarytenoid muscle
   C. Cricothyroid muscle
   D. Transverse arytenoid muscle

9. **The muscles of the larynx are supplied by:**
   A. Glossopharyngeal nerve
   B. Recurrent laryngeal nerve
   C. Internal laryngeal nerve
   D. Hypoglossal nerve

10. **The cricothyroid muscle is supplied by:**
    A. External laryngeal nerve
    B. Internal laryngeal nerve
    C. Recurrent laryngeal nerve
    D. Glossopharyngeal nerve

11. **The mucous membrane of the trachea is lined by:**
    A. Simple squamous cells
    B. Simple columnar cells
    C. Stratified columnar cells
    D. Pseudostratified ciliated columnar cells

12. **In adults the trachea bifurcates (in standing position) at the level of:**
    A. $T_1$ vertebra
    B. $T_2$ vertebra
    C. $T_4$ vertebra
    D. $T_6$ vertebra

13. **Which of the following statements is incorrect regarding the pleura?**
    A. Lungs are placed inside the pleural cavity
    B. The pressure inside the pleural cavity is negative
    C. Costodiaphragmatic recess is the most dependent part of the pleural cavity
    D. Mediastinal pleura is part of the parietal pleura

14. **Each bronchopulmonary segment is areated by:**
    A. Principal bronchus
    B. Tertiary bronchus
    C. Terminal bronchiole
    D. Respiratory bronchiole

15. **The apex of the heart is formed by:**
    A. Right atrium
    B. Left atrium
    C. Left auricle
    D. Left ventricle

16. **Following structures are related to the base of the heart *except*:**
    A. Left pair of pulmonary veins
    B. Right pair of pulmonary veins
    C. Thoracic aorta
    D. Esophagus

17. **Which of these chambers of heart is not partly overlapped by lungs at cardiac notch?**
    A. Right atrium
    B. Right ventricle
    C. Left ventricle
    D. Left atrium

18. **Which of these structures does not occupy the left posterior coronary sulcus of the heart?**
    A. Coronary sinus
    B. Terminal part of the great cardiac vein
    C. Circumflex branch of left coronary artery
    D. Small cardiac vein

19. **Fossa ovalis is present in the:**
    A. Anterior wall of the right atrium
    B. Posterior wall of the right atrium
    C. Septal wall of the right atrium
    D. None of the above

20. **The right branch of the atrioventricular bundle traverses:**
    A. Supraventricular crest
    B. Septomarginal trabecula
    C. Crista terminalis
    D. Right fibrous trigone

21. **Which of these valves is under most strain in a normal heart?**
    A. Aortic valve
    B. Mitral valve
    C. Pulmonary valve
    D. Tricuspid valve

22. **Posterior interventricular artery is accompanied by:**
    A. Middle cardiac vein
    B. Great cardiac vein
    C. Small cardiac vein
    D. Anterior cardiac vein

23. **The AV node is located in:**
    A. Upper part of the crista terminalis
    B. Triangle of Koch
    C. Fossa ovalis
    D. Limbus fossa ovalis

24. **Following are the branches of internal thoracic artery except:**
    A. Superior epigastric artery
    B. Anterior intercostal artery
    C. Musculophrenic artery
    D. Inferior epigastric artery

25. **The left ascending lumbar vein joins with left subcostal vein to form:**
    A. Lumbar azygos vein
    B. Azygos vein
    C. Hemiazygos vein
    D. Accessory hemiazygos vein

26. **Following are the direct branches arising from coeliac trunk except:**
    A. Right gastric artery
    B. Splenic artery
    C. Common hepatic artery
    D. Left gastric artery

27. **External iliac artery continues to form:**
    A. Internal iliac artery
    B. Common iliac artery
    C. Femoral artery
    D. Obturator artery

28. **The normal portal pressure is about:**
    A. 1–5 mm Hg
    B. 5–15 mm Hg
    C. 20–25 mm Hg
    D. 25–35 mm Hg

29. **Portal vein is formed:**
    A. At the porta hepatis
    B. Posterior to the duodenum
    C. Posterior to the neck of the pancreas
    D. Posterior to the spleen

30. **Portal vein terminates in:**
    A. Hepatic vein
    B. Liver
    C. Inferior vena cava
    D. Spleen

31. **Which of these arteries is not a branch of the thyrocervical trunk?**
    A. Superficial cervical artery
    B. Deep cervical artery
    C. Inferior thyroid artery
    D. Suprascapular artery

32. **Following are the branches of facial artery except:**
    A. Ascending pharyngeal artery
    B. Ascending palatine artery
    C. Tonsillar artery
    D. Submental artery

33. **Which of the following types of teeth is found in the permanent but not in the deciduous dentition?**
    A. Incisor
    B. Premolars
    C. Canines
    D. Molars

34. **The soft palate separates**
    A. Nasal cavity from oral cavity
    B. Nasopharynx from oropharynx

C. Nasopharynx from oral cavity

D. Nasal cavity from oropharynx

**35. Which of these bones contribute to the hard palate?**

A. Horizontal plate of palatine bone

B. Perpendicular plate of palatine bone

C. Pyramidal process of the palatine bone

D. None of the above

**36. Which of these structures is present on the roof of the nasopharynx?**

A. Opening of the auditory tube

B. Tubal tonsil

C. Pharyngeal recess

D. Pharyngeal bursa

**37. The lateral surface of the palatine tonsil is related to**

A. Superior constrictor muscle

B. Middle constrictor muscle

C. Inferior constrictor muscle

D. Buccinator muscle

**38. Piriform fossa is related to:**

A. Internal laryngeal nerve

B. External laryngeal nerve

C. Recurrent laryngeal nerve

D. Glossopharyngeal nerve

**39. The auditory tube connects:**

A. Nasal cavity and anterior wall of the middle ear

B. Nasopharynx and posterior wall of the middle ear

C. Nasopharynx and anterior wall of the middle ear

D. Oropharynx and posterior wall of the middle ear

**40. The second normal constriction of esophagus is where it is crossed by:**

A. Arch of aorta

B. Right bronchus

C. Left bronchus

D. Trachea

**41. Following are the parts of the mucous membrane of the alimentary tract except:**

A. Lining epithelium

B. Lamina propria

C. Muscularis externa

D. Muscularis mucosa

**42. Which of these structures is not present in the hilum of the kidney?**

A. Ureter

B. Renal arteries

C. Renal veins

D. Renal pelvis

**43. Which of these structures is not directly related to the anterior surface of the right kidney?**

A. Liver

B. Stomach

C. Jejunum

D. Duodenum

**44. Following are the parts of nephron except:**

A. Bowman's capsule

B. Convoluted tubules

C. Collecting tubules

D. Loop of Henle

**45. The pelvi-ureteric junction corresponds to the level of:**

A. Tip of the transverse process of $L_5$ vertebra

B. Tip of the transverse process of $L_1$ vertebra

C. Ischial spine

D. Tip of the transverse process of $L_3$ vertebra

**46. Uvula vesicae is produced by:**

A. Seminal vesicle

B. Median lobe of the prostate

C. Terminal part of the ductus deferens

D. Terminal part of the ureter

**47. Stenosis (constriction) of the sphincter of ampulla (Oddi) would interfere with:**

A. Transport of bile and pancreatic juice

B. Secretion of mucus

C. Passage of chyme into the small intestine

D. Peristalsis

**48. The dartos is a layer of smooth muscle fibers found within the:**

A. Scrotum

B. Penis

C. Epididymis

D. Prostate

**49. Spermatozoa are stored prior to emission and ejaculation in the:**

A. Epididymis

B. Seminal vesicles

C. Spongy urethra

D. Prostate

**50. Urethral glands**

A. Secrete mucus

B. Produce nutrients

C. Secrete hormones

D. Regulate spermatozoa production

51. **Fertilization normally occurs in the:**
    A. Isthmus of uterine tube
    B. Ampulla of the uterine tube
    C. Infundibulum of the uterine tube
    D. Fundus of the uterus

52. **The secretory phase of the endometrium corresponds to which of the following ovarian phases?**
    A. The follicular phase
    B. Ovulation
    C. The luteal phase
    D. The menstrual phase

53. **Which of the following statements about oogenesis is true?**
    A. Oogonia, like spermatozoa form continuously during postnatal life
    B. Primary oocytes are haploid
    C. Meiosis is completed prior to ovulation
    D. In ovulation, secondary oocytes are released from tertiary ovarian follicles.

## Short Note Questions (3 marks)

1. Nasal septum
2. Respiratory mucosa
3. Trachea
4. Cartilages of larynx
5. Inlet of the larynx
6. Tricuspid valve
7. Mitral valve
8. Arch of aorta
9. Left ventricle of the heart
10. Left atrium of the heart
11. Soft palate
12. Piriform fossa
13. Auditory tube
14. Jejunum and ileum
15. Parotid gland
16. Pancreas
17. Coverings of the kidney
18. Ureter
19. Trigone of the urinary bladder
20. Female urethra
21. Ductus deferens
22. Seminal vesicle
23. Uterine tube
24. Spermatogenesis
25. Oogenesis
26. Corpus luteum
27. Graafian follicle
28. Fertilization
29. Papillae of tongue

## Brief Essays (5 or 6 marks)

1. Give an account of paranasal air sinuses
2. Give an account of the pluera
3. Give an account of the pericardium
4. Write briefly on vocal cords
5. Write briefly on the cavity of the larynx
6. Enumerate the muscles of larynx
7. Give an account of the microscopic structure of the lung.
8. Write briefly on nerve supply to the heart.
9. Give an account of the venous drainge of the heart.
10. Write briefly about the normal constrictions of esophagus.
11. Give an account of the possible position of appendix. Add a note on its clinical significance.
12. Enumerate the general features of the large intestine.
13. Give an account of the extrahepatic biliary apparatus.
14. Write briefly about the microscopic structure of small intestine.
15. Give an account of the interior of the anal canal.
16. Write briefly about the structure of a nephron.
17. Give an account of the extension, constrictions and arterial supply of ureter.
18. Enumerate the parts of male urethra.
19. Give an account of the structures stabilizing the uterus.
20. Give a brief account of the ovary.
21. Give an account of the germ layers of the embryo. List the structures derived from them.
22. Write briefly about the structure and nerve supply of the dorsum of the tongue.

## Major Questions (10 marks)

1. Describe the lateral wall of the nasal cavity under the following headdings:
   A. Bones and cartilages forming
   B. Conchae and meatuses                    (4+6)
2. Give an account of the external features of the lung. Draw a neat labelled diagram of the medial surface of right/left lung showing their relations       (5+5)

3. Define bronchopulmonary segments. List their name in each lung. Add a note on its clinical significance. (3+4+3)
4. Give an account of the external features of the heart.
5. Enumerate the interior of the right atrium.
6. Enumerate the interior of the right ventricle
7. Give an account of the roof and lateral wall of the nasopharynx. Write briefly about palatine tonsil (5+5)
8. Give an account of the parts, relations, blood supply of the stomach. Add a note on structure of a gastric gland. (2+3+2+3)
9. Enumerate the general features of small intestine. Write briefly on duodenum. (6+4)
10. Give an account of the position, parts and relations of liver. Explain the microscopic structure of liver. (1+2+3+4)
11. Describe the kidney under the following headings:
   A. Position
   B. Parts and relations
   C. Macroscopic structure
   D. Blood supply (1+5+3+1)
12. Describe the urinary bladder under the following headings:
   A. Position
   B. Parts and relations
   C. Interior
   D. Nerve supply (1+4+2+3)
13. Name the parts of male reproductive system. Give an account of the position, macroscopic and microscopic structure of testis. Add a note on its blood supply. (1+4+4+1)
14. Give an account of the prostate gland under the following headdings:
   A. Position and coverings
   B. Lobes
   C. Microscopic structure
   D. Applied anotomy (2+4+2+2)
15. Discuss the uterus under the following headings:
   A. Normal axis
   B. Parts and relations
   C. Structure
   D. Arterial supply (2+4+2+2)
16. Discuss the blood supply to the heart in detail. Add a note on its clinical significance.

## Answers to Single Best Response Questions

| | | | | |
|---|---|---|---|---|
| 1. C | 12. D | 23. B | 34. B | 45. D |
| 2. B | 13. A | 24. D | 35. A | 46. B |
| 3. D | 14. B | 25. C | 36. D | 47. A |
| 4. B | 15. D | 26. A | 37. A | 48. A |
| 5. A | 16. A | 27. C | 38. A | 49. A |
| 6. A | 17. B | 28. B | 39. C | 50. A |
| 7. B | 18. D | 29. C | 40. A | 51. B |
| 8. A | 19. C | 30. B | 41. C | 52. C |
| 9. B | 20. B | 31. B | 42. A | 53. D |
| 10. A | 21. A | 32. A | 43. B | |
| 11. D | 22. A | 33. D | 44. C | |

# Nervous System, Endocrines and Special Senses

1. Name the meninges (coverings) of the brain
2. Name the dural folds present in the cranial cavity with dural venous sinuses present/related to them
3. List the dural venous sinuses in the cranial cavity and to explain cavernous sinus in brief
4. Name the coverings of the spinal cord and be able to explain the anatomy of epidural anesthetization and lumbar puncture
5. Be able to explain the external features of the spinal cord
6. To list the ascending and descending tracts of the spinal cord
7. Be able to explain the anatomy of the corticospinal and posterior column tracts
8. To list the parts of the brainstem and to name the major cranial nerve nuclei present in each of them
9. Be able to explain the external features of the medulla oblongata, pons and midbrain
10. Be able to explain the external features of the cerebellum and to list its functions
11. Be able to explain the major sulci and gyri on the superolateral and medial surface of the cerebrum
12. Be able to explain major functional areas of cerebrum (motor, sensory, speech, visual and auditory) and to give their arterial supply.
13. To explain the parts and function of corpus callosum
14. To explain the Internal capsule under location, parts, important fibers passing through each part and effect of vascular lesion.
15. Be able to list the parts of the basal nuclei and give their anatomical location and functions
16. Be able to explain the anatomical location and functions of thalamus and hypothalamus
17. To explain the formation, circulation, absorption, functions and applied aspects of CSF
18. Be able to locate the anatomical positions of lateral, third and fourth ventricle.
19. Be able to explain the major branches and distribution of internal carotid and vertebral arteries
20. Be able to explain the circle of Willis with the help of a diagram
21. To list the cranial nerves and to explain their functions in brief
22. To explain the pituitary gland under location, parts, functions, blood supply and applied anatomy
23. To explain the thyroid gland under location, parts, functions, blood supply and applied anatomy
24. To explain the suprarenal gland under location, parts, functions, blood supply and applied anatomy
25. To explain the anatomy of the middle ear and list its contents
26. With the help of a cross-sectional diagram of the eyeball identify all its layers
27. To explain cornea and retina in brief

# Coverings of the Brain and Dural Venous Sinuses

## 26

**M**eninges are connective tissue membranes covering brain and spinal cord. There are three layers of meninges which are named from outside to inside.

- Dura mater
- Arachnoid mater
- Pia mater

The space between the endosteum of the skull and outer dura mater is negligible, as endosteal layer of the dura mater forms inner periosteum. However, in the vertebral canal there is an extradural or epidural space between the dura meter covering the spinal cord and periosteum of the vertebral canal.

### I. DURA MATER

The dura mater is the outermost covering of the brain. *It is thick and tough fibrous membrane and is made up of two layers.*

- Outer endosteal layer
- Inner meningeal layer

The outer endosteal layer forms the inner periosteum of the skull bones. Meningeal blood vessels pass deep to this layer.

Most of the places the endosteal and meningeal layers are fused together (Fig. 26.1). However, at certain places meningeal layer is separated from the endosteal layer. This space between the endosteal and meningeal layers of the dura mater is occupied by endothelial-lined spaces, which drain venous blood from the brain and meninges. These spaces are called **dural venous sinuses.**

The meningeal layer of the dura mater projects inwards to form folds (or projections), which are called 'Dural folds'. They divide the cranial cavity into compartments.

### Dural Folds

#### 1. Falx cerebri

It is a sickle-shaped fold in the median sagittal plane and occupies in the median longitudinal fissure of the cerebrum. It has two ends, two margins and two surfaces (Fig. 26.2).

The anterior end is narrow and attached to the crista galli of ethmoid bone. The posterior end is broad and blends with upper surface of the tentorium cerebelli in the median plane.

The upper convex margin is attached to the inner aspect of the cranial vault. The lower margin is concave and free. It is related to the upper surface of the corpus callosum of the brain.

The right and left surfaces of the falx cerebri face the medial surfaces of the cerebrum. Following dural venous sinuses are related to falx cerebri.

a. *Superior sagittal sinus:* Along its upper attached convex margin. It presents plenty of arachnoid granulations.

b. *Inferior sagittal sinus:* Along its lower free margin.

c. *Straight sinus:* At the posterior end of the falx cerebri where it blends with upper surface of the tentorium cerebelli.

#### 2. Tentorium Cerebelli

It is a broad tent shaped dural fold placed horizontally between cerebrum above and the cerebellum below.

It has a posterior attached margin and an anterior free margin. It has upper and lower surfaces.

The attached margin is attached to occipital bone and upper border of petrous temporal bone. The anterior free margin forms a U-shaped notch, which is occupied by brainstem. Its upper surface is related to occipital lobes of the cerebrum and lower surface is related to cerebellum.

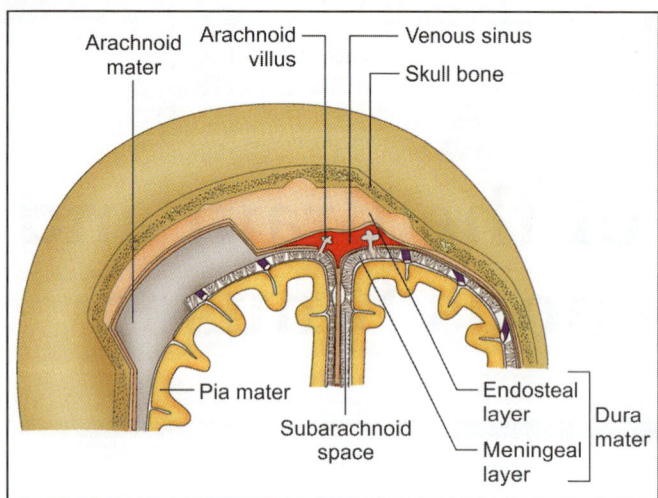

**Fig. 26.1:** Meningeal layers

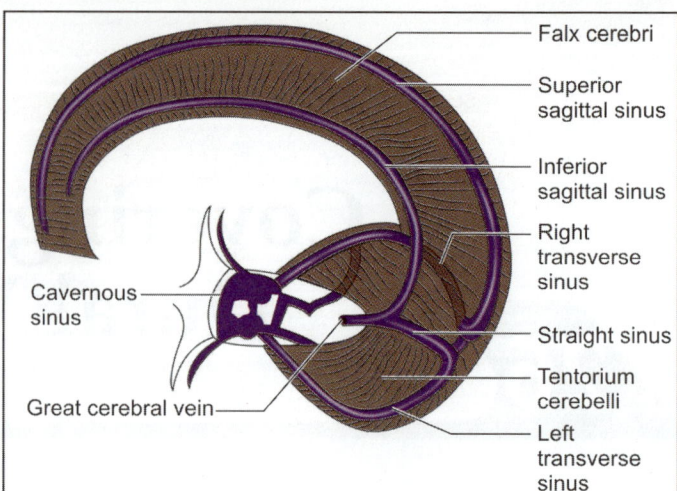

**Fig. 26.2:** Falx cerebri and tentorium cerebelli

Following dural venous sinuses are related to tentorium cerebelli (Figs 26.2 and 26.6).

a. *Straight sinus* is placed along the upper surface of tentorium cerebelli at the attachment of falx cerebri.

b. *Transverse sinus* is placed along its attachment to the occipital bone.

c. *Superior petrosal sinus* is situated along its attachment to the upper border of the petrous temporal bone.

### 3. Diaphragm Sellae

It is a horizontally placed dural fold forming the roof of pituitary fossa (sella turcica) and it is traversed in the centre by the stalk of the pituitary gland.

### 4. Falx Cerebelli

It is a dural fold, which lies below the tentorium cerebelli. It has occipital sinus along its attachment to the internal occipital crest of the occipital bone.

These meningeal folds are supplied by blood vessels and nerve fibers.

## II. ARACHNOID MATER

The arachnoid mater is closely applied to the inner surface of the dura mater with a potential space between them called subdural space.

The arachnoid mater is separated from the inner pia mater by a wider subarachnoid space, traversed by trabeculae and is filled with cerebrospinal fluid (CSF).

## SUBARACHNOID CISTERNS

These are enlarged subarachnoid spaces at the base of the brain and around the brainstem. These cisternae are traversed by cerebral blood vessels.

**Following are the subarachnoid cisternae** (Fig. 26.3)

a. *Cerebellomedullary cistern (cisterna magna):* It lies between the dorsal surface of medulla and inferior surface of cerebellum. The cerebrospinal fluid from the IV ventricle escapes into this cistern through an opening (foramen of Magendie).

b. *Cisterna pontis:* It lies on the ventral aspect of the pons and contains basilar artery. The CSF from the fourth ventricle escapes into this cistern through two lateral apertures (foramen of Luschka).

c. *Interpeduncular cistern:* It lies in base of the brain at interpeduncular fossa. It contains arterial circle of Willis.

## Arachnoid Granulations

Arachnoid granulation is made up of numerous arachnoid villi. Each villus is an extension of arachnoid mater into dura mater. Arachnoid villi are most numerous along the superior sagittal sinus. Arachnoid villi serve as sites where the cerebrospinal fluid diffuses into the bloodstream. The arachnoid is connected to the pia mater across the subarachnoid space by delicate strands of fibrous tissue. This arachnoid granulation helps in absorption of CSF into superior sagittal sinus (Fig. 26.1).

## III. PIA MATER

The pia mater is the innermost, thin vascular membrane and invests the brain closely. It extends into indentation like fissures and sulci. The pia mater consists of outer epi-pia and inner pia-intima. The bilaminar fold of pia mater in the ventricles of the brain is called 'tela choroidea'. The tela choroidea contains blood vessels called choroid plexus, which produces CSF (Fig. 26.2).

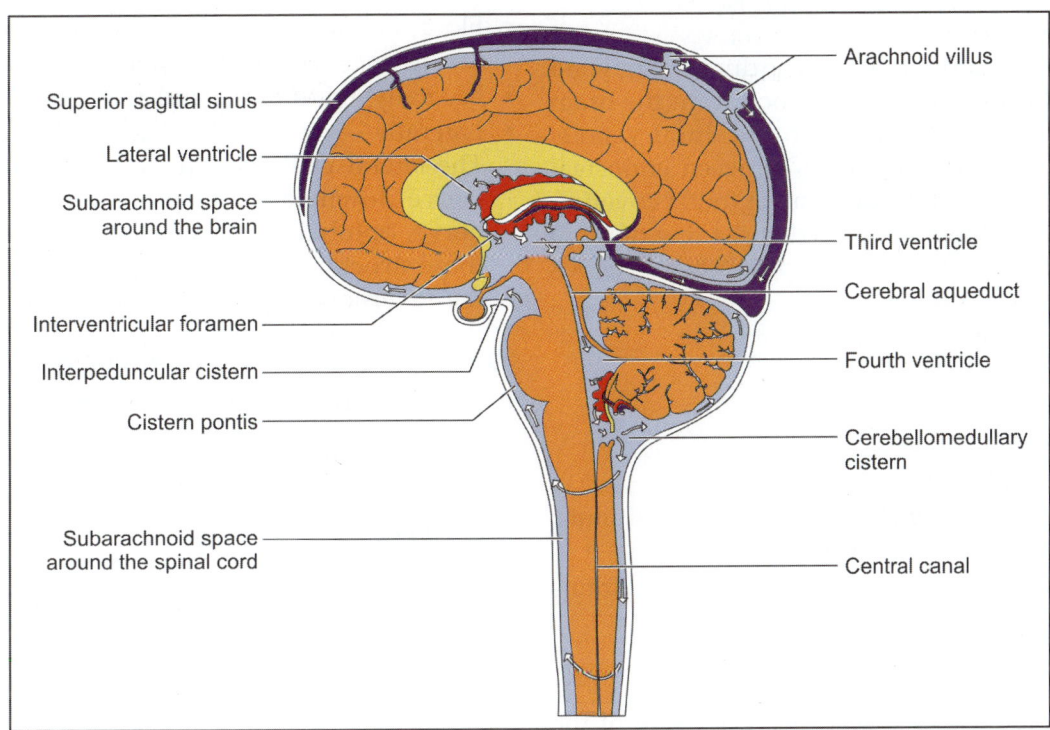

**Fig. 26.3:** Subarachnoid cisterns and CSF circulation

*Meningitis:* Meningitis is an inflammation of the meninges, usually caused by certain bacteria or viruses. The arachnoid mater and the pia mater are the two meninges most frequently affected. Meningitis is accompanied by high fever and severe headache. Complications may cause sensory impairment, paralysis or mental retardation. Untreated meningitis generally results in coma and death.

## MIDDLE MENINGEAL ARTERY

It is one of the major arteries supplying the cranial meninges. Along with the vein, it traverses on the outer surface of the dura mater (Fig. 26.3).

*Origin:* It arises from first part of the maxillary artery in the infratemporal fossa through foramen spinosum.

*Course*
- In the cranial cavity, the artery groove on the squamous part of the temporal bone and then divides into frontal (anterior) and posterior (parietal) branches.
- The frontal branch crosses the greater wing of the sphenoid and the parietal bone (close to its antero-inferior angle). Thereafter it divides into many branches. One of the branch ascends along the inner surface of the parietal bone coinciding with precentral sulcus of the cerebrum. This branch is placed about 1.25 cm behind and parallel to the coronal suture of the skull.

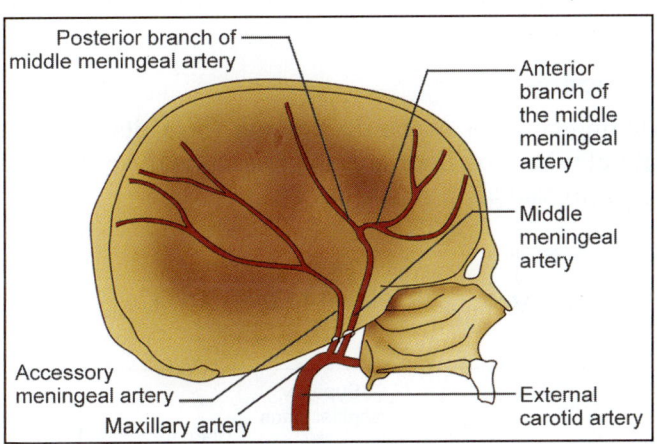

**Fig. 26.4:** Middle meningeal artery

- The parietal branch arches backwards on the squamous temporal bone and then crosses the parietal bone giving many branches.

*Epidural (extradural hematomas):* A severe blow to the temporal region or automobile accidents involving temporal region is likely to tear the middle meningeal artery. The blood gradually accumulates in the extradural space. Clinically it is manifested by irritability, confusion and later signs of cerebral compression may develop. Hematoma involving the frontal trunk can compress overlying motor area, which can lead to paralysis of the muscles of the opposite side of the body. Involvement of the posterior branch causes contralateral deafness, compressing auditory area.

26

## DURAL VENOUS SINUSES

These are venous spaces present in the dura mater, lined by endothelial cells. The venous blood from the brain and cranial cavity is drained into the dural venous sinuses. These sinuses are spaces between endosteal and meningeal layers of the dura mater (outer covering of brain). Some of them are paired and a few of them are unpaired. The following are the paired dural venous sinuses present around the brain:

- Cavernous sinuses
- Transverse sinuses
- Sigmoid sinuses
- Superior petrosal sinuses
- Inferior petrosal sinuses

The unpaired sinuses include superior sagittal sinus, straight sinus and inferior sagittal sinus.

The venous blood from these sinuses finally drains into the internal jugular vein (Fig. 26.5).

## CAVERNOUS SINUSES

These are paired sinuses placed on either side of the body of the sphenoid. The interior of the cavernous sinus shows many trabecular tissue giving a spongy appearance.

## Formation

Meningeal layer of the dura mater forms its roof and lateral wall. The floor and the medial wall are formed by endosteal layer of the dura mater.

## Relations

- Roof/above—it is related to optic tract

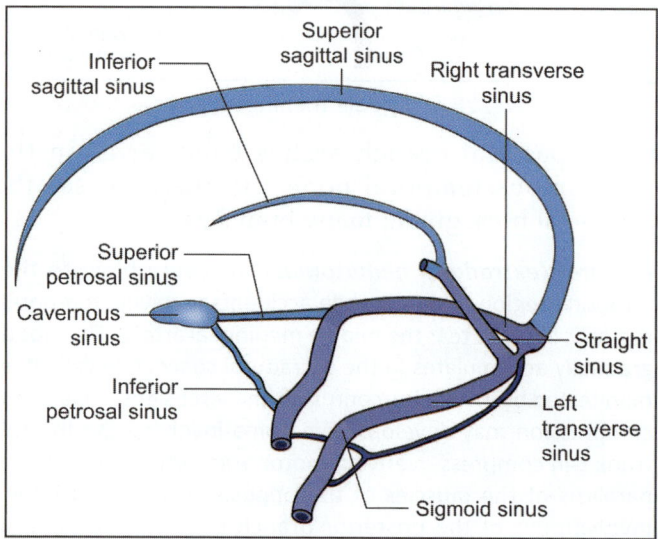

**Fig. 26.5:** Dural venous sinuses

- Floor/below—it is formed by the junction of body and greater wing of the sphenoid bone.
- Medially—pituitary gland and sphenoidal air sinus.
- Laterally—it is related to uncus of the temporal lobe. The lateral wall presents following structure from above downwards: Oculomotor nerve, trochlear nerve, ophthalmic nerve, and maxillary nerve. All these structures are separated from the blood inside the cavernous sinus by an endothelial layer.

### Structures Inside the Cavernous Sinus

1. Internal carotid artery with sympathetic plexus and venous plexus around it.
2. Abducent nerve.

### Tributaries

#### From the Orbit

- Superior ophthalmic vein
- A tributary of inferior ophthalmic vein
- Central vein of retina

#### From the Brain

- Superficial middle cerebral vein
- Inferior cerebral veins

#### From the Meninges

- Sphenoparietal sinus
- Anterior trunk of the middle meningeal vein

The superior and inferior hypophyseal veins also opens into cavernous sinus.

### Communications

1. The right and left cavernous sinuses are connected by anterior and posterior intercavernous sinuses.
2. Cavernous sinus is connected with facial vein through deep facial vein, pterygoid plexus of veins, emissary veins and also through superior ophthalmic vein (Fig. 26.6).
3. It is connected with transverse sinus through superior petrosal sinus and with internal jugular vein through inferior petrosal sinus.

### Other Venous Sinuses

The *superior sagittal sinus* is present along the upper convex margin of the falx cerebri. It presents number of arachnoid granulations, which drain the CSF back into the circulation.

The *inferior sagittal sinus* is present along with the lower free margin of the falx cerebri. It joins with great cerebral vein to form straight sinus, which is placed between the falx and tentorium cerebelli.

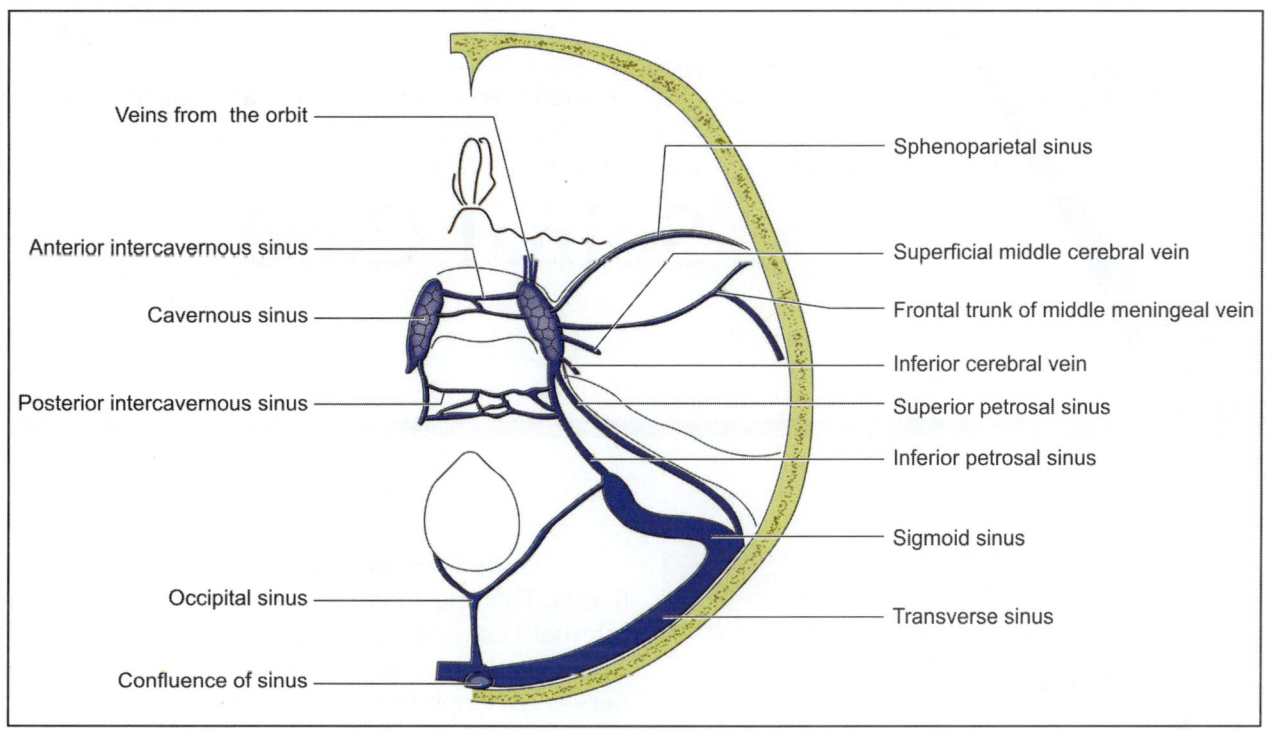

**Fig. 26.6** Tributaries and communications of cavernous sinus

The *right transverse sinus* is formed by the continuation of superior sagittal sinus.

The *left transverse sinus* is the continuation of straight sinus.

Each *sigmoid sinus* is the continuation of transverse sinus. It passes into the jugular foramen and continues as internal jugular vein.

The cranial cavity is divisible into anterior, middle and posterior cranial fossae. Accumulation of the blood (hematoma) due to rupture of blood vessels, slow growing tumors, defective CSF circulations can raise the intracranial pressure which can compress the brain tissue.

# Spinal Cord

## COVERINGS OF THE SPINAL CORD

Spinal cord is covered by following meninges from outside to inside (Fig. 27.1). They are:

- Dura mater
- Arachnoid mater
- Pia mater

### DURAMATER

The spinal dura mater is the continuation of meningeal layer of cranial dura mater. It extends from the foramen magnum to the lower border of second sacral vertebra. The spinal dura provides tubular sheaths on each side for the roots and the trunks of the spinal nerves.

### Epidural Space

The epidural or extradural space intervenes between the spinal dura mater and the periosteum lining the vertebral canal.

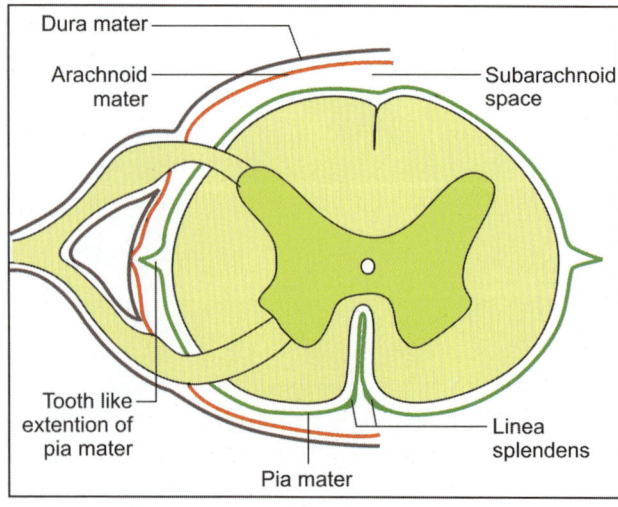

**Fig. 27.1:** Coverings of the spinal cord

*Labels:* Dura mater; Arachnoid mater; Tooth like extention of pia mater; Pia mater; Subarachnoid space; Linea splendens

It extends from the foramen magnum to the sacral hiatus. This space contains loose areolar tissue, fat and internal vertebral venous plexus.

The epidural space is traversed by the roots of spinal nerves enveloped by spinal meninges. Anesthetic fluid can be injected into the epidural space through the sacral hiatus to produce segmental or regional anesthesia (e.g. for painless childbirth).

### ARACHNOID MATER

The spinal arachnoid mater is thin, transparent membrane, which loosely invests the spinal cord. It extends up to the lower border of second sacral vertebra.

*Subarachnoid space:* It is the space deep to the arachnoid mater (between arachnoid and pia mater).

*Spinal cistern:* It is a wide subarachnoid space lying distal to the termination of spinal cord. It extends from the level of $L_1$ to $S_2$ vertebra. The space contains CSF and the roots of lower spinal nerves forming cauda equina and the filum terminale.

*Lumbar puncture:* It is a procedure in which the spinal cistern is approached for aspiration of CSF. It is usually performed between $L_3$ and $L_4$ spines, since this part of the vertebral canal is not occupied by the spinal cord (Fig. 27.2).

### SPINAL PIA MATER

Spinal pia mater is thicker and less vascular than the cerebral pia mater. The pia mater closely invests the spinal cord. The spinal cord terminates at the level of lower border of $L_1$ vertebra, however, this pia mater continues downwards as 'filum terminale'.

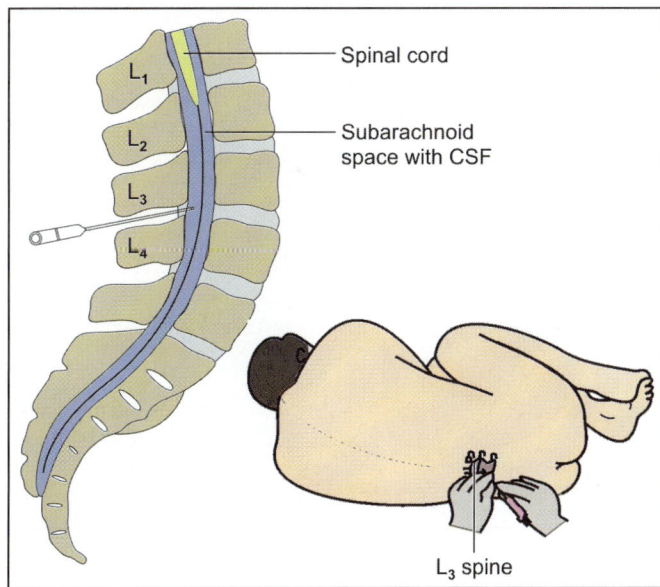

**Fig. 27.2:** Lumbar puncture

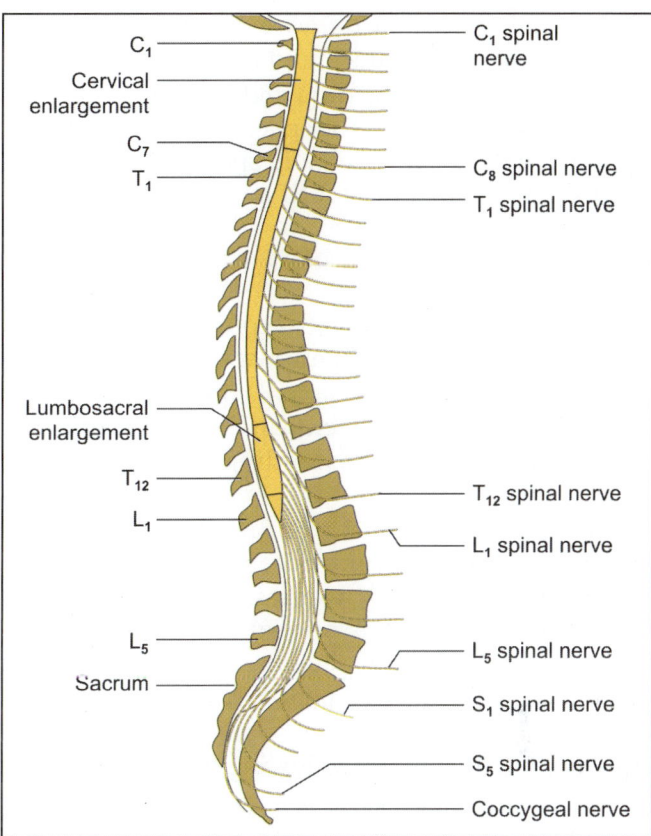

**Fig. 27.3:** Vertebral spines and spinal segments

## Special Features of Spinal Pia Mater

### a. Filum terminale

It is the extension of spinal pia mater beyond the termination of spinal cord. It extends up to the dorsal surface of first coccygeal vertebra. Filum terminale is about 15–20 cm in length. It provides better anchorage to the spinal cord.

### b. Linea splendens

Pia mater, which invests the anterior median fissure of the spinal cord, thickens to form a glistening band called linea splendens. This median longitudinal band continuous below with the filum terminale.

### c. Ligamentum denticulatum

It is a vertical thickening of pia mater on either side of spinal cord between the ventral and dorsal roots of the spinal nerves. It has 21 teeth-like processes on either side (hence the name). Each of this tooth-like processes passes laterally and is attached to the dura mater thereby provides better anchorage for the spinal cord. The site of attachment of ligamentum denticulatum guides the neurosurgeons to locate the lateral spinothalamic tract and pyramidal tract for selective tractotomy operation.

## EXTERNAL FEATURES OF SPINAL CORD

- It is about 45 cm in length and occupies the upper 2/3rds of the vertebral canal.
- The lower end of the spinal cord ends at the lower border of first lumbar vertebra in adults (when vertebral column is extended).

- In newborn, the cord terminates at the level of third lumbar vertebra.
- It gives 31 pairs of spinal nerves.
- The part of the spinal cord giving origin to rootlets of one pair of spinal nerves constitutes one spinal segment (total 31 segments). The spinal segment does not correspond to the corresponding vertebra.
- The cylindrical spinal cord presents 2 enlargements
  – Cervical enlargement accommodates motor neurons to supply upper limb muscles.
  – Lumbosacral is for lower limb muscles.
- The lower tapering end of the spinal cord is called 'conus medullaris'.
- The surface of the spinal cords is divided completely into two symmetrical halves by
  – Anterior median fissure
  – Posterior median sulcus
    Each half of the spinal cord further shows anterolateral and posterolateral sulci.
- The anterolateral sulcus provides attachment to the rootlets of ventral nerve roots of the spinal nerve.
- The posterolateral sulcus provides attachment to the rootlets of dorsal nerve roots of the spinal nerve.

- The spinal cord is surrounded by three meninges. Outer dura, middle arachnoid and inner pia mater.
- The space between the dura and arachnoid mater is called subdural space. The space between arachnoid and pia mater is subarachnoid space, which is filled with cerebrospinal fluid (CSF).

## INTERNAL STRUCTURE OF SPINAL CORD

- The cross section of the spinal cord shows H-shaped central grey matter and peripheral white matter.
- The white matter of the spinal cord on each half is divided into anterior, lateral and posterior columns (funiculi), which has ascending and descending tracts.
- Each half of the grey matter is divisible into a ventral horn which contains motor neurons, a dorsal horn which contains sensory neurons. In addition, a lateral or intermediate horn is present in the thoracic and upper two lumbar segments of the spinal cord. Neurons of this horn constitute preganglionic sympathetic neurons.
- The grey matter shows following types of neurons:
  a. *Motor neurons:* These are multipolar neurons which innervate the muscles, e.g. alpha, beta and gamma motor neurons.
  b. *Interneurons:* They connect the different types of neurons within the grey matter of the spinal cord. They are concerned with reflex activities.

## TRACTS OF THE SPINAL CORD

The white matter of the spinal cord is made up of nerve fibers with supporting cells. The groups of nerve fibers are termed as **tracts** (or fasciculus/funiculus), which include both ascending and descending. The white matter is divided into three columns. They are posterior, lateral and anterior (Fig. 27.4).

The positions and functions of these ascending and descending tracts of spinal cord are briefly mentioned below. A tract can be defined as collection of nerve fibers which has same origin, course, termination and function (Fig. 27.5).

1. **Descending or motor tracts**
   a. Pyramidal (corticospinal) tract
   b. Extrapyramidal tracts
      - Rubrospinal
      - Tectospinal
      - Vestibulospinal
      - Olivospinal
      - Reticulospinal

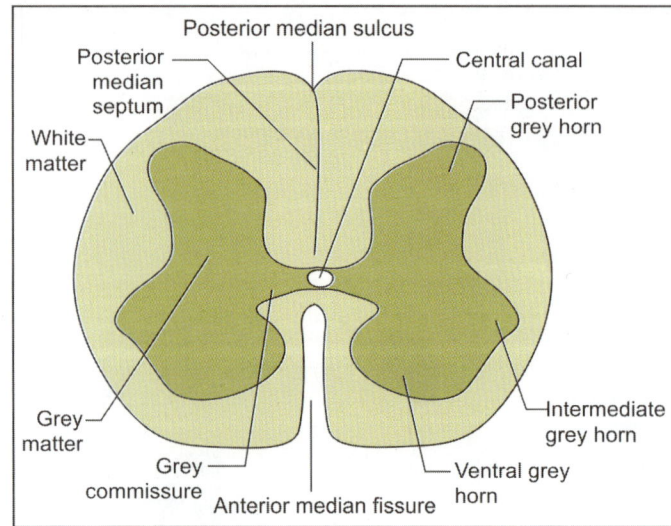

**Fig. 27.4:** Internal features of the spinal cord

2. **Ascending or sensory tracts**
   a. Fasciculus gracilis and cuneatus
   b. Spinothalamic tracts
   c. Spinocerebellar tracts

## PYRAMIDAL (CORTICOSPINAL) TRACT (Fig. 27.6)

- The fibers of this tract arise from the neurons (upper motor neurons) located in the cerebral cortex areas 4, 6 and 3, 1, 2.
- Axons from these neurons descend successively through the corona radiata, posterior limb of the internal capsule, crus cerebri of the midbrain, basilar part of the pons and pyramids of the medulla oblongata.
- In the lower part of the medulla oblongata, about 80% fibers decussate and enter into the opposite (contralateral) side and descend as lateral corticospinal tract. These fibers finally synapse with the neurons of the anterior horn cells (lower motor neurons) of the spinal cord.
- The remaining uncrossed fibers descend in the anterior part of the spinal cord as anterior corticospinal tract. However, these fibers also cross to the opposite side before terminating in the anterior horn cells of the spinal grey matter.
- This tract controls the voluntary movements of opposite half of the body.

## EXTRAPYRAMIDAL TRACTS

### a. Rubrospinal Tract

Fibers of this tract arise from red nucleus in the midbrain. After crossing to the opposite side in the midbrain, the fibers descend in the brainstem and spinal

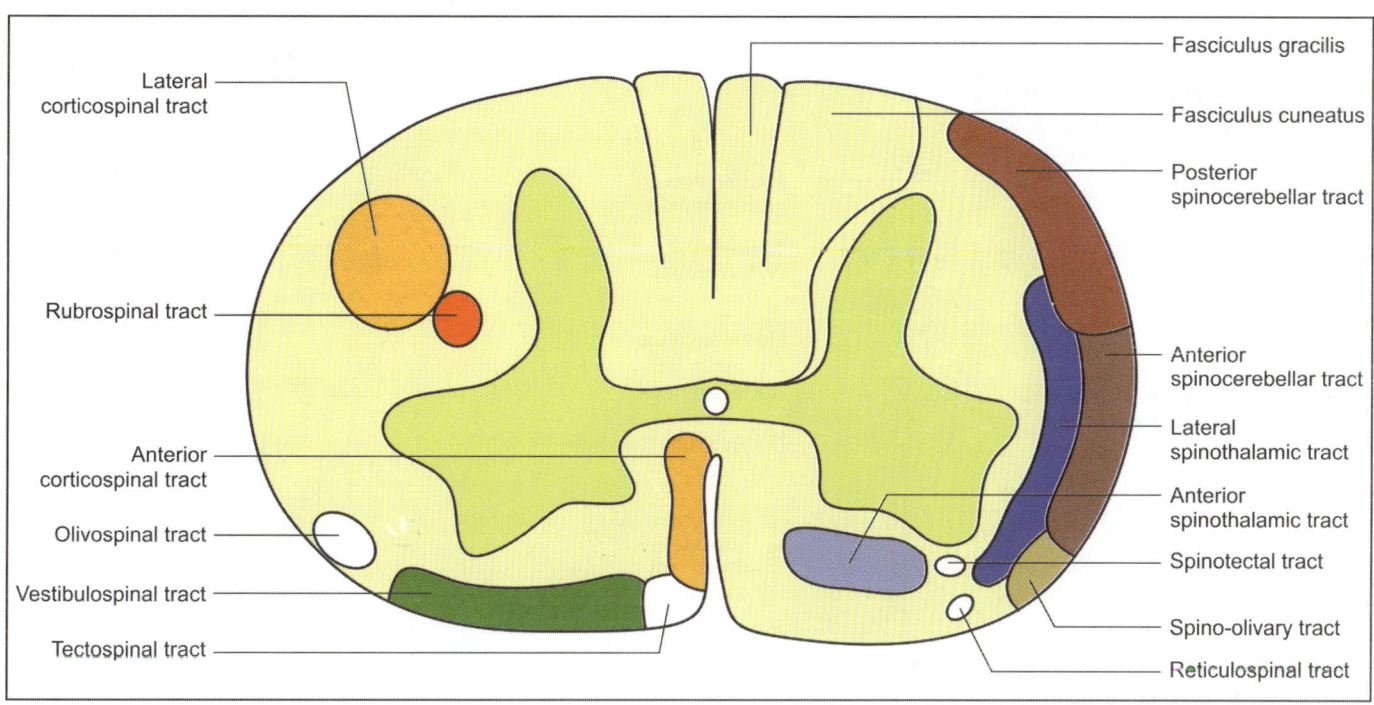

**Fig. 27.5:** Cross section of the spinal cord showing ascending and descending tracts

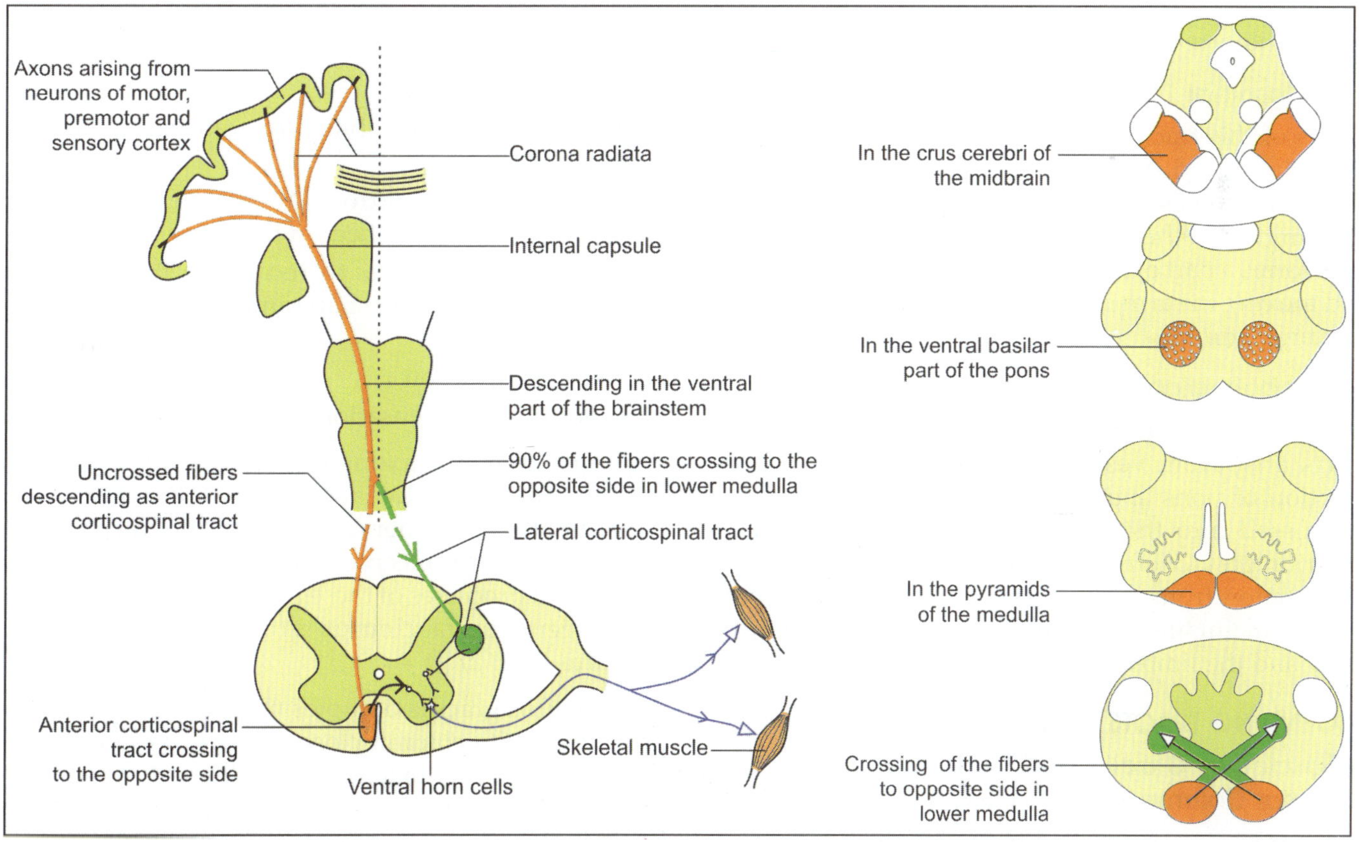

Lateral corticospinal tract

Rubrospinal tract

Anterior corticospinal tract

Olivospinal tract

Vestibulospinal tract

Tectospinal tract

Fasciculus gracilis

Fasciculus cuneatus

Posterior spinocerebellar tract

Anterior spinocerebellar tract

Lateral spinothalamic tract

Anterior spinothalamic tract

Spinotectal tract

Spino-olivary tract

Reticulospinal tract

Axons arising from neurons of motor, premotor and sensory cortex

Corona radiata

Internal capsule

Descending in the ventral part of the brainstem

Uncrossed fibers descending as anterior corticospinal tract

90% of the fibers crossing to the opposite side in lower medulla

Lateral corticospinal tract

Anterior corticospinal tract crossing to the opposite side

Ventral horn cells

Skeletal muscle

In the crus cerebri of the midbrain

In the ventral basilar part of the pons

In the pyramids of the medulla

Crossing of the fibers to opposite side in lower medulla

**Fig. 27.6:** Corticospinal (pyramidal) tract

27

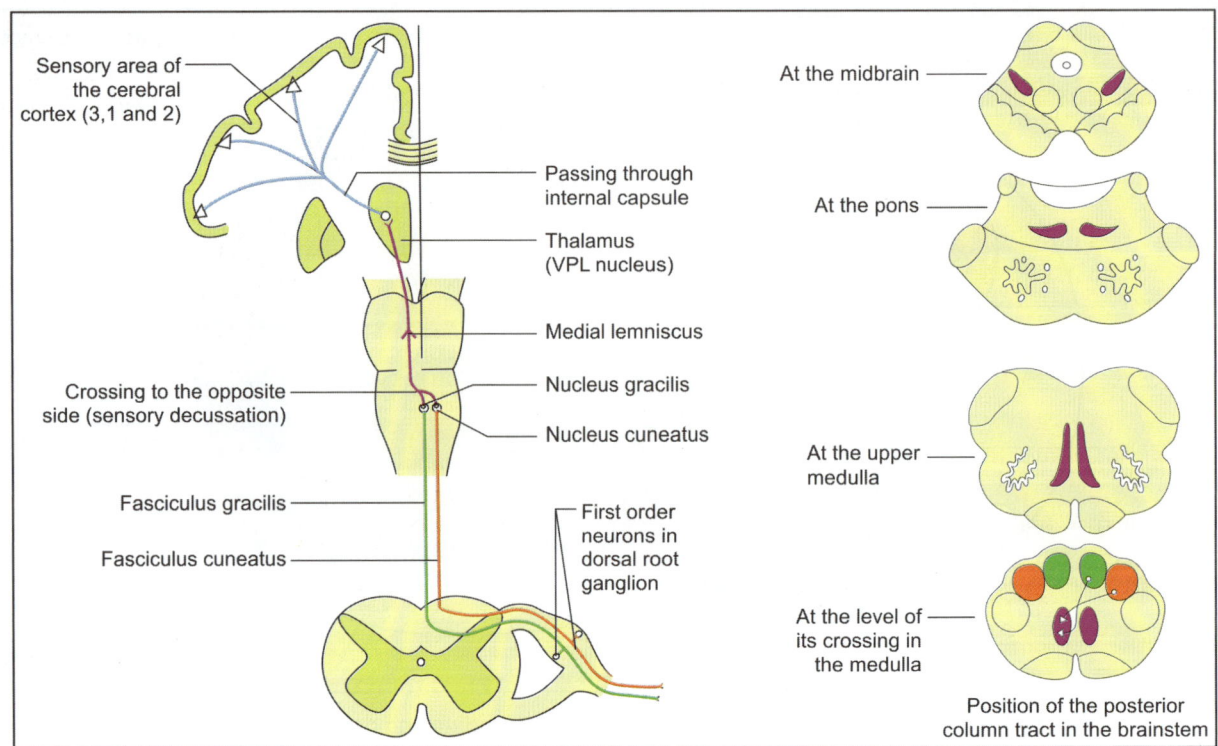

**Fig. 27.7:** Posterior column tract

cord to terminate in its grey matter. Red nucleus receives fibers from motor area (area 4) of the cerebral cortex and cerebellum.

### b. Tectospinal Tract

Fibers of this tract arise from neurons of the superior colliculus of midbrain. These fibers cross to the opposite side and then descend in the brainstem and spinal cord to terminate in the neurons of anterior grey horn. This tract forms a part of reflex pathway for turning the head and moving the arm in response to visual and auditory (hearing) stimuli.

### c. Vestibulospinal Tract

It consists of two parts: Lateral and medial. Both these tracts arise from vestibular nuclear complex (at the junction of pons and medulla). These tracts descend uncrossed into the spinal cord to terminate in the anterior grey column. The vestibular nuclei receive information from internal ear and through the spinal cord, it maintains the equilibrium and posture of the body and the limbs.

### ASCENDING TRACTS OF THE SPINAL CORD

### a. Fasciculus Gracilis and Cuneatus/
### Posterior Column Tract (Fig. 27.7)

These tracts are also called tract of Gall and Burdach. These are the main ascending tracts carrying several modalities of sensation from the entire body except the head and neck area. They carry:

  i. Fine touch
 ii. Pressure
iii. Tactile localization (ability to locate exactly the part touched)
 iv. Tactile discrimination (ability to localize two separate points touched on the skin)
  v. Stereognosis (ability to recognize the objects of common use by their shape and size with eye closed, held in hand)
 vi. Sense of vibration
vii. Proprioceptive sensation

These tracts are axons (central processes) of the neurons (pseudounipolar) placed in the dorsal root ganglia of the spinal nerves. Their peripheral processes innervate sensory receptors to bring the information. The central processes of these neurons enter spinal cord and ascend as fasciculus gracilis and fasciculus cuneatus (Fig. 27.7).

**Fasciculus gracilis** occupies more medial part of the posterior white column close to the posterior median septum. This tract extends along the entire length of the spinal cord and carries sensory information from lower limb and part of the trunk below the midthoracic level.

**Fasciculus cuneatus** occupies lateral to fasciculus gracilis on each side. This tract is prominent in the upper part of the spinal cord and conveys sensory information from the trunk above the midthoracic level including upper limb.

Fibers of these tracts end in the nucleus gracilis and nucleus cuneatus placed in the medulla oblongata. Axons arising from the neurons of these nuclei cross to the opposite side (sensory decussation) forming internal arcuate fibers and then ascends as **'medial lemniscus'** in the brainstem and reach ventral posterolateral nucleus of thalamus. Fibers arising from these neurons of thalamus terminate in the sensory area of the cerebral cortex (areas 3, 1 and 2) after passing through internal capsule, for integration of conscious sensation.

In this way major sensory information from the body is conveyed to opposite cerebral hemisphere.

### b. Spinothalamic Tracts

The **anterior spinothalamic tract** is located in the anterior white column of the spinal cord. The axons (central processes) of the neurons (pseudounipolar) placed in the dorsal root ganglia of the spinal nerves terminate in posterior grey horn of the spinal cord. Axons arising from the neurons in the posterior grey horn crosses to the opposite side and then ascends in the spinal cord. **They carry crude touch and pressure sensation** from the body. In the brainstem it joins the medial lemniscus and terminates along with it (Fig. 27.8).

The **lateral spinothalamic tract** is located in the lateral white column of the spinal cord. The axons of the neurons placed in the dorsal root ganglia of the spinal nerves terminate in posterior grey horn of the spinal cord. Fibres arising from the neurons of posterior grey horn cross to the opposite side close to the central canal and ascend in the lateral white column as lateral spinothalamic tract. They carry **pain and temperature** sensation from the opposite half of the body. They ascend in the brainstem as 'spinal lemniscus' and reach ventral posterolateral nucleus of thalamus (Fig. 27.8).

### c. Spinocerebellar Tracts

**The posterior spinocerebellar tract** begins at the level of 2nd or 3rd lumbar segments of the spinal cord. These tracts ascend in the lateral white column of the spinal cord and in medulla it passes through inferior cerebellar peduncle to reach cerebellum. This tract conveys unconscious proprioceptive sensation and also touch and pressure sensation from lower limb and lower half of the body to the cerebellum. It is concerned with fine coordination of individual lower limb muscles during posture and movements (Fig. 27.9).

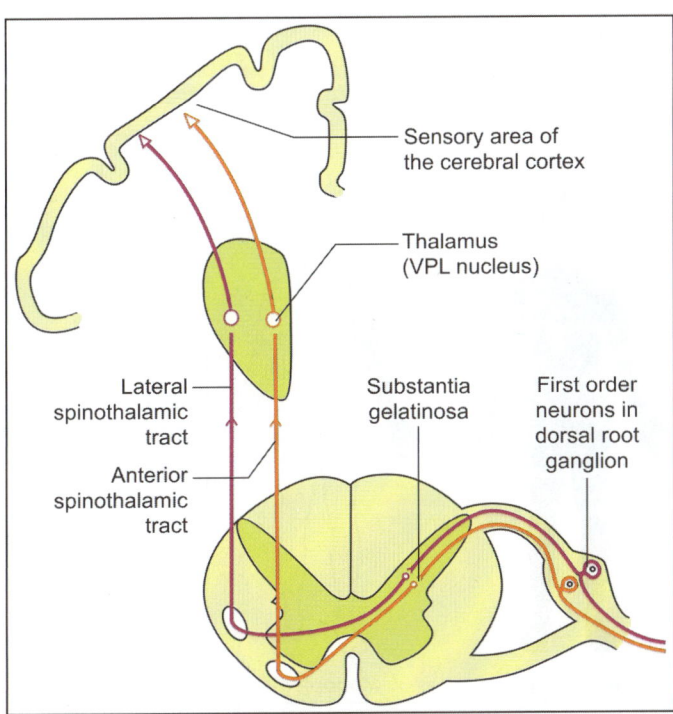

**Fig. 27.8:** Spinothalamic tracts

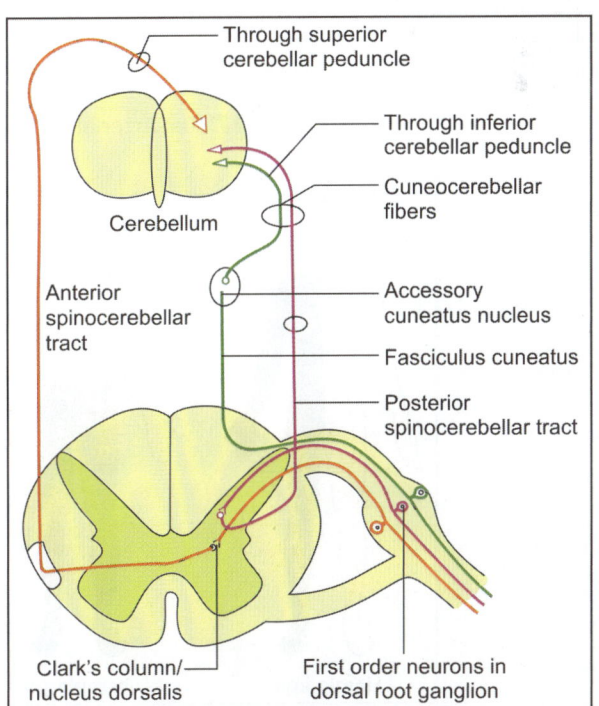

**Fig. 27.9:** Spinocerebellar tracts

27

**The anterior spinocerebellar tract** is located in the lateral white column of the spinal cord. It ascends through the brainstem. In the upper part of the pons it enters the superior cerebellar peduncle and enters the cerebellum. This tract transmits unconscious proprioceptive and exteroceptive information from the lower limb and lower part of the body. It is concerned with general status of posture and movements of the lower limb (Fig. 27.9).

### Blood Supply to Spinal Cord

*Arterial Supply*

a. **Anterior spinal artery:** Each anterior spinal artery arises from vertebral artery inside the cranial cavity.

The right and anterior spinal artery join to form single anterior spinal artery which descends in anterior median fissure.

b. **Two posterior spinal arteries:** They also arise from vertebral artery and descend along the attachment of dorsal nerve roots.

c. **Radicular arteries** from spinal branches of vertebral artery, ascending cervical artery, posterior intercostal arteries and lumbar arteries (Fig. 27.10). The spinal branches enter the vertebral canal through intervertebral foramina and divides into anterior and posterior radicular branches. In a cross section of the spinal cord anterior 2/3rds is supplied by anterior radicular branches while posterior 1/3rd by posterior

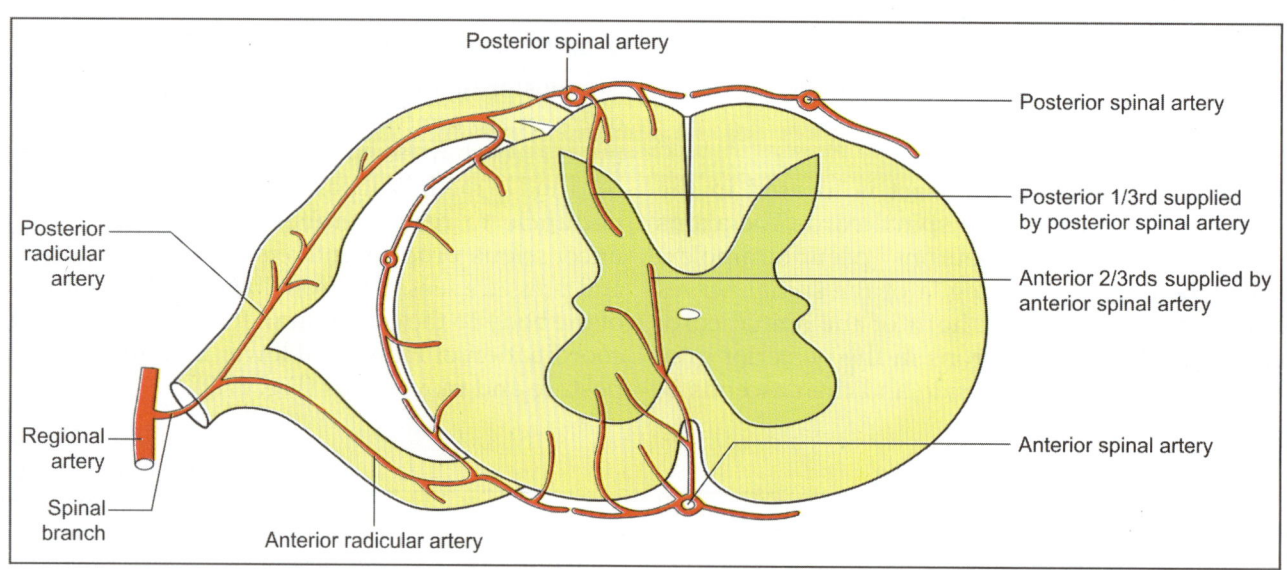

**Fig. 27.10a:** Arterial supply to spinal cord—cross-sectional view

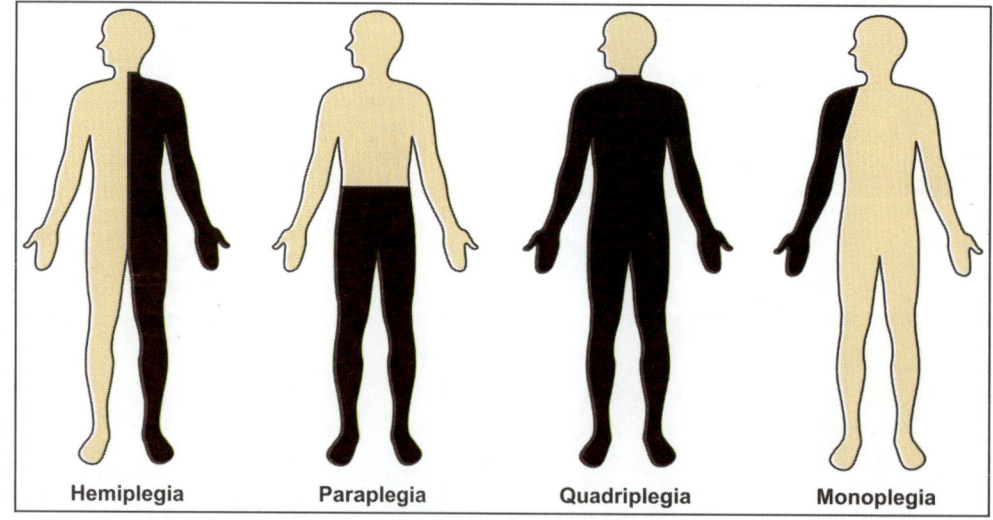

**Fig. 27.10b:** Spinal cord lesions affecting motor system

radicular branches. One of the anterior radicular branch arising from 11th posterior intercostal artery is large and called 'Arteria radicularis magna'. The veins drain into vertebral venous plexus.

## Venous Drainage

Veins from spinal cord drain into 6 tortuous longitudinal channels. These channels communicate freely with each other. The blood from these veins drain into internal vertebral venous plexus placed outside the spinal dura mater within the vertebral canal.

## Applied Anatomy

Spinal cord injuries may result from impairment of blood supply, infection, tumours, trauma and demyelinating disorders.

1. Thrombosis of the anterior spinal artery affects ventral portion of the spinal cord, which includes anterior grey column, corticospinal, and spinothalamic tracts. Hence, thrombosis of the anterior spinal artery in the upper thoracic segment produces flaccid paralysis (lower motor neuron paralysis) and also loss of pain and temperature sensation.

2. **Poliomyelitis:** It is a viral disease selectively affecting the anterior horn cells of the spinal cord (lower motor neurons) and also motor neurons of the brainstem. This condition is manifested by segmental paralysis of voluntary muscles with loss of all reflexes. In this condition, muscle tone is decreased.

3. **Upper motor neuron lesion:** This is due to the lesion in motor cortex or corticospinal tract (pyramidal tract). When the lesion takes place above the pyramidal decussation of medulla, the voluntary muscles of the opposite half are paralysed (contralateral). If the lesion is located below the decussation, then muscles of the same side are affected (ipsilateral).

   Note the following terminologies (Fig. 27.10b) in this lesion
   **Hemiplegia:** Paralysis of upper and lower extremities on one side. The most common cause for hemiplegia is stroke. The site of lesion is usually in internal capsule.
   **Quadriplegia:** When all four limbs are involved. This occurs due to complete transection of the cord above the level of C5 (remember C5 to T1 supplies upper limb).

**Monoplegia:** Loss of movement of one limb. The lesion may be anterior part of the posterior limb of the internal capsule
**Paraplegia:** Bilateral (both sides) paralysis of lower extremities. It occurs due to transection between cervical and lumbosacral enlargements (lesion in thoracic region)

4. The partial transection (hemisection) of the spinal cord results in **Brown-Séquard's syndrome**. It is clinically manifested by:
   a. Bilateral loss of pain and temperature sensation at the level of injury.
   b. Contralateral loss of pain and temperature sensation below the level of injury.
   c. Ipsilateral loss of line touch and proprioception sensation at the level as well as below the level of injury.
   d. Involvement of pyramidal tract produces spastic paralysis and destruction of ventral roots of spinal nerve produces flaccid paralysis.

5. Demyelination of nerve fibers in the posterior column of the spinal cord results in loss of sense of position, discriminative touch and vibration.

6. **Tabes dorsalis:** In this condition posterior white column is affected (e.g. in syphilis) The patient walks with broad base with the legs apart, eyes are fixed to the ground for correcting the steps. The muscle tone will be decreased with loss of tendon reflexes.

7. **Syringomyelia:** In this condition there is a dilatation of central canal of the spinal cord, which involve the crossing fibers of the lateral spinothalamic tract. This leads to loss of pain and temperature sensation in the affected side.

8. **Amyotrophic lateral sclerosis (ALS):** It is a bilateral degenerative disease involving motor system. It affects corticospinal tract (upper motor neuron lesion) and anterior horn cells (lower motor neuron lesion). Fasciculations (twitching of the muscle as it loses innervation) are characteristic of lower motor neuron lesions in ALS. It is characterized by progressive weakness in the muscle, difficulty in speaking, difficulty in breathing and difficulty in swallowing.

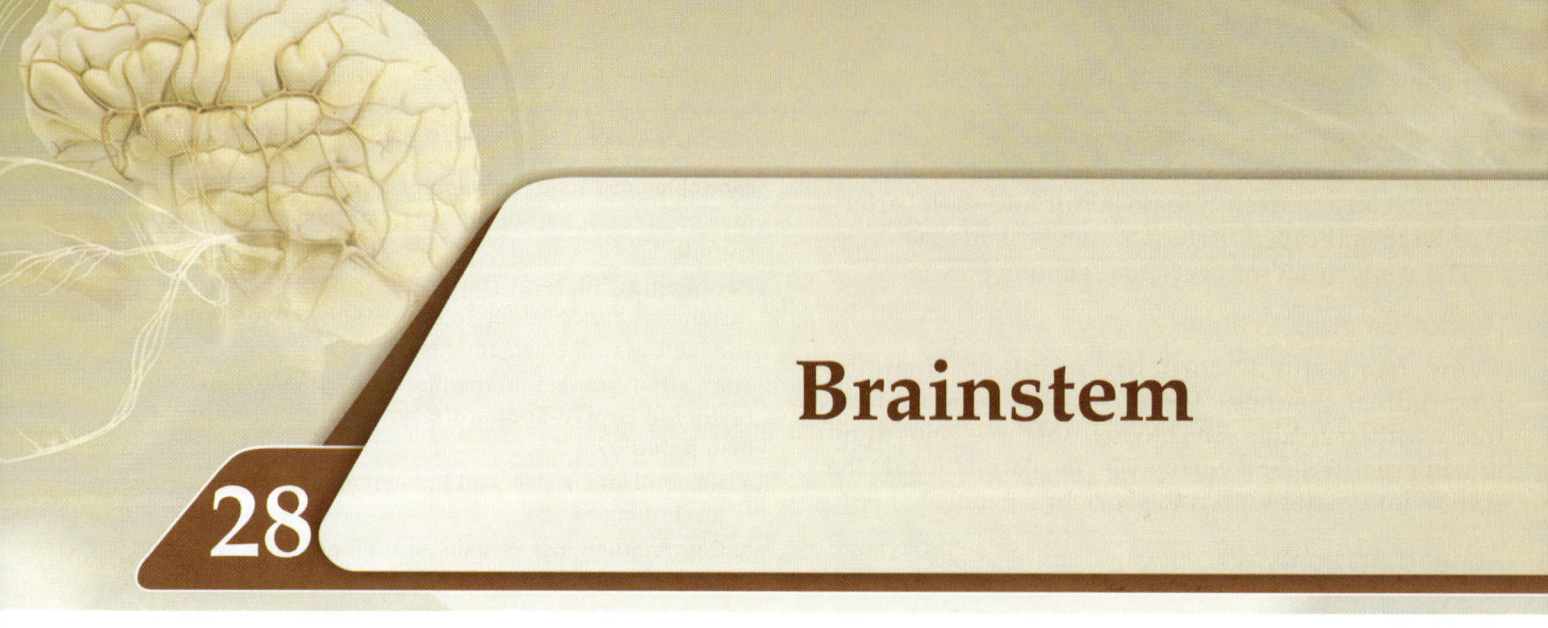

# Brainstem

Brainstem connects cerebrum and spinal cord. It has following parts from below upwards:
- Medulla oblongata
- Pons
- Midbrain

The brainstem has ascending and descending tracts of the central nervous system. It contains the nuclei of the cranial nerves and reticular nuclei (Fig. 28.1).

Three pairs of peduncles connect the cerebellum to the brainstem. The inferior peduncles with medulla, the middle pediculus with pons and the superior peduncles with the midbrain.

## MEDULLA OBLONGATA

Medulla oblongata is the lower part of the brainstem and intervenes between the upper end of the spinal cord and pons. It is about 3 cm in length and has two parts. The lower 'closed part' containing central canal and upper 'open part', which forms the floor of the fourth ventricle.

### External Features

The anterior portion of the medulla presents two prominent bulgings on either side of the anterior median fissure. These are called pyramids, which contain corticospinal fibers.

The area lateral to pyramids presents an oval elevation called olive produced by underlying inferior olivary nucleus.

On each side, the posterolateral portion of the upper part presents inferior cerebellar peduncle (ICP) through which it is connected with cerebellum (Fig. 28.2).

The posterior area of the medulla shows two elevations. Fasciculus gracilis on the medial side (either side of posterior median sulcus) and fasciculus cuneatus lateral to it. The upper parts of these fasciculi show elevations called gracile and cuneate tubercles respectively. They contain nuclei of same name beneath them.

The following cranial nerve roots emerge from medulla oblongata.

a. *Abducent nerve:* Emerges at the junction of pyramid and pons.

b. *Facial nerve:* Emerges at the junction of olive and pons.

c. *Vestibulocochlear nerve:* Emerges at the junction of pons and inferior cerebellar peduncle (at ponto-cerebellar junction).

d. *Hypoglossal nerve:* Emerges at the sulcus between pyramid and olive.

e. *Glossopharyngeal, vagus and cranial part of the accessory nerves* emerge successively one below the other at the area lateral to olive.

### Internal Features

The central grey matter is disrupted into smaller masses called nuclei. The following important nuclei are located within the medulla.

#### 1. Nucleus Gracilis and Cuneatus

Fasciculus gracilis and cuneatus terminate in the neurons present in these nuclei. Fibers arising from them (internal arcuate fibers) cross to the opposite side (sensory decussation) and ascend as medial lemniscus. Functions of these tracts are explained in earlier chapter.

#### 2. Hypoglossal Nucleus

Fibers arising from them form the hypoglossal nerve, which supplies the muscles of the tongue.

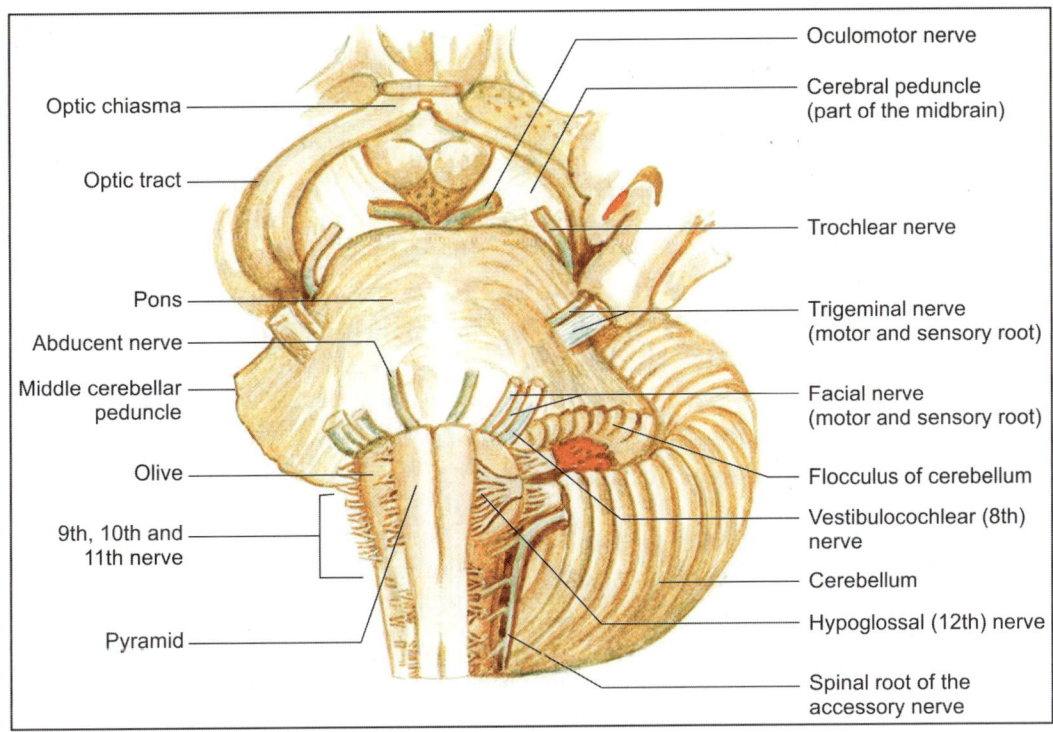

**Fig. 28.1:** Brainstem—anterior view

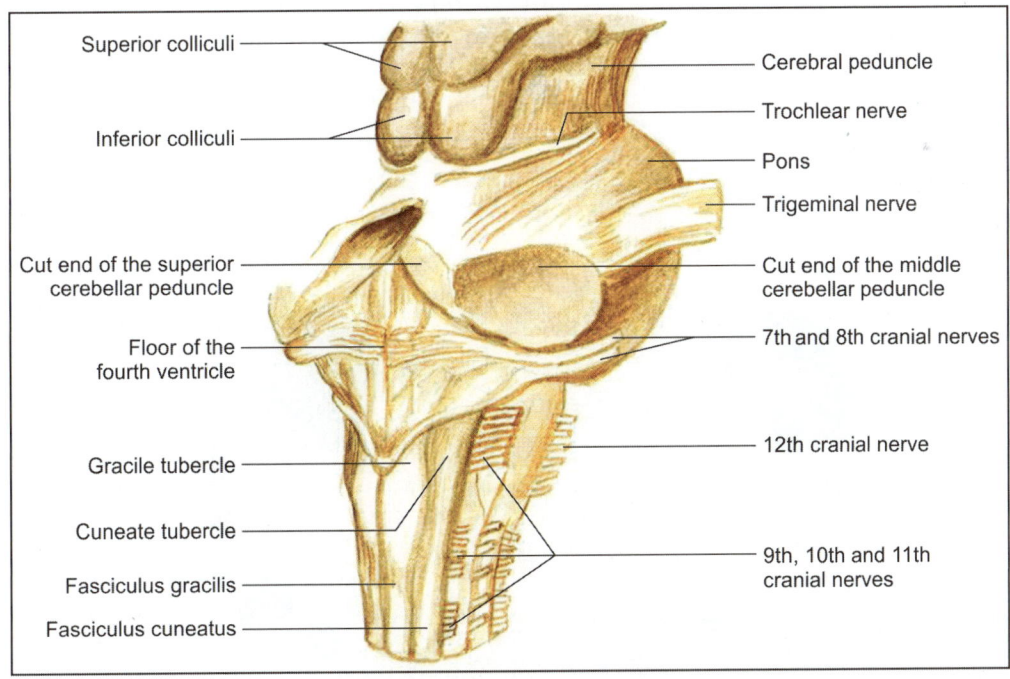

**Fig. 28.2:** Brainstem—posterolateral view

### 3. *Dorsal Nucleus of the Vagus*

Fibers arising from this nucleus are parasympathetic fibers to the heart, lungs and abdominal organs.

### 4. *Solitary Nucleus (nucleus of tractus solitarius)*

It receives gustatory (taste) fibers from the tongue through facial, glossopharyngeal and vagus nerves.

### 5. Spinal Nucleus of the Trigeminal Nerve

It receives pain and temperature sensation from the head (face).

### 6. Nucleus Ambiguus

Fibers arising from this nucleus supplies muscles of palate, pharynx and larynx, through vagus nerve.

### 7. Inferior Olivary Nucleus

It is connected with cerebellum reciprocally and it also sends fibers to spinal cord as olivospinal tract.

### 8. Vestibular Nucleus

It consists of four groups and is located at the junction of medulla oblongata and pons. It receives vestibular nerve carrying information from the internal ear. This nucleus is also connected with cerebellum reciprocally and sends fibers to spinal cord as vestibulospinal tract.

The internal features of medulla can be studied by taking transverse sections at various levels. Identify the nuclei, tracts, motor and sensory decussation in Figs 28.3 to 28.5.

Apart from these nuclei two major events occur at medulla oblongata

a. *Pyramidal decussation (motor decussation):* About 80% of the pyramidal tract fibers (corticospinal fibers) cross to the opposite side in the lower part of the medulla oblongata. Then they descend in the lateral white column of the spinal cord as lateral corticospinal tract. The uncrossed pyramidal fibers descend in the anterior white column of the spinal cord as anterior corticospinal tract, but they also cross to the opposite side in the spinal cord.

b. *Sensory decussation:* Fibers arising from nuclei gracilis and cuneatus proceed forward as internal arcuate fibers to cross to the opposite side. This crossing is referred as sensory decussation. After crossing to the opposite side the fibers ascend as medial lemniscus to reach the thalamus.

Three other nuclei within the medulla oblongata function as autonomic centers for controlling vital visceral functions. The nuclei are:

• Cardiac center
• Vasomotor center
• Respiratory center

### Arterial Supply

Each half of the medulla oblongata is supplied by anterior spinal artery, direct branches from vertebral artery and posterior inferior cerebellar artery from medial to lateral side.

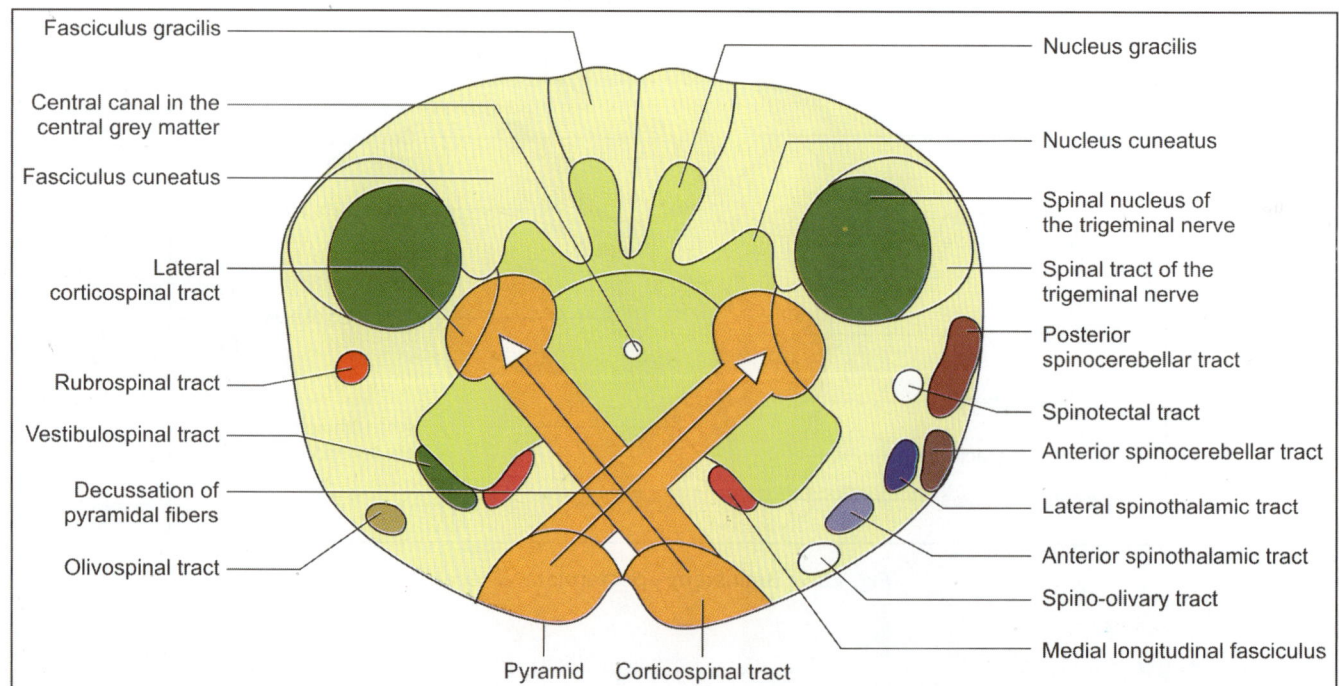

**Fig. 28.3:** Cross-section of the lower medulla (at the level of motor decussation)

Labels:
- Fasciculus gracilis
- Central canal in the central grey matter
- Fasciculus cuneatus
- Lateral corticospinal tract
- Rubrospinal tract
- Vestibulospinal tract
- Decussation of pyramidal fibers
- Olivospinal tract
- Nucleus gracilis
- Nucleus cuneatus
- Spinal nucleus of the trigeminal nerve
- Spinal tract of the trigeminal nerve
- Posterior spinocerebellar tract
- Spinotectal tract
- Anterior spinocerebellar tract
- Lateral spinothalamic tract
- Anterior spinothalamic tract
- Spino-olivary tract
- Medial longitudinal fasciculus
- Pyramid
- Corticospinal tract

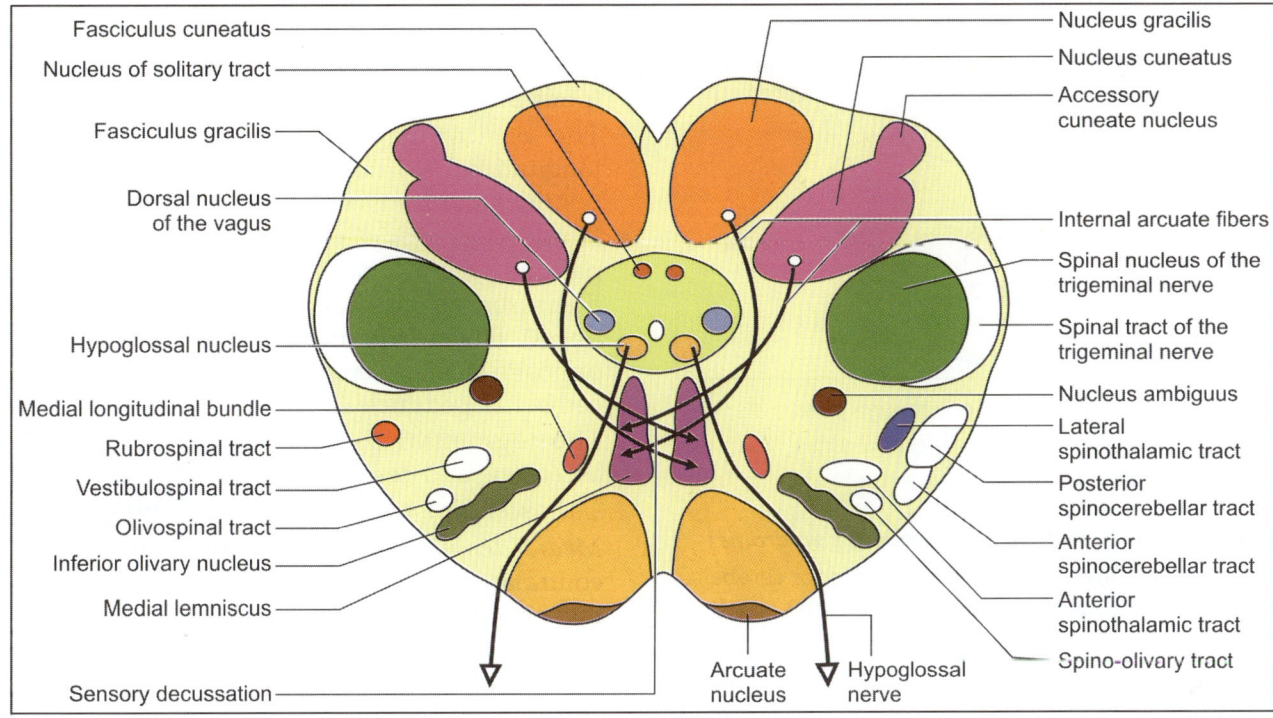

**Fig. 28.4:** Cross-section of the medulla (at the level of sensory decussation)

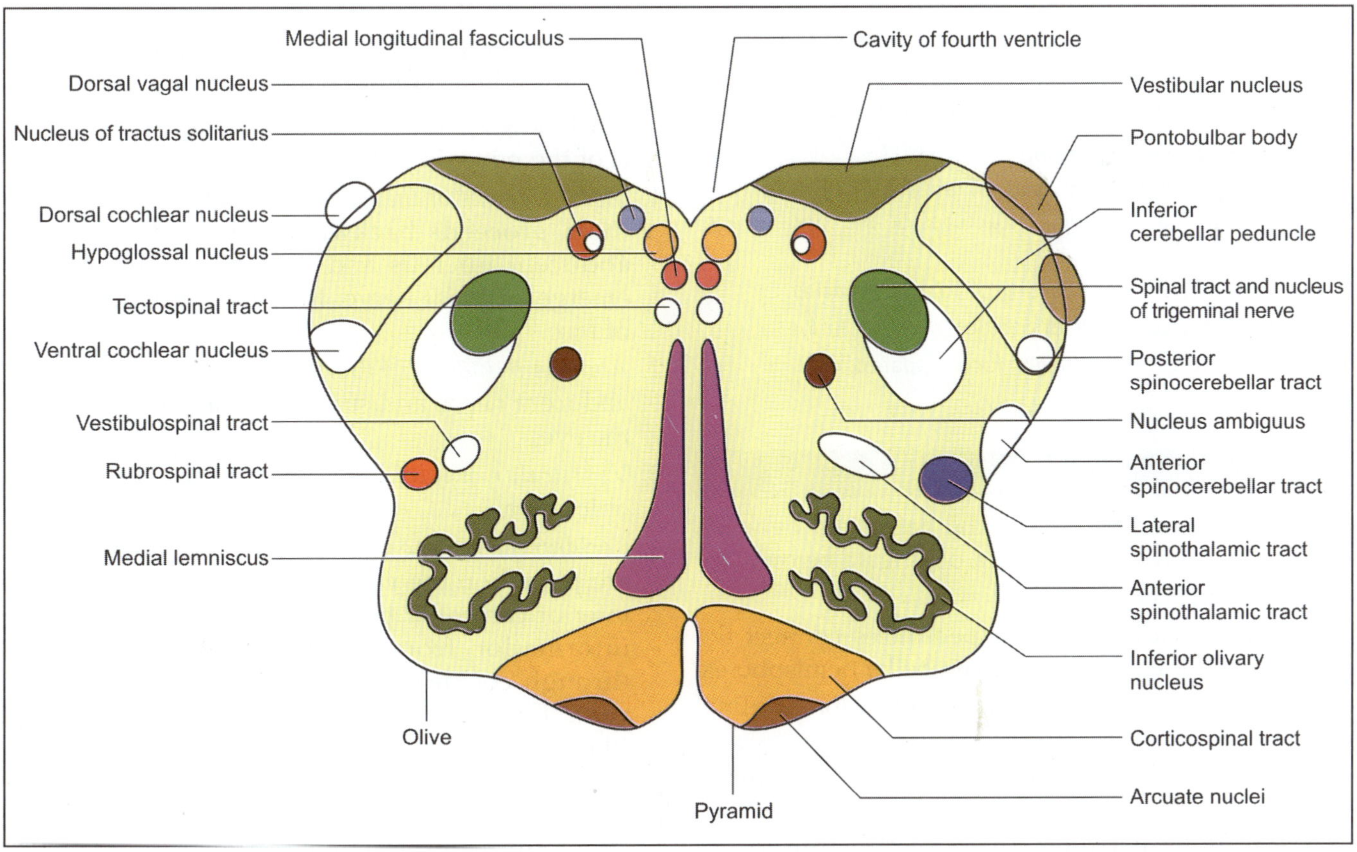

Labels (Fig. 28.4), left side:
- Fasciculus cuneatus
- Nucleus of solitary tract
- Fasciculus gracilis
- Dorsal nucleus of the vagus
- Hypoglossal nucleus
- Medial longitudinal bundle
- Rubrospinal tract
- Vestibulospinal tract
- Olivospinal tract
- Inferior olivary nucleus
- Medial lemniscus
- Sensory decussation

Labels (Fig. 28.4), right side:
- Nucleus gracilis
- Nucleus cuneatus
- Accessory cuneate nucleus
- Internal arcuate fibers
- Spinal nucleus of the trigeminal nerve
- Spinal tract of the trigeminal nerve
- Nucleus ambiguus
- Lateral spinothalamic tract
- Posterior spinocerebellar tract
- Anterior spinocerebellar tract
- Anterior spinothalamic tract
- Spino-olivary tract

Labels (Fig. 28.4), bottom:
- Arcuate nucleus
- Hypoglossal nerve

**Fig. 28.5a:** Cross-section of the upper part of the medulla (at the level of inferior olivary nucleus)

Labels (Fig. 28.5a), left side:
- Medial longitudinal fasciculus
- Dorsal vagal nucleus
- Nucleus of tractus solitarius
- Dorsal cochlear nucleus
- Hypoglossal nucleus
- Tectospinal tract
- Ventral cochlear nucleus
- Vestibulospinal tract
- Rubrospinal tract
- Medial lemniscus

Labels (Fig. 28.5a), right side:
- Cavity of fourth ventricle
- Vestibular nucleus
- Pontobulbar body
- Inferior cerebellar peduncle
- Spinal tract and nucleus of trigeminal nerve
- Posterior spinocerebellar tract
- Nucleus ambiguus
- Anterior spinocerebellar tract
- Lateral spinothalamic tract
- Anterior spinothalamic tract
- Inferior olivary nucleus
- Corticospinal tract
- Arcuate nuclei

Labels (Fig. 28.5a), bottom:
- Olive
- Pyramid

28

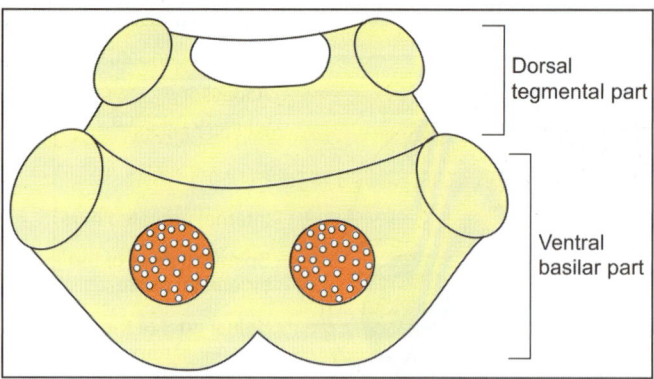

**Fig. 28.5b:** Cross-section through pons

## Applied Aspects

1. *Lateral medullary syndrome (Wallenberg's syndrome)*

This is due to the thrombosis of posterior inferior cerebellar artery supplying medulla. The structures affected and their clinical manifestations are listed below.

a. Nucleus ambiguus—difficulty in swallowing (dysphagia) and hoarseness.

b. Spinal nucleus and tract of 5th cranial nerve—loss of pain and temperature sensation from face (same side), loss of corneal reflex.

c. Inferior cerebellar peduncle—ataxia of the limbs.

d. Vestibular nuclei—vertigo, vomiting, nystagmus.

e. Lateral spinothalamic tract—loss of pain and temperature sensation of the trunk and limbs (opposite side).

2. *Medial medullary syndrome*

This is due to the thrombosis of anterior spinal artery supplying medulla. Following structures of the medulla are involved.

a. Hypoglossal nucleus—wasting of tongue muscles.

b. Medial lemniscus—loss of position sense in limbs.

c. Pyramidal tract—hemiplegia, face is spared.

## PONS

- Pons is the middle part of the brainstem between midbrain above and medulla oblongata below.
- It is about 2.5 cm long.
- Laterally middle cerebellar peduncles connect the pons with the corresponding cerebellar hemispheres.
- Ventral surface of the pons presents a longitudinal sulcus which is occupied by basilar artery.
- Dorsal surface of the pons forms the upper part of the floor of the fourth ventricle.
- The rootlets of trigeminal nerve emerge at the junction of middle cerebellar peduncle and pons.

## Internal Features

- Internally pons is divided into a ventral basilar part (pons proper) and a dorsal tegmental part.
- The basilar part is occupied by number of longitudinal (corticospinal, corticonuclear, cortico-pontine) and transverse (pontocerebellar) fibers.
- Scattered groups of neuronal masses in this basilar part are 'pontine nuclei'. These pontine nuclei receive fibers from all parts of cerebral cortex (corticopontine fibers). Fibers from the pontine nuclei cross to the opposite side and enter cerebellum through middle cerebellar peduncle.
- The tegmental part of the pons shows many ascending and descending tracts (Figs 28.6 and 28.7). The ascending tracts form many lemnisci.

*Medial lemniscus:* It consists of fibers arising from contralateral nucleus gracilis and nucleus cuneatus in the medulla oblongata. It ascends in the brainstem to reach thalamus.

*Trigeminal lemniscus:* The fibers arising from the spinal nucleus of the fifth cranial nerve crosses to the opposite side then ascend as trigeminal lemniscus.

*Spinal lemniscus:* It is the upward continuation of lateral spinothalamic tract.

*Lateral lemniscus:* It is part of the auditory pathway discussed later in this chapter.

The following important nuclei occupy the tegmental part of the pons (Figs 28.6 and 28.7):

1. *Motor nucleus of the facial nerve:* Fibers arising from them proceeds backwards to wind around the abducent nucleus and then passes forwards to emerge as facial nerve. It mainly supplies muscles of face.

2. *Abducent nucleus:* Fibers arising from them form abducent nerve and supply lateral rectus muscle of the eye.

3. *Vestibular nuclei:* It is explained in medulla oblongata.

4. *Cochlear nuclei:* The ventral and dorsal cochlear nuclei are placed on the ventral and dorsal aspects of the inferior cerebellar peduncle. They receive auditory information from organ of Corti (internal ear) through cochlear nerve. Fibers arising from the ventral cochlear nucleus cross to the opposite side (these fibers form trapezoid body) and most of them terminate in superior olivary nucleus. Fibers arising from superior olivary nucleus ascend as lateral lemniscus, which terminates in inferior colliculus of the midbrain.

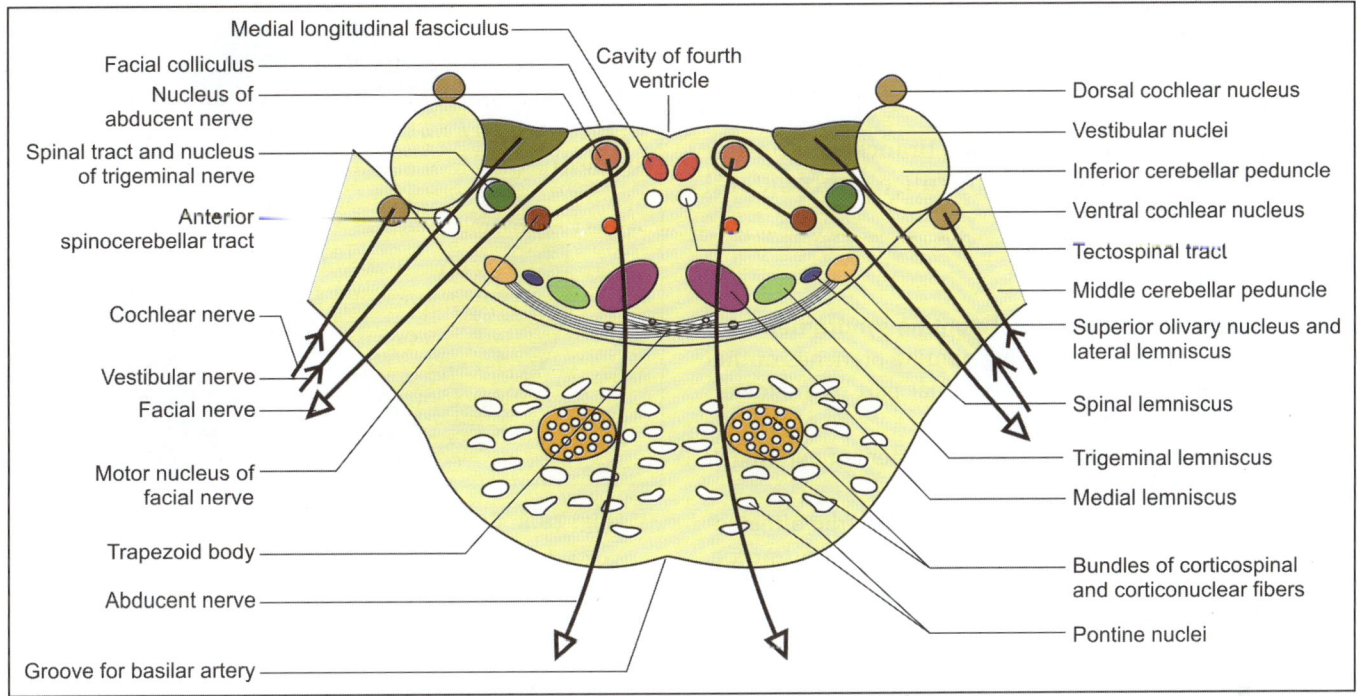

**Fig. 28.6:** Cross-section of the pons (lower part)

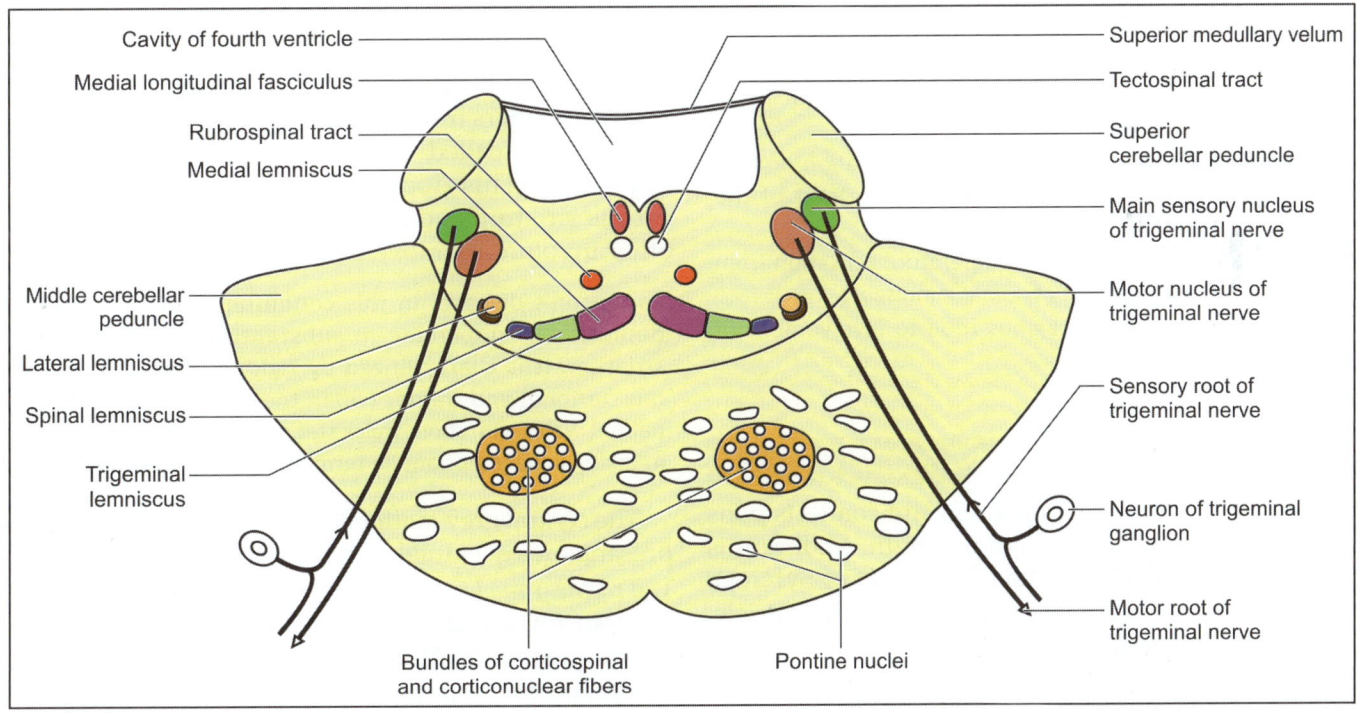

**Fig. 28.7:** Cross-section of the pons (upper part)

5. *Spinal nucleus of trigeminal nerve:* It is explained in medulla oblongata.
6. *Motor nucleus of the trigeminal nerve:* The fibers of this nucleus give origin to motor root of the trigeminal nerve (which later joins the mandibular nerve) and supplies muscles of mastication, mylohyoid, anterior belly of digastric, tensor tympani and tensor veli palatini muscles.

7. *Chief sensory nucleus of the trigeminal nerve:* It receives touch and pressure sensation from the face.

## Arterial Supply

Pons is mainly supplied by pontine branches of basilar artery. Pontine hemorrhage can cause contralateral hemiplegia.

## Applied Anatomy

**Millard Gubler syndrome (medial pontine syndrome):** It is due to the vascular lesion involving pontine branches of the basilar artery. It usually affects the basilar part of the lower pons. The clinical manifestations are:
- Contralateral hemiplegia (due to involvement of pyramidal tract)
- Paralysis of the facial muscle (facial palsy) on the affected side (due to involvement of fibers arising from motor nucleus of the facial nerve)
- Internal squint (due to involvement of abducent nerve fibers which supplies lateral rectus muscle)

**Lateral inferior pontine syndrome (AICA syndrome):** It occurs due to a vascular lesion affecting anterior inferior cerebellar artery. It affects the lateral portion of the lower pons, hence sometimes referred as lateral inferior pontine syndrome. It is also referred as alternating trigeminal hemiplegia. The major clinical manifestations area:
- Ipsilateral facial paralysis (due to involvement of facial nucleus)
- Ipsilateral loss of pain and temperature sensation on face (due to involvement of spinal nucleus and tract of the trigeminal nerve)
- Contralateral loss of pain and temperature sensation from body (due to involvement of spinal lemniscus)
- Vertigo, nausea and nystagmus (due to involvement of vestibular nucleus)

---

## MIDBRAIN

It is the upper part of the brainstem and connects pons and cerebrum. It is about 2 cm in length. Midbrain is traversed by cerebral aqueduct (aqueduct of Sylvius), which connects the third ventricle with fourth ventricle. A horizontal line passing through the cerebral aqueduct divides the midbrain into a dorsal part—the tectum and ventral part—cerebral peduncle (Fig. 28.8).

The right and left cerebral peduncles are further divided into 3 parts from anterior to posterior side. They are:
- Crus cerebri
- Substantia nigra
- Tegmentum

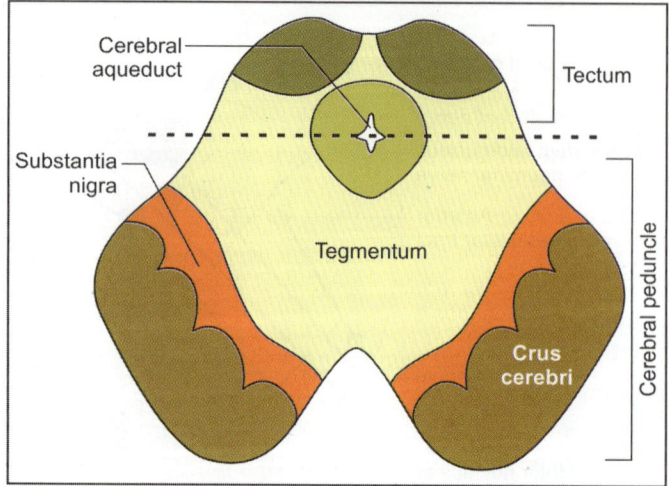

**Fig. 28.8:** Cross-section of midbrain and its division

*Crus cerebri:* It is the anterior most part of each cerebral peduncle. It has bundles of nerve fibers arising from cerebral cortex. It includes:
- Corticopontine fibers
- Corticospinal fibers
- Corticonuclear fibers

*Substantia nigra:* It is a layer of grey matter consisting of pigmented nerve cells. The neurons are rich in dopamine and are connected to the corpus striatum. The nerve fibers from substantia nigra reaching corpus striatum are called 'nigrostriate fibers', which carry **dopamine**. This dopamine is known to inhibit the corpus striatum and by which it prevents tremor and other involuntary movements during voluntary acts.

**Parkinson's disease:** In this condition there is a marked depletion of dopamine in substantia nigra and corpus striatum. It is characterized by rigidity (due to increased muscle tone) and tremor (when the subject is at rest). The patient walks with short, quick steps and experiences difficulty in taking initial steps and in terminating the movements.

The central grey matter around the cerebral aqueduct presents many cranial nerve nuclei, which include:
1. *Trochlear nucleus in the lower part:* Fibers arising from them form tochlear nerve which supply superior oblique muscle of the eye.
2. *Oculomotor nucleus in the upper part:* Fibers arising from this nucleus form oculomotor nerve which supply all the extraocular muscles of the eye except superior oblique and lateral rectus. It also carries parasympathetic fibers from Edinger-Westphal nucleus for visual reflexes (pupillary light and accommodation reflex). They supply sphincter pupillae and ciliaris muscles.

3. *Mesencephalic nucleus of the trigeminal nerve:* It receives proprioceptive fibers from muscles of mastication, muscles of face and extraocular muscles of the eye.

4. *Red nucleus:* A pair of red nuclei located in tegmentum in the upper part of midbrain. The red nucleus is slightly pinkish in color when freshly cut and is rich in iron content. It receives fibers from cerebellum and motor area of the cerebral cortex. Its main output forms rubrospinal tract (extra-pyramidal tract).

The posterior (tectum) part of the midbrain presents two pairs of elevations.

a. A pair of **superior colliculi** in the upper part. Grey matter deep to each colliculus is concerned with visual reflexes and it is connected to lateral geniculate body (LGB) of the thalamus (Fig. 28.9).

b. A pair of **inferior colliculi** in the lower part. Each is a part of the auditory (hearing) pathway. It receives lateral lemniscus from the pons (see pons). Inferior colliculus is connected to medial geniculate body (MGB) of the thalamus. The auditory fibers from the thalamus reach the auditory area of the cerebral cortex (Fig. 28.10).

Midbrain is connected with cerebellum through a pair of superior cerebellar peduncles.

*Argyll-Robertson pupil:* This condition is due to the lesion is the pre tectal nucleus of midbrain. This nucleus is involved in light reflex. In this condition light reflex is lost but the accommodation reflex remains intact. This condition can occur in tertiary syphilis.

*Weber's syndrome:* This occurs due to a vascular lesion affecting the crus cerebri involving corticospinal tract and oculomotor nerve. It usually involves branches from posterior cerebral artery. It is characterized by contralateral hemiplegia (UMN paralysis) due to the involvement of the corticospinal tract. Involvement of oculomotor nerve fibers results in ipsilateral paralysis of eye muscles supplied by it. The eye looks down and out (external strabismus) due to unopposed action of superior oblique and lateral rectus muscle. The involvement of parasympathetic fibers results in fixed (loss of accommodation reflex) and dilated pupil. Involvement of levator palpebrae superioris causes ptosis (remember in Horner's syndrome there will be a ptosis with constriction of pupil).

## Reticular Formation

It is a complex network of nuclei and nerve fibers within the brainstem that functions as the 'reticular activating system' (RAS) in arousing the cerebrum. The reticular formation contains ascending and descending fibers from most of the structures within the brain. Nuclei

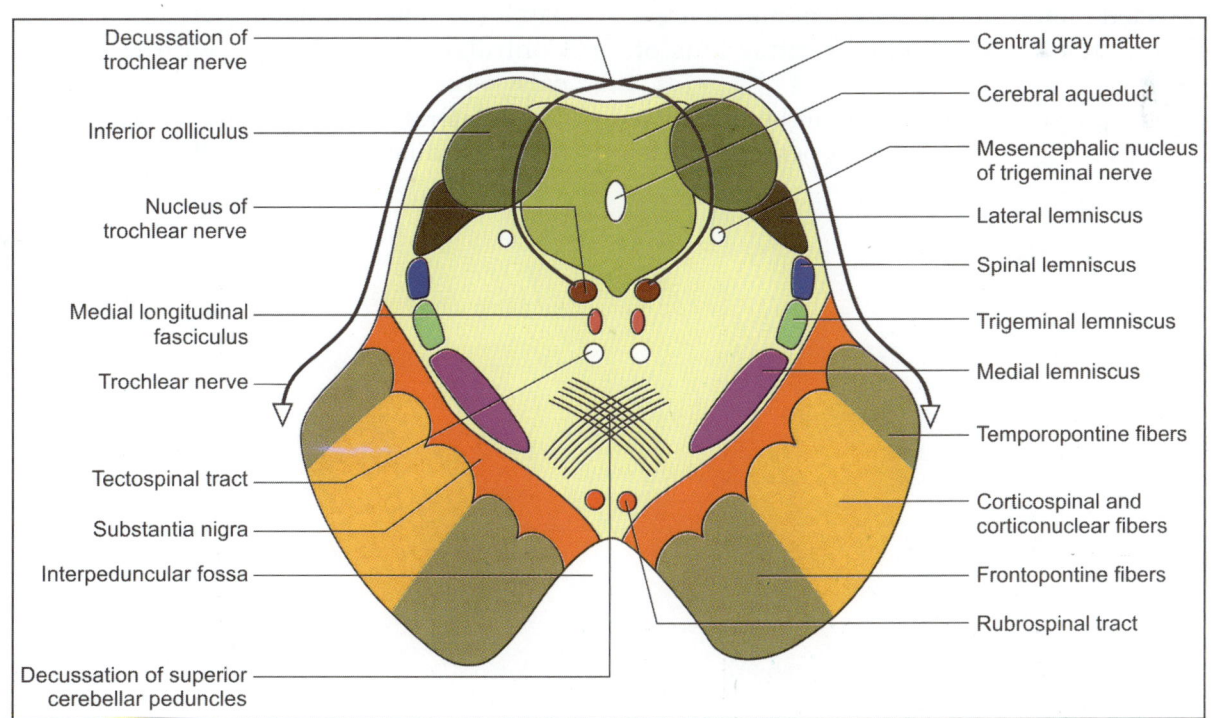

**Fig. 28.9:** Cross-section of the midbrain—at the level of inferior colliculus

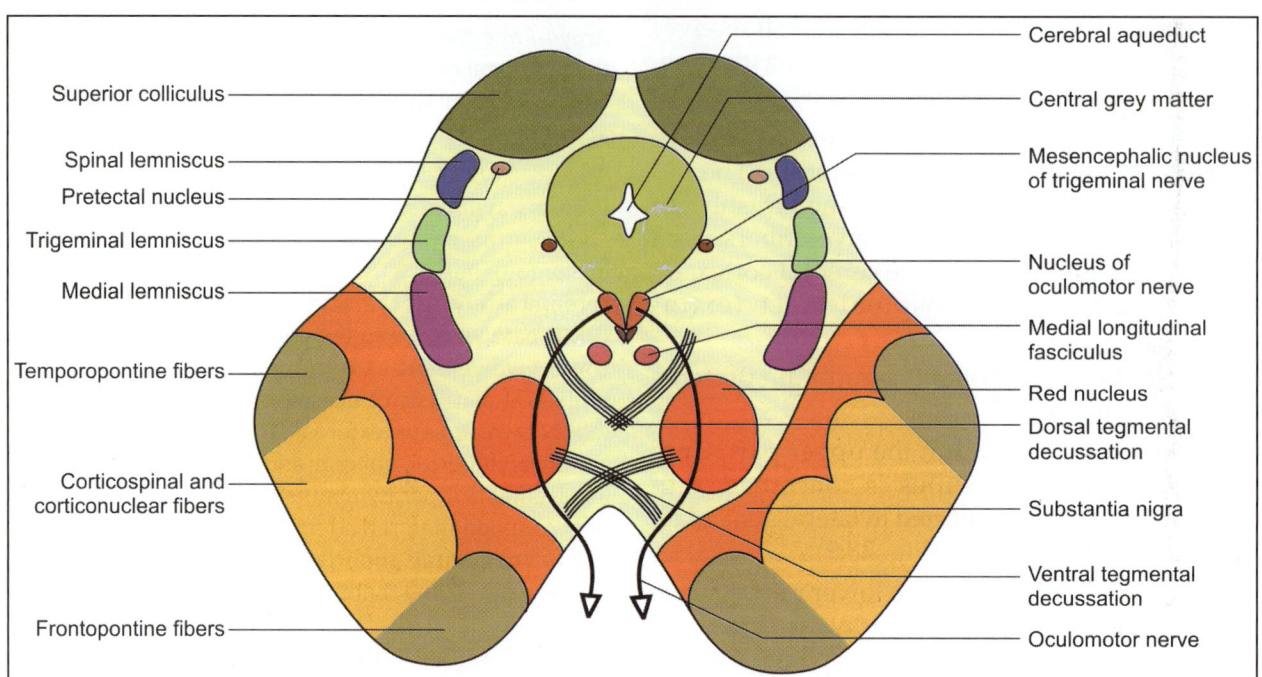

Superior colliculus

Spinal lemniscus

Pretectal nucleus

Trigeminal lemniscus

Medial lemniscus

Temporopontine fibers

Corticospinal and corticonuclear fibers

Frontopontine fibers

Cerebral aqueduct

Central grey matter

Mesencephalic nucleus of trigeminal nerve

Nucleus of oculomotor nerve

Medial longitudinal fasciculus

Red nucleus

Dorsal tegmental decussation

Substantia nigra

Ventral tegmental decussation

Oculomotor nerve

**Fig. 28.10:** Cross-section of the midbrain—at the level of superior colliculus

within the reticular formation generate a continuous flow of impulses unless they are inhibited by other parts of the brain. The principle functions of the RAS are to keep the cerebrum in a state of alert consciousness and to selectively monitor the sensory impulses perceived by the cerebrum. The RAS also helps the cerebellum to activate selected motor units to maintain muscle tone and produce smooth, coordinated contractions of skeletal muscles.

The sleep response is thought to occur because of a decrease in the activity within the RAS, perhaps due to the secretion of specific neurotransmitters. A blow to the head or certain drugs and diseases may damage RAS, causing unconsciousness.

### Note the Lesion Affecting Brainstem

- Contralateral hemiplegia with tongue muscle paralysis—medulla oblongata.
- Contralateral hemiplegia with ipsilateral facial palsy—pons.
- Contralateral hemiplegia, eye muscle paralysis with fixed and dilated pupil—midbrain.

# Cerebellum

Cerebellum lies in the posterior cranial fossa behind the pons and medulla oblongata and below the tentorium cerebelli. Cerebellum is separated from the pons and medulla by the cavity of the fourth ventricle. Cerebellum is connected to the brainstem by three pairs of peduncles (Fig. 29.1):

- Superior cerebellar peduncles with midbrain
- Middle cerebellar peduncles with pons
- Inferior cerebellar peduncles with medulla oblongata

## External Features

- The cerebellum consists of outer grey matter forming cerebellar cortex and inner white matter.
- The outer cerebellar cortex shows numerous transverse folds called 'folia', separated by fissures. This type of folding of cortex provides large surface area for accommodation of numerous neurons in a limited space.
- Anatomically cerebellum consists of two cerebellar hemispheres, connected by a median worm-like structure called 'vermis'.
- The cerebellum is divided into three lobes by two fissures.
- The posterolateral fissure separates the flocculo-nodular lobe from the remaining main part of the cerebellum called 'corpus cerebelli'.

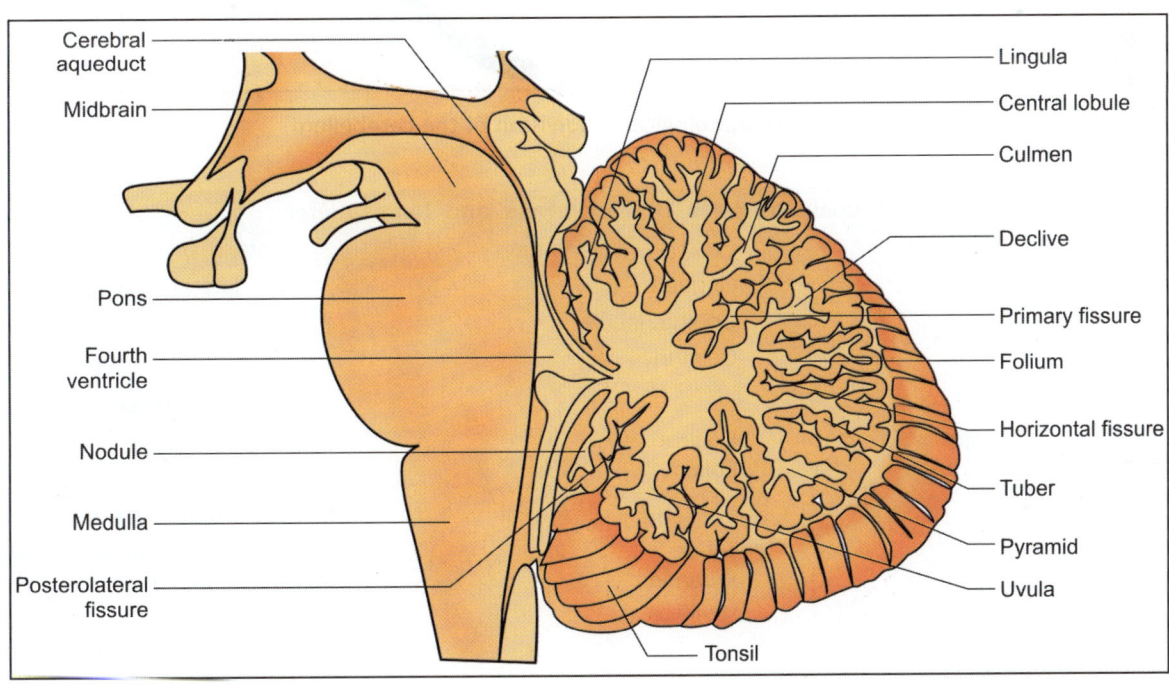

**Fig. 29.1:** Sagittal section through cerebellum showing parts of the vermis

307

- The corpus cerebelli is further divided into anterior and posterior (or middle) lobes by a 'primary fissure'.
- A horizontal fissure demarcates the superior surface of the cerebellum from its inferior surface.
- The vermis connecting the two cerebellar hemispheres is divided into many parts extending from superior to inferior surface.
- Each part of the vermis has lateral extensions, which form the cerebellar hemispheres, which are mentioned in Fig. 29.2.

## MORPHOLOGICAL SUBDIVISION OF CEREBELLUM

On phylogenetic criteria (evolutionary basis) the cerebellum is divided into three parts (Fig. 29.2):

### Archicerebellum (Fig. 29.3)

- First to appear in evolution
- It is formed by flocculonodular lobe and lingula.
- It receives fibers from vestibular nuclei and concerned with the maintenance of equilibrium, muscle tone and posture of the trunk.

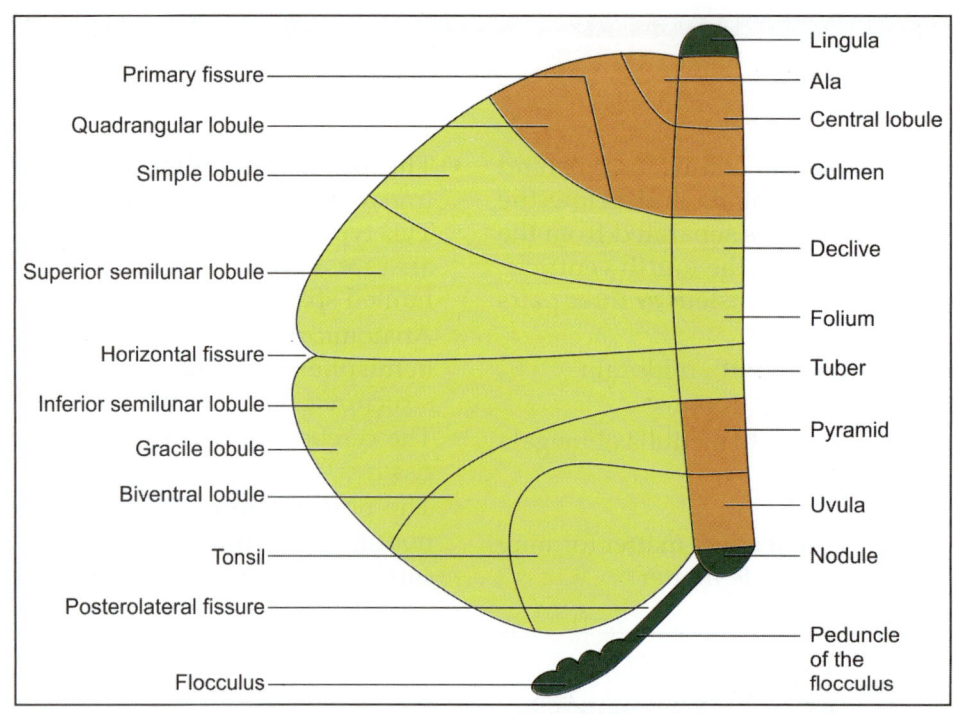

**Fig. 29.2:** Morphological subdivision of the cerebellum

| Cerebellum—parts of the vermis and hemispheres | | |
|---|---|---|
| | *Parts of the vermis* | *Lateral part of the hemisphere* |
| 1. Anterior lobe | Lingula | No lateral projection |
| | Central lobule | Ala |
| | Culmen | Quadrangular lobule |
| | | **Primary fissure** |
| 2. Posterior lobe (middle) | Declive | Simple lobule |
| | Folium | Superior semilunar lobule |
| | | **Horizontal fissure** |
| | Tuber | Inferior semilunar lobule |
| | Pyramid | Biventral lobule |
| | Uvula | Tonsil |
| | | **Posterolateral fissure** |
| 3. Floculonodular lobe | Nodule | Flocculus |

## Paleocerebellum (Fig. 29.4)

- It consists of anterior lobe (except lingula), pyramid and the uvula.
- It receives input from spinal cord (spinocerebellar tract).
- Functionally, it is concerned with muscle tone and posture of the limbs.

## Neocerebellum (Fig. 29.5)

- It includes remaining part of the cerebellum (post/middle lobe except pyramid and uvula)

- It receives input from cerebral cortex via corticopontine, pontocerebellar fibers, inferior olivary nucleus, visual and auditory pathways. These inputs are processed in the cerebellum and integrated into the motor system by means of motor cortex, red nucleus, vestibular nuclei and brainstem reticular formation. Corticospinal, rubrospinal, vestibulospinal and reticulospinal tracts are involved in expressing the cerebellar activities on motor mechanism.

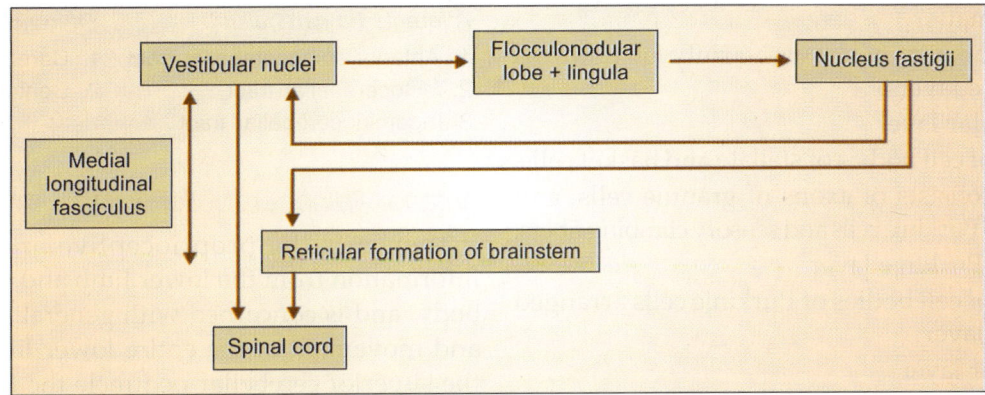

**Fig. 29.3:** Connections of archicerebellum

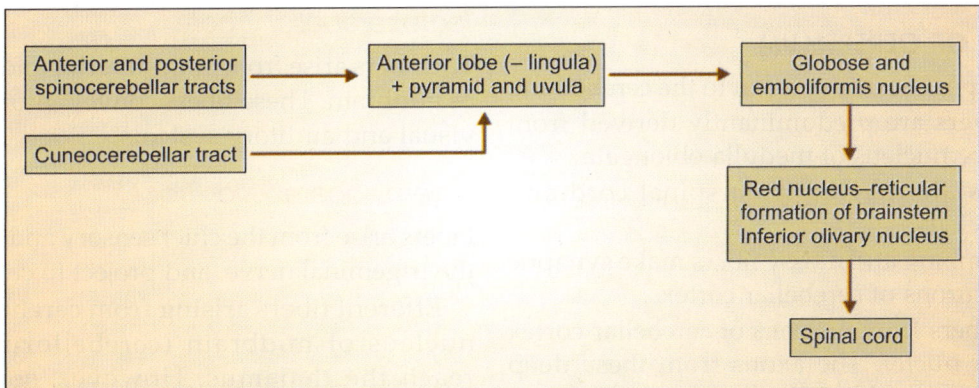

**Fig. 29.4:** Connections of paleocerebellum

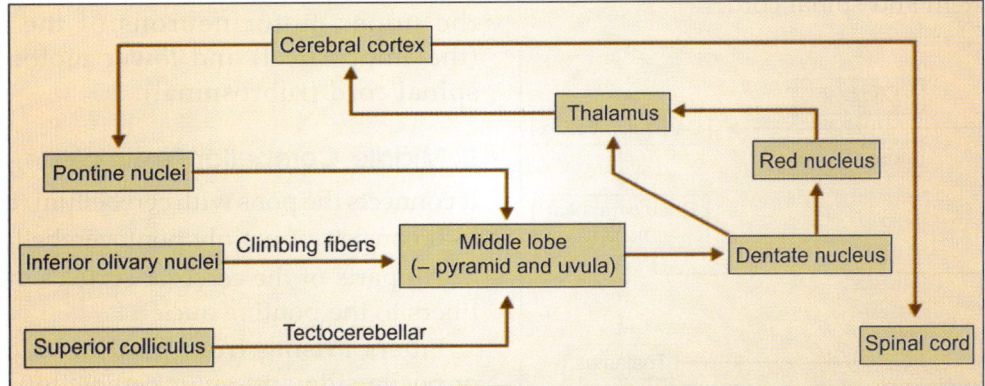

**Fig. 29.5:** Connections of neocerebellum

29

## DEEP CEREBELLAR NUCLEI

Embedded in the white matter of cerebellum are four bilateral cerebellar nuclei, which are named from lateral to medial side as:

- Dentate nucleus
- Nucleus emboliformis
- Nucleus globosus
- Nucleus fastigii

## MICROSCOPIC STRUCTURE OF CEREBELLUM

Cerebellum presents an outer cortex (grey matter) and an inner white matter.

The cerebellar cortex shows variety of neurons arranged in three layers.

a. Outer molecular layer
   - It consists of cell bodies of stellate and basket cells.
   - It mainly consists of axons of granule cells, and dendrites of Purkinje cells and sensory climbing fibers.
b. Intermediate Purkinje layer
   - It consists of cell bodies of Purkinje cells arranged in a single layer.
c. Inner granular layer
   - It consists of cell bodies of granule cells, Golgi cells and their processes and sensory mossy fibers.

## CONNECTIONS OF CEREBELLUM

There are two types of sensory input to the cerebellum.
1. **Climbing fibers** are predominantly derived from inferior olivary nucleus of medulla oblongata.
2. **Mossy fibers** are derived from spinal cord and vestibular nucleus.

Both these climbing and mossy fibers make synaptic contacts with neurons of cerebellar cortex.

The output fibers from neurons of cerebellar cortex reach cerebellar nuclei. The axons from these deep cerebellar nuclei are considered as final output pathway and they traverse the cerebellar peduncles and reach thalamus, brainstem and spinal cord.

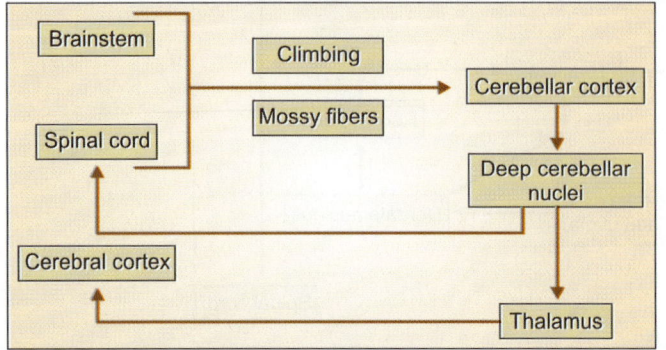

**Schematic representation of cerebellar connections**

## CEREBELLAR PEDUNCLES

Three pairs of cerebellar peduncles connect the cerebellum with different parts of brainstem.

### 1. Superior Cerebellar Peduncle (Brachium Conjunctivum)

It connects the midbrain and cerebellum. The right and left superior cerebellar peduncles are connected by superior medullary velum.

Fibers present in them are:

| Afferents (to cerebellum) | Efferents (from cerebellum) |
| --- | --- |
| 1. Anterior spinocerebellar tract | 1. Cerebellorubral fibers |
| 2. Tectocerebellar tract | 2. Dentatothalamic fibers |
| 3. Trigeminocerebellar tract | |

### *Anterior Spinocerebellar Tract*

It transmits the proprioceptive and exteroceptive information from the lower limb and lower part of the body, and is concerned with general status of posture and movement of the entire lower limb. On reaching the superior cerebellar peduncle the fibers of the tract cross the middle line.

### *Tectocerebellar Tract*

The fibers arise from both superior and inferior colliculi of midbrain. These fibers convey information from the visual and auditory systems.

### *Trigeminocerebellar Tract*

Fibers arise from the chief sensory and spinal nucleus of the trigeminal nerve, and project to cerebellum.

Efferent fibers arising from cerebellum end in red nucleus of midbrain (cerebellorubral) and then reach the thalamus. However, some fibers from cerebellum directly reach thalamus through superior cerebellar peduncle. These tracts influence the upper motor neurons of the cerebral cortex (thalamocortical) and lower motor neurons of the spinal cord (rubrospinal).

### 2. Middle Cerebellar Peduncle

It connects the pons with cerebellum (brachium pontis).

It consists of mainly pontocerebellar fibers.

All parts of the cerebral cortex send corticopontine fibers to the pontine nuclei.

Fibers arising from pontine nuclei cross to the opposite side and enter cerebellum through middle cerebellar peduncle.

## 3. Inferior Cerebellar Peduncle (Restiform Bodies)

It connects the medulla oblongata and cerebellum

*Vestibulocerebellar tract:* Fibers arise form medial and inferior vestibular nuclei, pass through inferior cerebellar peduncle and project to flocculonodular lobe, uvula and lingula.

*Olivocerebellar tract:* The fibers arise from the inferior olivary nucleus, cross the middle line and project to the contralateral cerebellum as climbing fibers.

*Reticulocerebellar tract:* Fibers arise from lateral reticular and paramedian nuclei of the medulla.

*Posterior spinocerebellar tract:* It arises from the thoracic nucleus (Clarke's column) of the spinal cord and conveys proprioceptive and exteroceptive senses from hind limb area.

*Cuneocerebellar tract (posterior external arcuate fibers):* Fibers arise from the accessory cuneate nucleus of medulla, convey proprioceptive and exteroceptive information from the upper limb.

*Rostral spinocerebellar tract:* It arises from the posterior grey column of the cervical and upper thoracic segments of the spinal cord. It transmits sensations from the upper limb and upper part of the trunk, and corresponds functionally with the anterior spino-cerebellar tract.

*Anterior external arcuate fibers:* It arises from the arcuate nuclei of both sides, pass along the superficial surface of the inferior cerebellar peduncle. The arcuate nuclei are displaced pontine nuclei, and form part of cortico-pontocerebellar pathway.

*Parolivocerebellar tract:* The fibers arise from the medial and dorsal accessory olivary nuclei.

*Cerebellovestibular fibers:* Fibers derived from flocculo-nodular lobe and fastigial nuclei. These fibers project into 4 vestibular nuclei.

*Cerebelloreticular fibers:* They take origin from fastigial nuclei and are distributed to pontine and medullary reticular formation.

## BLOOD SUPPLY TO CEREBELLUM

Cerebellum is supplied by following branches from the vertebral and basilar arteries.

a. Posterior inferior cerebellar artery—branch of the vertebral artery.
b. Anterior inferior cerebellar artery—branch of the basilar artery.
c. Superior cerebellar artery—branch of the basilar artery.

Veins from the cerebellum drain into straight, transverse, sigmoid and occipital dural venous sinuses.

## FUNCTIONS OF THE CEREBELLUM

1. Maintenance of equilibrium, muscle tone and posture
2. Co-ordination of skilful movements
3. Cerebellum controls the movements of same side of the body.
4. Cerebellum receives proprioceptive sensation from the limbs and trunk (muscles and joints). These sensory informations are integrated into motor system. This motor activity is expressed through vestibulospinal, rubrospinal and reticulospinal tracts.

### Applied Aspects

Cerebellar lesions can occur due to tumor, vascular occlusion or other pathological conditions.
1. Tumors affecting the vestibular portion of cerebellum (medulloblastoma in children) disturb the sense of equilibrium. The patient walks on a wide base and sways from side to side.

| Fibers present in the inferior cerebellar peduncle | |
|---|---|
| *Afferents (to cerebellum)* | *Efferents (from cerebellum)* |
| 1. Vestibulocerebellar tract | 1. Cerebellovestibular |
| 2. Olivocerebellar tract | 2. Cerebello-olivary |
| 3. Reticulocerebellar tract | 3. Cerebelloreticular |
| 4. Posterior spinocerebellar tract | |
| 5. Cuneocerebellar tract | |
| 6. Rostral spinocerebellar tract | |
| 7. Anterior external arcuate fibers | |
| 8. Parolivocerebellar tract | |

2. Neocerebellar syndrome: It is characterized by hypotonia (decreased muscle tone), dysnergia on the same side of lesion and intention tremors (while working)

   a. *Ataxia:* Inability to maintain equilibrium while standing or walking. The ataxia becomes worse with eyes closed and is referred as Romberg's sign. The person sways to the side of the lesion.

   b. *Dysmetria:* It is lack of coordinated movements, for example, when reaching the finger to the nose, the finger overshoots the nose.

   c. *Dysarthria:* Speech is scanned so that words are broken up into syllables. Speech becomes slurred.

   d. *Nystagmus:* It is conjugate usually rhythmic involuntary movements of the eyeballs. It occurs due to defective postural fixation of conjugate gaze.

   e. *Hypotonia:* It is due to decreased alpha and gamma motor neuron activity. It may be responsible for decreased tendon reflexes, ataxia and intention tremor.

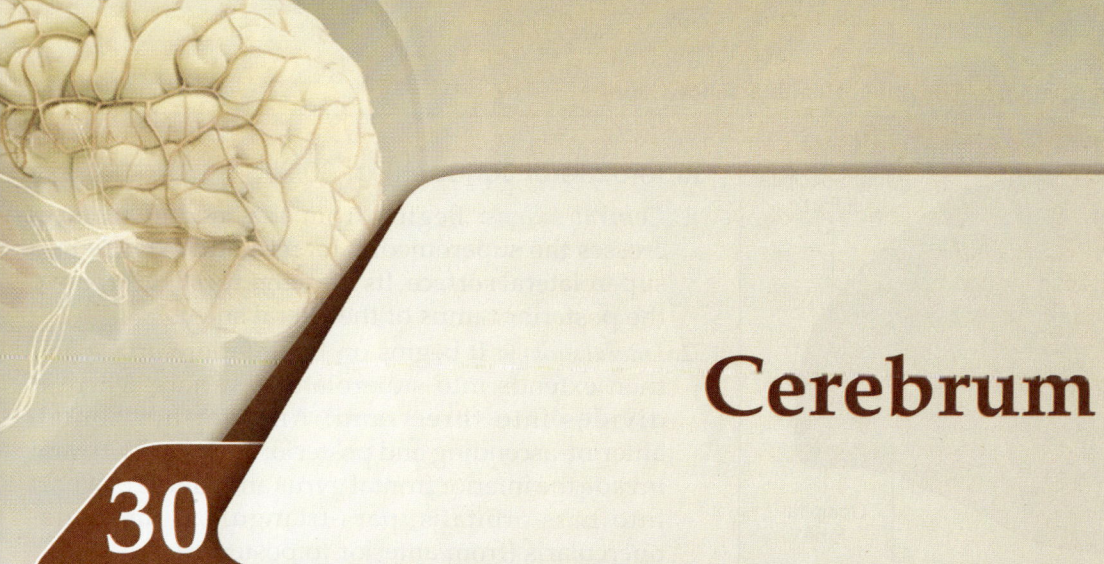

# Cerebrum

## 30

The right and left cerebral hemispheres are partially connected by a white matter called 'corpus callosum'. The narrow interval between the two cerebral hemispheres is the median longitudinal fissure, which is occupied by falx cerebri.

Each cerebral hemisphere has an outer cortex made up of mainly cell bodies of neurons and an inner white matter which consists of nerve fibers and some scattered grey matter (nuclei).

Each cerebral hemisphere presents three surfaces, three borders and three poles.

*The surfaces are*
- Superolateral
- Medial
- Inferior—which is further divided into an anterior orbital part and the posterior tentorial part.

*The borders include* (Fig. 30.1)
- Superomedial—which separates medial surface from the superolateral surface
- Inferolateral—which separates superolateral and inferior surface
- Inferomedial

The cerebral surfaces show elevations and depressions called gyri and sulci, respectively. Each hemisphere is divided into four lobes—frontal, parietal, occipital and temporal. These lobes are separated from each other by grooves present on the cerebral surface (Fig. 30.1).

### SUBDIVISION OF THE CEREBRAL HEMISPHERE

Cerebrum is divided into four lobes by the following sulci and two imaginary lines.

a. *The lateral sulcus:* It begins on the inferior surface (where it separates the orbital and tentorial part) and

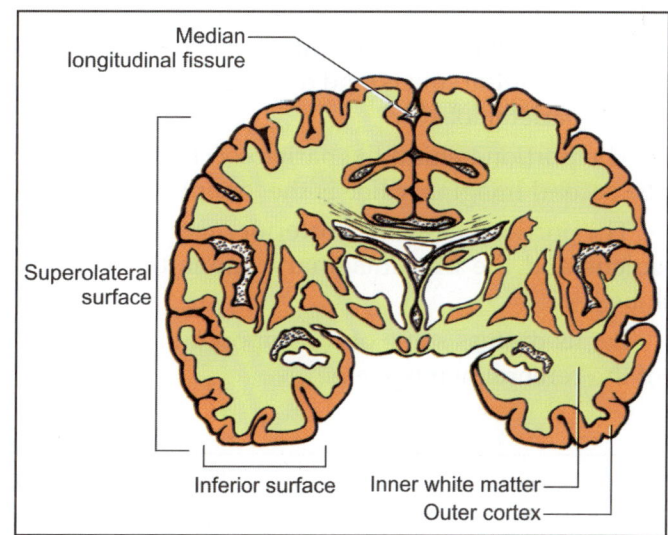

**Fig. 30.1:** Cerebral hemisphere—coronal view

then extends into superolateral surface where it divides into three rami (anterior-horizontal, anterior-ascending and posterior).

b. *The central sulcus:* It begins on the medial surface close to the superomedial border then runs on the superolateral surface to end just above the posterior ramus of the lateral sulcus.

c. *Parieto-occipital sulcus:* It is seen on the medial surface and partly extends into the superolateral surface.

Two imaginary lines complete the subdivision of cerebral hemisphere as follows:

The first imaginary line extends from parieto-occipital sulcus to pre-occipital notch (just in front of the occipital pole). The second imaginary line is an extension of posterior ramus of the lateral sulcus.

The portion of the cerebrum in front of the central sulcus and above the posterior ramus of the lateral sulcus is the 'frontal lobe' (Fig. 30.2).

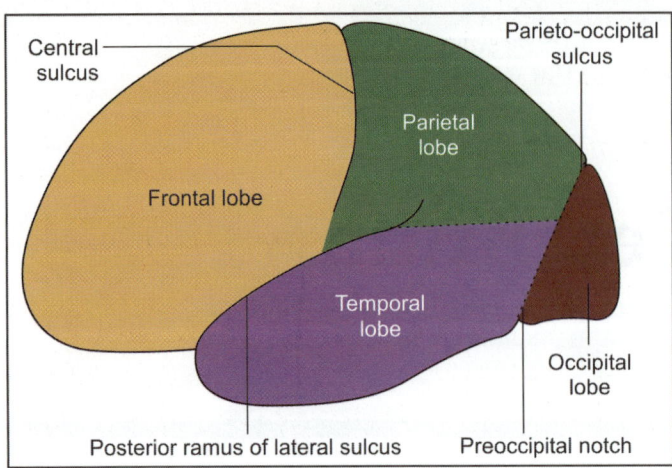

Fig. 30.2: Subdivision of cerebrum (lateral view)

The portion behind the central sulcus and in front of parieto-occipital sulcus (and the second imaginary line) is the 'parietal lobe'.

The portion behind the parieto-occipital sulcus and the second imaginary line is the 'occipital lobe'.

The portion below the posterior ramus of the lateral sulcus and the first imaginary line is the 'temporal lobe'.

Let us discuss some of the important sulci and gyri of the cerebral hemisphere.

## Superolateral Surface (Fig. 30.3)

1. *Central sulcus:* Begins from the medial surface, crosses the superomedial margin and extends into superolateral surface. Its lower end is slightly above the posterior ramus of the lateral sulcus.

2. *Lateral sulcus:* It begins on the inferior surface and then extends into superolateral surface where it divides into three rami: Anterior-horizontal, anterior-ascending and posterior. The first two rami invade the inferior frontal gyrus and divide that part into pars-orbitalis, pars-triangularis and pars-opercularis (from anterior to posterior).

3. *Parieto-occipital sulcus:* It begins from the medial surface and cuts the superomedial margin and appears partly on the superolateral surface where it is surrounded by a gyrus called 'arcus parieto-occipitalis'.

4. *Precentral sulcus:* It lies just in front and parallel to the central sulcus. The portion between the central and precentral sulcus is called 'precentral gyrus'.

5. *Superior frontal sulcus and inferior frontal sulcus:* These sulci extend forward from the precentral sulcus and divide the rest of the frontal lobe into superior, middle and inferior frontal gyri.

6. *Postcentral sulcus:* It lies just behind and parallel to the central sulcus. The portion between it and central sulcus is called 'postcentral gyrus'.

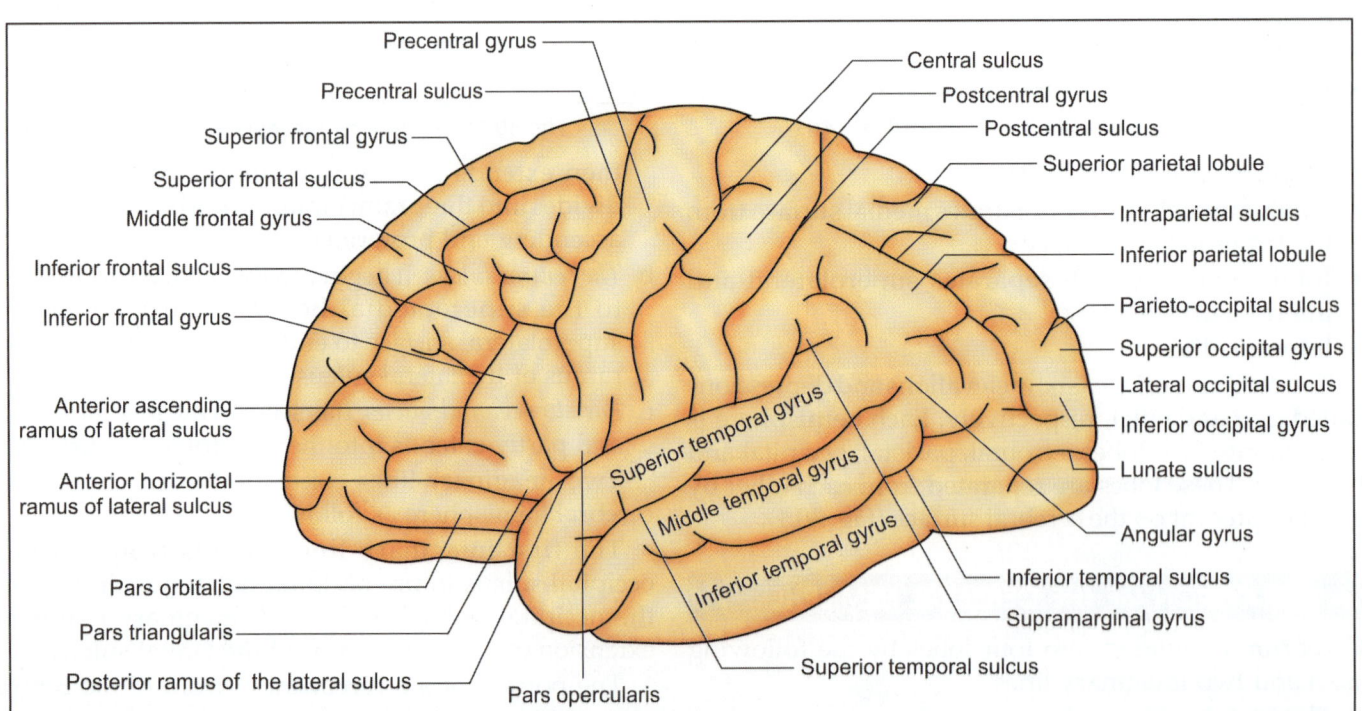

Fig. 30.3: Gyri and sulci of superolateral surface

7. *Transverse parietal sulcus:* This divides the parietal lobe into superior parietal lobule and inferior parietal lobule. The inferior parietal lobule is further divided into three parts by the posterior ends of the posterior ramus of the lateral sulcus, superior temporal sulcus and inferior temporal sulcus. The three parts are (from anterior to posterior): Supramarginal gyrus, angular gyrus and arcus temporo-occipitalis.

8. *Superior and inferior temporal sulcus:* These sulci divide the temporal lobe into superior, middle and inferior temporal gyri.

9. *Transverse occipital sulcus:* It extends from the supero-medial margin just behind the parieto-occipital sulcus and proceeds forward into the superolateral surface.

10. *Lateral occipital sulcus:* It extends horizontally and divides the occipital lobe into superior and inferior occipital gyri.

11. *Lunate sulcus:* It is a curved sulcus lies just in front of the occipital pole on the superolateral surface.

## Medial Surface (Fig. 30.4)

The medial surface of the cerebrum shows the corpus callosum, septum pellucidum, fornix, thalamus and hypothalamus (identify all these structures in Fig. 30.4).

1. *Cingulate sulcus:* It extends from the frontal lobe, proceeds backwards above and parallel to the corpus callosum. It divides that part of the frontal lobe into medial frontal gyrus (above the sulci) and cingulate gyrus (below the sulci).

2. The small portion surrounding the commencement of central sulcus on the medial surface is called 'para-central lobule'.

3. *Parieto-occipital sulcus:* It extends from the supero-medial margin about 5 cm in front of the occipital pole. It passes downwards and forwards and meets the anterior part of the calcarine sulcus.

4. *Calcarine sulcus:* It extends forwards from the occipital pole and joins the parieto-occipital sulcus, further proceeds forward below the splenium of the corpus callosum. The triangular area between it and parieto-occipital sulcus is called 'cuneus'. The portion in front of the cuneus and behind the paracentral lobule is called 'precuneus'.

## Inferior Surface (Fig. 30.5)

1. The stem of the lateral sulcus divides inferior surface into an anterior orbital and posterior tentorial part.

2. The orbital part of the inferior surface shows two sulci. (a) Olfactory sulcus: It is occupied by olfactory tract and (b) H-shaped sulcus, which divides the area into 4 orbital gyri.

3. The tentorial part shows collateral sulcus which runs in anteroposterior direction. The portion medial to it is called 'parahippocampal gyrus'.

## Base of the Brain

The base of the brain presents the following structure (Fig. 30.5):
- A pair of olfactory bulbs and tracts
- Optic chiasma

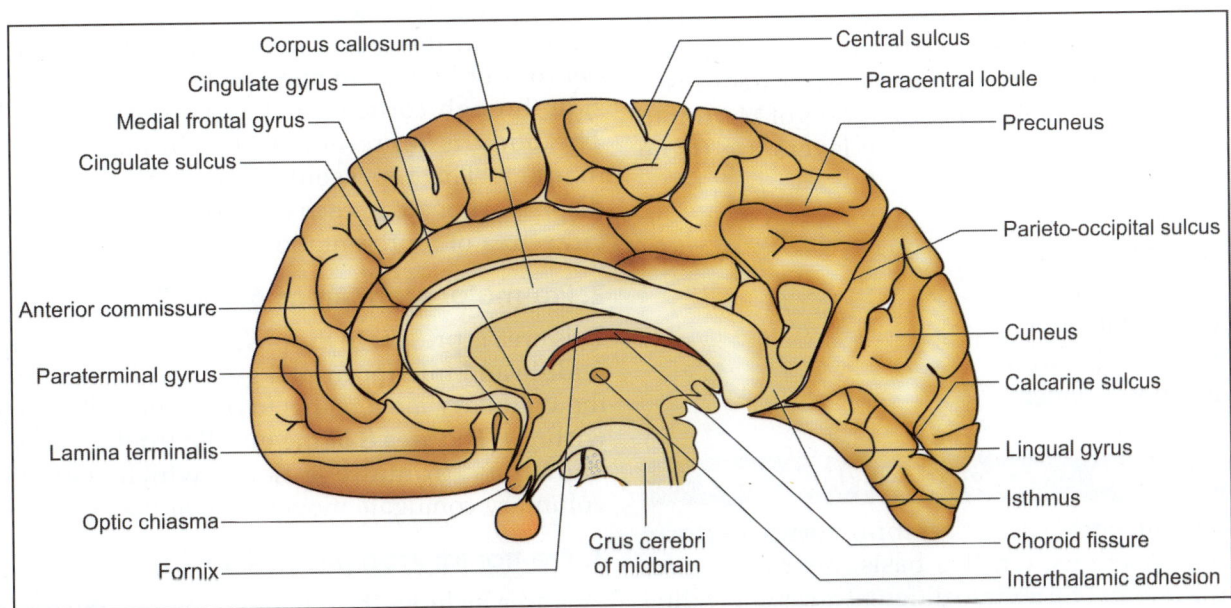

**Fig. 30.4:** Gyri and sulci on medial surface of cerebral hemisphere

Corpus callosum
Cingulate gyrus
Medial frontal gyrus
Cingulate sulcus
Anterior commissure
Paraterminal gyrus
Lamina terminalis
Optic chiasma
Fornix
Crus cerebri of midbrain
Central sulcus
Paracentral lobule
Precuneus
Parieto-occipital sulcus
Cuneus
Calcarine sulcus
Lingual gyrus
Isthmus
Choroid fissure
Interthalamic adhesion

30

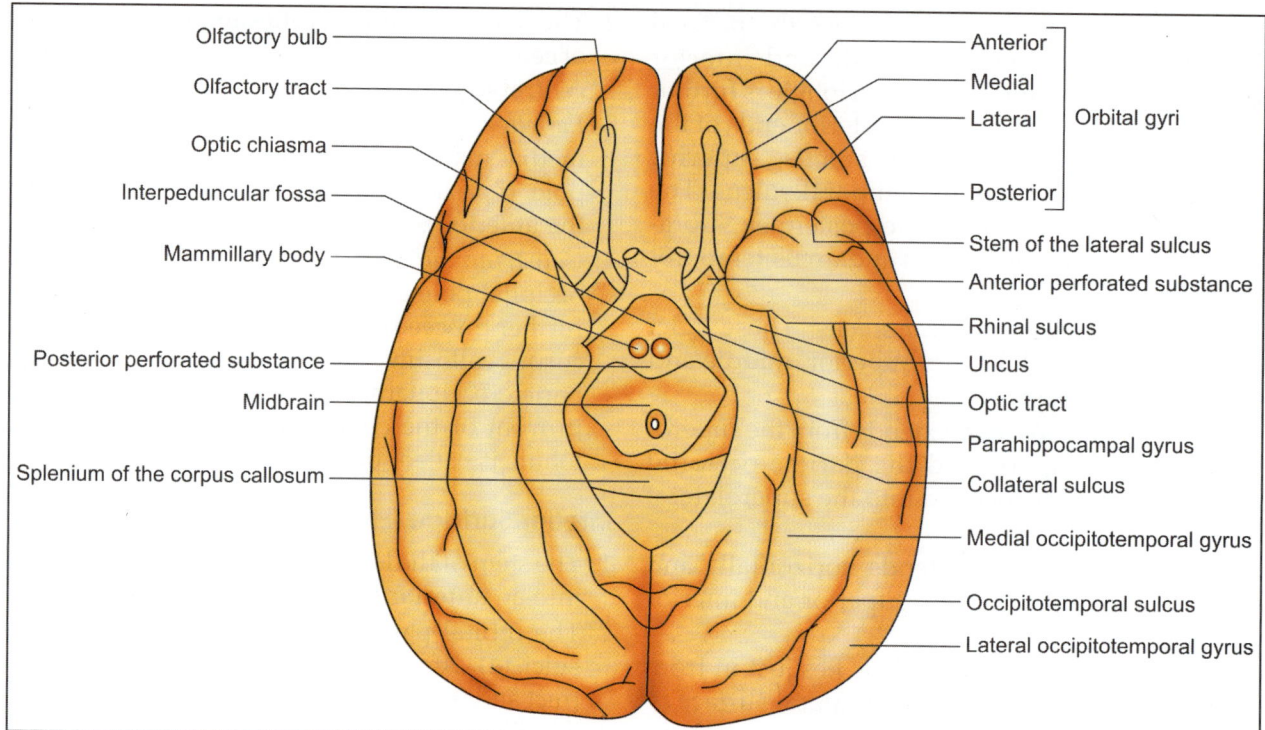

**Fig. 30.5:** Gyri and sulci of an inferior surface of the cerebrum

- Interpeduncular fossa
- An arterial circle of Willis
- A pair of mammillary bodies
- Stalk of the pituitary gland

## STRUCTURE OF CEREBRAL CORTEX

The thickness of the grey matter (cerebral cortex) varies from 1.5 to 4 mm. It is thick over the gyri and thin in the sulci. Structurally it shows 6 layers. All these layers mainly consist of the following types of neurons—pyramidal neurons, stellate neurons, cells of Martinotti and horizontal cells of Cajal. The layers are (from superficial to deep):

1. Molecular layer
2. Outer granular layer
3. Outer pyramidal layer
4. Inner granular layer
5. Inner pyramidal layer
6. Polymorphous layer

## FUNCTIONAL AREAS OF CEREBRAL CORTEX

The different parts of the cerebral cortex perform particular functions. On this basis, neurobiologists divide the cerebral cortex into different areas depending on the functions performed by those neurons. At present, Brodmann's area is accepted and used frequently (Fig. 30.6a and b).

### 1. Primary Motor Area (Area 4)

It includes precentral gyrus and also extends to the paracentral lobule on the medial surface. This area controls the voluntary movements of the opposite half of the body by innervating the skeletal muscles. The fibers from the motor area end in the lower motor neurons of brainstem and spinal cord of the opposite side through corticospinal and corticonuclear tracts. The body is represented here in an upside down manner. The representation of particular part is disproportionate to each other, hand and lips having a large area of representation.

### 2. Pre-motor Area (Areas 6 and 8)

This area is present in the posterior part of the superior, middle and inferior frontal gyrus. This area integrates the voluntary movements to perform skillful acts (like writing). The area 8 of the middle frontal gyrus is also known as 'frontal eye-field', which regulates the voluntary conjugate movements of the eyes.

### 3. Pre-frontal Area (Areas 9 to 12)

This area includes the remaining part of the frontal lobe anterior to the pre-motor area. The high qualities of

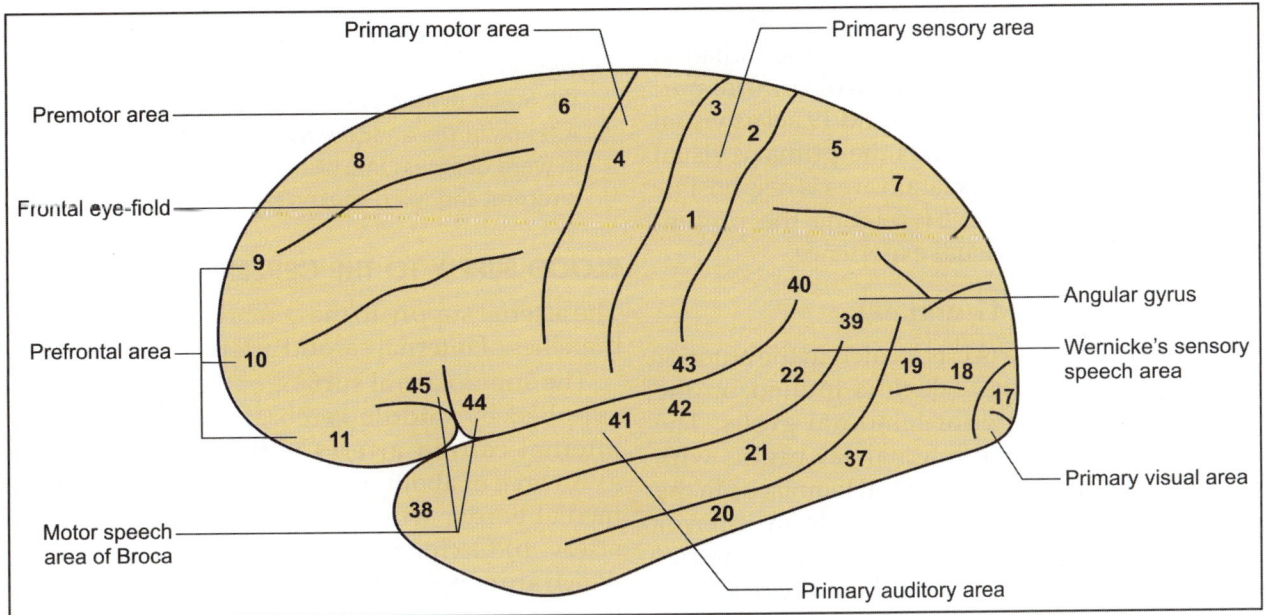

**Fig. 30.6a:** Functional areas of the superolateral surface

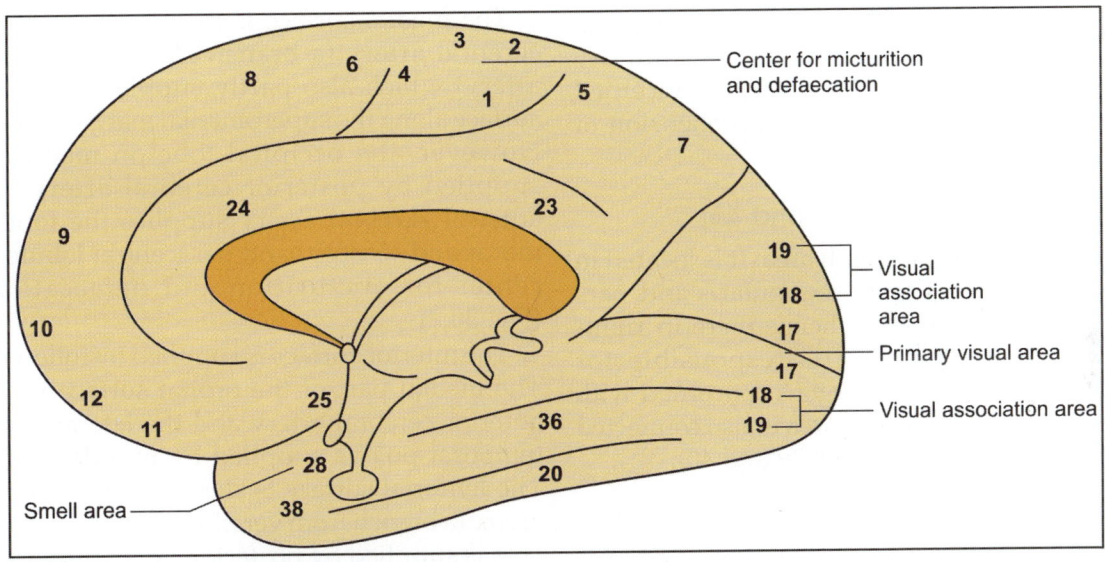

**Fig. 30.6b:** Functional areas of the medial surface

human behavior like abstract thinking, mature judgment, foresight and tactfulness are regulated by this area. It also regulates the depth of feeling of an individual.

### 4. Primary Sensory Area (Areas 3,1 and 2)

It is located in the postcentral gyrus and also extends into the medial surface in the paracentral lobule. This area receives majority of the sensory information (touch, pressure, position and vibratory senses) from the opposite half of the body through the thalamus. The areas of sensation are represented upside-down (head end below and leg end up).

### 5. Sensory Association Area (Areas 5 and 7)

It is located in superior parietal lobule and also partly in the supramarginal gyrus (area 40). This area receives fibers from thalamus and postcentral gyrus and it further processes the sensory information for perception or recognition of the general senses.

### 6. Visual Area (Areas 17 to 19)

It is located along the lips and walls of the calcarine sulcus (mainly on the medial surface, partly on the superolateral surface). The visual information from the retina passes through optic nerve, optic chiasma, optic

30

tract and lateral geniculate body of thalamus. The fibers from lateral geniculate body spread as optic radiation and reach this visual area through retrolentiform part of the internal capsule. The areas 18 and 19 act as visual association area, which surrounds the primary visual area (area 17). This visual association area is responsible for recognition of the object by relating the present impression with the past visual experience.

### 7. Auditory Area (Areas 41 and 42)

The primary auditory area (41) is located in the anterior transverse temporal gyrus, which is located on the upper surface of the superior-temporal gyrus. The auditory pathway from the internal ear begins with cochlear nerve then proceeds as lateral lemniscus in the brainstem. This lateral lemniscus ends in inferior colliculus of the midbrain and then into medial geniculate body of thalamus. From here fibers spread as auditory radiation which enters the primary auditory area through sublentiform part of internal capsule. The area 42 immediately behind the primary auditory area is considered as auditory association area. Area 22 (Wernicke's area) is considered as higher auditory association area. These areas (42 and 22) are concerned with interpretation of sounds and comprehension of spoken language.

### 8. Motor Speech Area (Areas 44 and 45)

It is also referred as Broca's speech area. It is located in the inferior frontal gyrus (pars triangularis and pars opercularis) of the left cerebral hemisphere in right-handed individual. This area is responsible for coordinated movements of the organs concerned with spoken speech. The motor speech area is also connected with sensory speech area (areas 22, 39 and 40).

### Lesions of Cerebral Cortex

A vascular lesion in different parts of cerebral cortex will be manifested like this:
1. A lesion in the primary motor cortex results in paralysis of all the muscles of the body of the opposite side.
2. A lesion in the pre-frontal area (areas 9 to 12) or its atrophy results in mental dysfunctions like lack of sense of responsibility in personal affairs, vulgarity in speech, clownish behavior.
3. A lesion affecting the sensory association area (area 40) produces tactile agnosia and tactile aphasia.
4. A lesion in the visual association area (area 39 of the dominant hemisphere) produces visual agonosia in which the patient exhibits inability to recognize the known object by vision. The patient also develops sensory aphasia or word blindness and is unable to recognize the written word even when written by the patient himself (also involving the lesion in area 22).
5. A lesion in the auditory association area (area 22) results in word deafness in which affected individual is unable to interpret the word spoken by himself or by others.

## BLOOD SUPPLY TO THE CEREBRUM

The arterial supply to the cerebrum is derived from the branches of internal carotid artery and vertebral artery.

The superolateral surface of the cerebrum is mainly supplied by middle cerebral artery (a branch from internal carotid artery) with following exceptions. a) An area of about one inch breadth along the supero-medial border which is supplied by anterior cerebral artery. b) Occipital lobe and inferior temporal gyrus, which are supplied by posterior cerebral artery. Hence, the middle cerebral artery supplies major part of the motor and sensory areas (except the foot area), the auditory area and speech area (Fig. 30.7).

The medial surface is mainly supplied by anterior cerebral artery (a branch from the internal carotid artery) which also partly supplies the superolateral surface along the superomedial margin of the cerebrum. However, the occipital lobe on medial surface is supplied by posterior cerebral artery. Hence, the anterior cerebral artery supplies the foot area (both motor and sensory) and paracentral lobule, which is a center for micturition and defaecation reflexes (Fig. 30.7)

The inferior surface is supplied by following arteries: The medial part of the orbital surface is supplied by anterior cerebral artery and the lateral part including temporal pole is supplied by middle cerebral artery. The tentorial surface is supplied by posterior cerebral artery (a branch from vertebral artery). Hence, the visual area is supplied by posterior cerebral artery (Fig. 30.7).

## WHITE MATTER OF THE CEREBRUM

The nerve fibers arising from the cerebral cortex passes deep to form the white matter. The white matter also contains fibers ending in different parts of the cortex. This white matter is classified into three types:
1. Association fibers
2. Commissural fibers
3. Projection fibers

### 1. Association Fibers

These fibers connect the cortical areas of the same cerebral hemisphere and are of two types:

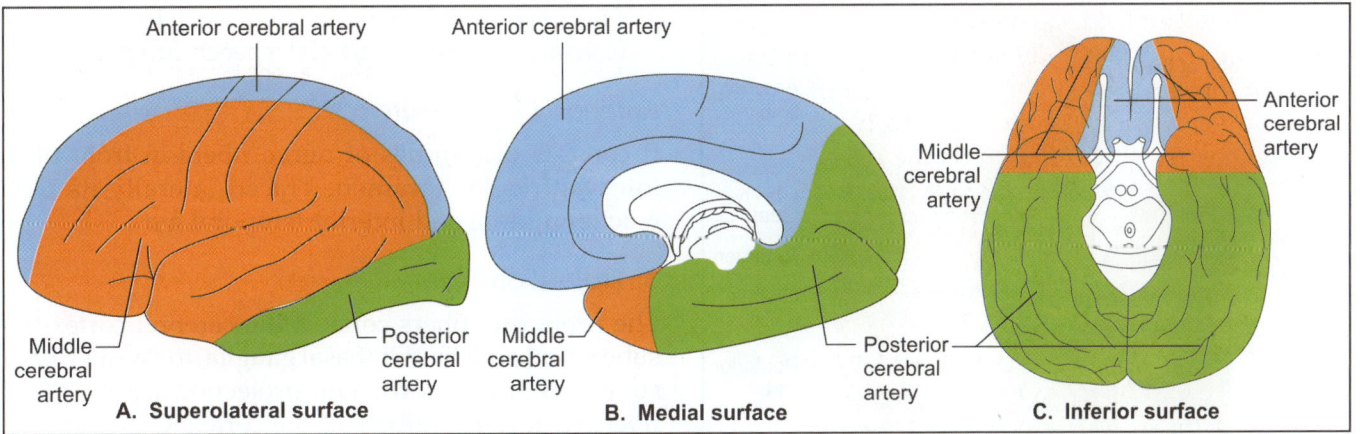

**Fig. 30.7:** Arteries of the cerebral hemisphere

a. *Short association fibers*—which connects the adjacent gyri.

b. *Long association fibers*—which connects the different lobes of the same cerebral hemisphere. Following are the some of the examples for long association fibers: Cingulum, uncinate fasciculus, superior longitudinal fasciculus, inferior longitudinal fasciculus and fronto-occipital fasciculus.

1. *Cingulum:* It is an arched bundle of nerve fibres lies within the cingulated gyrus. It forms the part of Papez circuit which is concerned with recent memory.

2. *Uncinate fasciculus:* It hooks around the floor of the stem of lateral sulcus, and connects the Broca's area (areas 44 and 45) and the orbital surface of the frontal lobe with temporal pole.

3. *Superior longitudinal fasciculus:* It extends between frontal region and occipital region. The visual cortex (area 17) of occipital lobe is connected with frontal eye field.

4. *Inferior longitudinal fasciculus:* It extends longitudinally along the lateral wall of posterior horn of lateral ventricle outside the fibers of optic radiation and tapetum of corpus callosum.

5. *Fronto-occipital fasciculus:* It extends from the frontal pole to occipitotemporal lobes.

## 2. Commissural Fibers

These fibres connect the two cerebral hemispheres across the midline. Most of the fibers connect the identical areas of the two hemispheres. Following are the examples for commissural fibers: Corpus callosum, anterior commissure, posterior commissure, habenular commissure, etc.

## Corpus Callosum (Fig. 30.8a)

- It is a band of commissural fibers connecting two cerebral hemispheres.
- About 300 million myelinated fibers are contained in the corpus callosum in human brain.
- It forms an arched band with upward convexity and it is about 10 cm in length.
- It has the following parts from behind-forwards: The splenium, body or trunk, genu and rostrum. The splenium is the posterior expanded part. Genu is the anterior part, which forms an abrupt bend to continue backward as rostrum.
- The upper surface of the corpus callosum forms the floor of the median longitudinal fissure and is related to anterior cerebral arteries, the lower margin of the falx cerebri with inferior sagittal sinus.
- The lower surface of the corpus callosum forms the roof of lateral ventricle (central part and anterior horn) and hence lined by ependymal cells. Its lower surface is in direct contact with the fornix and also gives attachment to the septum pellucidum.

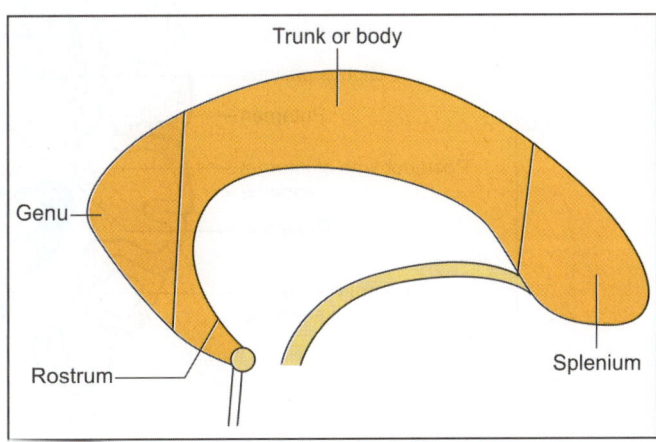

**Fig. 30.8a:** Corpus callosum—parts

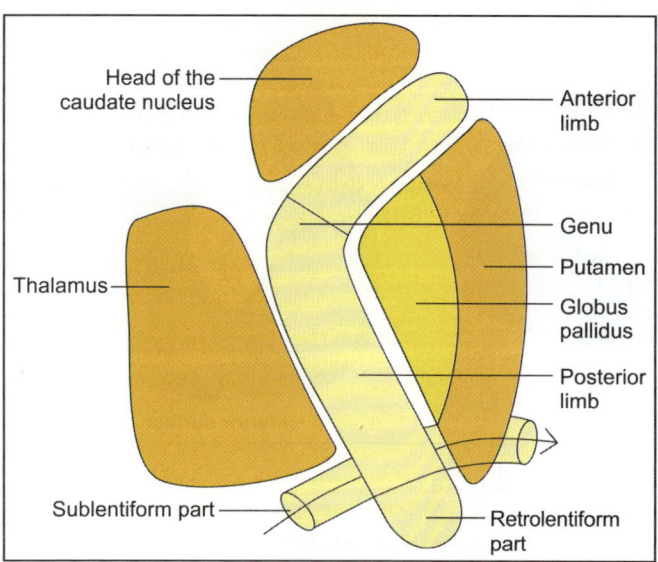

**Fig. 30.8b:** Parts of the internal capsule—schematic

- Forceps minor consists of fibers arising from the genu of the corpus callosum and connects the medial and lateral surfaces of the frontal lobes.
- Tapetum consists of fibers arising from the posterior part of the body. It forms the roof and lateral wall of the posterior horn of the lateral ventricle.
- Forceps major is made up of fibers arising from the splenium and connect the occipital lobes of the two cerebral hemispheres.

- The corpus callosum is involved in transfer of learning processes and also speech functions.

## Anterior Commissure

It consists of bundles of nerve fibers in front of the interventricular foramen. Traced laterally its fibers reaches middle and inferior temporal gyri.

## 3. Projection Fibers

The projection fibers connect the cerebral cortex with subcortical grey matter (basal ganglia, thalamus), brainstem and spinal cord. The projection fibers include fibers to and from fibers of the cortex. Corona radiata and internal capsule are the example for projection fibers.

## Internal Capsule

- It is a bundle of nerve fibers which includes fibers to the cortex as well as from the cortex.
- Traced above, it is continuous with corona radiata, which arises from the cerebral cortex. Traced below the internal capsule is continuous with the crus cerebri of the midbrain.
- The internal capsule is V-shaped in a horizontal section with concavity directed laterally (Fig. 30.8b).
- The internal capsule is bounded medially by head of the caudate nucleus and thalamus, and laterally by lentiform nucleus (Fig. 30.9).

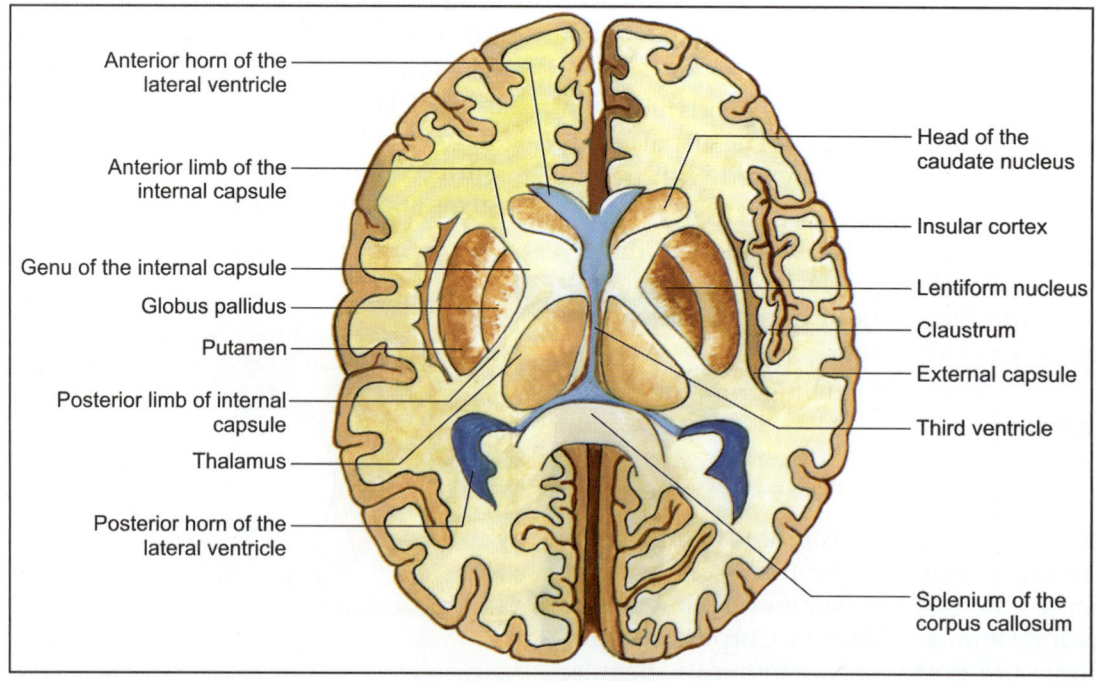

**Fig. 30.9:** Horizontal section of cerebrum showing internal capsule and its relations

- For the purpose of description, the internal capsule is divided into following parts from before backwards: Anterior limb, genu, posterior limb, sublentiform part and retrolentiform part.

- *Anterior limb* consists of following fibers: Frontopontine fibers, anterior thalamic radiation, and some corticostriate fibers.

- *Genu* consists of corticonuclear fibers (these are the fibres arising mainly from the motor and pre-motor areas to the motor nuclei of brainstem).

- *Posterior limb* of the internal capsule consists of many fibers of which the important ones are:
  - Corticospinal tracts (fibers mainly arising from the motor area of the cerebral cortex. They innervate the voluntary muscles of the opposite half of the body through ventral horn cells of the spinal cord. The fibers for the upper limb lying in front, for the trunk in the middle and lower limb behind.
  - Corticorubral fibers
  - Frontopontine and parietopontine fibers
  - Superior thalamic radiation: It consists of fibers mainly arising from ventral posterior group of nucleus of thalamus. The sensory information from the body in the form of many lemnisci (medial, spinal and trigeminal lemniscus) ends in the thalamus. Through the posterior limb of the internal capsule it passes mainly into sensory cortex.

- *Sublentiform part* of the internal capsule consists of auditory radiation. These fibers are derived from medial geniculate body of thalamus and after traversing the internal capsule project to the auditory cortex (areas 41 and 42). The sublentiform part also includes temporopontine and parietopontine fibers.

- *Retrolentiform part* of the internal capsule consists of optic radiation. These fibers are derived from lateral geniculate body of the thalamus and after traversing the internal capsule project to the visual cortex (areas 17 to 19). The retrolentiform part also consists of parietopontine and occipitaopontine fibers.

## Arterial Supply of Internal Capsule

### Anterior Limb

1. Striate branches from anterior cerebral artery
2. Striate branches of middle cerebral artery (Charcot's artery of cerebral hemorrhage)
3. Recurrent branch of anterior cerebral artery (artery of Heubner).

### Genu

1. Striate branch of middle cerebral artery
2. Direct branches from internal carotid artery.

### Posterior Limb

1. Striate branches from middle cerebral artery
2. Anterior choroid artery
3. Branches from posterior cerebral artery.

### Sublentiform Part

1. Anterior choroid artery
2. Posterior cerebral artery

### Retrolentiform Part

1. Posterolateral branches of posterior cerebral artery

## Applied Aspects

These arteries supplying the internal capsule are end arteries and may be involved in cerebrovascular injuries (thrombosis, embolism or hemorrhage) and are of immense clinical importance.

In the presence of high blood pressure, one of the arteries may rupture and cause hemorrhage in the substance of internal capsule producing a "stroke". The corticospinal and corticonuclear fibers of the internal capsule are affected and results in contralateral hemiplegia.

The brain of a newborn is sensitive to oxygen deprivation or excessive oxygen. If complications arise during childbirth and the oxygen supply from the mother's blood to the baby is interrupted while it is still in the birth canal, the infant may be stillborn or suffer brain damage that can result in cerebral palsy, epilepsy, paralysis or mental retardation. Excessive oxygen administered to a newborn may cause blindness.

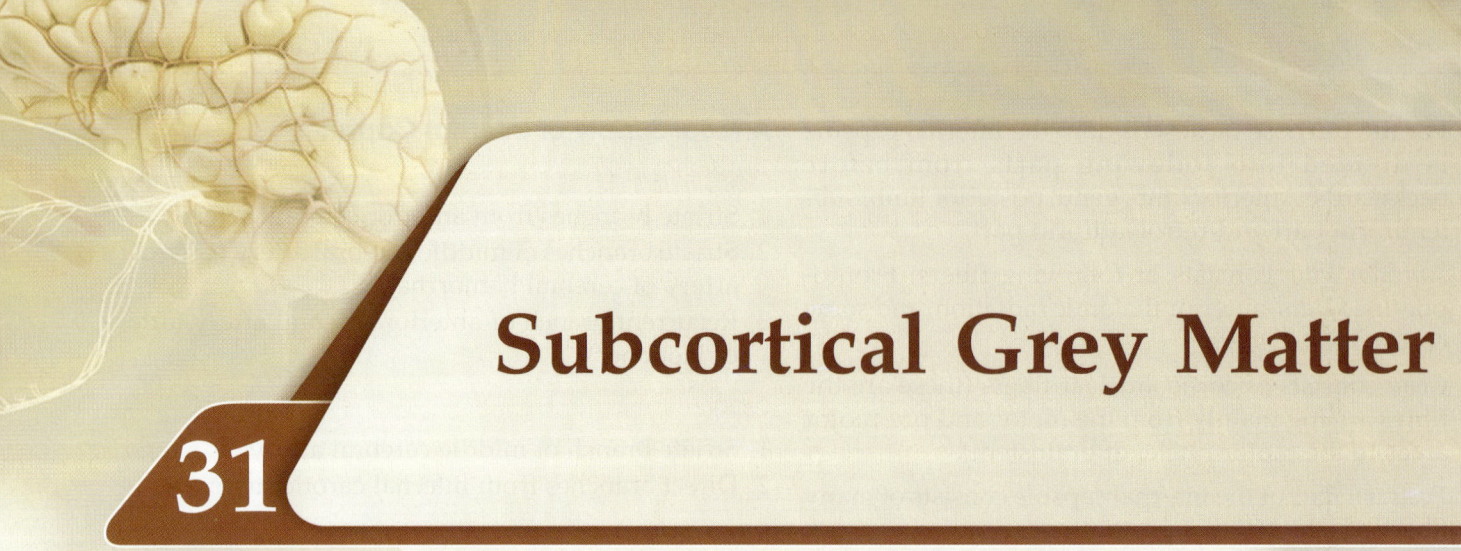

# Subcortical Grey Matter

## 31

As studied earlier, the cerebral cortex consists of outer grey matter (cerebral cortex) and inner white matter. Within the white matter of cerebrum, there are many masses of grey matter, which are referred as subcortical grey matter. It includes basal nuclei (basal ganglia), thalamus, hypothalamus and limbic system.

### BASAL NUCLEI

They consist of three parts:
1. Corpus striatum: It consists of two parts

- Caudate nucleus
- Lentiform nucleus: It is further divided into putamen and globus pallidus.
2. Claustrum
3. Amygdaloid body

### Caudate Nucleus (Figs 31.1 and 31.2)

- It is an arched mass of grey matter consisting of head, body and tail.
- The head is the anterior expanded part and forms the floor of anterior horn of lateral ventricle.

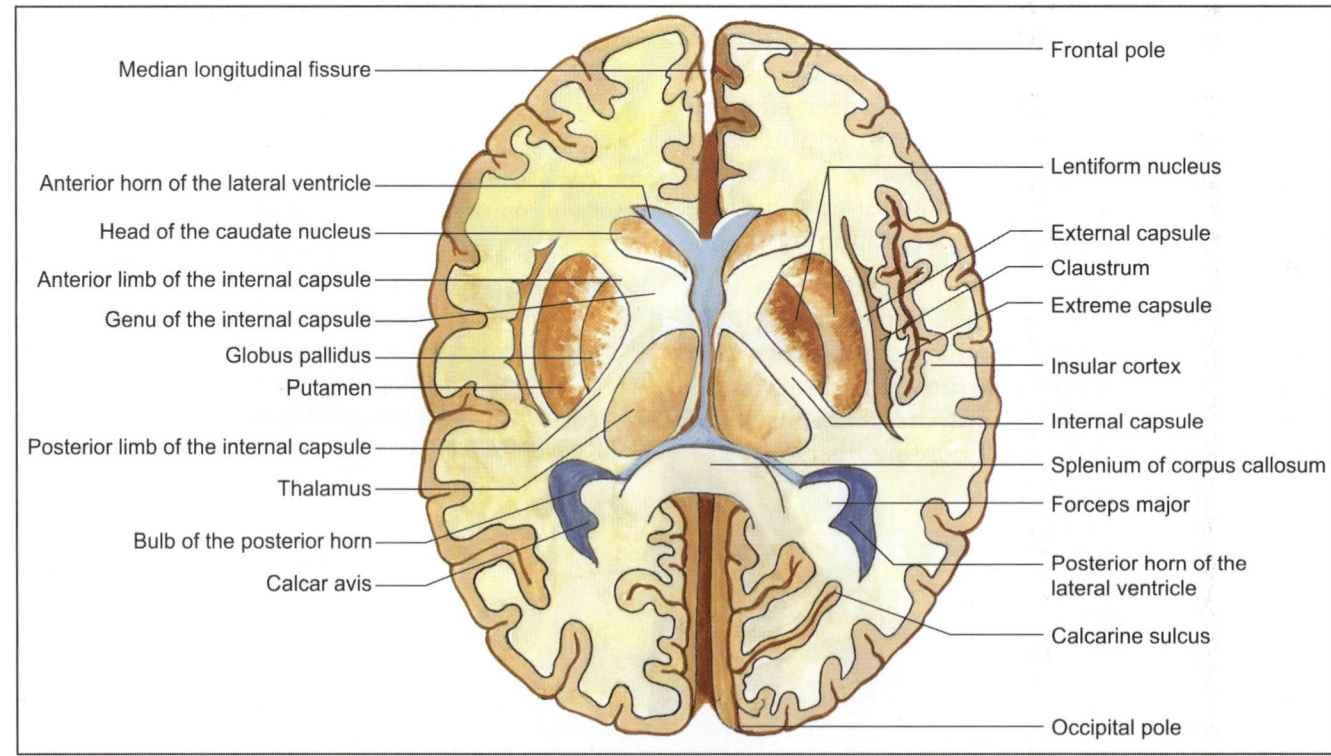

**Fig. 31.1:** Horizontal section of cerebrum at the level of the interventricular foramen (left half) showing parts of the basal ganglia

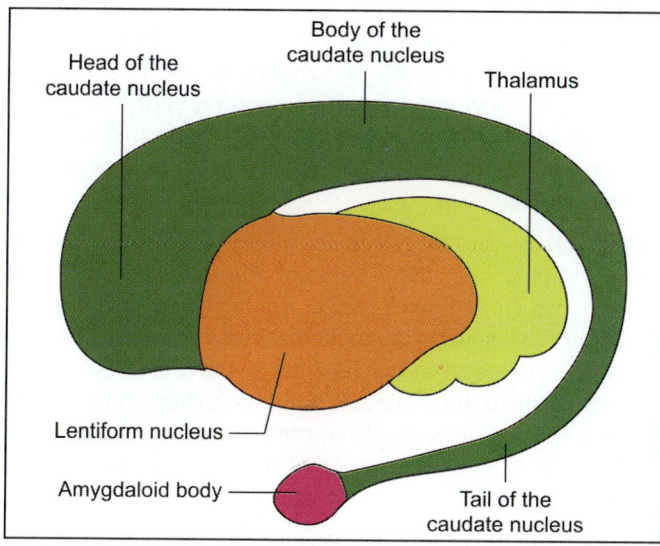

**Fig. 31.2:** Caudate nucleus and amygdaloid body

- The body extends backwards from head and it forms the floor of the central part of the lateral ventricle.
- The tail runs downwards and forwards along the roof of the inferior horn of lateral ventricle. The tail is continuous with amygdaloid body.

## Lentiform Nucleus

- It is a biconvex mass of grey matter placed lateral to the internal capsule.
- The lentiform nucleus is further divided into an outer (lateral) larger part called 'putamen' and inner (medial) smaller part called 'globus pallidus'.
- Lentiform nucleus is covered laterally by external capsule and medially by posterior limb of the internal capsule.
- Above it is related to corona radiata.
- Below it is separated from the inferior horn of the lateral ventricle by the external capsule, sub-lentiform

part of the internal capsule, tail of the caudate nucleus and stria terminalis.

### Claustrum (Fig. 31.1)

It is a thin sheet of grey matter placed lateral to the putamen.

### Amygdaloid Body (Fig. 31.2)

It is also a part of the limbic system and is present in the anterior part of the roof of inferior horn of lateral ventricle. The tail of the caudate nucleus is continuous with the amygdala.

## CONNECTIONS OF CORPUS STRIATUM

The stiatum (caudate nucleus and putamen) receives primarily afferent fibers from many sources but its efferents (output) are mainly to globus pallidus. The globus pallidus conveys information to the motor cortex (areas 4 and 6) through the thalamus and also influences the lower motor neurons, the red nucleus, reticular and other brainstem nuclei to produce integrated motor responses.

### Afferent Fibers to the Striatum

1. *Corticostriate fibers:* Most of the fibers are derived from the ipsilateral sensorimotor cortex. These fibers reach the striatum through external capsule and internal capsule.

2. *Thalamostriate fibers:* Fibers are derived from centromedian nucleus, intralaminar and midline nuclei.

3. *Nigrostriate fibers:* Fibers arise from pars compacta of substantia nigra and are projected to caudate nucleus, putamen and partly to globus pallidus. These fibers are dopaminergic and exert inhibitory influence to the striatal and pallidal neurons.

### Connections of basal ganglia

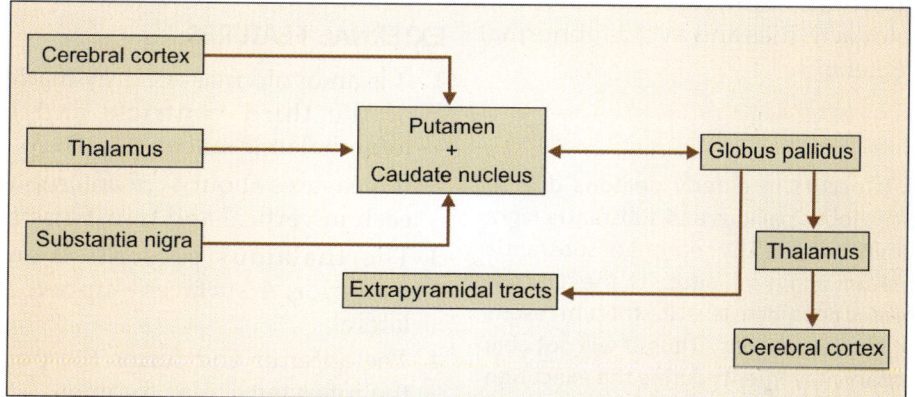

### Efferent Fibers from Striatum

1. Striopallidal fibers are connected to the globus pallidus.
2. Some fibers from the striatum enter the thalamus.
3. Strionigral fibers connect the striatal neurons with the pars reticularis of substantia nigra, and convey neurotransmitter substance GABA (gamma amino-butyric acid) which inhibits the dopaminergic neurons of the pars compacta of substantia nigra.

### Afferent Fibers to the Pallidum

1. The globus pallidus receives afferents mainly from the striatum and partly from the pars compacta of the substantia nigra.
2. The inner segment of the globus pallidus receives fibers from subthalamic nucleus.

### Efferents from the Pallidum

1. Fasciculus lenticularis
2. Ansa lenticularis

   These two efferent tracks joins to form fasciculus thalamicus to terminate in the ventral anterior and ventral lateral nuclei of thalamus.
3. Fasciculus subthalamicus

   It consists of both afferent and efferent fibers, and connects the globus pallidus with the subthalamic nucleus.
4. Pallidotegmental fibers

   These fibers terminate in the red nucleus of the midbrain, reticular nuclei of brainstem and inferior olivary nucleus of medulla. By these connections the basal ganglia exert influence on the lower motor neurons.

### Functions

1. Basal ganglia control the extrapyramidal motor pathway, which influences the lower motor neurons of brainstem and spinal cord.
2. Through its connections with cerebral cortex, it modulates the motor activities and avoids abnormal involuntary movements.

### Applied Aspects

**Parkinson's disease:** It occurs in elderly persons due to degenerative changes in globus pallidus and substantia nigra of midbrain. The dopamine secreted by neurons of substantia nigra is released in striatum and is inhibitory to the neurons of striatum. The diminished dopamine level in striatum results in excitatory actions of striatal neurons. Thus, it will not able to suppress the involuntary movements during the execution of purposeful acts. It is characterized with rigidity and tremor (when subject is at rest). The rigidity is due to increased muscle tone. Slowness in initiating and repeating voluntary movement is the characteristic feature of Prkinson's disease. All other clinical manifestation of basal nuclei are hyperkinetic and hypotonic.

**Chorea:** It is characterized by brisk, jerky, purposeless movements of the distal parts of the extremities. These movements are irregular, rapid, uncontrolled, involuntary. When chorea is severe, the movements may cause movement of the arms or legs that results in throwing whatever is in the hand or falling to the ground. Huntington's chorea occurs with massive bilateral loss of cells of the head of the caudate and putamen. It is due to decrease of GABA in the striatonigral neurons.

**Hemiballism:** It is usually characterized by involuntary violent flinging (throwing) motions (wild flail-like movements) of the limbs on one side (when both sides are involved, then called ballism). It occurs due to degenerative changes in the subthalamic neurons.

**Athetosis:** It is characterized by slow worm-like writhing (twisting) movements of the limbs. A constant succession of slow, writhing, involuntary movements of flexion, extension, pronation, and supination of the fingers and hands, and sometimes of the toes and feet. The lesion occurs at putamen.

## THALAMUS

The third ventricle divides the diencephalon into two symmetrical halves. A hypothalamic sulcus, extending from the interventricular foramen to the upper end of aqueduct of the midbrain, divides each half of the diencephalon into dorsal and ventral parts.

The dorsal part includes the thalamus, epithalamus (pineal body) and metathalamus (lateral and medial geniculate bodies).

The ventral part includes the hypothalamus and subthalamus.

### EXTERNAL FEATURES

1. It is an ovoid mass of grey matter in the lateral wall of the third ventricle and lies dorsal to the hypothalamic sulcus (Fig. 31.3).
2. It measures about 4 cm anteroposteriorly and 1.5 cm each in vertical and transverse measurements.
3. The thalamus presents 2 ends—anterior and posterior, 4 surfaces—upper, lower, medial, and lateral.
4. The anterior end forms the posterior boundary of the interventricular foramen.

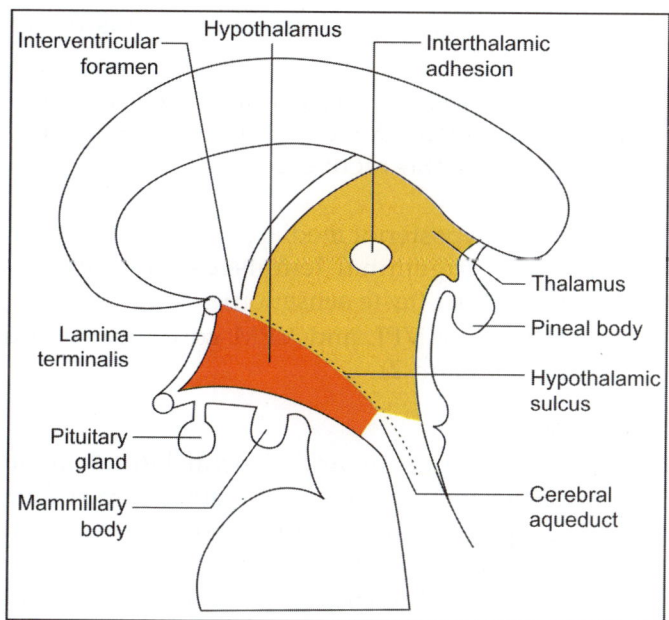

**Fig. 31.3:** Thalamus and hypothalamus

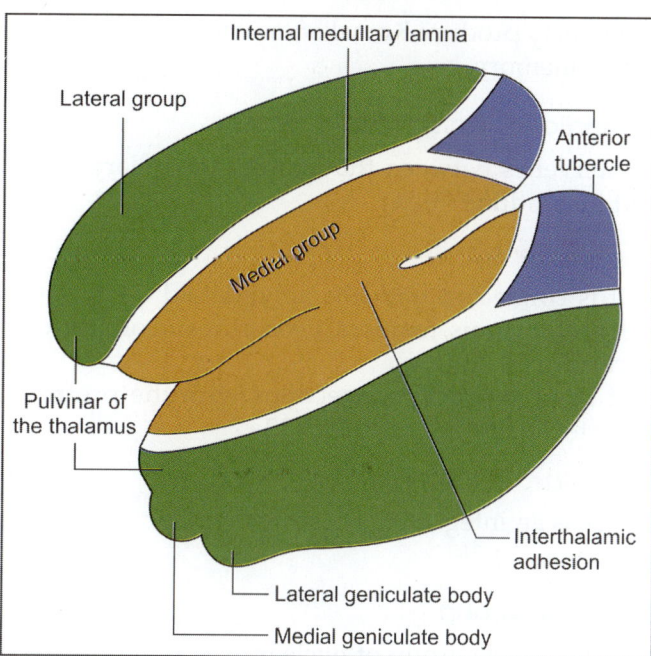

**Fig. 31.4:** Right and left thalamus

5. The posterior end is expanded to form pulvinar. It presents lateral geniculate body inferolaterally and medial geniculate body inferomedially.

The medial geniculate body is separated from the pulvinar by superior brachium.

6. The upper surface of the thalamus is covered by a thin sheet of white matter, the stratum zonale. The upper surface is divided into lateral and medial areas by the free margin of the body of the fornix. The lateral area forms the floor of the central part of the lateral ventricle and is covered by ependyma. Laterally it is related to stria terminalis (bundle of nerve fibers) and thalamostriate vein. The medial area of the upper surface is separated from the body of the fornix (*see* Fig. 32.2a) by the tela choroidea of the third ventricle.

7. The lower surface is related to zona incerta and sub-thalamic nucleus (subthalamus and hypothalamus).

8. The medial surface forms the lateral wall of the third ventricle. It is connected to the other thalamus by interthalamic adhesion (*see* Fig. 32.2a).

9. The lateral surface of thalamus is separated from the lentiform nucleus by the posterior limb of the internal capsule. This lateral surface is covered by a thin sheet of white matter called external medullary lamina.

## INTERNAL FEATURES OF THALAMUS

A vertical sheet of white matter, the internal medullary lamina divides the thalamus into medial and lateral nuclear masses; rostrally the lamina splits in Y-shaped manner to enclose the anterior group of nuclei.

The neurons (nuclei) of thalamus are divided into following groups, which have specific connections and functions (Fig. 31.4).

1. Anterior group
2. Medial group
3. Lateral group
4. Intralaminar group lie within the internal medullary lamina
5. Reticular group: It forms a thin sheet of nuclear mass which envelope the ventrolateral aspect of thalamus, and intervenes between the external medullary lamina and the posterior limb of internal capsule.
6. Midline group intervenes between the ependymal lining of third ventricle and the medial nucleus.

## 1. Anterior Group

It intervenes between the diverging limbs of the internal medullary lamina.

### Connections

- It has reciprocal connections with the mammillary body via mammillothalamic tract.
- It receives fibers from the column of the fornix.
- It is connected with hebanular nucleus through stria medullaris thalami.
- It is connected with cingulate gyrus.

### Functions

The anterior group is incorporated in the Papez circuit of limbic system, and a lesion affecting the anterior

31

group may produce Korsakoff's syndrome with loss of recent memory.

## 2. Medial or Dorso Medial Group

It intervenes between the internal medullary lamina and the midline nuclei.

### Connections

- It is connected with the amygdaloid body, lateral hypothalamus, temporal neocortex and orbitofrontal cortex.
- It has reciprocal connections with the prefrontal cortex including areas 9 to 12.

### Function

It acts as an integrating center for somatic and visceral impulses.

## 3. Lateral Group

It is the largest group of nuclear masses and its nuclei are arranged in ventral and dorsal parts.

The ventral part consists of ventral anterior, ventral lateral, ventral posterior—which is further divided into medial and lateral.

The dorsal part presents lateral dorsal, lateral posterior and pulvinar.

### Connections

1. *Ventral anterior*
   It receives fibers from substantia nigra, globus pallidus, brainstem of the reticular formation.
   It sends fibers to pre motor cortex, orbitofrontal cortex.
2. *Ventral lateral*
   It receives fibers from dentate nucleus of cerebellum, red nucleus of midbrain, globus pallidus, substantia

nigra. Its efferents go to precentral gyrus (motor area).

3. *Ventral posterior*
   1. The ventral posterior lateral (VPL) receives fibers from the medial lemniscus and spinal lemniscus.
   2. The ventral posterior medial (VPM) receives fibers from the trigeminal lemniscus and solitario-thalamic tract (taste sensation).

The efferents of VPL and VPM go to post-central gyrus (areas 3, 1 and 2).

### Functions

1. The ventral anterior and ventral lateral nuclei receives information from motor areas of the frontal lobe, corpus striatum and substantia nigra. In degenerative lesions of the basal ganglia, the thalamic nuclei discharge abnormally and give rise to dyskinesia.
2. The ventral lateral nucleus convey impulses from the cerebellum and basal ganglia to the motor cortex and exerts its role as a prime mover of the motor pathway. Surgical ablation of VL may abolish the tremor and rigidity of Parkinson's disease.
3. The ventral posterior nucleus acts as the largest specific somatosensory relay nucleus of the thalamus.

## Medial Geniculate Body (MGB)

- It receives auditory input from both ears from lateral lemniscus through inferior colliculus.
- Most of its fibers are projected to the primary auditory cortex through sublentiform part of the internal capsule.

**Connections of thalamus**

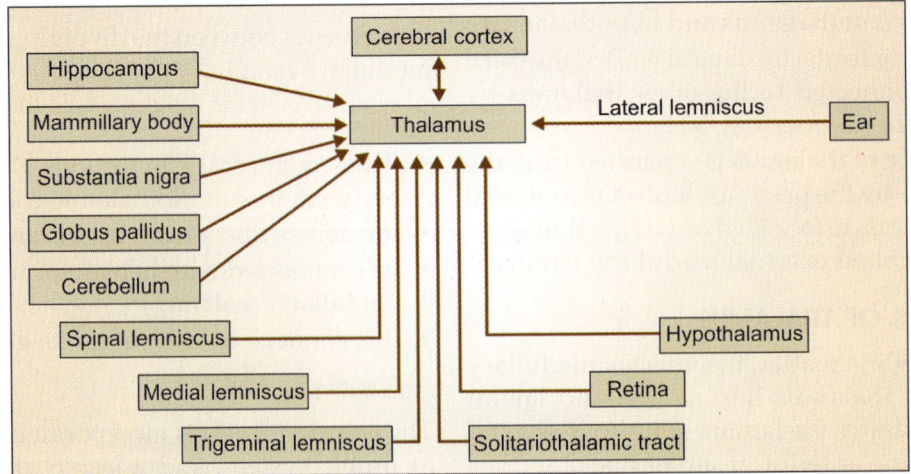

## Lateral Geniculate Body (LGB)

- It receives fibers from optic tract (retinofugal fibers). Crossed fibers of the tract terminate in layers 1, 4, 6 and uncrossed fibers in layers 2, 3, 5.
- The output fibers form optic radiation, which project into primary visual cortex of the occipital lobe through retrolentiform part of the internal capsule.

## Functions of Thalamus

- All the sensory informations are processed and integrated in the thalamus before reaching the cerebral cortex.
- Through the reticular system (ascending reticular activating system) it is responsible for wakefulness and alertness.
- Thalamus is concerned with interpretation of crude sensations like pain and temperature.
- Thalamus also regulates the motor activity by its connections with motor cortex, cerebellum and globus pallidus.

## Applied Aspects

**Thalamic syndrome**

It occurs due to the vascular lesion of the thalamus. The threshold for sensation like touch, pain and temperature is raised (exaggerated) on the opposite side. A pin-prick may be felt as intolerable pain. The patient with eyes closed is unable to locate the position of a limb.

### HYPOTHALAMUS

This mass of grey matter is placed ventral to the thalamus on either side of third ventricle.

- Anteroinferiorly the hypothalamus forms the floor of the third ventricle and has the following structures from before backward, optic chiasma, stalk of the pituitary gland and mammillary bodies.
- The neurons (nuclei) of hypothalamus are also divided into many groups depending on their location, connection and functions. Some of these nuclei are preoptic, supraoptic and paraventricular.
- *Preoptic region:* It is located just caudal to and along the lamina terminalis.
- *Supraoptic region:* It lies above the optic chiasma and is continuous with preoptic area. This region presents following nuclei—supraoptic, paraventricular, anterior and suprachiasmatic.
- *Tuberal region:* It lies above the tuber cinerium, is widest in extent.

- *Mammillary region:* It includes a pair of mammillary bodies.
- *Medial forebrain bundle:* It forms the major pathway of the hypothalamus. It consists of ascending and descending fibers to and from the hypothalamus. The ascending fibers arise from the midbrain and project to the lateral hypothalamic and preoptic nuclei. The descending fibers extend from the orbitofrontal cortex, septal area, olfactory tubercle and piriform cortex to lateral hypothalamic zone and preoptic nuclei.
- *Locus coeruleus:* It is an area rich in norepinephrine neurons in the upper part of the floor of the fourth ventricle. The major output pathway from this neuronal mass ascends into cerebellum and cerebrum. Fibers on its way to cerebrum give collateral fibers to thalamus, hypothalamus, hippocampus. These projections modify the behavior of arousal and alertness.
- Serotonin is another brain amine from the raphe nuclei of pons and lower midbrain terminates in hypothalamus. They regulate the sleep-wake cycle, because total insomnia develops when the serotonin levels are depleted.
- Fibers from hippocampus and septal area mainly terminate in mammillary nucleus and preoptic nucleus.
- The mammillothalamic tract connects with the anterior nuclei of thalamus and projected to the cingulate gyrus thus forming a part of the Papez circuit.
- Fibers from amygdaloid body and piriform cortex reach the hypothalamus by stria terminalis.
- Hypothalamo-hypophyseal tract is composed of 100,000 unmyelinated fibers and is derived from the axons of supraoptic and paraventricular nuclei of the hypothalamus. The fibers of the tract pass to neurohypophysis (posterior lobe of pituitary) through the infundibular stem.

The cells of the supraoptic and paraventricular nuclei secrete vasopressin (anti-diuretic hormone—ADH) and oxytocin and these hormones are conveyed to the posterior lobe of the pituitary gland.

### Functions

- The hypothalamo-hypophyseal tract has axons of the neurons derived from supraoptic and paraventricular nuclei of hypothalamus. Neurons of supraoptic nucleus secrete 'vasopressin' which regulates the water reabsorption from the distal convoluted tubules of nephrons. The neurons of paraventricular group secrete 'oxytocin' which

**Connections**

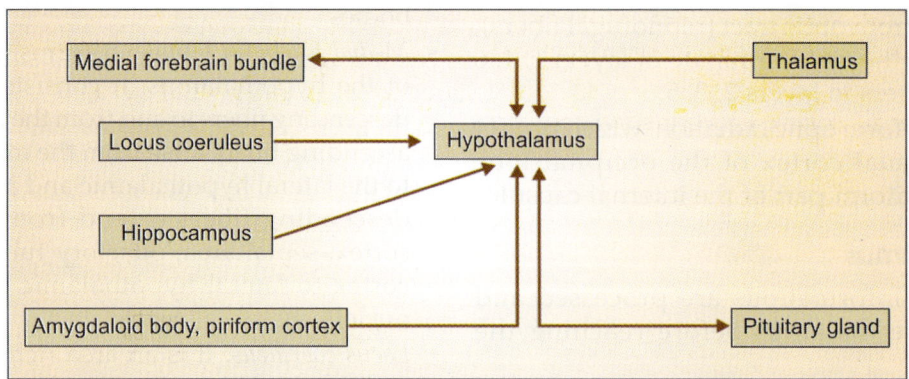

stimulates the contraction of myoepithelial cells surrounding the alveoli of lactating mammary gland (milk ejection) and also acts on musculature of uterus.

- Hypothalamus controls both components (sympathetic and parasympathetic) of autonomic nervous system and thus helps in maintaining the constant body environment (homeostasis).
- Hypothalamus regulates the body temperature.
- Hypothalamus regulates the food and water intake response. The hunger, thirst and satiety centers are located in the hypothalamus.
- Hypothalamus regulates the sexual behavior.
- Physical expression of emotion is mediated by hypothalamus (physical expression involves aggressive and fear response, feeling of pleasure and displeasure, etc.).
- Hypothalamus maintains the circadian rhythm (sleep-wake cycle).

## LIMBIC SYSTEM

Emotional behavior of the human being is dependent on olfaction, vision, hearing, taste and influence of psychic cortex. Broca introduced the name 'limbic system' for a series of structures, which are involved in higher functions of human beings like movement for procuring food, aggression for self defense, sex urge for mating, rearing the younger generation, etc.

Following are the parts of the limbic system:
1. *Hippocampal formation:* It includes indusium griseum (with longitudinal striae and gyrus fasciolaris), dentate gyrus and hippocampus.
2. Amygdaloid body and its efferent pathway—stria terminalis.
3. Olfactory pathway and olfactory area
4. Cingulate gyrus, septal area

5. Hypothalamus
6. Pyriform lobe (including uncus and entorhinal area)
7. Some parts of the thalamus and midbrain.

### HIPPOCAMPUS

It presents an elongated mass of grey matter along the floor of the inferior horn of the lateral ventricle. The anterior end of the hippocampus presents an enlarged mass with oblique grooves called pes hippocampi. The ventricular surface of the hippocampus is lined by ependymal cells.

The hippocampus is produced by the complex infoldings of dentate gyrus, cornu ammonis and subiculum. On cross section, the hippocampus is C-shaped in outline.

The axons of the pyramidal cells of the hippocampus form a thin sheet of white matter called 'alveus'. The fibers of alveus converge along the medial margin of hippocampus and form fimbria of the hippocampus. Fimbria precedes backwards overlapping dentate gyrus and on reaching the splenium of corpus callosum is continuous with fornix.

### Connections of Hippocampus

1. It receives fibers from cingulate gyrus, septal nuclei and from the entorhinal area (parahippocampal gyrus).
2. The major efferent (output) fibers from hippocampus are the fornix. The fornix begins as continuation of alveus and fimbria and is formed mainly by the axons of the pyramidal cells of hippocampus. On reaching the splenium of the corpus callosum, the fibers of the fimbria sweeps forwards below the splenium and form of a pair of crura of the fornix. The crura proceed forward and converge to form the body of the fornix. On reaching the interventricular foramen the body of the fornix diverges into a pair

of columns of fornix. Some fibers descend in front of the anterior commissure and are called pre-commissural fornix. It terminates in paraterminal gyrus.

The postcommissural fornix descends behind the anterior commissure to reach the mammillary body.

Thus, a neuronal circuit is established, as postulated by Papez, and includes the following:

- Hippocampus—fimbria and fornix
- Mammillary body—anterior nucleus of thalamus
- Cingulate gyrus—hippocampus.

This circuit is presumably responsible for emotional integration and for recent memory trace.

## Amygdaloid Body

- It is a collection of nuclear masses and lies in the roof of the inferior horn of the lateral ventricle. It is continuous behind with the tail of the caudate nucleus.
- It receives input from olfactory system via lateral olfactory stria and also from parahippocampal gyrus.
- The fibers of stria terminalis form the major output fibers from the amygdala, which proceeds backwards along the roof of the inferior horn of the lateral ventricle. Then the stria turns forward and runs along the floor of the central part of the lateral ventricle. Finally the fibers of the stria terminalis terminates in septal nuclei and hypothalamus.

## Olfactory Pathway and Olfactory Area

It includes olfactory nerves, bulbs, tracts and striae, pyriform area, anterior perforated substance and septal area in the paraterminal gyrus.

- The gyrus ambiens and the lateral olfactory gyrus form together the pre-pyriform region.
- The pre-pyriform region and entorhinal area (area 28) are collectively known as the pyriform lobe.
- Primary olfactory cortex—anterior perforated substance, lateral olfactory gyrus, gyrus ambiens and corticomedial part of the amygdaloid body.
- Secondary olfactory cortex—entorhinal area.

## Functions of Limbic System

- Along with hypothalamus and brainstem, limbic system is required for self-defensive responses, which is necessary for the survival of the individual as well as the species. It includes:
- Procuring food and drink
- Aggressive, defensive and flight responses
- Sex urge for mating (reproduction of species), rearing of the young.
- The higher functions of human brain like feeling of fear, anger, pleasure and physical expression of these status.

Hippocampus of the limbic system is involved in retaining the recent memory. A condition called 'Korsakoff's syndrome' in which there is loss of recent memory due to lesions in hippocampus or in Papez circuit.

# Ventricles of the Brain

- Ventricles are the cavities of brain lined by ependymal cells and filled with cerebrospinal fluid (CSF). Each cerebral hemisphere presents a C-shaped cavity called 'lateral ventricle'.
- A midline cavity between the two thalami is called 'third ventricle'.
- Another cavity posterior to the pons and upper part of medulla and anterior to cerebellum is called 'fourth ventricle' (Fig. 32.1).

The cerebrospinal fluid (CSF) presents inside these cavities circulates into subarachnoid space around brain and spinal cord.

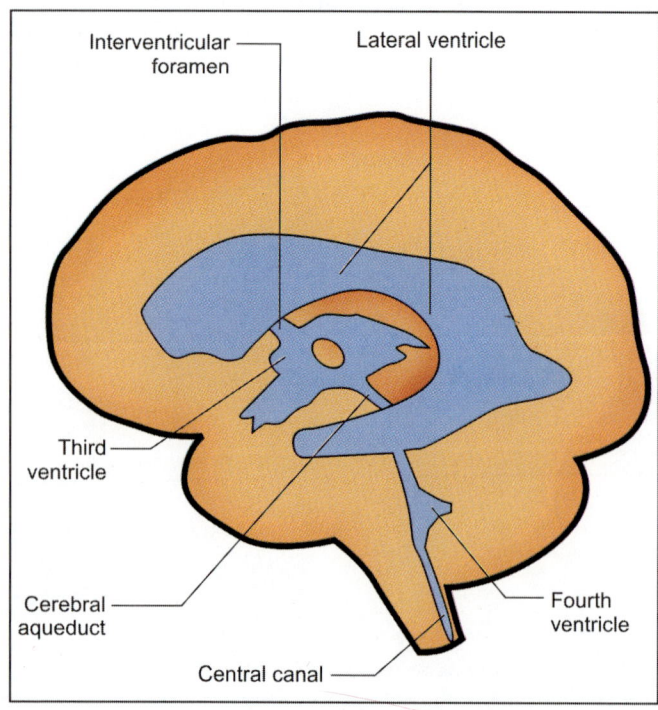

**Fig. 32.1:** Ventricles of the brain

## LATERAL VENTRICLE

Each lateral ventricle is a roughly C-shaped cavity in the cerebral hemisphere. The right and left lateral ventricles are separated by a membranous partition called 'septum pellucidum'. Each lateral ventricle communicates below with third ventricle through interventricular foramen (foramen of Monro). Each lateral ventricle consists of body (central part) and three horns—anterior, posterior and inferior (Fig. 32.1).

1. *The central part* (body) is triangular in coronal section. It extends from interventricular foramen to the splenium of the corpus callosum. It has following boundaries (Fig. 32.2a).

*Roof:* Under surface of the body of the corpus callosum.

*Floor:* It slopes downwards and medially. It is formed by (lateral to medial).

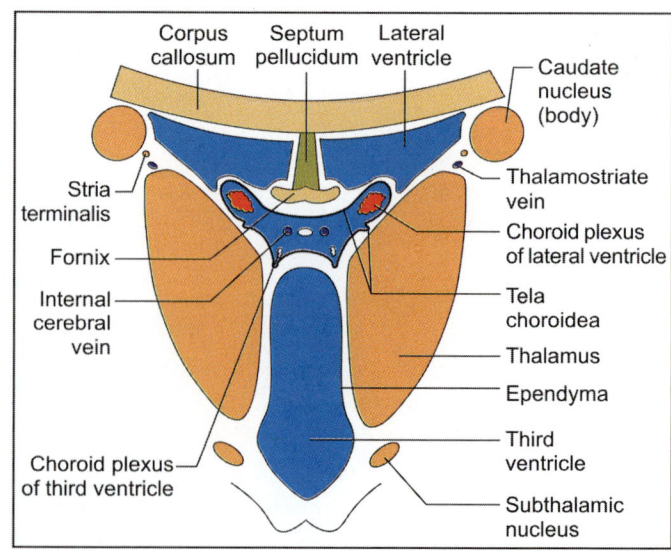

**Fig. 32.2a:** Central part of the lateral ventricle (coronal section)

330

a. Body of the caudate nucleus

b. Upper surface of thalamus

Stria terminalis and thalamostriate vein occupying between them.

*Medially:* Anterior part of the septum pellucidum, but more behind roof and floor meet because the body of the corpus callosum comes in direct contact with the body of the fornix.

Choroid plexus projects into the body of lateral ventricle through a choroid fissure between the upper surface of the thalamus and lower border of the body of the fornix.

2. *The anterior horn* is an extension into the frontal lobe. On coronal section, it is also triangular in shape (Fig. 32.2b).

*Roof:* Under surface of anterior part of corpus callosum.

*Floor:* Formed by rostrum of the corpus callosum medially and head of the caudate nucleus laterally.

*Medially:* Septum pellucidum.

*Anteriorly:* Genu of the corpus callosum.

3. *The posterior horn* is the backward extension into the occipital lobe (Fig. 32.2c).

*Roof and lateral wall:* Tapetum (fibers of corpus callosum), which separates optic radiation from the lateral wall of the posterior horn.

*Medial wall and floor:* It shows two elevations.

The upper elevation is called **bulb of the posterior horn** and it is produced by forceps major (fibers of splenium of the corpus callosum).

The lower elevation is called **calcar avis** and it is formed by anterior part of the calcarine sulcus.

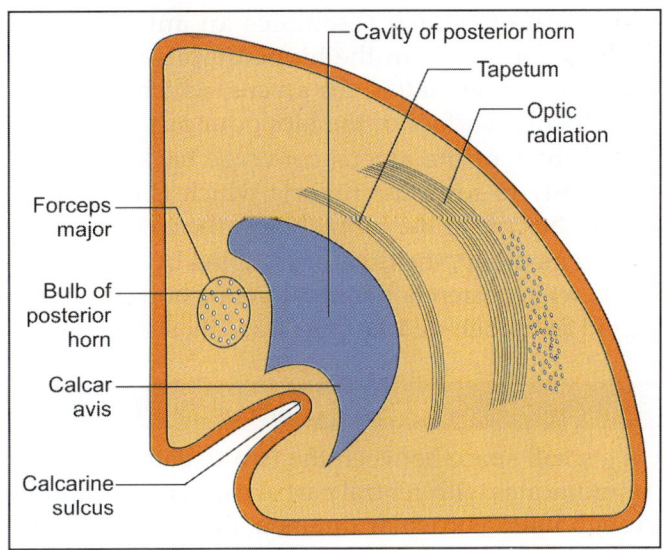

**Fig. 32.2c:** Posterior horn of the lateral ventricle (coronal section)

4. *The inferior horn* is the downward and forward extension into the temporal lobe. It presents roof and floor (Fig. 32.2d).

*Roof:* Tapetum of corpus callosum on the lateral side and tail of caudate nucleus, amygdaloid body and stria terminalis on the medial side.

*Floor:* It shows two structures.

a. An elevation on the lateral side called 'collateral eminence', which is produced by inward projection of the intermediate part of the collateral sulcus.

b. Hippocampus is a prominent longitudinal elevation and lies medial to the collateral eminence. Hippocampus is a part of limbic system. Its enlarged anterior end with oblique grooves is known as pes

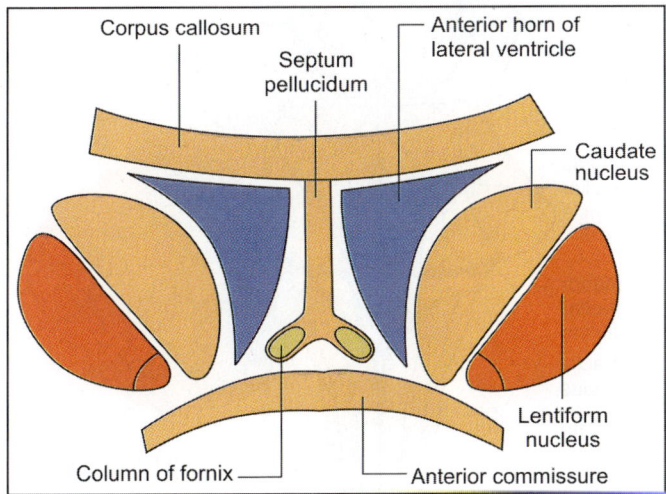

**Fig. 32.2b:** Anterior horn of the lateral ventricle (coronal section)

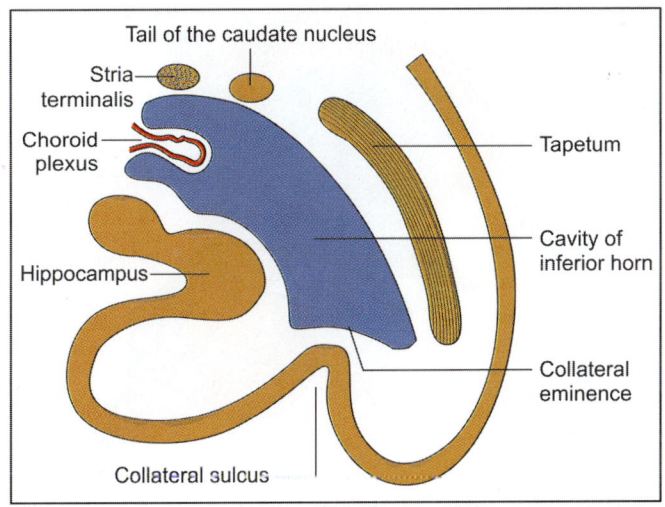

**Fig. 32.2d:** Inferior horn of the lateral ventricle (coronal section)

hippocampi which resembles an animal's paw. Fibers derived from the hippocampus form a thin sheet of white matter, the alveus, which covers the ventricular surface of the hippocampus.

c. The fibers of the alveus converge backwards and medially to form the fimbria which is continuous with the crus of the fornix below the splenium.

Most medially, the floor is occupied by the choroid plexus which extends into the inferior horn through a choroid fissure between the fimbria and the stria terminalis.

## THIRD VENTRICLE

It is a small space between the two thalami. Above, it communicates with central part of each lateral ventricle through interventricular foramen. Below it communicates with the fourth ventricle through cerebral aqueduct of the midbrain. The third ventricle presents roof, floor, anterior and posterior walls and two lateral walls (Fig. 32.3).

The roof is formed by a double-layered pia mater (tela choroidea), which is lined below by ependymal cells. The choroid plexus projects downwards from the roof. The floor presents from before backwards

a. The optic chiasma
b. Tuber cinereum and infundibulum
c. A pair of mammillary bodies
d. Posterior perforated substance
e. Subthalamus (upper extension of tegmentum of midbrain)

*Anterior wall:* It is limited by a membrane called lamina terminalis, which extends from the optic chiasma below to the rostrum of the corpus callosum above.

*Posterior wall:* It presents stalk of the pineal gland and commencement of cerebral aqueduct. The stalk of the pineal gland is divided into upper and lower laminae by pineal recess. The upper lamina contains habenular commissure and lower lamina posterior commissure. Each lateral wall is formed by medial surface of thalamus and hypothalamus. These two structures are demarcated by 'hypothalamic sulcus'.

## FOURTH VENTRICLE

- It is the cavity of hindbrain located anterior to the cerebellum and posterior to the pons and upper part of medulla oblongata (Fig. 32.4a and b).
- The fourth ventricle is roughly diamond-shaped and presents roof (dorsal wall), floor (ventral wall), and two lateral angles—superior and inferior.
- The superior angle is continuous with cerebral aqueduct of midbrain. The inferior angle continuous with central canal of lower part of medulla. Each lateral angle is prolonged laterally behind the inferior cerebellar peduncle. At its lateral end, it presents an opening called foramen of Luschka (lateral aperture). Through this opening the cerebrospinal fluid from the fourth ventricle passes into subarachnoid space.
- The roof (dorsal surface) is tent shaped. The upper part of the roof is formed by two superior cerebellar peduncles and 'superior medullary velum' between them. The lower part of the roof is formed by enpendymal cells lining pia mater (ventral lamina of tela choroidea of fourth ventricle).

The lower part of the roof presents a median aperture, the foramen of Magendie through, which CSF

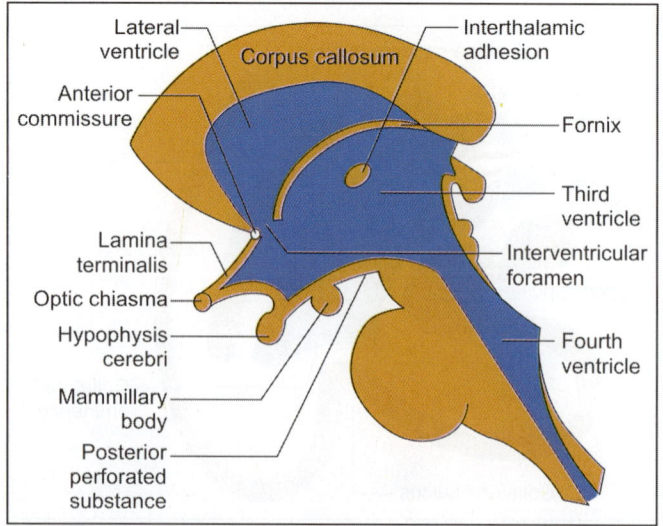

**Fig. 32.3:** Third ventricle—lateral view

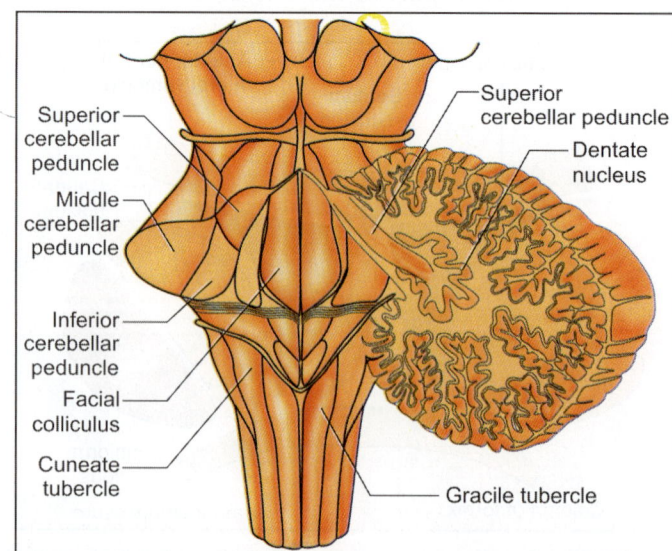

**Fig. 32.4a:** Fourth ventricle—superolateral boundary

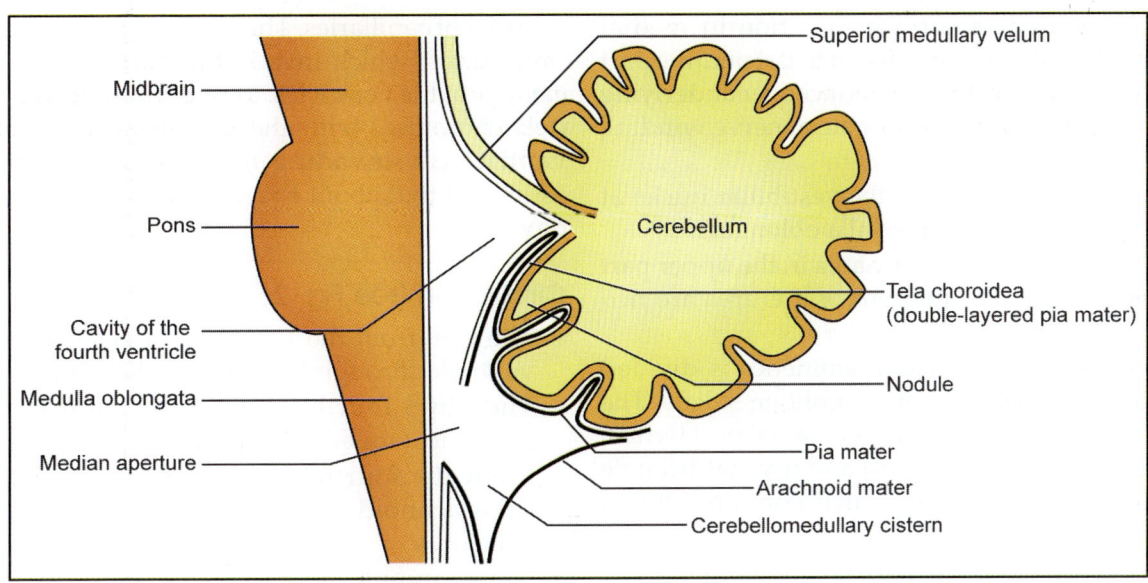

**Fig. 32.4b:** Fourth ventricle—mid-sagittal section

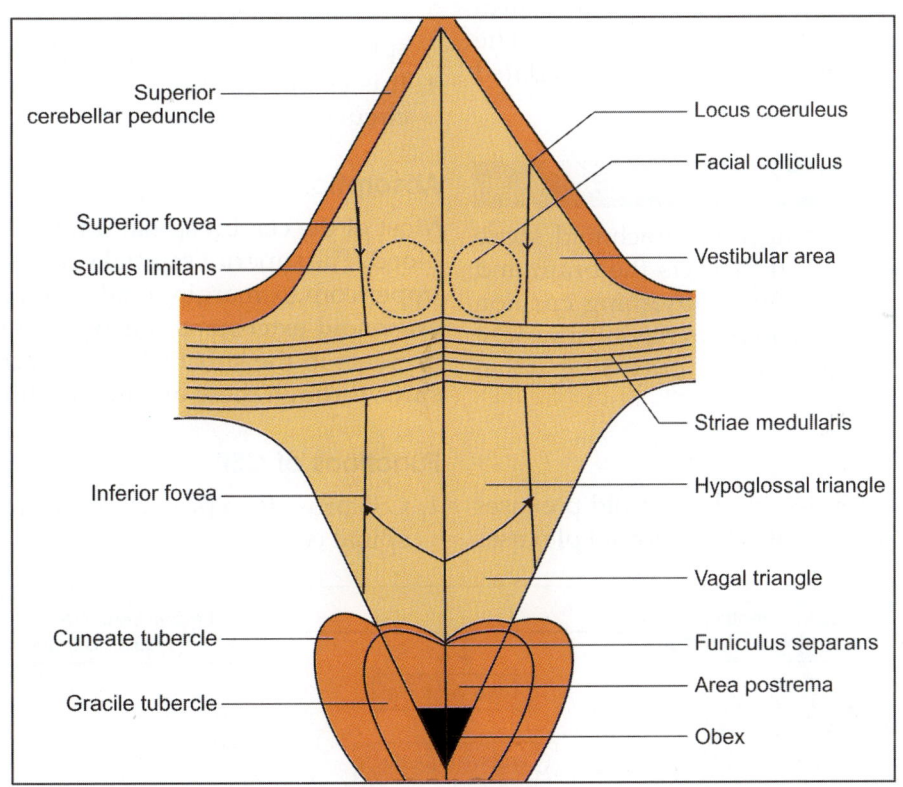

**Fig. 32.5:** Floor of the fourth ventricle

passes into subarachnoid space. The floor (ventral wall) of the fourth ventricle is also called **rhomboid fossa** (since it is diamond-shaped in outline) (Fig. 32.5).
1. The floor is divided into right and left symmetrical halves by a 'median sulcus', which extends from superior to inferior angle.

2. Each half is further divided by 'sulcus limitans' sinto a medial area called medial eminence and a lateral vestibular area. The sulcus limitans shows two depressions above and below called the superior and inferior foveae.

3. Facial colliculus is a surface elevation in medial eminence opposite superior fovea in the pontine part of the floor. This elevation is produced by underlying abducent nucleus and fibers of facial nerve winding around it.
4. The vestibular area overlies the vestibular nuclei at the junction of pons and medulla oblongata.
5. Locus coeruleus is bluish grey area in the upper part of sulcus limitans. The neurons of this area are rich in norepinephrine.
6. The lower part of the medial eminence is divided into two triangular areas by an oblique sulcus. The hypoglossal triangle in the upper medial part (which contains hypoglossal nucleus) and a vagal triangle in the lower lateral part (which contains dorsal nucleus of vagus).
7. Stria medullaris are a few horizontally placed white fibers crossing the floor of the ventricle from the median sulcus.
8. Area postrema is an area in the floor of the fourth ventricle inferolateral to the vagal triangle. The vomiting and respiratory centers are closely related to this area.

## CEREBROSPINAL FLUID (CSF)

Cerebrospinal fluid is present in subarachnoid space and ventricles of the brain. It protects the brain and spinal cord by providing a shock-absorbing cushion around them. The adult human brain having a weight of about 1500 g in air will weigh only 50 g when suspended in CSF.

### Formation

Cerebrospinal fluid is formed by the choroid plexuses of lateral, third and fourth ventricles. Choroid plexuses are tufts of capillaries. They present numerous villi-like projections, which invade the pia mater to enter the cavities of the ventricles. This double-layered pia mater (tela choroidea) with choroid plexus projects into the ventricle by invading the ependymal lining. It is estimated that about 600–700 ml of CSF is formed per day.

### Circulation (see Fig. 26.2)

- The CSF from the lateral ventricles pass into third ventricle through interventricular foramina.
- Then into fourth ventricle through the cerebral aqueduct (aqueduct of Sylvius).
- From the fourth ventricle, CSF escapes into the subarachnoid space through lateral and median apertures.
- Some amount of CSF passes into central canal of spinal cord.
- After entering the subarachnoid space, it passes into cranial subarachnoid space (around the brain) and spinal subarachnoid space (Fig. 32.6).
- It is estimated that about 135 ml of CSF will be in circulation at a time.

### Absorption

Most of the cerebrospinal fluid is drained into venous blood. The superior sagittal venous sinus present in the upper convex margin of falx cerebri receives plenty of arachnoid extensions called 'arachnoid villi'. The CSF presents in the subarachnoid space enters the venous sinus through these arachnoid villi (see Fig. 26.1).

### Functions of CSF

1. CSF provides a protective coat around the brain and spinal cord.

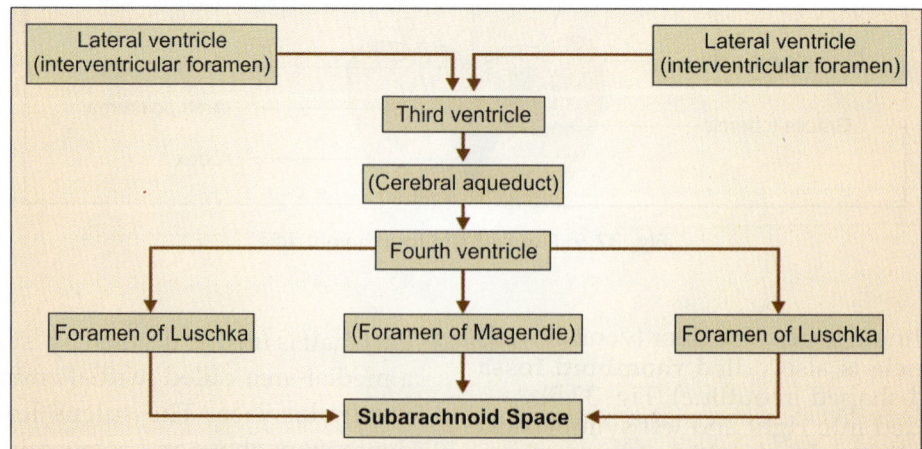

**Fig. 32.6:** CSF circulation—schematic

2. The analysis of CSF provides information about the diseases of the central nervous system.

3. It regulates the volume of cranial cavity.

## Applied Aspects

**Hydrocephalus** (Fig. 32.7)

In this condition there is excessive accumulation of cerebrospinal fluid in subarachnoid space or within the ventricles of brain. In case of occlusion of foramen of Magendie and Luschka, the ventricles enlarge due to obstruction in CSF circulation. CT scan and MRI scan will reveal such conditions.

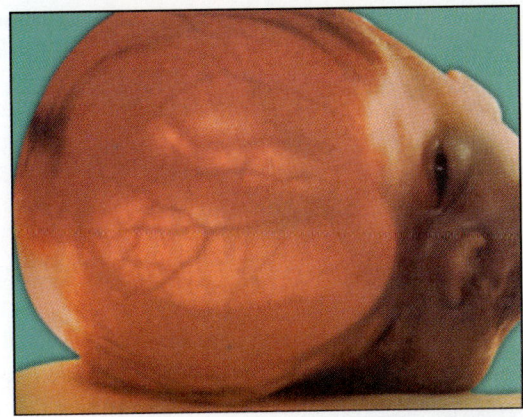

**Fig. 32.7:** Hydrocephalus

# Blood Supply to the Brain

The brain receives about one sixth of the cardiac output and one-fifth of the oxygen consumed by the body at rest. An acute arrest of circulation to brain results in loss of consciousness. A vascular lesion affecting a brain for a minute can leads to loss of tremendous number of neurons. About 750 ml of blood circulates through the brain of average weight per minute. This would explain the importance of the blood supply to the brain. Hypertension, atherosclerosis and diabetes are the common causes for cerebrovascular accidents.

Brain is supplied by two sets of arteries—carotid and vertebral.

## INTERNAL CAROTID ARTERY

It is one of the terminal branches of the common carotid artery given at the level of upper border of the lamina of the thyroid cartilage in the neck.

- It ascends in the neck without giving any branch. It enters the cranial cavity by passing through the petrous part of the temporal bone (it passes through lower and upper carotid openings of carotid canal).
- Within the petrous part of the temporal bone it forms an S-shaped curvature which is referred as carotid siphon in angiogram X-rays.
- Then it enters the cavernous sinus and finally terminates by giving anterior and middle cerebral arteries.

The internal carotid artery gives the following branches:

### 1. Superior and Inferior Hypophyseal Arteries

These arteries supply the pituitary gland.

### 2. Ophthalmic Artery

It enters the bony orbit through optic canal along with optic nerve. It gives many branches (lacrimal artery, long and short posterior ciliary arteries, supraorbital, supratrochlear and dorsal nasal branches). All these branches supply structures present in the orbit, ethmoidal air sinuses and nasal cavity. One of the branches called 'central artery of retina' traverses the substance of the optic nerve with central vein of retina. It supplies the deeper layers of retina. Functionally it is an end artery; hence occlusion of this artery results in blindness.

### 3. Anterior Choroid Artery

It provides choroid plexus to the lateral ventricle.

### 4. Posterior Communicating Artery

It connects the internal carotid artery with posterior cerebral artery. It contributes to completion of the 'circle of Willis'.

### 5. Anterior Cerebral Artery

Each anterior cerebral artery passes anteriorly towards median longitudinal fissure, where the two arteries are connected by anterior communicating artery. Then it proceeds over the superior surface of the corpus callosum. Anterior cerebral artery supplies mainly the medial surface of the cerebrum (except occipital lobe) and also part of the superolateral surface along the superomedial margin (Fig. 33.1).

Among the branches of the anterior cerebral artery, the recurrent branch is of immense clinical significance.

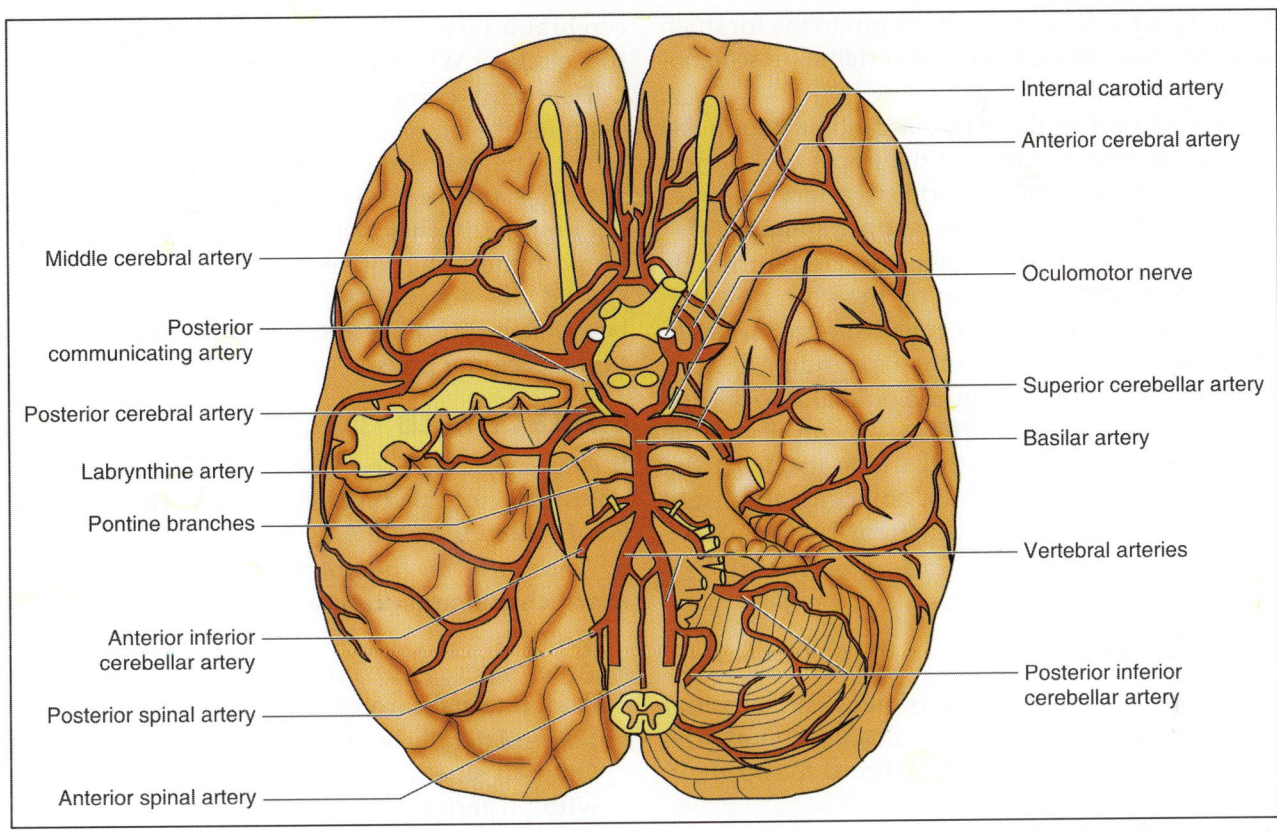

Middle cerebral artery

Posterior communicating artery

Posterior cerebral artery

Labrynthine artery

Pontine branches

Anterior inferior cerebellar artery

Posterior spinal artery

Anterior spinal artery

Internal carotid artery

Anterior cerebral artery

Oculomotor nerve

Superior cerebellar artery

Basilar artery

Vertebral arteries

Posterior inferior cerebellar artery

**Fig. 33.1:** Arteries at the base of the brain

Occlusion of anterior cerebral artery involves paracentral lobule; hence it can result in paralysis of the lower limb muscles below the knee on the opposite side, altered sensorium in the opposite limb and urinary incontinence. Involvement of the recurrent branch can result in contralateral paralysis of the upper limb, tongue and weakness in the contralateral lower facial muscles; this is due to the involvement of the genu of the internal capsule.

## 6. Middle Cerebral Artery

On each side it passes into the stem of the lateral sulcus (between tentorial and orbital part of the inferior surface of the cerebrum) and then appears on the superolateral surface of the cerebrum in posterior ramus of the lateral sulcus. It supplies mainly the superolateral surface of the cerebrum except the area along the superomedial margin and occipital lobe (Fig. 33.1).

Among the branches of the middle cerebral artery, lenticulostriate arteries are of immense clinical significance.

### Lenticulostriate Arteries

They are arranged in medial and lateral striate branches and pierce the anterior perforated substance.

The medial lenticulostriate arteries ascend through the lentiform nucleus and supply internal capsule, caudate nucleus and lentiform nucleus.

The lateral lenticulostriate arteries ascend through the external capsule and then turn medially through the lentiform nucleus to supply the caudate nucleus and part of the internal capsule.

Occlusion of the middle cerebral artery supplying the cortex involves major portion of the motor and sensory areas and also motor speech area. Hence, it can result in paralysis of trunk, upper limb and lower part of the face on the contralateral side and an altered sensorium in the same area.

One of the striate artery is long and slender and is vulnerable to rupture in the presence of high blood pressure hence called **artery of cerebral hemorrhage** (Charcot's artery). Occlusion of lenticulostriate artery involves internal capsule which can cause contralateral hemiplegia also involving lower half of the facial muscles and altered sensorium.

## VERTEBRAL ARTERY

It is a branch from the first part of the subclavian artery given off in the neck. It supplies brainstem, cerebellum and occipital lobes of the cerebrum. The artery has four parts (Fig. 33.1).

i. The first part ascends from its origin to the foramen transversarium of sixth cervical vertebra (in scaleno-vertebral triangle).

ii. The second part of the artery ascends through the foramina transversaria of all the upper six cervical vertebrae. This part of the vertebral artery provides many spinal branches, which supply spinal cord.

iii. The third part appears in the suboccipital triangle where it appears by passing on the posterior arch of the atlas vertebra. Then it enters the cranial cavity by passing through the foramen magnum.

iv. The fourth part appears in the cranial cavity. The right and left vertebral arteries ascend along the ventral surface of the medulla oblongata. At the junction of pons and medulla oblongata, the right and left vertebral arteries join to form 'basilar artery'.

Before forming the basilar artery, each vertebral artery gives following branches:

### a. Anterior Spinal Artery

The two anterior spinal arteries (of right and left side) join to form a single trunk, which descends along the anterior median fissure of the spinal cord to supply it.

### b. Posterior Spinal Artery

On each side it descends separately along the postero-lateral sulcus of the spinal cord to supply it.

### c. Posterior Inferior Cerebellar Artery

It supplies medulla oblongata and part of the cerebellum.

### THE BASILAR ARTERY

It is formed by the union of two vertebral arteries at the junction of pons and medulla oblongata. It ascends on the ventral surface of the pons in basilar sulcus. It gives many pontine branches supplying pons and a labyrinthine artery, which enters internal acoustic meatus. It also gives anterior inferior cerebellar artery and superior cerebellar arteries supplying the cerebellum. The basilar artery terminates at the level of upper border of pons by dividing into two posterior cerebral arteries (Fig. 33.1).

### Posterior Cerebral Artery

On each side it passes laterally and backwards winding around the crus cerebri of midbrain to reach the under surface of the splenium of corpus callosum. It gives many cortical branches supplying occipital lobe of the cerebrum. The posterior communicating artery connects the internal carotid artery with posterior cerebral artery on each side and helps in completing the 'circle of Willis'.

Posterior cerebral artery through its branches supplies thalamus, occipital and part of the temporal lobes. The calcarine branch is important because it supplies the primary visual cortex (area 17). An occlusion of this artery produces contralateral homonymous hemianopia. Macular vision is often spared due to anastomosis of the cortical branches between the posterior and middle cerebral arteries close to the occipital pole.

### CIRCLE OF WILLIS

It is an arterial circle presents at the base of the brain within the interpeduncular cistern. The arterial circle is formed in the following way:

- Anteriorly by the anterior communicating artery, which connects the right and left anterior cerebral arteries.
- Anterolaterally by anterior cerebral arteries arising from internal carotid artery.
- Posterolaterally by posterior communicating arteries: On each side it connects the internal carotid artery with posterior cerebral artery.
- Posteriorly the two posterior cerebral arteries (Fig. 33.2).

The branches arising from this arterial circle provide many central (perforating) branches which perforate the base of the brain (anterior and posterior perforated substances) to supply the deeper structures like basal ganglia, thalamus, hypothalamus and limbic system.

This communication between vertebral and carotid system of arteries provides an alternate route of blood supply to the brain in case of occlusion of any of these arteries.

> **Berry aneurysm:** This is a dilatation (out pouching) affecting one of the components of circle of Willis, usually at the junction of anterior cerebral and anterior communicating arteries. An increase in the blood pressure may cause its rupture and bleeds inside the subarachnoid space (interpeduncular cistern).

### VENOUS DRAINAGE

The veins of the brain are thin-walled and devoid of valves.

Most of them drain into dural venous sinuses after piercing arachnoid and meningeal layer of the dura mater.

The veins are arranged in 3 sets—cerebral, brainstem and cerebellum.

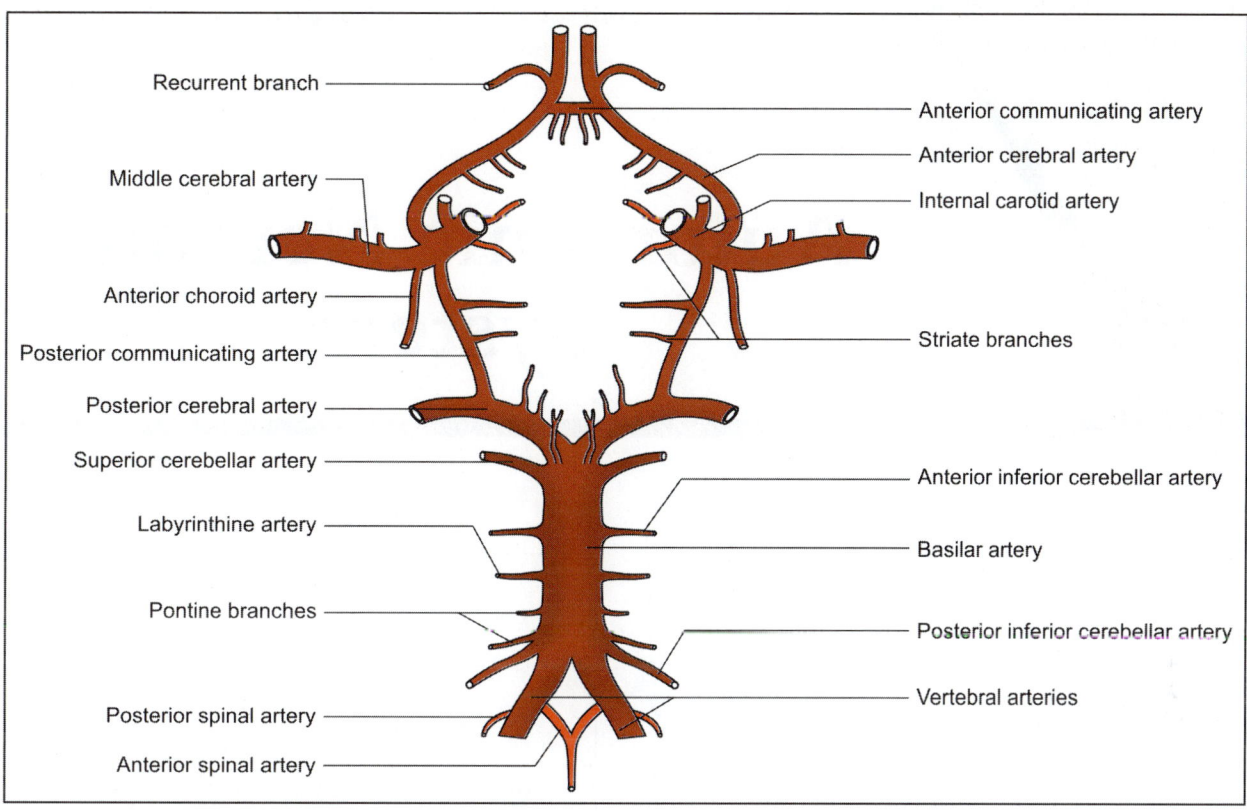

Recurrent branch

Middle cerebral artery

Anterior choroid artery

Posterior communicating artery

Posterior cerebral artery

Superior cerebellar artery

Labyrinthine artery

Pontine branches

Posterior spinal artery

Anterior spinal artery

Anterior communicating artery

Anterior cerebral artery

Internal carotid artery

Striate branches

Anterior inferior cerebellar artery

Basilar artery

Posterior inferior cerebellar artery

Vertebral arteries

**Fig. 33.2:** Arteries of the brain with circle of Willis—schematic

## Cerebral Veins

It consists of superficial and deep groups.

The superficial veins include:

1. Superior cerebral veins—about 8–10 in number on superolateral surface. They drain into superior sagittal sinus. These thin-walled veins cross the subdural space. Rupture of these veins cause subdural hematoma.
2. Superficial middle cerebral veins drains the blood from the superolateral surface. It drains into cavernous sinus.
3. Inferior cerebral veins drain the inferior surface.

The deep veins include:

1. *Internal cerebral veins:* Each vein is formed close to the interventricular foramen by the union of thalamostriate vein and choroids veins. Both the vein pass below the splenium of the corpus callosum and join to form great cerebral vein of Galen.
2. *Basal veins:* Each basal vein is formed in the region of the anterior perforated substance by the union of

anterior cerebral vein, deep middle cerebral vein and striate veins. Each basal vein terminates in great cerebral vein.

3. *Great cerebral vein of Galen:* It is formed by the union of two internal cerebral veins below the splenium of the corpus callosum. It terminates at the anterior end of the straight sinus.

## CEREBRAL ANGIOGRAPHY

It is the radiographic investigation demonstrating the blood vascular system of the brain. The method consists of injecting an iodine containing radiopaque solution into the internal carotid or vertebral artery, followed by serial X-ray photography at intervals. The arteries are visualized within 2 seconds after the injection, and during this period an angiogram is taken. The dye reaches the veins within the next 2 seconds, when a venogram may be made. Cerebral angiography is useful in localizing vascular malformations, aneurysms and space-occupying intracranial masses.

# Autonomic Nervous System

Autonomic nervous system along with endocrine glands maintains the constant internal environment (both of them are under the influence of hypothalamus). The maintenance of the constant internal environment (homeostasis) is performed by regulating the body temperature, blood pressure, cardiorespiratory rate, gastrointestinal motility and glandular secretion. They supply cardiac and smooth muscles (e.g. smooth muscles of the viscera, blood vessels, erector pylorum muscle and intrinsic muscles of the eye and many glands).

Autonomic nervous system has two components.

a. Sympathetic
b. Parasympathetic

## SYMPATHETIC NERVOUS SYSTEM

Functionally this system is 'sympathetic' to the body and its nerve is considered as 'nerve of emergency'. Sympathetic system has two components.

### I. MOTOR COMPONENT

The preganglionic sympathetic neurons are derived from intermediate (or lateral) horn cells of all thoracic and upper two lumbar segments of the spinal cord. This is often referred as 'thoracolumbar outflow'.

The fibers from these neurons pass through ventral motor root of the spinal nerve, then into the mixed spinal nerve. They leave the spinal nerve and reach sympathetic ganglion by white rami communicantes (preganglionic) and relay in the sympathetic ganglion (Fig. 34.1). However, some fibers without relaying can ascend or descend in the sympathetic chain.

Neurons of sympathetic ganglion act as post-ganglionic neurons.

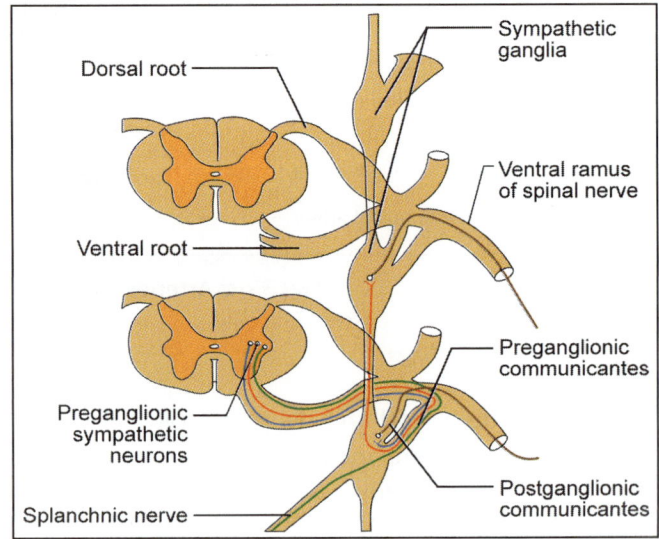

**Fig. 34.1:** Sympathetic outflow

Postganglionic fibers from the sympathetic ganglion can

a. Again join the spinal nerve through grey rami communicantes (postganglionic).
b. Emerge as 'splanchnic nerves'.

### GANGLIONATED SYMPATHETIC CHAIN

- There are two sympathetic chains (right and left), which occupies in front and sides of the vertebral bodies (Fig. 34.2).
- They extend from the base of the skull to the first piece of coccygeal vertebra where both chains unite to form a median ganglion called 'ganglion impar'.
- Each chain presents about 22 ganglia (3 cervical, 11 thoracic, 4 lumbar and 4 sacral).
- All the thoracic and upper two lumbar sympathetic ganglia are connected with corresponding spinal

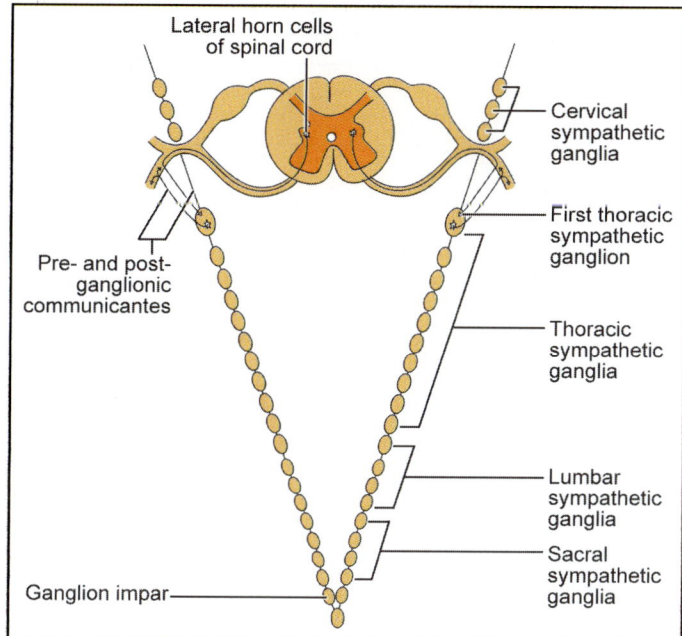

Fig. 34.2: Ganglionated sympathetic chain (schematic)

**Table 34.1:** Sympathetic distribution

| Structures | Spinal segment of sympathetic innervation |
|---|---|
| 1. Upper limb | $T_1$ to $T_4$ or $T_5$ |
| 2. Head and neck | $T_1$ to $T_3/T_4$ |
| 3. Lower limb | $T_{10}$ to $L_2$ |
| 4. Heart | $T_1$ to $T_5$ |
| 5. Lungs | $T_2$ to $T_4$ |
| 6. Stomach | $T_6$ to $T_9$ |
| 7. Small intestine | $T_9$ to $T_{10}$ |
| 8. Large intestine | $T_{11}$ to $L_1$ |
| 9. Urinary bladder | $T_{11}$ to $L_2$ |
| 10. Uterus | $T_{12}$ to $L_1$ |

nerves by both pre- and postganglionic communicantes. However, other ganglia send only postganglionic communicantes to the corresponding spinal nerve.
- Structurally the ganglia consist of multipolar neurons with supporting cells.
- Sympathetic system liberates noradrenaline at the postganglionic endings.

## II. SENSORY COMPONENT OF THE SYMPATHETIC SYSTEM CONVEYS VISCERAL PAIN SENSATION

They carry visceral pain sensation. These fibers without relaying in the sympathetic ganglia enter the spinal cord through dorsal root. The communication between the sensory fibers arising from the body wall with pain fibers arising from the viscera in the dorsal root mixed which explain why visceral pain is referred in the body wall. For example, appendix receives sympathetic fibers from $T_{10}$ segment of the spinal cord. In appendicitis, the pain fibers enter the spinal cord through dorsal root ganglion of $T_{10}$ spinal nerve which also brings sensory information around the umbilicus. This is why there will be a referred pain around the umbilicus in appendicitis.

## EFFECTS OF SYMPATHETIC STIMULATION

- Cutaneous blood vessels undergo vasoconstriction but skeletal and coronary blood vessels dilate.
- Heart rate is accelerated, blood pressure is raised.
- Pupils dilate

- Bronchioles dilate
- Gastric motility (peristalsis) is suppressed and sphincters constrict (closes them).

*Horner's syndrome:* A lesion affecting the preganglionic fibers from $T_1$ & $T_2$ segments of the spinal cord cause Horner's syndrome. The site of injury could be ventral ramus of 1st thoracic nerve or upper thoracic sympathetic ganglion or any of the three cervical sympathetic ganglia. An aneurysm of internal carotid or common carotid artery, thyroid enlargement, presence of cervical rib, tumors affecting the apex of the lung, lymph node enlargement can cause Horner's syndrome. It is manifested by:
a. *Miosis:* Constriction of the pupil (dilator papillae supplied by the sympathetic fibers is involved, hence sphincter papillae constrict the pupil, which is supplied by parasympathetic fibers through oculomotor nerve).
b. *Ptosis:* Drooping of the upper eyelid due to paralysis of superior tarsal muscle.
c. *Enophthalmos:* Retraction of the eyeball into the orbit due to paralysis of the orbitalis muscle that spans the inferior orbital fissure, supplied by sympathetic fibers.
d. *Unhydrosis:* Loss of sweating in the face and head on the affected side.

## PARASYMPATHETIC NERVOUS SYSTEM

This system also has motor and sensory components.

## I. THE MOTOR COMPONENT

The pre-ganglionic parasympathetic neurons are located mainly in a few cranial nerve nuclei and also in sacral segments of the spinal cord (craniosacral outflow).

Parasympathetic fibers are distributed through third, seventh, ninth and tenth cranial nerves. The parasympathetic system liberates acetylcholine at the postganglionic endings.

### Effects of Parasympathetic Stimulation

- Heart rate is diminished and blood pressure falls.
- Pupils are constricted
- Gastric motility is stimulated
- Glandular secretion of the gastrointestinal tract is promoted.
- Urinary bladder and rectum are evacuated.

The parasympathetic distribution through various cranial nerve is discussed below (Table 34.2).

### 1. Oculomotor Nerve

- The parasympathetic fibers concerned with visual reflexes (light and accommodation reflex) arise from Edinger-Westphal nucleus of midbrain.
- The fibers pass through oculomotor nerve and relay in ciliary ganglion present in the orbit.
- The postganglionic fibers reach the target structures (sphincter pupillae and ciliaris muscles) through short ciliary nerves (Fig. 34.3).

### 2. Facial Nerve (Fig. 34.4)

- It carries parasympathetic secretomotor fibers to lacrimal gland and submandibular and sublingual salivary glands.

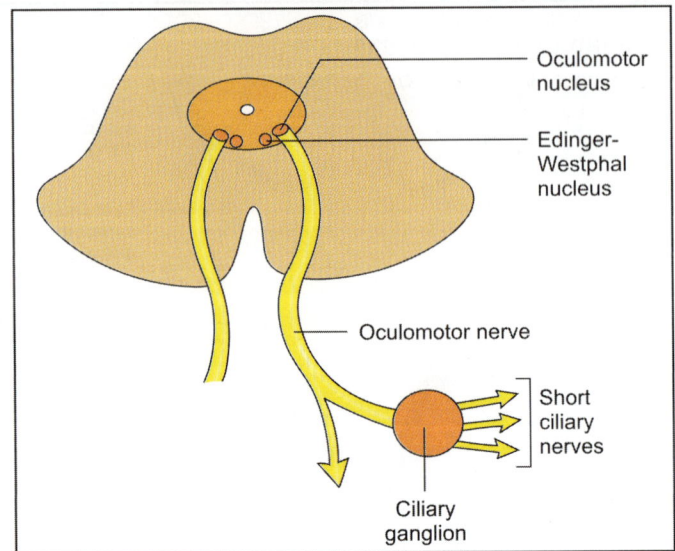

**Fig. 34.3:** Ciliary ganglion and parasympathetic fibers (schematic)

- The parasympathetic fibers for the lacrimal gland are derived from lacrimatory nucleus of brainstem. Fibers pass through facial nerve, its branch greater petrosal nerve to reach pterygopalatine ganglion. Postganglionic fibers reach the lacrimal gland through maxillary, its zygomatic branch and lacrimal nerve.

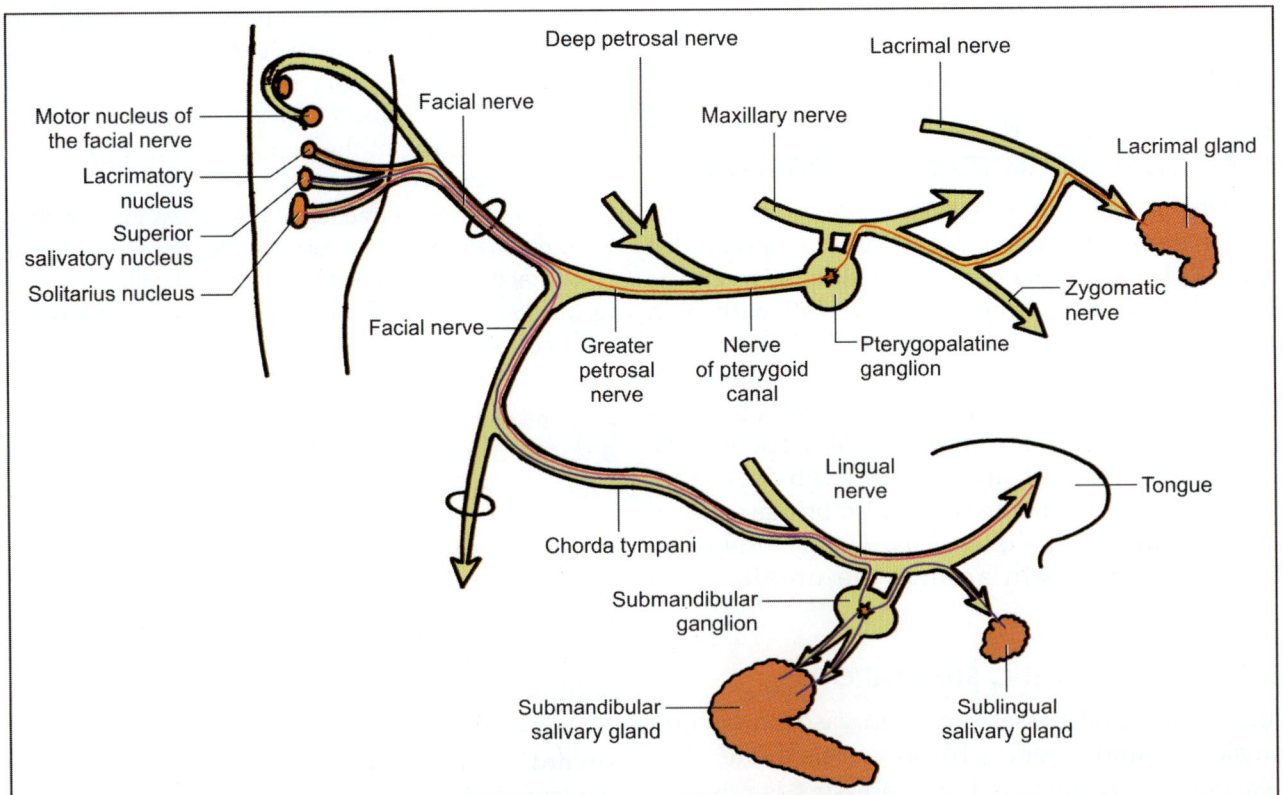

**Fig. 34.4:** Parasympathetic fibers in facial nerve

- The parasympathetic fibers to submandibular and sublingual salivary glands are derived from superior salivatory nucleus of brainstem. Fibers pass through facial nerve and its branch chorda tympani nerve to reach the lingual nerve.

- The fibers relay in submandibular ganglion. The postganglionic fibers reach the target structures through lingual nerve.

### 3. *Glossopharyngeal Nerve* (Fig. 34.5)

- It carries parasympathetic fibers to parotid salivary gland.

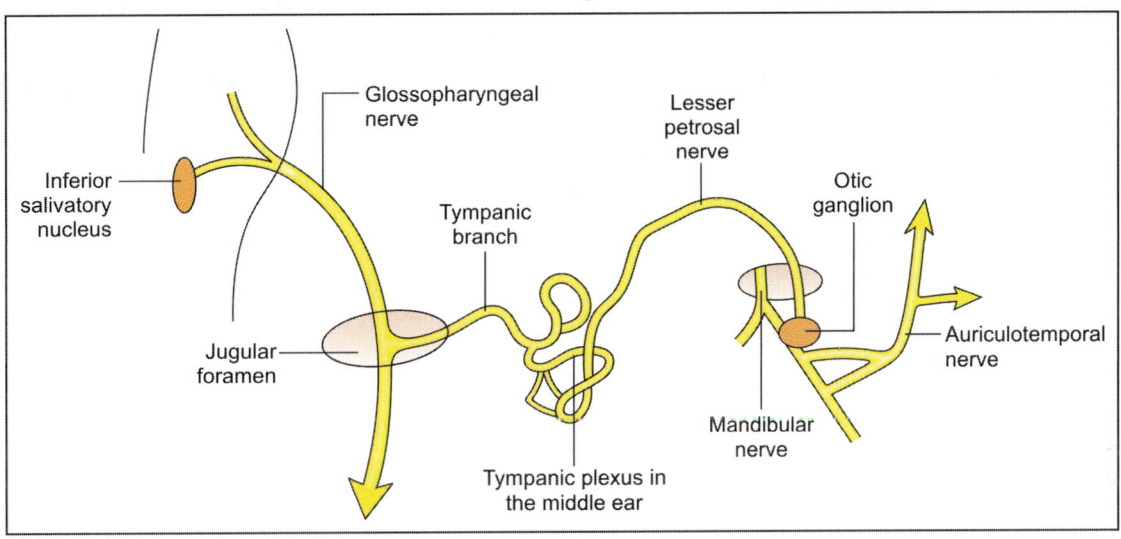

**Fig. 34.5:** Parasympathetic fibers in glossopharyngeal nerve—schematic

**Table 34.2:** Distribution of parasympathetic fibers—schematic

| Preganglionic parasympathetic neurons | Cranial nerves | Parasympathetic ganglia | Target structure |
|---|---|---|---|
| Edinger-Westphal nucleus of midbrain | **Oculomotor nerve** | Ciliary ganglion | Sphincter pupillae / Ciliaris muscle |
| Lacrimatory nucleus of pons Superior salivatory nucleus of pons | Greater petrosal nerve | Pterygopalatine ganglion | Lacrimal gland and glands of nasal cavity |
| | **Facial nerve** Chorda tympani nerve | Submandibular ganglion | Submandibular and sublingual salivary glands |
| Inferior salivatory nucleus | **Glossopharyngeal nerve** (Lesser petrosal nerve) | Otic ganglion | Parotid salivary gland |
| Dorsal nucleus of vagus | **Vagus nerve** | Ganglia are located close to the target structure | Heart, lungs, stomach. Intestine (up to right 2/3rds of transverse colon), etc. |
| Anterior horn cells of the 2nd, 3rd and 4th sacral segments of the spinal cord | **Pelvic splanchnic nerve** | Ganglia are located close to the target structure | Distal part of the GIT, urinary bladder, uterus, uterine tube, etc. |

- The fibers are derived from inferior salivatory nucleus of brainstem and pass through glossopharyngeal nerve and its branch (tympanic branch, tympanic plexus and lesser petrosal nerve) to reach otic ganglion.
- The postganglionic fibers reach the parotid gland through auriculotemporal nerve.

### 4. Vagus Nerve

- It carries parasympathetic fibers to heart, lungs, stomach, intestine and abdominal organs.
- The fibers are derived from dorsal nucleus of vagus.

- Vagotomy is a procedure performed in some people with chronic ulcers to reduce the production of HCl, because HCl secreting parietal cells are mainly controlled by vagus.

### 5. Pelvic Splanchnic Nerve

- It carries fibers from ventral horn cells of second to fourth sacral segments of the spinal cord.
- These parasympathetic fibers supply pelvic organs like urinary bladder, uterus, uterine tubes, rectum, anal canal, etc.

# Cranial Nerves

## 35

Cranial nerves are those, which arise (passes into) from the brain. There are 12 pairs of cranial nerves.

1. Olfactory
2. Optic
3. Oculomotor
4. Trochlear
5. Trigeminal
6. Abducent
7. Facial
8. Vestibulocochlear
9. Glossopharyngeal
10. Vagus
11. Accessory
12. Hypoglossal

Each cranial nerve will have central connections (nuclei of origin) within the brain and has peripheral connections.

### 1. OLFACTORY NERVE (1ST CRANIAL NERVE)

This is a sensory nerve carrying sense of smell from the nose. The roof, upper part of the septum and lateral wall of the nasal cavity is lined by olfactory epithelium. The epithelium consists of bipolar olfactory neurons.

The central processes of these olfactory cells form olfactory nerves, which pass through the cribriform plate of the ethmoid bone and terminate in the neurons of the olfactory bulb (Fig. 35.1).

Axons arising from these neurons (olfactory bulb) form olfactory tract, which terminates in anterior part of the temporal lobe.

### 2. OPTIC NERVE (2ND CRANIAL NERVE)

It is the nerve of vision. The rods and cones of retina act as photoreceptors. The rods are concerned with dim

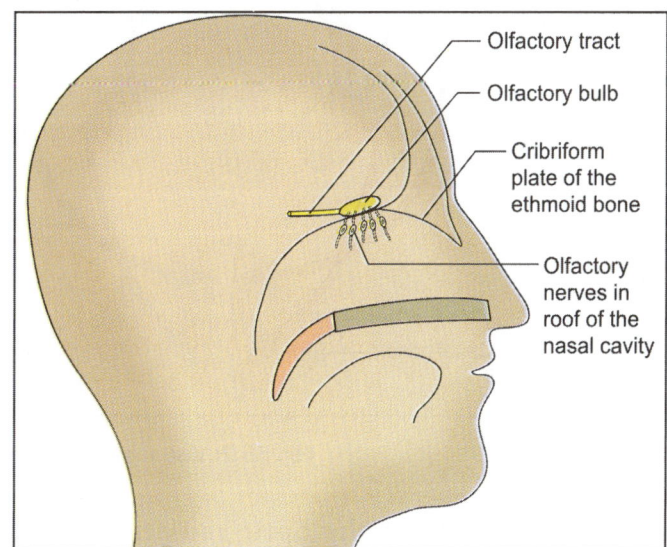

**Fig. 35.1:** Olfactory nerve

light and black and white vision. It is estimated that about 120 millions of rods are present in each human retina. The cones are concerned with bright light and color vision. Each retina comprises about 7 millions of cones.

Impulses from rods and cones are carried by bipolar neurons of retina. The axons of these bipolar neurons make synaptic contacts with ganglion cells of retina. **The axons of these ganglionic cells form the optic nerve.**

The optic nerve emerges from the eyeball and leaves the orbit through optic canal. The two optic nerves decussate to form optic chiasma. After decussation, it continues (on each side) as optic tract. Each optic tract contains temporal (lateral) fibers of same retina and nasal (medial) fibers of opposite retina (Fig. 35.2).

The optic tract ends in the lateral geniculate body of thalamus. Fibers from the lateral geniculate body

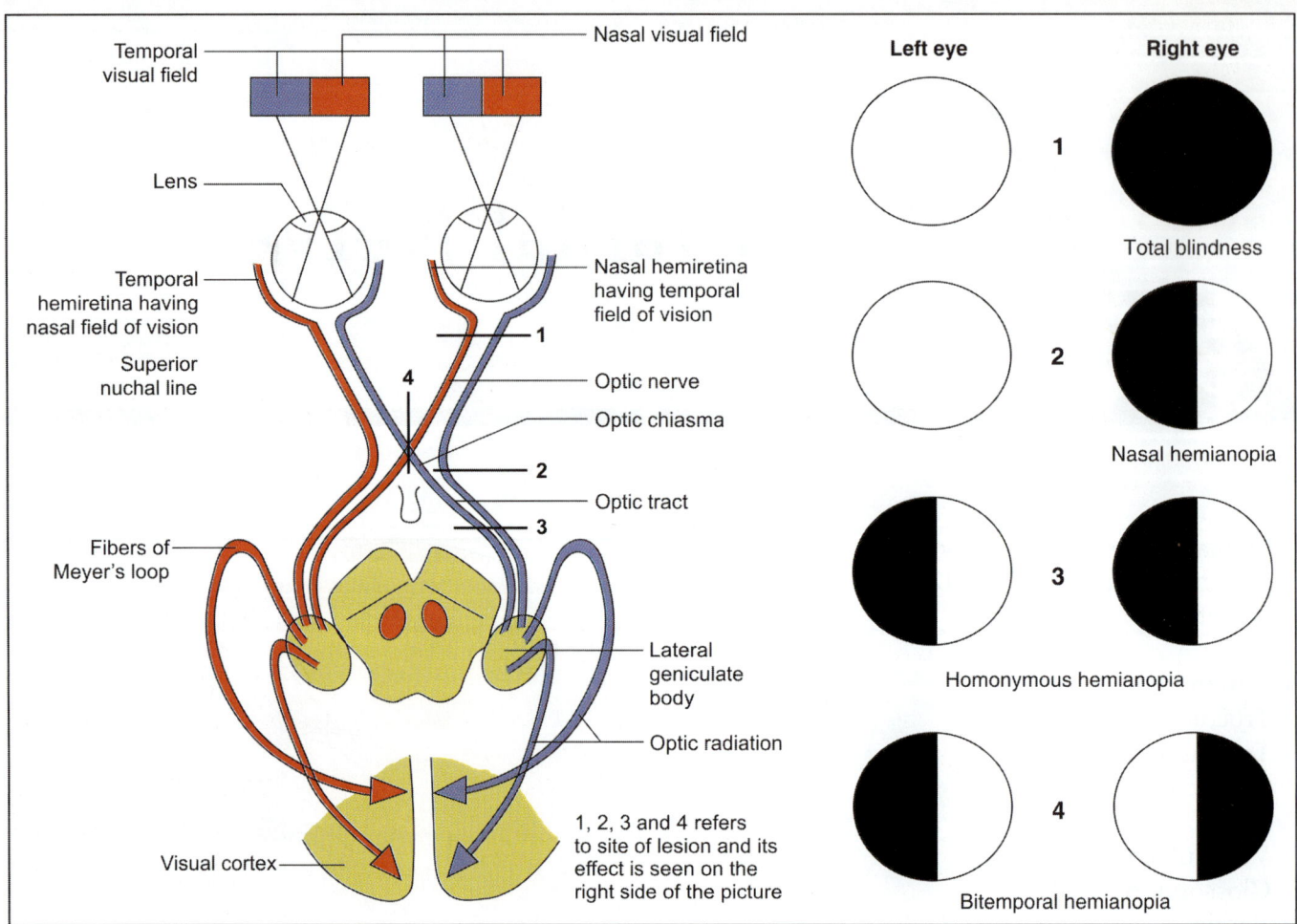

**Fig. 35.2:** Visual pathway and effect of lesion at various sites

spreads out to form the optic radiation in the retrolentiform part of the internal capsule and reach primary visual cortex (area 17) around the calcarine sulcus of occipital lobe.

Optic nerve is traversed in the center by central artery and vein of retina. This central artery of retina is an end artery. Occlusion of this artery leads to blindness.

### Applied Aspects

a. Complete lesion of the optic nerve is manifested by total blindness.
b. A midline lesion of the optic chiasma will produce bitemporal hemianopia (heteronymous). The patient is able to see the objects placed in the nasal visual field but not the temporal visual field (Fig. 35.2)
c. Unilateral complete lesion of optic tract, lateral geniculate body or optic radiation produces contralateral homonymous hemianopia.

Hemianopia: Loss of vision in one half (right or left) of the visual field.

Homonymous: Same half of the visual field is affected in both eyes.

Heteronymous: Different halves of the visual field are affected in both eyes.

### 3. OCULOMOTOR NERVE (3RD CRANIAL NERVE)

This cranial nerve supplies most of the extraocular muscles and also carries preganglionic parasympathetic fibers concerned with visual reflexes.

### Nuclei of Origin

a. The fibers of the oculomotor nerve arise from the oculomotor nucleus located in the ventral part of the cerebral aqueduct of midbrain. Fibers from this nucleus form oculomotor nerve, which supplies all the extraocular muscles except superior oblique and lateral rectus.
b. The parasympathetic fibers are derived from the Edinger-Westphal nucleus of midbrain for

accommodation reflex. The nerve also receives fibers from pretectal nucleus for pupillary light reflex.

## Course (Fig. 35.3)

Oculomotor nerve emerges from the medial side of the crus cerebri of midbrain and runs in the lateral wall of the cavernous venous sinus. It enters the orbit through superior orbital fissure by dividing into upper and lower divisions, and supplies following extraocular muscles.

- Inferior oblique
- Superior rectus
- Medial rectus
- Inferior rectus
- Levator palpebrae superioris

(All the extraocular muscles of eye are supplied by oculomotor nerve except superior oblique, which is supplied by 4th cranial nerve [SO4] and lateral rectus by 6th cranial nerve [LR6]).

## Pupillary Light Reflex

When eye is exposed to bright light, pupil will constrict reflexly. The impulses from retina pass successively through optic nerve, optic chiasma, optic tract and to the pre-tectal nucleus of midbrain. From the pre-tectal nucleus fibers pass to Edinger-Westphal nuclei of both sides. Preganglionic fibers from this nucleus pass through oculomotor nerve and relay in ciliary ganglion in the orbit. Postganglionic fibers from the ganglion pass through the short ciliary nerves, which supply sphincter pupillae and ciliaris muscles.

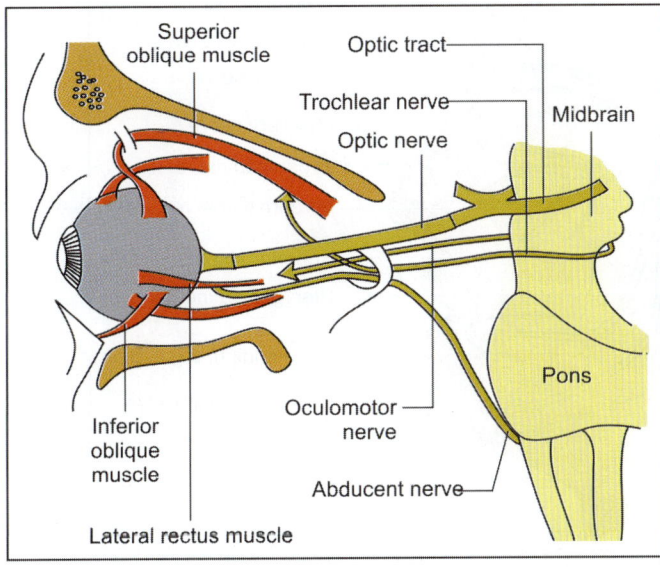

**Fig. 35.3:** Nerves supplying extraocular muscles

## Accommodation Reflex (for Near Vision)

Accommodation of the eye for near vision requires three actions:

a. Convergence of the eyes by contraction of medial rectus muscle.

b. Constriction of the pupil by sphincter pupillae muscle

c. Thickening of lens, produced by ciliaris muscle which relaxes the suspensory ligament of lens (bulging of lens)

The pathway includes optic nerves, optic chiasma, optic tract, lateral geniculate bodies, optic radiation, visual cortex, frontal eye field, oculomotor nuclear complex (for medial rectus muscle) and Edinger-Westphal nucleus (for ciliaris and sphincter pupillae muscle).

Injury to the oculomotor nerve (midbrain lesion, compression by the arteries accompanying it or by cavernous sinus thrombosis) results paralysis of most of the extraocular muscles. The eye looks "down and out" due to unopposed action of superior oblique and lateral rectus muscles. In addition to ptosis (drooping of the upper eyelid because of levator palpebrae superiosis), the pupil will be fixed and dilated.

## TROCHLEAR NERVE (4TH CRANIAL NERVE)

This cranial nerve supplies only one muscle—superior oblique.

## Nuclear Origin

Fibers of the trochlear nerve emerges from trochlear nucleus of midbrain.

## Course (Fig. 35.3)

The nerve emerges from the dorsal surface of the midbrain. After decussating the nerve winds forward around the crus cerebri. After traversing the lateral wall of the cavernous sinus it enters the orbit through superior orbital fissure and supplies superior oblique muscle.

In case of injury to the trochlear nerve or in paralysis of superior oblique muscle of the eye, depression of the eye is possible when the eye is looking straight due to intact inferior rectus muscle, but when the eye is adducted superior oblique is the only muscle responsible for depression. Hence, diplopia occurs when the eye is depressed and adducted (reading newspaper).

## TRIGEMINAL NERVE (5TH CRANIAL NERVE)

It is the largest of all the cranial nerves. It has both motor and sensory components.

### Nuclei of Origin

a. *Spinal nucleus of the 5th nerve:* This nucleus is present in the pons, medulla and extends up to the cervical part of the spinal cord. It receives pain and temperature sensation from the head area. The cell bodies of neurons bringing this information are located in trigeminal ganglion.

b. *Principal sensory nucleus:* It lies in the pons and receives the general sensation from the trigeminal area (skin of face and scalp as far as vertex, teeth, mucosa of gums, oral and nasal cavities with paranasal sinuses, cornea and conjunctiva and most of the dura mater). The cell bodies of the neurons bringing this information are located in trigeminal ganglion.

c. *Motor nucleus of the 5th nerve:* It is situated in the pons and fibers arising from this nucleus form motor root of the trigeminal nerve and supply muscles of mastication and a few other muscles.

d. *Mesencephalic nucleus:* It is situated in the central grey matter of the midbrain. It receives proprioceptive sensation from muscles of mastication, facial expression and extraocular muscles.

### Course (Fig. 35.4)

The sensory and motor roots of the trigeminal nerve are attached to the ventral surface of the pons at its junction with the middle cerebellar peduncle. The sensory root is formed by the central processes of neurons of the 'trigeminal ganglion'. This ganglion contains unipolar (pseudounipolar) neurons. The peripheral processes of these neurons form ophthalmic, maxillary and mandibular divisions of the trigeminal nerve. The smaller motor root is distributed through mandibular division.

### Ophthalmic Nerve

After emerging from the trigeminal ganglion, the nerve traverses the lateral wall of the cavernous sinus and enters the orbit through superior orbital fissure where it divides into three terminal branches.

a. Frontal nerve—which further divides into supra-trochlear and supraorbital nerves, which supply the skin of scalp and forehead.

b. Nasociliary nerve—this nerve brings sensation from ciliary body, iris and cornea through its long ciliary branches. It gives infratrochlear nerve, anterior and posterior ethmoidal nerves.

c. Lacrimal nerve—it supplies lacrimal gland after receiving secretomotor fibers through zygomatico-temporal nerve (from pterygopalatine ganglion).

The ophthalmic nerve supplies cornea, conjunctiva, upper eyelid, forehead, anterior part of the scalp and the nose.

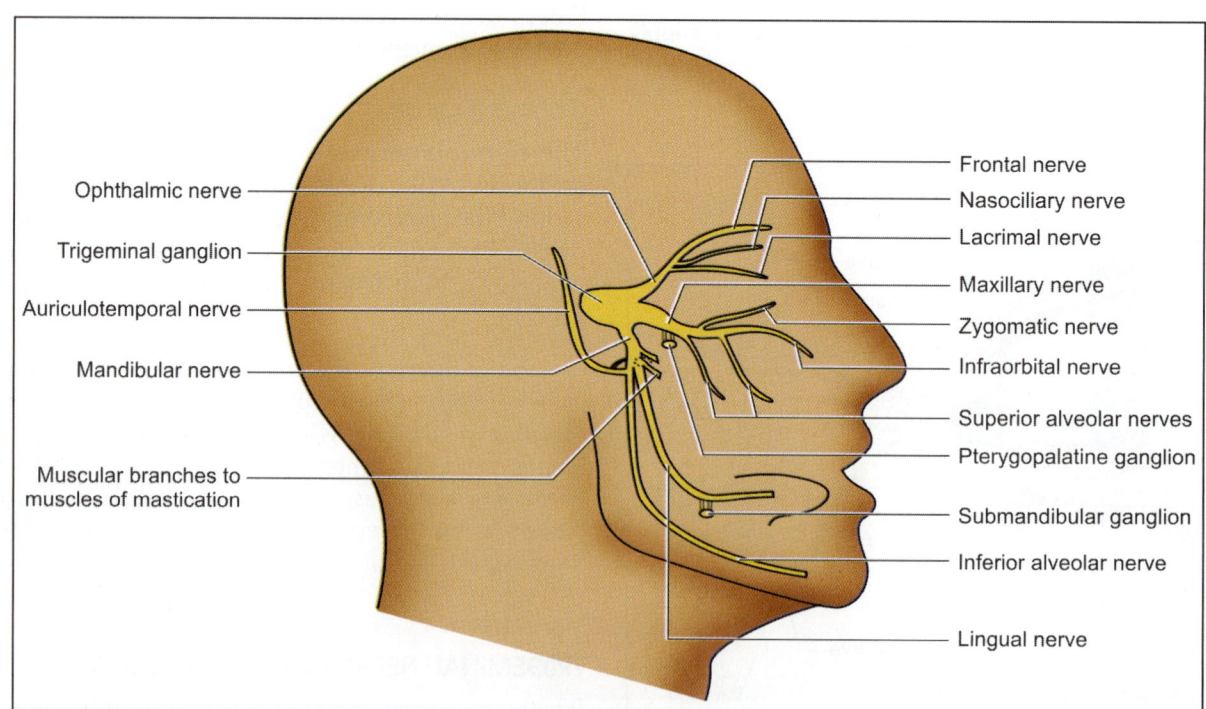

**Fig. 35.4:** Branches of trigeminal nerve

## Maxillary Nerve

After emerging from the trigeminal ganglion the nerve proceeds forward in the lateral wall of the cavernous sinus. Then it enters the pterygopalatine fossa through the foramen rotundum. In the pterygopalatine fossa the maxillary nerve suspends pterygopalatine ganglion. Maxillary nerve gives following branches:

a. Meningeal branches
b. Zygomatic nerve which further divides into zygomaticotemporal and zygomaticofacial nerves
c. Posterior superior alveolar nerve.
d. Infraorbital nerve: It is the continuation of maxillary nerve and terminates in the face. It gives anterior and middle superior alveolar nerves.

Maxillary nerve also distributed through branches of the pterygopalatine ganglion. It includes:

- Orbital branches—bring sensory fibers from orbit.
- Paltine branches—bring sensory fibers from palate.
- Nasal branches—bring sensory fibers from nasal cavity.
- Pharyngeal branch—bring sensory information from nasopharynx.

## Mandibular Nerve

It is a mixed nerve, having both sensory and motor distribution. The sensory root of the mandibular nerve emerges from trigeminal ganglion and proceeds towards foramen ovale in the base of the skull where it joins the motor root. Just below the foramen ovale in the infratemporal fossa the mandibular nerve divides into anterior and posterior divisions.

The main trunk gives the following branches:

a. Meningeal branch
b. Nerve to medial pterygoid muscle, which also supplies tensor tympani and tensor palati muscles.

The anterior division gives the following branches

a. Masseteric nerve—supplying masseter muscle and temporomandibular joint.
b. Deep temporal nerves—supplying temporalis muscle
c. Nerve to lateral pterygoid muscle
d. Buccal nerve: It is a sensory nerve which pierces buccal pad of fat, buccopharyngeal fascia and buccinator muscle and supplies mucous membrane lining the cheek and also skin over the cheek.

The posterior division gives the following branches:

a. *Auriculotemporal nerve:* This nerve ascends in front of the auricle and supplies the skin of auricle and temporal region. Auriculotemporal nerve receives a communicating branch from the otic ganglion, which gives secretomotor fibers to the parotid salivary gland.
b. *Inferior alveolar nerve:* This nerve enters the mandibular canal after passing through the mandibular foramen. It supplies all the lower teeth and adjacent gum. Finally the nerves emerge at the mental foramen as mental nerve to supply the skin of the chin. Before entering the mandibular foramen, the inferior alveolar nerve gives mylohyoid branch, which supplies mylohyoid muscle and anterior belly of digastric muscle.
c. *Lingual nerve:* This nerve brings general sensation from the mucous membrane of the anterior 2/3rds of the dorsum of the tongue and floor of the mouth. However, lingual nerve is joined by a branch of facial nerve called 'chorda tympani' for carrying taste sensation from the anterior 2/3rds of the dorsum of the tongue and also gives secretomotor fibers to submandibular and sublingual salivary glands.

## TRIGEMINAL NEURALGIA

This condition usually affects adults over 40 years of age. The patient suffers severe pain triggered by contact with the lip, tongue, or gums. The pain arrives with a sudden shocking intensity and then disappears. Usually only one side of the face is involved.

## ABDUCENT NERVE (6TH CRANIAL NERVE)

This cranial nerve supplies only one muscle—lateral rectus. Paralysis of lateral rectus muscle results in medial squint. Diplopia (double vision) occurs due to the change in the visual axis of the affected eyeball.

### Nuclei of Origin

Fibers of the abducent nerve emerge from the abducent nucleus in pons.

### Course (Fig. 35.3)

The nerve emerges at the lower border of the pons and just above the pyramid of the medulla. After traversing the cavernous sinus, the nerve enters the orbit through superior orbital fissure and supplies lateral rectus muscle.

Paralysis of lateral rectus muscle results in medial squint. Diplopia (double vision) occurs due to the change in the visual axis of the affected eyeball.

## FACIAL NERVE (7TH CRANIAL NERVE)

This is a mixed nerve and consists of motor and sensory components.

35

### Nuclei of Origin

a. *Motor nucleus of the facial nerve:* It is located in the pons. Fibers arising from it first pass backward to wind around the abducent nucleus and then proceed forward to emerge as motor root. The abducent nucleus and motor fibers of facial nerve around them form a surface elevation in the floor of the fourth ventricle called facial colliculus.

b. *Superior salivatory nucleus:* Fibers arising from this nucleus travel in the sensory root and supply secretomotor fibers to submandibular and sublingual salivary glands.

c. *Lacrimatory nucleus:* Fibers arising from it join the sensory root of facial nerve and supply lacrimal gland.

d. *Nucleus of tractus solitarius:* This nucleus receives taste sensation from the anterior 2/3rds of the dorsum of the tongue.

### Course (Fig. 35.5)

Facial nerve emerges at the junction of pons and olive (of medulla) by a motor and sensory root (nervus intermedius). Along with the 8th cranial nerve, it enters the internal acoustic meatus. The facial nerve passes above the vestibule of the internal ear, reaches the medial wall of the middle ear and then turns backwards abruptly forming a genu. Then the nerve proceeds backwards and downwards and finally emerges through stylomastoid foramen. The above course of the facial nerve is inside a bony canal in the middle ear. The genu shows an enlargement called 'geniculate ganglion'. After emerging from the stylomastoid foramen, the facial nerve enters the parotid salivary gland and divides into its terminal branches, which appear on the face.

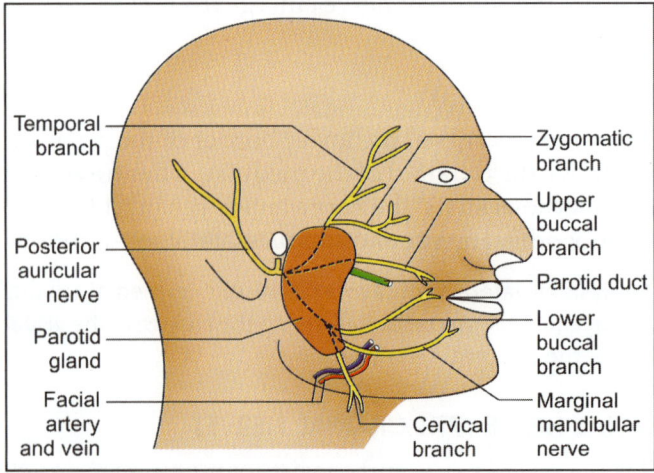

**Fig. 35.5:** Branches of the facial nerve

Temporal branch
Posterior auricular nerve
Parotid gland
Facial artery and vein
Cervical branch
Zygomatic branch
Upper buccal branch
Parotid duct
Lower buccal branch
Marginal mandibular nerve

### Branches and Distribution

Branches within the petrous part of the temporal bone.

a. *Greater petrosal nerve:* It carries secretomotor fibers to the lacrimal gland, and glands of nasal cavity and soft palate.

b. *Nerve to stapedius:* This nerve supplies stapedius muscle. Paralysis of the stapedius muscle produces hyperacusis.

c. *Chorda tympani nerve:* This nerve enters the infratemporal fossa and joins the lingual nerve. It gives secretomotor fibers to the submandibular and sublingual salivary glands. It also brings taste sensation from anterior 2/3rds of the dorsum of the tongue.

### Branches below the Stylomastoid Foramen

a. Posterior auricular nerve: It supplies the occipital belly of the occipitofrontalis muscle.

b. Muscular branches to the posterior belly of the digastric and stylohyoid muscle.

c. Terminal branches emerge from under cover of the anterior border of the parotid gland on the face and supply muscles of facial expression (also frontal belly of occipitofrontalis muscle and platysma of the neck). The terminal branches are:

- Temporal branch
- Zygomatic branch
- Buccal branch
- Marginal mandibular branch
- Cervical branch

### Applied Aspects

a. *Supranuclear paralysis:* It involves the motor area of the cerebral cortex or corticonuclear fibers. This results in impairment or loss of movement of the lower facial muscles of the opposite side. The upper facial muscles escape because dorsal part of the motor facial nerve nucleus receives corticonuclear fibers from both sides of the cerebrum.

b. *Infranuclear paralysis (Bell's palsy):* This occurs due to the lesion in facial nerve itself. All facial muscles on the affected (same) side are paralysed. The face becomes asymmetrical and is manifested by:

- Transverse wrinkles of the forehead disappear.
- Eyebrow droops.
- The patient is unable to close his eyelids and the tears roll over the check.
- During smiling the angle of the mouth is fixed on the affected side but the other angle moves upward and laterally (mouth becomes triangular).
- Food accumulates in the vestibule (due to paralysis of buccinator muscle).

## VESTIBULOCOCHLEAR NERVE (8TH CRANIAL NERVE)

It has two components:
1. Vestibular component—concerned with maintenance of equilibrium.
2. Cochlear component—concerned with hearing.

### Vestibular Nerve (Fig. 35.6)

- This nerve arises from vestibular ganglion of the internal ear.
- The peripheral processes of the bipolar neurons of vestibular ganglion arise from maculae of saccule and utricle (for static equilibrium) and ampullary crests of 3 semicircular ducts (for kinetic equilibrium).
- The central processes of bipolar neurons of the vestibular ganglion form vestibular nerve.
- Along with the cochlear nerve, the vestibular nerve traverses the internal acoustic meatus.
- Then it is attached to the brainstem at the junction of pons and olive.
- Fibers of vestibular nerve terminate in four groups of vestibular nuclei located at the junction of pons and medulla oblongata.
- The vestibular nuclei are further connected with cerebellum and spinal cord for maintaining equilibrium.

### Cochlear Nerve (Fig. 35.6)

- This nerve arises from the spiral ganglion of the internal ear.
- The spiral ganglion consists of bipolar neurons. The peripheral processes of these neurons bring information from 'organ of Corti' (its hair cells are receptors for hearing).
- The central processes of these bipolar neurons form cochlear nerve, which traverses the bony internal acoustic meatus along with vestibular and facial nerve.
- Cochlear nerve is attached to the brainstem at the junction of pons and medulla.
- The fibers of the cochlear nerve terminate in the ventral and dorsal cochlear nuclei, which are located at the ventral and dorsal surfaces of inferior cerebellar peduncle.
- Fibers from these ventral and dorsal cochlear nuclei pass to the opposite side in the pons forming 'trapezoid body' and terminate in superior olivary nucleus of pons.
- Fibers arising from superior olivary nucleus ascend as lateral lemniscus, which terminate in the inferior colliculs of midbrain.
- Fibers from inferior colliculus enter medial geniculate body of thalamus and then into auditory area of the cerebral cortex (areas 41 and 42) through internal capsule.

## GLOSSOPHARYNGEAL NERVE (9TH CRANIAL NERVE)

It is a mixed nerve supplying mainly tongue and pharynx.

### Nuclei of Origin

a. *Nucleus ambiguus:* Fibers arising from this nucleus supply stylopharyngeus muscle.
b. *Inferior salivatory nucleus:* Fibers arising from this nucleus give secretomotor fibers to the parotid salivary gland.
c. *Nucleus solitarius:* Taste fibers from vallate papillae, posterior 1/3rd of tongue and palate are relayed here.
d. *Spinal nucleus of 5th nerve:* It receive general sensation from posterior 1/3rd of tongue.

### Course

The glossopharyngeal nerve emerges from medulla oblongata at the junction of inferior cerebellar peduncle and olive. It leaves the cranial cavity by passing through jugular foramen where it presents two ganglia. The nerve passes deep to the styloid process and winds around the stylopharyngeus muscle. After giving branches on the wall of the pharynx, the nerve proceed forward deep to hyoglossus muscle of tongue. The nerve terminates by supplying posterior part of the tongue.

### Branches and Distribution

1. *Tympanic branch:* This nerve enters middle ear and supplies mucous membrane by forming 'tympanic

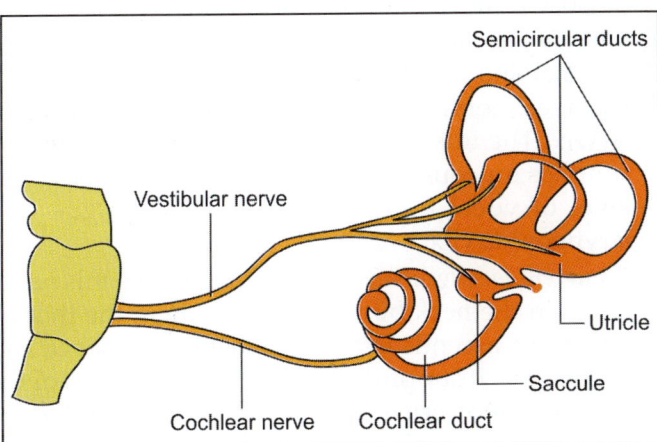

Fig. 35.6: Vestibulocochlear nerve

Semicircular ducts

Vestibular nerve

Utricle

Saccule

Cochlear nerve    Cochlear duct

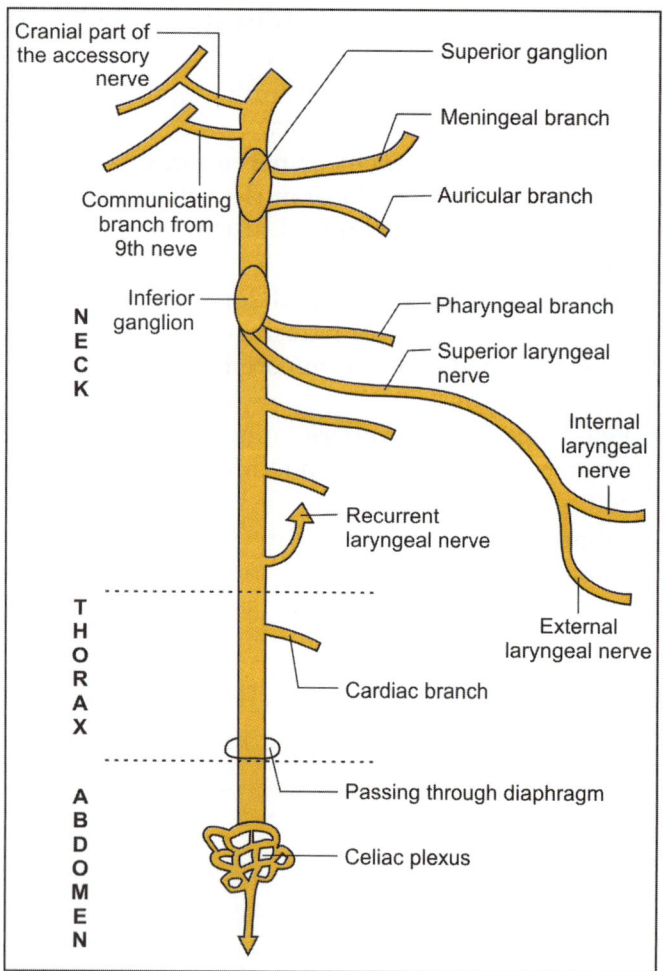

**Fig. 35.7:** Vagus nerve and its branches

## Nuclei of Origin

a. *Nucleus ambiguus:* Fibers arising from it supply muscles of larynx and a few pharyngeal muscles.

b. *Dorsal nucleus of vagus:* Fibers arising from it give parasympathetic fibers to heart, lungs, and abdominal part of the gastrointestinal tract.

c. *Nucleus of tractus solitarius:* It receives taste fibers from posterior most part of the tongue.

d. *Spinal nucleus of trigeminal nerve:* It receives cutaneous sensation from the external ear and tympanic membrane.

## Course

Vagus nerve emerges from the posterolateral sulcus of the medulla oblongata. It descends through the jugular foramen where it presents two ganglia. Vagus nerve descends within the carotid sheath between internal and common carotid arteries and internal jugular vein. Vagus nerve enters the thorax through root of the neck. In the thorax it descends posterior to the hilum of the lung. Further it descends on either side of the oesphagus. It enters the abdomen by passing through esophageal opening of diaphragm.

The right and left vagus nerves terminate as posterior and anterior gastric nerves respectively. These gastric nerves terminate by forming plexus around the celiac trunk and further distributed through it.

## Branches and Distributions

1. Meningeal branch

2. Auricular branch supplying the skin of the auricle and tympanic membrane.

3. Pharyngeal branches carry motor fibers from cranial part of the accessory nerve (11th cranial nerve) and supply muscles of pharynx and soft palate. It also contributes to the pharyngeal plexus, which carries sensory information from pharynx.

4. *Superior laryngeal nerve:* This nerve divides into external and internal laryngeal nerves. The external laryngeal nerve supplies cricothyroid muscle of the larynx. The internal laryngeal nerve is sensory and supplies mucous membrane of the larynx above the level of vocal fold, vallecula of the tongue and laryngopharynx.

5. *Recurrent laryngeal nerve:* On the right side this nerve arises in the neck but on the left side in the thorax. The nerve ascends in a groove between trachea and esophagus. It supplies all the intrinsic muscles of the larynx except cricothyroid (which is supplied by external laryngeal nerve). It also supplies mucous membrane of the larynx below the vocal folds.

plexus'. From this plexus a branch called 'lesser petrosal nerve' arises and passes through foramen ovale along with mandibular nerve. The lesser petrosal nerve carries secretomotor fibers to the parotid salivary gland through otic ganglion and auriculotemporal nerve.

2. Muscular branch supplies stylopharyngeus muscle.

3. Pharyngeal branches contribute to the pharyngeal plexus on the wall of the pharynx, through which it gives sensory branches to the mucous membrane of the pharynx.

4. Carotid branch terminates in carotid body and sinus to regulate the blood pressure and heart rate.

5. Terminal branches supply mucous membrane of the posterior 1/3rd of the dorsum of the tongue, palatine tonsil and also soft palate.

## VAGUS NERVE (10TH CRANIAL NERVE)

Vagus is a mixed nerve and distributes in the neck, thorax and abdomen. It carries parasympathetic fibers to the heart, lungs and many abdominal organs.

35

6. *Cardiac branches:* The cardiac branches, arise in neck as well as thorax. They terminate in the cardiac plexuses. They provide parasympathetic fibers to the heart (cardioinhibitory).

   It also provides parasympathetic fibers to lungs (bronchoconstriction) through pulmonary plexus.

7. Branches arising from celiac plexus provide parasympathetic fibers to the stomach, small intestine and part of the large intestine. Functionally they are motor to the musculature, secretomotor to the glands and inhibitory to the sphincter.

> **Vagotomy:** Section of the vagus nerve is sometimes performed to reduce production of hydrochloric acid from the parietal cells in patients with peptic ulcers. Injuries to the external and recurrent laryngeal nerves are possible during thyroid surgeries and can cause hoarseness.

## ACCESSORY NERVE (11TH CRANIAL NERVE)

It is entirely a motor nerve and it consists of cranial and spinal parts.

### 1. The Cranial Part

The fibers of cranial part of the accessory nerve are derived from nucleus ambiguus of medulla oblongata. It emerges from the posterolateral sulcus of the medulla along with 9th and 10th cranial nerves. The nerve passes towards the jugular foramen where it is joined by spinal part of the nerve. However, the cranial part soon separates and joins the vagus nerve in the jugular foramen. Through the vagus nerve, the cranial part of the accessory nerve supplies muscles of soft palate (except tensor veli palatini muscle) and pharynx (except stylopharyngeus).

### 2. The Spinal Part

The spinal part of the accessory nerve arises from the anterior grey horn of the upper 5 cervical segments of the spinal cord. The rootlets of this nerve arise from the spinal cord between ventral and dorsal roots of upper 5 cervical spinal nerves. These rootlets unite to form an ascending spinal root, which enters the cranial cavity through foramen magnum and joins with cranial part of the accessory nerve. It again separates and descends from the cranial cavity through jugular foramen. It traverses the digastric and upper part of the carotid triangle to enter the substance of the sternocleidomastoid muscle. It emerges from the midpoint of the posterior border of the sternocleido-mastoid muscle to traverse the posterior triangle (as a content) to terminate in the trapezius muscle. It supplies

• Sternocleidomastoid muscle
• Trapezius muscle

## HYPOGLOSSAL NERVE (12TH CRANIAL NERVE)

It is a motor nerve supplying the muscles of tongue.

### Nuclei of Origin

Fibers of the hypoglossal nerve arises from the hypoglossal nucleus in the medulla oblongata.

### Course

The nerve emerges from the surface of the medulla oblongata between pyramid and olive. The nerve leaves the cranial cavity by passing through the hypoglossal canal. It receives a communicating branch from ventral ramus of first cervical nerve. The hypoglossal nerve terminates by supplying muscles of tongue (Fig. 35.8).

### Distribution

a. Hypoglossal nerve supplies all the muscles of tongue except palatoglossus.
b. The ventral ramus of first cervical nerve ($C_1$) supplies geniohyoid and thyrohyoid muscles and forms the superior root of ansa cervicalis.

> A unilateral lesion of hypoglossal nerve results in paralysis of tongue muscles on the affected side. Upon protrusion, the tip of the tongue deviates **to the side of the lesion** due to opposite genioglossus action.

### Miscellaneous

#### Phrenic Nerve ($C_{3,4,5}$)

This nerve descends in front of the scalenus anterior muscle in the root of the neck. In the thorax it descends in front of the root of the lung. It is the motor nerve supplying the diaphragm. In addition, it also supplies

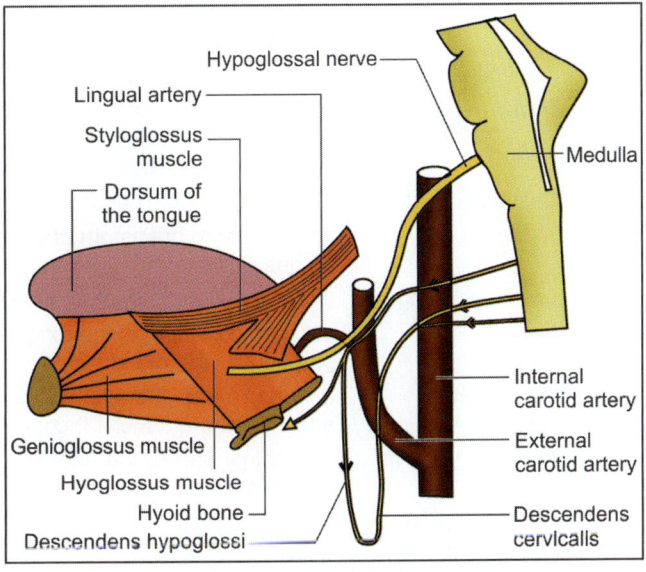

**Fig. 35.8:** Hypoglossal nerve

35

sensory fibers to the fibrous pericardium of heart, parietal pleura and peritoneum lining under surface of the diaphragm. Involvement of any of these structures can cause referred pain in the shoulder region on the affected side. This is because skin over the shoulder is supplied by supraclavicular nerve having similar root value $C_3$ and $C_4$.

### Ansa Cervicalis

It is a nerve loop located in front of the carotid sheath of the neck. It is formed by two roots.

a. *Superior root (descendens hypoglossi):* A branch from the ventral ramus of first cervical nerve ($C_1$) joins the hypoglossal nerve and after a short-course leaves that nerve as superior root of ansa cervicalis.

b. *Inferior root (descendens cervicalis):* This nerve is formed by branches from ventral rami of second and third cervical ($C_2$, $C_3$) nerves.

The superior and inferior root joins to form 'ansa cervicalis'.

The superior root supplies superior belly of the omohyoid muscle. The loop of the ansa cervicalis gives muscular branches to inferior belly of omohyoid, sternothyroid and sternohyoid muscles.

### Thoracic Spinal Nerves

There are 12 pairs of thoracic spinal nerves. The ventral rami of first ($T_1$) to eleventh ($T_{11}$) thoracic nerves run in the spaces between the ribs and are called 'intercostal nerves'. These nerves traverse the intercostal spaces (spaces between the ribs).

The ventral ramus of 12th thoracic nerve lies below the 12th rib and is called 'subcostal nerve'.

### Typical Intercostal Nerves

The 3rd to 6th intercostal nerves are considered as 'typical', because they are confined only to the thoracic wall (the first two thoracic nerves supply upper limb and lower 6 thoracic nerves supply abdominal wall in addition to thoracic wall).

| No. | Name of the cranial nerve | Functions |
|---|---|---|
| | | **Cranial nerves and their distributions** |
| 1. | Olfactory nerve | It conveys smell sensation from the roof of the nasal cavity to the olfactory cortex of the cerebrum. |
| 2. | Optic nerve | It conveys visual information from the eye to the visual cortex of the cerebrum. |
| 3. | Oculomotor nerve | It conveys motor fibres to most of the extra ocular muscles (except superior oblique and lateral rectus). It also carries parasympathetic fibres to ciliaris and sphincter pupillae muscles of the eye for visual reflexes. |
| 4. | Trochlear nerve | It conveys motor fibers to superior oblique muscle of the eyeball. |
| 5. | Trigeminal nerve | Through its three divisions (ophthalmic, maxillary and mandibular), it carries sensory information from major parts of the head and neck (anterior quadrant of the scalp, face, nasal cavity, paranasal air sinuses, palate, oral cavity and nasopharynx). It also supplies muscles of mastication through its mandibular division. |
| 6. | Abducent nerve | It conveys motor fibers to lateral rectus muscle of the eyeball. |
| 7. | Facial nerve | It conveys motor fibers to muscles of facial expression and stapedius muscle of the ear. It carries parasympathetic secretomotor fibers to the lacrimal, submandibular and sublingual glands. It also carries taste sensation from the anterior part of the dorsum of the tongue. |
| 8. | Vestibulocochlear nerve | The vestibular part of the nerve carries information from saccule, utricle and semicircular ducts of internal ear to brainstem and cerebellum to maintain the equilibrium. The cochlear part of the nerve carries auditory impulses from the organ of Corti of internal ear to brainstem. |
| 9. | Glossopharyngeal nerve | It conveys motor fibers to stylopharyngeus muscle and carries sensory information from posterior part of the dorsum of the tongue and oropharynx. It conveys parasympathetic secretomotor fibers to parotid salivary gland. |
| 10. | Vagus nerve | It carries motor fibers to muscles of larynx, pharynx and palate and sensory information from larynx and skin of the auricle. It conveys parasympathetic fibers to heart, lungs and abdominal organs. |
| 11. | Accessory nerve | The spinal part of the accessory nerve supplies trapezius and sternocleidomastoid muscles. The cranial part supplies muscles of palate and pharynx through vagus nerve. |
| 12. | Hypoglossal nerve | It carries motor fibers to muscles of the tongue |

## Course of a Typical Intercostal Nerve

1. After emerging from the intervertebral foramen, the nerve enters the 'costal groove' of the corresponding rib.
2. In the posterior part of the intercostal space, the nerve lies between pleura and internal intercostal membrane.
3. Then the nerve proceeds between internal intercostal and innermost intercostal muscles.
4. The intercostal nerve lies below the posterior intercostal vessels.
5. In the anterior part of the intercostal space, the intercostal nerve pierces internal intercostal muscle and other superficial muscles.
6. It terminates as anterior cutaneous nerve of the thorax.

## Branches and Distribution

1. Muscular branches supply the intercostal muscles, transversus thoracis muscle.
2. Collateral branch arising near the angle of rib also supply muscles of the intercostal space.
3. Lateral cutaneous branch arises near the angle of the rib, pierces the muscles and becomes cutaneous in the midaxillary line.
4. Anterior cutaneous branch (termination of intercostal nerve) emerges on the side of the sternum to supply the overlying skin.

## Subcostal Nerve

The 12th thoracic nerve enters the abdomen by passing deep to the lateral arcuate ligament of diaphragm. It supplies anterior abdominal wall muscles including rectus abdominis and pyramidalis muscle.

# Endocrine Glands

**36**

Endocrine glands are those (ductless glands), which pour their secretions directly into the blood. Secretions of these endocrine glands are called hormones.

The different endocrine glands and tissues of the body are:

1. Hypophysis cerebri (pituitary)
2. Thyroid and parathyroid glands
3. Suprarenal gland (adrenal)
4. Pineal gland
5. Islets of Langerhans in pancreas
6. Interstitial cells of the testes
7. Follicles and corpus luteum of ovaries
8. Some cells of kidney, placenta and lining epithelium of GIT.

## HYPOPHYSIS CEREBRI (PITUITARY GLAND)

It regulates the activity of many other endocrine glands; hence it is called the master gland.

### Situation

It is situated in the hypophyseal fossa of the body of sphenoid bone and is suspended from floor of the third ventricle. It measures about 12 mm in breadth and 8 mm in length.

### Parts

It has two parts, which differ from each other structurally and developmentally (Fig. 36.1).

1. *Adenohypophysis:* Which is further divided into pars anterior, pars intermedia and pars tuberalis.
2. *Neurohypophysis:* Which is divided into pars nervosa, infundibular stem and the median eminence.

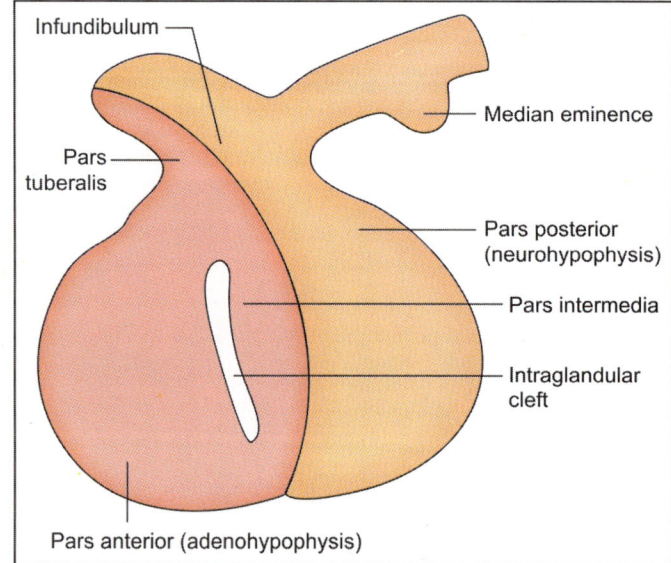

**Fig. 36.1:** Parts of the pituitary

### Microscopic Structure

The cells of the adenohypophysis are classified into chromophobes (they take less stain because of less number of cellular organelles) and chromophils (they take stain). The chromophil cells are further classified into acidophils and basophils depending on staining character. These acidophil and basophil cells are further classified into variety of cells on the basis of type of hormones they secrete.

### Anterior Lobe (pars anterior)

Anterior lobe (pars anterior) consists of a clusters of cells supported by reticular fibers, permeated by sinusoids and fenestrated capillary plexus. They secrete following hormones.

- *Somatotrophs:* It secrete somatotrophic hormone (STH or growth hormones). The hormone promotes proliferation of cartilage cells in the epiphysis of the growing bone.
- *Mammotrophs:* It secrete prolactin or lactogenic hormone (LTH). More numerous in females than males and most numerous during pregnancy. The hormone stimulates the growth and secretory activities of a lactating mammary gland.
- *Thyrotrophs:* They produce thyroid stimulating hormone (TSH), which stimulates the activity of the thyroid gland.
- *Corticotrophs:* They produce corticotropic hormones, also called adrenocorticotropic hormones (ACTH). The hormone stimulates the cells of the adrenal cortex.
- *Gonadotrophs:* They produce follicular stimulating hormone (FSH), which stimulates the growth of ovarian follicles in females and regulate the spermatogenesis in males.
- *Luteotrophs:* It secretes the luteinizing hormone (LH). It stimulates the ovulation and conversion of graafian follicle into corpus luteum in females. In males, it (ICSH) stimulates interstitial cells of Leydig to produce testosterone.

### Intermediate Lobe (pars intermedia)

The cells of this lobe called melanotrophs, secrete melanocyte stimulating hormone (MSH). It causes increased pigmentation of the skin.

### Posterior Lobe (pars nervosa)

Consists of nonmyelinated nerve fibers, fenestrated plexus of blood capillaries and special types of neuroglial cells called pituicytes (Fig. 36.2).

Posterior lobe is connected with hypothalamus through the **hypothalomohypophyseal tract**, arising from the supraoptic and paraventricular nuclei of hypothalamus. Supraoptic nucleus of the hypothalamus synthesizes vasopressin and paraventricular nucleus oxytocin. These hormones pass through the hypothalamohypophyseal tract and reach the sinusoids of the posterior lobe (Fig. 36.2). The posterior lobe therefore does not synthesize the hormones, but acts as storage and releasing center.

- *Vasopressin/antidiuretic hormone (ADH):* It increases the water reabsorption in the distal convoluted tubules of the kidney, and produces concentrated urine. In the absence of ADH, large volumes of water will be excreted in the urine (polyuria) and is associated with excessive thirst. This uncommon condition is called diabetes insipidus.

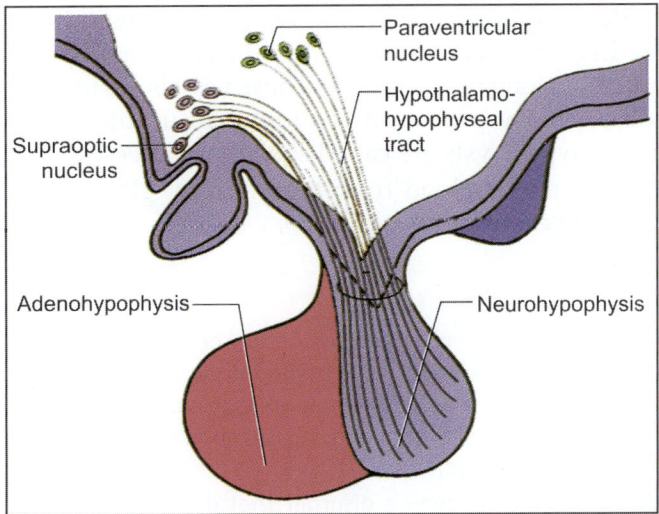

**Fig. 36.2:** Hypothalamohypophyseal tract

- *Oxytocin:* It stimulates the alveoli of the mammary gland for milk ejaculation. It also causes contraction of uterine musculature during final stage of delivery.

### Blood Supply

It is mainly supplied by the superior and inferior hypophyseal arteries, which are the branches of the internal carotid artery (Fig. 36.3).

1. Superior hypophyseal artery terminates by forming capillary plexus in the median eminence and lower part of the infundibulum.
2. Inferior hypophyseal artery gives a few direct branches to the posterior lobe and some of them terminate in the capillary plexus in the lower part of the infundibulum.

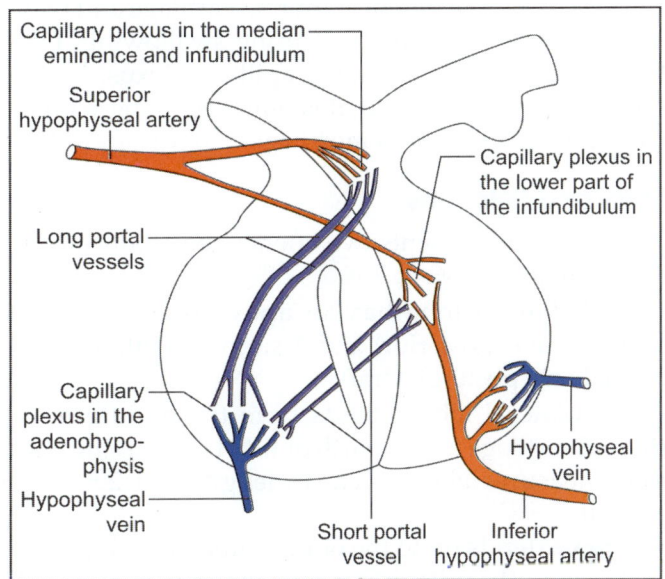

**Fig. 36.3:** Blood supply to the pituitary gland

Vessels arising from the capillary plexus in the median eminence draining into the adenohypophysis are called long portal vessels. Those vessels arising from the capillary plexus in the lower infundibulum to adenohypophysis are called short portal vessels.

The venous blood from the pituitary gland drains into cavernous sinus.

### Applied Aspects

1. A tumor of the pituitary is generally detected easily as it begins to grow and interfere with hormonal activity. If the tumor grows superiorly it may compress optic chiasma to cause bitemporal hemianopia (temporal field of vision is lost in both eyes)
2. Diabetes insipidus—a disorder that develops when the posterior pituitary no longer releases adequate amounts of ADH.

## THYROID GLAND

### Situation

It is an endocrine gland situated in front and sides of the trachea at the lower part of the neck. It is mainly concerned with metabolic activities of all the cells and also calcium metabolism.

### Coverings

Thyroid gland is externally covered by an inner true capsule and outer false capsule. The false capsule is derived from pretracheal fascia, which is attached to hyoid bone and cricoid cartilage. Its attachment to cricoid cartilage is thick and forms 'ligament of Berry'. Because of its attachment to thyroid cartilage and hyoid bone, thyroid gland moves during swallowing. Deep to the true capsule is dense capillary plexus. During removal of thyroid gland, it is removed along with the true capsule to avoid hemorrhage.

### Parts and Relations

Thyroid gland presents two lateral lobes connected by an isthmus (Fig. 36.4).

Each lateral lobe has an apex, base, 2 borders (anterior and posterior) and 3 surfaces (anterolateral, medial and posterolateral).

Each lateral lobe extends from the middle of the thyroid cartilage to the fourth or fifth tracheal ring. Each lobe measures about 5 cm in length and 2.5 cm in breadth.

- **Apex** extends up to the oblique line in the lamina of the thyroid cartilage. It is related to superior thyroid artery in front and external laryngeal nerve behind.

- **The base** extends up to 4th or 5th tracheal ring and is related to inferior thyroid artery and recurrent laryngeal nerve.
- **The anterolateral surface** is related to strap muscles of the neck (sternohyoid, sternothyroid and superior belly of the omohyoid).
- **The posterolateral surface** is related to carotid sheath and its contents (common carotid artery, internal jugular vein and vagus nerves).
- **The medial surface** is related to trachea and esophagus (2 tubes), cricothyroid and inferior constrictor muscle of the pharynx (2 muscles) and two nerves (external laryngeal and recurrent laryngeal nerve).
- **The anterior border** is related to anterior descending branch of the superior thyroid artery.
- **The posterior border** is related to anastomoses between the posterior descending branch of superior thyroid artery and ascending branch of the inferior thyroid artery.

Isthmus connects the 2 lateral lobes and is about 1.25 cm in both vertical and transverse diameters. Occasionally a pyramidal lobe extend from the upper part of the isthmus (Fig. 36.4).

### Blood Supply

*Arterial Supply* (Figs 36.5a and b)

A. *Superior thyroid artery:* It is a branch of external carotid artery. It reaches the gland close to the apex of the lateral lobe where it divides into anterior and posterior branches. The anterior branch descends along the anterior border of the lateral lobe then along the upper border of the isthmus. Where it

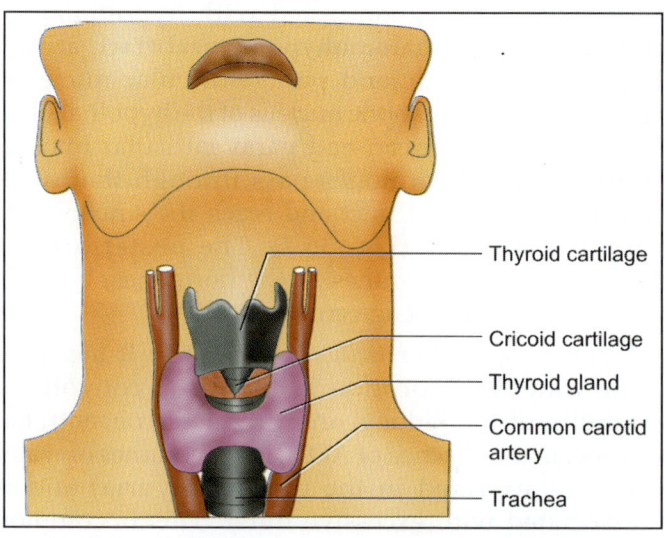

Thyroid cartilage

Cricoid cartilage

Thyroid gland

Common carotid artery

Trachea

**Fig. 36.4:** Thyroid position—anterior view

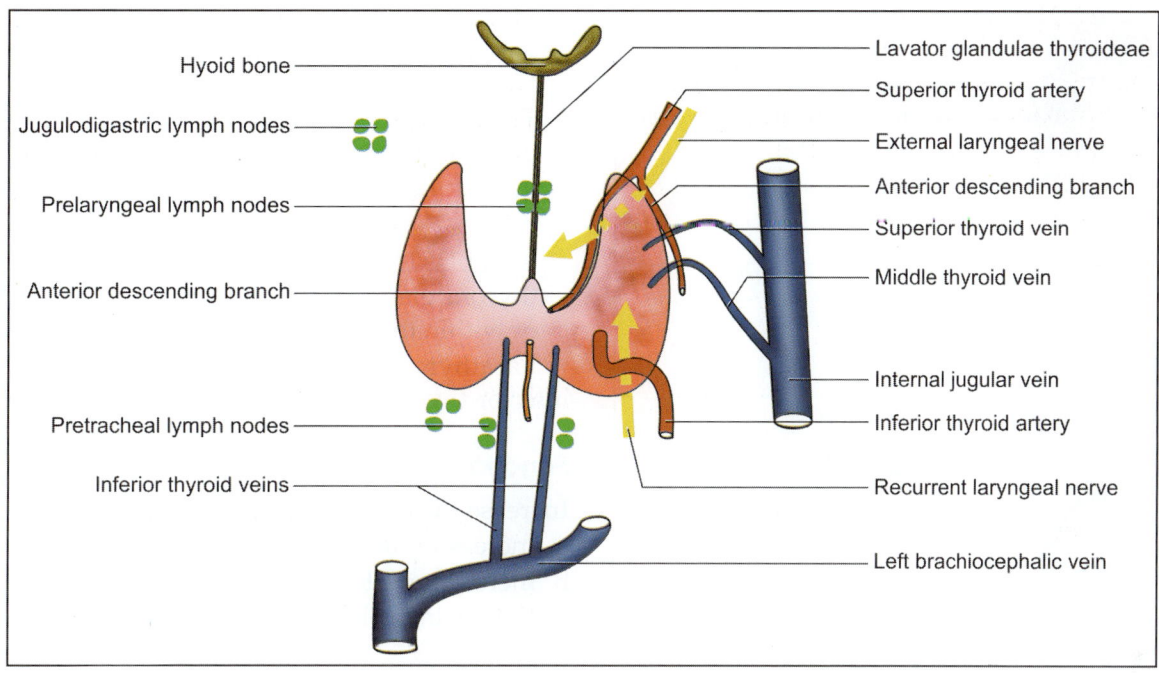

**Fig. 36.5a:** Blood supply and lymphatic drainage of thyroid gland

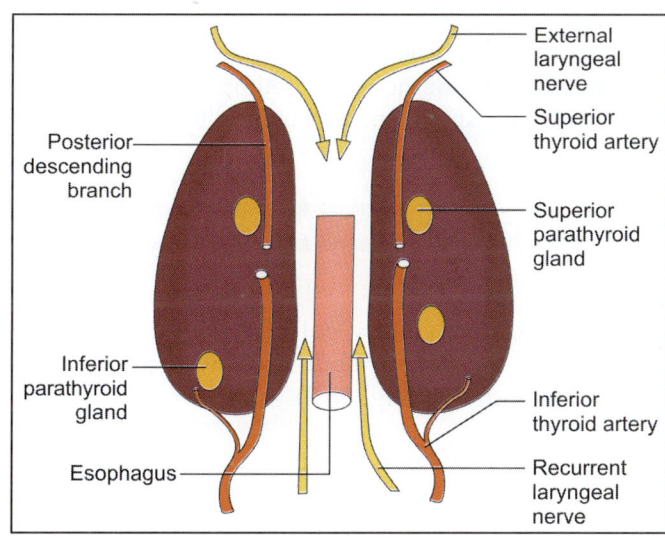

**Fig. 36.5b:** Arterial supply—posterior view

anastomose with similar artery of the opposite side. The posterior branch descends along the posterior border and anastomoses with ascending branch of the inferior thyroid artery.

B. *Inferior thyroid artery:* It is a branch from the thyrocervical trunk of the subclavian artery. It ascends towards the base of the thyroid gland where it gives many direct branches to the gland. One of the branches called ascending branch ascends along the posterior border to anastomose with posterior branch of superior thyroid artery.

C. Thyroid gland is supplied by many accessory arteries (tracheal and esophageal arteries).

## Venous Drainage

A pair of superior thyroid veins drains into internal jugular veins or common facial vein. Another pair of middle thyroid veins drains into internal jugular veins. Inferior thyroid vein(s) emerging from the lower part of the isthmus often drains into left brachiocephalic vein.

## Microscopic Structure

Human thyroid gland consists of about 3 millions of thyroid follicles. These thyroid follicles are lined by cuboidal cells during moderate activity of the gland (Fig. 36.6). However, it can be columnar during high activity or flattened when inactive. These cells are involved in synthesis of a protein called thyroglobulin. Iodine derived from the food substances reaches the thyroid follicles by blood vessels and is taken into the lumen of the follicle, where thyroglobulin is iodinated to form colloid. It is acted upon by certain enzymes and released as thyroxin hormone triiodothyronine ($T_3$) and tetraiodothyronine ($T_4$) to the bloodstream. Thyroxin hormone increases rate of protein synthesis and rate of energy release from carbohydrates. It regulates the rate of growth and stimulates maturity of nervous system.

36

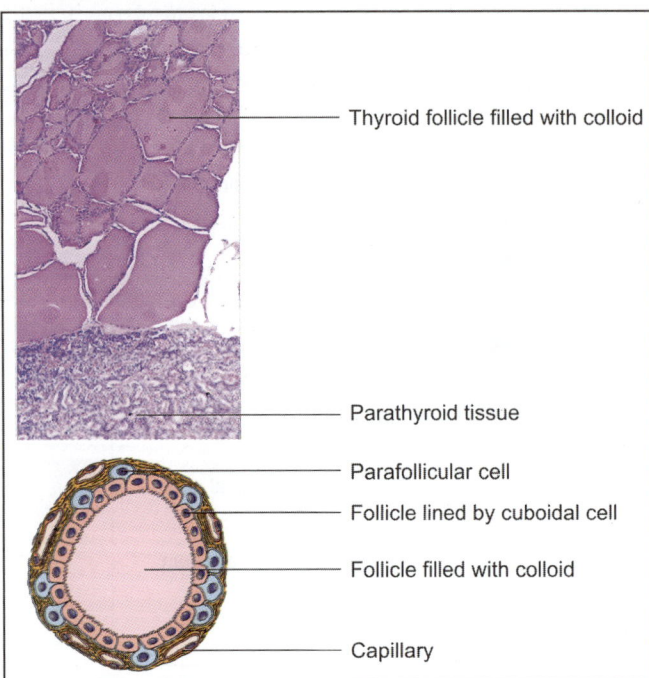

**Fig. 36.6:** Microscopic structure of thyroid and parathyroid

## PARAFOLLICULAR CELLS (C-CELLS/CLEAR CELLS)

Cells are polyhedral, with oval eccentric nuclei. The parafollicular cells, which are present between the base of the follicular cell and basement membrane, secrete "thyrocalcitonin". This hormone regulates the calcium metabolism. It tends to withdraw the serum calcium by depositing it in the bone.

### Applied Aspects

1. An enlargement of thyroid gland is called goiter. In the absence of sufficient dietary iodine, the thyroid cannot produce adequate amounts of $T_4$ and $T_3$. The resulting lack of negative feedback inhibition causes abnormally high levels of TSH secretion (from pituitary), which in turn, stimulates the abnormal growth of the thyroid (a goiter).
2. Hypothyroidism causes cretinism in infants, and myxedema in adults (subcutaneous swelling, dry skin, hair loss low body temperature).
3. Hyperthyroidism (thyrotoxicosis) is characterized by tachycardia, tremors and exophthalmos.

## PARATHYROID GLANDS

- They are yellowish brown lentiform bodies (size of a split pea).
- Their number varies, usually (in 80%) 4 in number and arranged in superior and inferior pairs.
- Their secretion is called parathormone.

- The superior pair of parathyroids is also called parathyroid IV and the inferior pair called parathyroid III.
- The position of the superior parathyroid is constant and is placed along the posterior border of the lateral lobe of thyroid (at the level of cricoid cartilage).
- However, the position of inferior parathyroid is variable. It can be placed close to the base of the thyroid gland (inside or out side the false capsule) or within the substance of thyroid gland (Fig. 36.5b).

Parathyroid glands are supplied by superior and inferior thyroid arteries.

### Functions of Parathormone

Increase the serum calcium level by:

a. Increasing bone resorption through osteoclasts.
b. Increasing calcium reabsorption from renal tubules.
c. Enhancing calcium absorption of the gut.

### Applied Aspects

**Hyperparathyroidism:** Increased removal of calcium from bone, calcium level in blood increases and increased urinary excretion of calcium (causes stones of the urinary tract),
**Hypoparathyroidism:** Increased neuromuscular irritability causing muscular spasm and convulsions (tetany).

## SUPRARENAL GLANDS (ADRENAL GLANDS)

### Location

These are golden yellow colored endocrine glands situated on the posterior abdominal wall at the upper poles of the kidneys (Fig. 36.7).

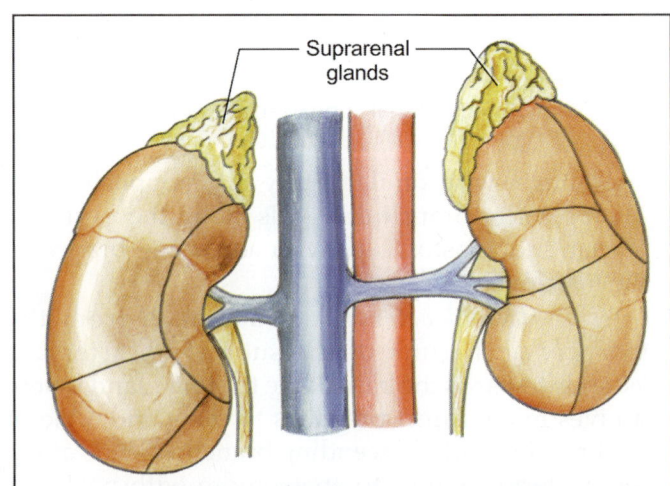

**Fig. 36.7:** Position of the suprarenal glands

## External Features and Relations

- Each suprarenal gland occupies upper pole of the kidney at the level of vertebral end of 12th rib.
- They are retroperitoneal organs and enclosed within the renal fascia which also encloses the kidney
- The right suprarenal gland is pyramidal in shape and left suprarenal gland is semilunar in shape.
- Each gland is about 50 mm in length and 30 mm in width.

## Blood Supply

Suprarenal glands are highly vascular. Each gland is supplied by 3 separate sets of arteries.

- *Superior suprarenal artery:* Branch from inferior phrenic artery
- *Middle suprarenal artery:* Branch from abdominal aorta
- *Inferior suprarenal artery:* Branch from renal artery

The right suprarenal vein drains into inferior vena cava. The left suprarenal vein drains into left renal vein.

## Microscopic Structure

The suprarenal gland presents an outer cortex and inner medulla (Fig. 36.8).

### Cortex

The cells of the cortex are arranged in 3 zones from outside inwards

1. Zona glomerulosa
2. Zona fasciculata
3. Zona reticularis

### 1. Zona glomerulosa

It forms the outer 1/5th of the cortex. Cells are arranged in inverted columns.

They secrete the mineralocorticoid hormone—**aldosterone**.

They influence the electrolyte and water balance of the body (increased $Na^+$ uptake in exchange of $K^+$ or $H^+$ in kidney).

The secretion of aldosterone is influenced by renin from the juxtaglomerular cells of kidney, and partly by the pituitary.

### 2. Zona fasciculata

It forms the middle 3/5th of the cortex. Cells are arranged in vertical columns with sinusoid in between them.

They secrete glucocorticoids **cortisol**. They influence the carbohydrate and protein metabolism of the body.

Cortisol is diabetogenic, delays wound healing (diminishes the activity of fibrocytes), is antiallergic in response, and diminishes antibody formation.

### 3. Zona reticularis

Irregularly arranged clusters of cells, separated by capillaries and sinusoids.

They secrete sex hormones estrogen and androgens.

These hormones regulate the secondary sex characters.

### Medulla

Medulla forms 1/10th of the gland and consists of chromaffin cells.

They secrete noradrenaline and adrenaline.

This secretion takes place mainly at times of stress. The effects are similar to that of the sympathetic stimulation.

## Applied Aspects

1. *Addison's disease:* Deficiency of mineralocorticoids (muscular weakness, low blood pressure, anemia)
2. *Cushing's syndrome:* Excessive secretion of glucocorticoids (obesity, diabetes and hypogonadism)
3. *Pheochromocytoma:* A tumor of the medulla, produces hypertension due to excessive secretion of catecholamines.

## PINEAL GLAND (EPIPHYSIS CEREBRI)

It is attached to the roof of the third ventricle by a stalk. The stalk consists of superior (habenular commissure) and inferior (posterior commissure) laminae. The pineal gland projects below the splenium of corpus callosum and above the tectum of the midbrain. Pineal body is rich in melatonin, serotonin and norepinephrine. The pineal gland suppresses the gonadal development before puberty.

***Other endocrine tissues and hormones***

a. Growing ovarian follicle inside the ovary—estrogen
b. Corpus luteum—progesterone and estrogen
c. Interstitial cells of Leydig in testis—testosterone
d. Islets of Langerhans in pancreas—insulin and glucagon
e. Some cells of lining epithelium of the stomach and intestine—serotonin, gastrin, somatostatin, secretin cholecystokinin, etc.

# Special Senses

The human body has a special ability to sense change in its internal and external environment, which enables it to maintain a state of homeostasis which is required for survival. The 5 sense organs are:

1. Eye—for sight
2. Ear—for hearing
3. Nose—for smell
4. Tongue—for taste
5. Skin—for touch

The ear and eye is explained in this chapter. The skin is explained in Chapter 3.

## EAR

Ear is an organ of hearing and also maintains equilibrium of the body (Fig. 37.1).

### Parts

1. External ear
2. Middle ear
3. Internal ear

### 1. External Ear

It collects and conducts the sound waves from the air to the tympanic membrane.

i. *Pinna/auricle:* It is made up of elastic cartilage and connective tissue, covered by skin.
ii. *External acoustic (auditory) meatus:* It is about 24 mm in length.

### 2. Middle Ear (Tympanic Cavity/Tympanum)

It is a bony cavity within the petrous part of the temporal bone lined by mucous membrane and filled

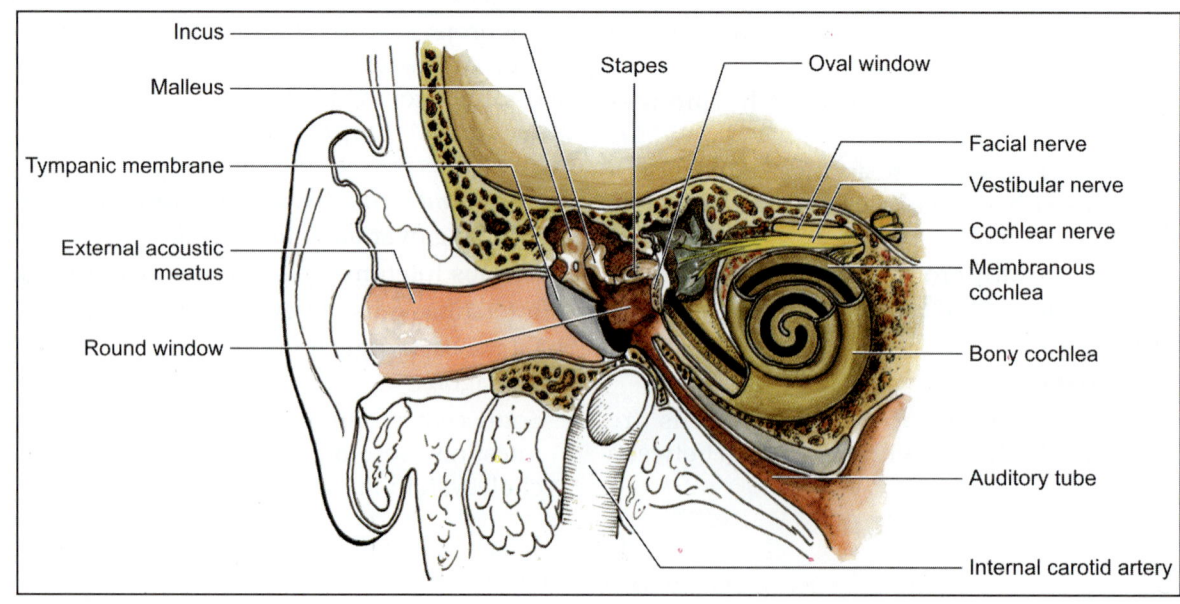

**Fig. 37.1:** Parts of the ear

with air. It intensifies the force of sound vibrations, without altering the amplitude, conveys the vibration from the tympanic membrane to the fenestra vestibuli (vestibule of internal ear), by the movements of the ear ossicles (malleus, incus and stapes—Fig. 37.2).

The middle ear cavity is like a match box having 6 walls. The vertical and anteroposterior diameters are about 15 mm. Following are the walls of the middle ear:

a. *Roof:* A thin bony plate called tegmen tympani forms roof.

b. *Floor* It is formed by a thin plate of bone which separate the middle ear from superior bulb of the internal jugular vein

c. *Anterior wall (carotid wall)* (Fig. 37.3)

   i. The upper part of the anterior wall presents the canal for tensor tympani muscle.

   ii. The middle part has the opening of auditory tube.

   iii. The lower part is separated from the internal carotid artery by a thin plate of bone.

d. *Posterior wall (mastoid wall)* (Fig. 37.3)

   i. The upper part of the posterior wall presents an opening (aditus) to communicate with 'mastoid antrum'.

   ii. Fossa incudis is a depression, which lodges the short process of the incus.

   iii. Pyramid is a conical bony projection. The opening at its apex transmits the tendon of stapedius muscle.

e. *Lateral wall* is formed by tympanic membrane.

***Tympanic membrane:*** It is a trilaminar membrane and separates the tympanic cavity from the external acoustic meatus. Its maximum diameter is about 9–10 mm. The membrane is placed obliquely at an angle of 55° with the floor of the external acoustic meatus. The circumference of the membrane is attached to the tympanic sulcus (in the tympanic bone). The sulcus is deficient above, from the 2 ends of which, the anterior and posterior malleolar folds converge to the lateral process of the malleus (Fig. 37.3).

### Parts

   i. *Pars flaccida:* It is small triangular area between the two-malleolar folds.

   ii. *Pars tensa:* It is a large area of the tympanic membrane, which is taut by the attachment of the handle of the malleus.

The tympanic membrane has an outer concave surface, and an inner convex surface, and the point of maximum convexity, is called UMBO at the attachment of the handle of the malleus.

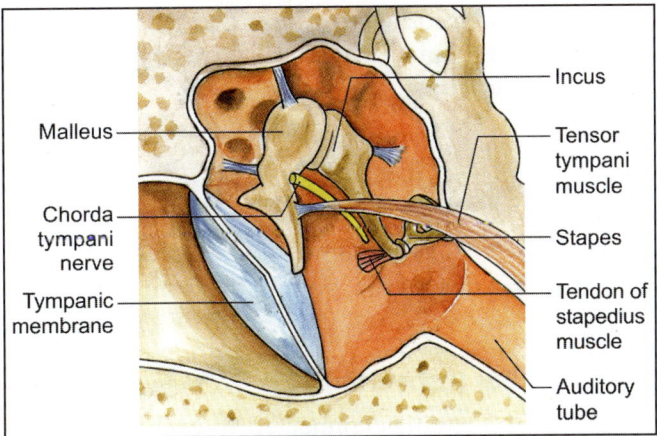

**Fig. 37.2:** Middle ear

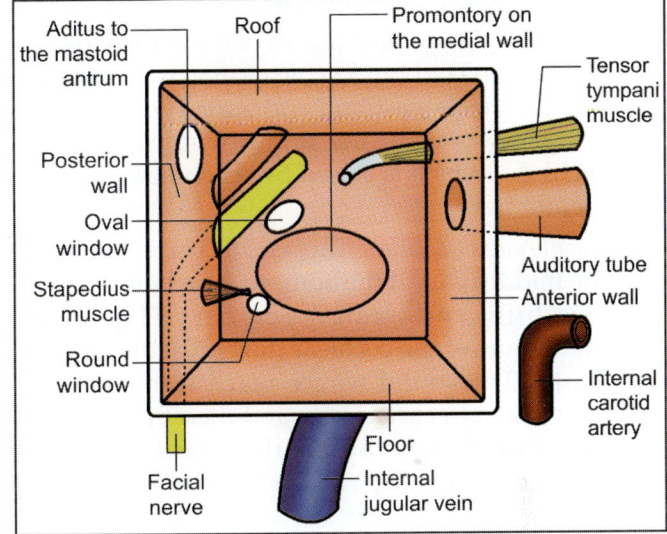

**Fig. 37.3:** Middle ear (lateral view after opening the tympanic membrane—schematic)

f. *Medial (labyrinthine) wall:* It separates the middle ear from the internal ear (Fig. 37.3). It presents the following features.

   i. **Promontory:** A rounded bulging produced by first turn of the cochlea.

   ii. **Fenestra vestibuli (oval window):** It leads to vestibule of the internal ear and is closed by the foot plate of the stapes.

   iii. **Fenestra cochleae (round window):** It opens into the scala tympani of the cochlea.

   iv. **Bony canal** for the facial nerve.

### Communications of Middle Ear

*Anteriorly:* The middle ear cavity communicates with the nasopharynx through the auditory tube, by which it maintains an equal pressure on either side of the tympanic membrane.

*Posteriorly:* The middle ear cavity communicates with the mastoid antrum and air cells through the aditus to the mastoid antrum.

### Contents of the Middle Ear

a. Ear ossicles—malleus, incus and stapes {three small bones}.
b. Muscles—tensor tympani and stapedius.
c. Vessels and nerves that supply the tympanic cavity.
d. Air.

### 3. Int nal Ear (Labyrinth) (Figs 37.1 and 37.4a)

It consists of 3 cavities connected to each other. Each cavity is having an outer bony labyrinth and inner membranous labyrinth.

1A Bony cochlea resembles the shell of a common snail. This bony canal makes two and three quarter (2¾) turns. The bony cochlear canal is divided into 2 parts—scala vestibuli and scala tympani. Scala tympani opens at the round window (fenestra cochleae) which is closed by secondary tympanic membrane.

1B *Membranous cochlea:* This cochlear duct occupies the middle part of the bony cochlea between scala vestibuli and scala tympani. The basilar membrane of the cochlear duct presents 'organ of Corti'. The sound waves reach from tympanic membrane to ear ossicles and then through scala vestibuli reach the basilar membrane. The auditory receptors, viz, the hair cells of 'ogan of

Corti' are stimulated. This organ of Corti is innervated by peripheral processes of the bipolar neurons of spiral ganglion. The central processes of these neurons form **cochlear nerve** (Fig. 37.4b)

2A *Bony vestibule:* It is the central part of the internal ear medial to the middle ear. The lateral wall of the bony vestibule opens into the middle ear at oval window (fenestra vestibuli) which is closed by foot-plate of the stapes. The medial wall of the bony vestibule presents internal acoustic meatus. Saccule and utricle occupy the bony vestibule.

2B *Saccule and utricle:* The saccule is connected with membranous cochlear duct. Posteriorly the saccule connected with utricle. Utricle receives 3 semicircular ducts through 5 openings.
The wall of the saccule and utricle present a specialized structure called 'macula'. Maculae are concerned with static equilibrium (gives information about the position of the head)

3A *Bony semicircular canals:* They lie posterosuperior to the bony vestibule. The 3 bony semicircular canals are anterior, posterior and lateral. These 3 bony canal opens into bony vestibule by 5 openings.

3B *Membranous semicircular ducts:* The 3 semicircular ducts occupy the corresponding bony canals.
Each duct has an enlargement called 'ampulla' where it opens into utricle.
The wall of the ampulla presents a specialized structure called 'cristae'.

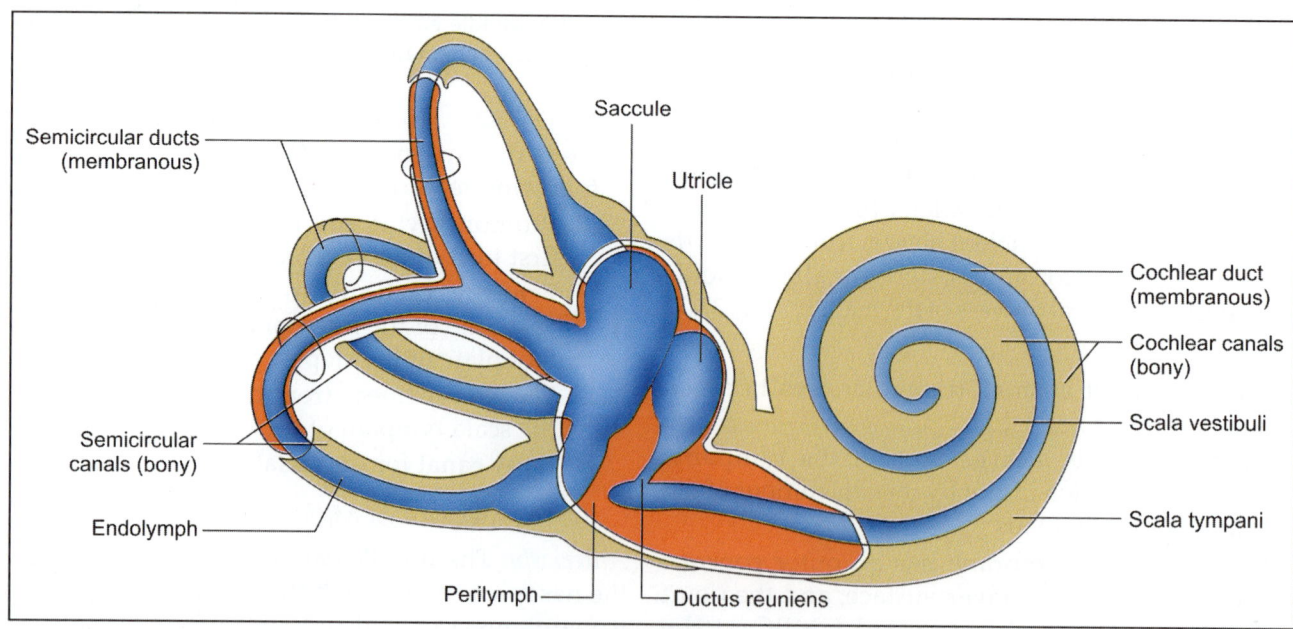

**Fig. 37.4a:** Internal ear—schematic

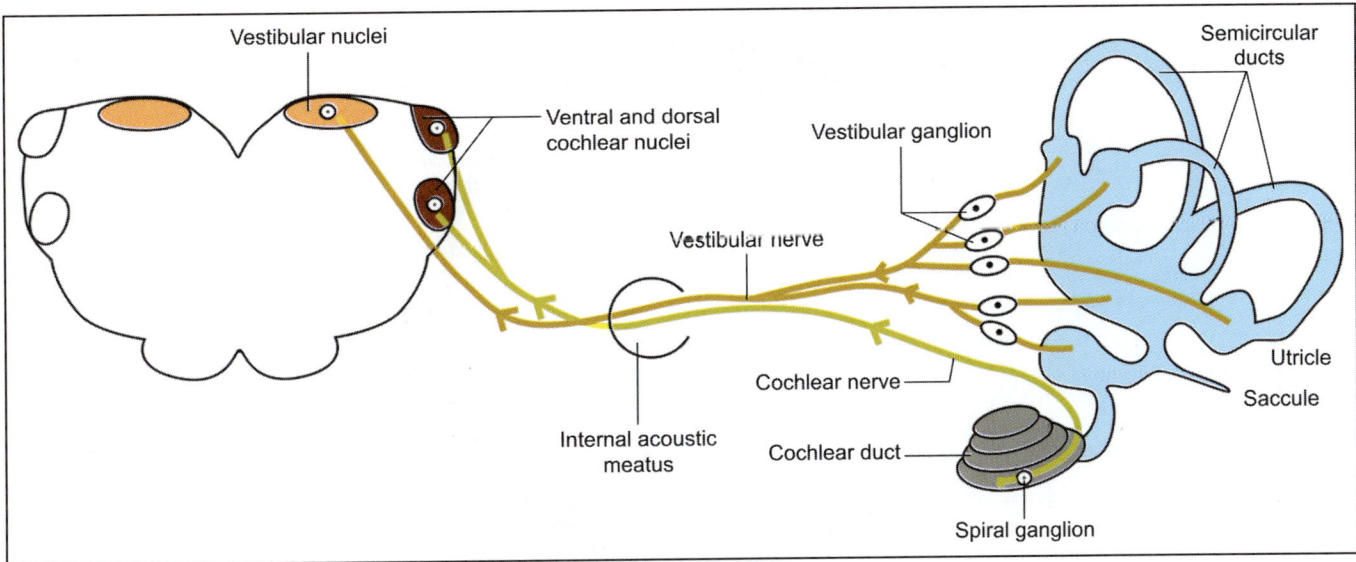

**Fig. 37.4b:** Origin of the vestibulocochlear nerve

Cristae are concerned with kinetic equilibrium (respond to pressure changes in the endolymph caused by movements of the head).

The 'maculae' of the saccule and utricle and 'cristae' of the semicircular ducts are innervated by peripheral processes of bipolar neurons of the vestibular ganglion. The central processes of these neurons form **vestibular nerve** (Fig. 37.4b).

> **Otitis media:** The infection in the middle ear is called otitis media. It can spread from nasopharynx through auditory tube. It can also spread into mastoid antrum and air cells and cause mastoiditis

## EYEBALL

The eyeball is the organ of sight. It is almost spherical in shape, and has a diameter of about 2.4 cm. It is placed in the bony orbit and externally covered with a well defined fascial sheath called Tenon's capsule. The globe of the eye moves within this Tenon's capsule by extra ocular muscles which are attached to the outer coat of the eyeball.

It is made up of 3 concentric coats.
a. *Outer fibrous coat* comprises the sclera and the cornea.
b. *Middle vascular coat* (uveal tract) consists of choroid, ciliary body and the iris.
c. *Inner nervous coat* is retina.

### Sclera

- It is opaque and forms the posterior 5/6th of the eyeball.
- It is firm and maintains the shape of the eyeball.
- Anteriorly it continues with the cornea at the limbus (sclerocorneal junction).
- Sclera gives attachments to the extra ocular muscles.
- Externally sclera is separated from bulbar fascia by episcleral space. Eyeball moves in the episcleral space.

### Cornea

- It is transparent and forms the anterior 1/6th of the eyeball.
- Cornea is a convex and an avascular structure, and is sensitive to pain.
- It is separated from the iris by a space called the anterior chamber of the eye.
- Cornea is supplied by ophthalmic nerve (sensitive to touch).

The transparency of the cornea is due to:
i. Absence of blood vessels.
ii. Uniform organization of collagen fibers.

*Structure of the cornea:* It is made up of following layers (Fig. 37.5a) (from superficial to deep)
i. Corneal epithelium is the conjunctiva of the eye. It is lined by stratified squamous non-keratinized epithelium.
ii. Bowman's membrane
iii. Substantia propria which is made up of bundles of collagen fibres.
iv. Descemet's membrane
v. Endothelium

Cornea is nourished by lacrimal fluid and aqueous humor.

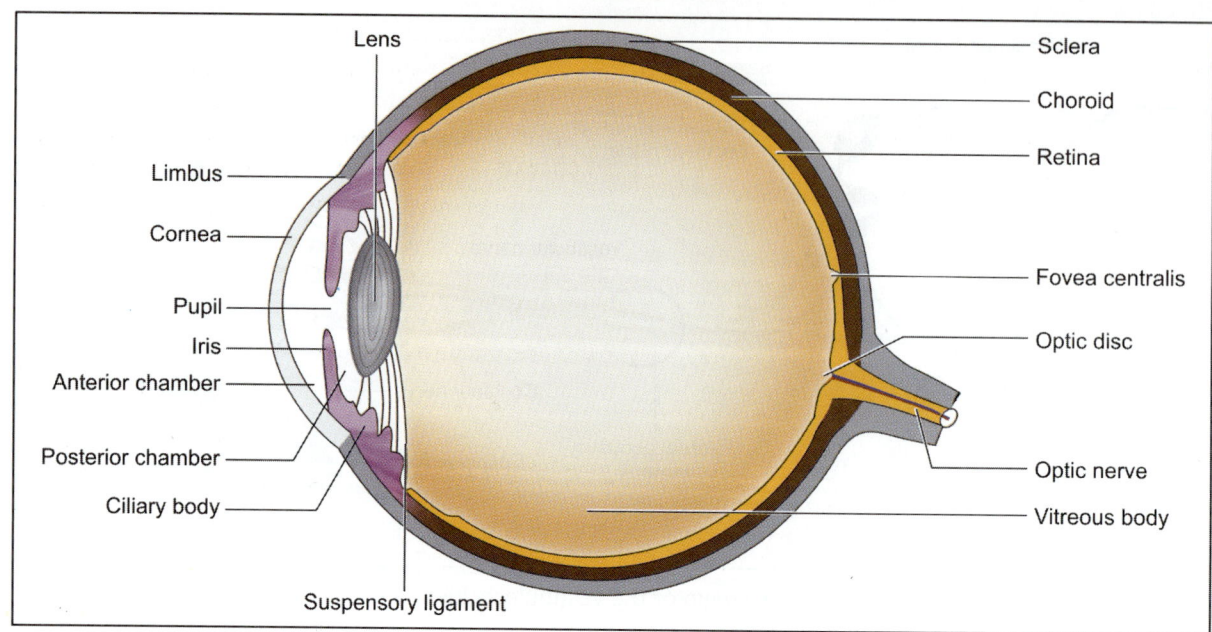

**Fig. 37.5a:** Section of the eyeball showing all the layers

### Choroid

- It is a pigmented layer, which separates the posterior part of the sclera from retina.
- Anteriorly it ends at ciliary body.

### Ciliary Body

- It is a thickened part of the uveal tract.
- Anteriorly it continues with the iris and posteriorly with choroid.
- Ciliary body is triangular in section with its apex joining the choroid (Fig. 37.5b).
- The inner surface of the ciliary body presents ciliary processes, which give attachment to the suspensory ligament of the lens.
- The ciliaris muscle present within the ciliary body is supplied by parasympathetic nerve for accommodation reflex. When ciliaris muscle contracts suspensory ligament of the lens is relaxed and allows the lens to bulge to adjust the eye for near vision.

### Iris

- It is a circular diaphragm and forms the anterior part of the uveal tract. It presents a circular opening in the center called the 'pupil'.
- The iris contains the sphincter pupillae and dilator pupillae muscles. These muscles adjust the size of the pupil, and control the amount of light entering the eye. The color of the iris is determined by the number pigments present in it.

- Sphincter pupillae is supplied by parasympathetic fibers for constriction of the pupil and accommodation reflex.
- Dilator pupillae is supplied by sympathetic fibers.

### Retina

- It is the inner delicate layer of the eyeball.
- Externally it is attached to the choroid and internally separated from vitreous body by the hyaloid membrane.
- Retina extends anteriorly up to ora serrata.
- Structurally retina consists of many sensory neurons and supporting cells, which are arranged in ten layers.
- Rods and cones are the photoreceptors present in the retina. Rods are concerned with dim light and cones are concerned with bright and color vision. These photoreceptors of the retina receive an inverted image of the object.
- There are about 120 million rods and 7 million cones in the retina of each eye.
- The other neurons of the retina include Bipolar cells, horizontal cells, amacrine cells, ganglion cells, etc.
- Optic nerve arises as axons of ganglionic cells (about 1 million ganglion cell nerve fibers form each optic nerve).

*Optic disc:* It is a circular area situated superomedial to the posterior pole of the eyeball where the optic nerve

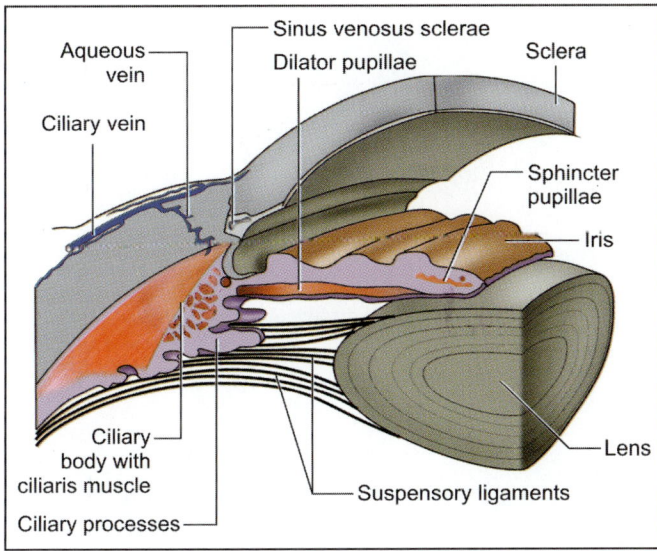

**Fig. 37.5b:** Sclerocorneal angle

begins. The optic disc is devoid of rods and cones and is called blind spot.

*Macula lutea:* It is an area at the posterior pole of the eyeball with a central depression called 'fovea centralis'. Only cones are present in the fovea and is concerned with discriminative vision.

*Lens:* It is a transparent biconvex structure, present behind the iris. It is suspended from the ciliary body by suspensory ligament. Lens can adjust its curvature on its anterior surface for near or distant vision. With age lens becomes hard with loss of accommodation power.

## Aqueous Humor

Aqueous humor is a (protein free plasma) clear fluid which fills anterior (between cornea and iris) and posterior chamber (between iris and lens) of the eye. It is secreted in the posterior chamber by capillaries of ciliary body. It moves into the anterior chamber through pupil where it is drained into veins through 'sinus venosus sclerae' (venous space at the sclerocorneal junction/limbus)

Aqueous humor provides nutrition to the cornea and lens. It maintains the intraocular pressure (normal pressure is about 15–20 mm of Hg)

## Vitreous Body

It is a colorless jelly like transparent mass, which fills the posterior segment of the eyeball. The vitreous body is covered by a transparent hyaloid membrane.

## Applied Anatomy

1. *Glaucoma:* Increase in the intraocular pressure causes 'glaucoma'. It occurs due to blockage in the drainage of aqueous humor. Increased pressure can damage retina and lead to blindness.

2. *Cataract:* The transparency of the lens depends on a precise combination of structural and biochemical characteristics. When the balance becomes disturbed, the lens loses its transparency and the opaque lens is known as cataract. As aging proceeds the lens becomes less elastic and the individual has difficulty in focussing on nearby objects (far-sight)

3. The anteroposterior, transverse and vertical diameters of normal adult eyeball measure about 2.4 cm. An increase in anteroposterior diameter is 'myopia' and decrease is called 'hypermetropia'

4. *Corneal transplants:* The cornea has a very restricted ability to repair itself. So corneal injuries must be treated immediately to prevent serious vision losses. Corneal replacements are probably the most common form of transplant surgery. It can be performed between unrelated individuals because of its avascularity.

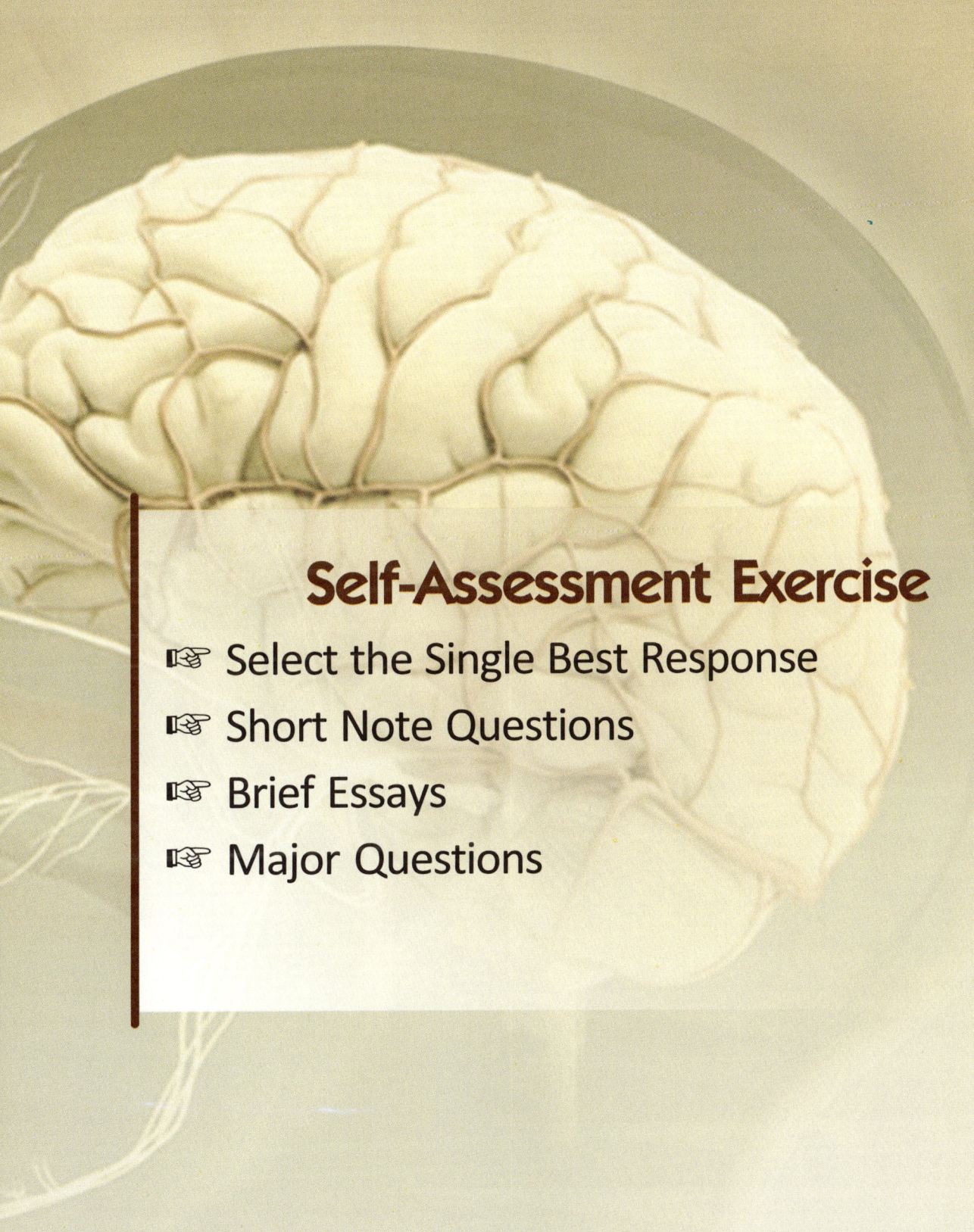

# Self-Assessment Exercise

☞ Select the Single Best Response

☞ Short Note Questions

☞ Brief Essays

☞ Major Questions

## Select the Single Best Response

1. **Which of these venous sinus is related to falx cerebri?**
   A. Sigmoid sinus
   B. Superior petrosal sinus
   C. Straight sinus
   D. Transverse sinus

2. **Which of these venous sinus is related to tentorium cerebelli?**
   A. Straight sinus
   B. Transverse sinus
   C. Superior petrosal sinus
   D. All of the above

3. **Arachnoid granulations are more numerous in:**
   A. Superior sagittal sinus
   B. Straight sinus
   C. Transverse sinus
   D. Sigmoid sinus

4. **The cerebrospinal fluid (CSF) from the foramen magnetic of fourth ventricle enters into:**
   A. Cisterna pontis
   B. Cisterna magna
   C. Cisterna of the lateral sulcus
   D. Interpedencular cisterna

5. **The lumbar puncture is performed at the level of:**
   A. $L_3$ and $L_4$ spine
   B. $L_1$ and $L_2$ spine
   C. $L_2$ and $L_3$ spine
   D. $L_4$ and $L_5$ spine

6. **The bilateral paralysis of lower limb is referred as:**
   A. Hemiplegia
   B. Quadriplegia
   C. Monoplegia
   D. Paraplegia

7. **Which of the following statements is incorrect regarding the fasciculus gracilis and cuneatus?**
   A. The first order neurons are located in the dorsal root ganglion of the spinal nerve.
   B. Fasciculus cuneatus carry sensory information from the upper limb.
   C. In the brainstem they ascend as lateral lemniscus
   D. They cross to the opposite side in medulla oblongata.

8. **The posterior column tract carry following sensation from the body except:**
   A. Proprioceptive sensation
   B. Stereognosis
   C. Pain
   D. Pressure

9. **Which of these tracts of the spinal cord is responsible for turning the head in response to visual and auditory stimuli?**
   A. Rubrospinal tract
   B. Tectospinal tract
   C. Vestibulospinal tract
   D. Corticospinal tract

10. **The lower end of the adult spinal cord ends at the level of:**
    A. Lower border of $L_3$ vertebra
    B. Lower border of $L_5$ vertebra
    C. Lower border of $S_1$ vertebra
    D. Lower border of $L_1$ vertebra

11. **Which of the following structures is a modification of spinal pia mater?**
    A. Conus medullaris
    B. Filum terminale
    C. Cauda equina
    D. None of the above

12. **Following are the parts of the vermis of the cerebellum except:**
    A. Culmen
    B. Tuber
    C. Pyramid
    D. Tonsil

13. **Which of these cranial nerves emerge at the junction of pons and pyramid of medulla oblongata?**
    A. Hypoglossal nerve
    B. Abducent nerve
    C. Facial nerve
    D. Glossopharyngeal nerve

14. **The nerve supply to the muscles of palate, pharynx and larynx is derived from:**
    A. Nuclues ambiguus
    B. Superior olivary nucleus
    C. Inferior olivary nucleus
    D. Vestibular nucleus

15. **Following are the clinical symptoms of Wallenberg's syndrome except:**
    A. Dysphagia
    B. Hemiplegia
    C. Ataxia of the limbs
    D. Loss of pain and temperature sensation from face.

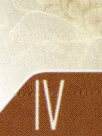

IV

16. **Lateral lemniscus is the:**
    A. Upward continuation of fasciculus gracilis and cuneatus
    B. Upward continuation of lateral spinothalamic tract
    C. Part of the auditory pathway
    D. Part of the visual pathway

17. **The neurons of substantia nigra are rich in:**
    A. Dopamine
    B. Norepinephrine
    C. Serotonin
    D. None of the above

18. **Which of these cranial nerve nuclei is present inside the pons?**
    A. Oculomotor
    B. Hypoglossal
    C. Abducent
    D. Cochlear

19. **The red nucleus is located in:**
    A. Midbrain
    B. Pons
    C. Medulla oblongata
    D. All of the above

20. **Which of the following parts of the cerebellum belongs to paleocerebellum?**
    A. Uvula
    B. Lingula
    C. Folium
    D. Tuber

21. **Following are the neuronal masses present in the cerebellum except:**
    A. Olivary nucleus
    B. Dentate nucleus
    C. Nucleus emboliformis
    D. Nucleus globosus

22. **Climbing fibers to the cerebellum are mainly derived from**
    A. Inferior olivary nucleus
    B. Vestibular nucleus
    C. Red nucleus
    D. Superior olivary nucleus

23. **The precentral gyrus is located in:**
    A. Frontal lobe
    B. Parietal lobe
    C. Occipital lobe
    D. Temporal lobe

24. **The triangular area of the occipital cortex between parieto-occipital sulcus and calcarine sulcus is**
    A. Precuneus
    B. Cuneus
    C. Paracentral lobule
    D. Isthmus

25. **The areas 3,1 and 2 refer to:**
    A. Primary motor area
    B. Premotor area
    C. Primary sensory area
    D. Visual area

26. **The 'foot area' of the cerebral cortex is supplied by:**
    A. Posterior cerebral artery
    B. Anterior cerebral artery
    C. Middle cerebral artery
    D. Circle of Willis

27. **The visual area of the cerebral cortex is located at the floor of the**
    A. Parieto-occipital sulcus
    B. Lateral sulcus
    C. Cingulate sulcus
    D. Calcarine sulcus

28. **Which of these functional areas is located in the inferior frontal gyrus?**
    A. Auditory area
    B. Motor speech area
    C. Wernickes speech area
    D. Visual area

29. **The visual area of the cerebral cortex is supplied by:**
    A. Anterior cerebral artery
    B. Middle cerebral artery
    C. Posterior cerebral artery
    D. Circle of Willis

30. **The posterior expanded part of the corpus callosum is called:**
    A. Rostrum
    B. Trunk
    C. Splenium
    D. Genu

31. **Following are the fibers arising from the corpus callosum except:**
    A. Forceps major
    B. Forceps minor
    C. Corona radiata
    D. Tapetum

32. **Which of the following statements is incorrect regarding the internal capsule?**
    A. Its anterior limb is placed between the thalamus and the body of the caudate nucleus
    B. The corticospinal fibers traverse its posterior limb
    C. The auditory radiation passes through its sublentiform part
    D. It has fibers from thalamus, passing into cerebral cortex.

33. **The bulb of the posterior horn of the lateral ventricle is produced by:**
    A. Tapetum
    B. Forceps major
    C. Forceps minor
    D. Calcarine sulcus

34. **Following structures bound the inferior horn of the lateral ventricle** *except*:
    A. Stria terminalis
    B. Tapetum
    C. Hippocampus
    D. Stria medullaris

35. **The facial colliculus of the IV ventricle is produced by:**
    A. Motor nucleus of the facial nerve
    B. Abducent nucleus with fibers from motor nucleus of facial nerve
    C. Spinal nucleus of the trigeminal nerve
    D. None of the above

36. **The neurons of the locus coeruleus are rich in**
    A. Dopamine
    B. Norepinephrine
    C. Serotonin
    D. GABA

37. **The respiratory center is closely related to:**
    A. Superior fovea
    B. Facial colliculus
    C. Vestibular area
    D. Area postrema

38. **The III ventricle communicates with IV ventricle through:**
    A. Interventricular foramen
    B. Foramen Magendi
    C. Cerebral aqueduct
    D. Foramen Luschka

39. **Following are the parts of the basal ganglia** *except*:
    A. Putamen
    B. Globus pallidus
    C. Hippocompus
    D. Caudate nucleus

40. **The optic tract terminates at:**
    A. Medial geniculate body
    B. Lateral geniculate body
    C. Optic chiasma
    D. Visual vortex

41. **Complete lesion affecting optic tract of one side results in:**
    A. Contralateral homonymous hemianopia
    B. Bitemporal heteronymous hemianopia
    C. Bitemporal homonymous hemianopia
    D. Ipsilateral homonymous hemianopia

42. **Following cranial nerve nuclei are connected with oculomotor nerve** *except*:
    A. Oculomotor nucleus
    B. Edinger-Westphal nucleus
    C. Pretectal nucleus
    D. Abducent nucleus

43. **Trochlear nerve supplies:**
    A. Superior rectus muscle
    B. Superior oblique muscle
    C. Lateral rectus muscle
    D. Inferior oblique muscle

44. **The mandibular nerve supplies following muscles** *except*:
    A. Tensor palati muscle
    B. Mylohyoid muscle
    C. Masseter muscle
    D. Buccinator muscle

45. **The vestibular nerve carries information from:**
    A. Maculae of saccule and utricle
    B. Organ of Corti
    C. Ear ossicles
    D. Tympanic membrane

46. **The glossopharyngeal nerve supplies following** *except*:
    A. Mucous membrane of the posterior part of the tongue
    B. Stylopharyngeus muscle
    C. Mucous membrane of the larynx
    D. Mucous membrane of the pharynx

47. **Following are the effects of the sympathetic stimulation** *except*:
    A. Constriction of bronchioles
    B. Suppression of gastric motility

C. Dilatation of pupils

D. Increased heart rate

**48. Following are the effects of parasympathetic stimulation** *except:*

A. Emptying of urinary bladder

B. Gastric motility is supressed

C. Pupils constrict

D. Heart rate is diminished

**49. Which of the following cranial nerves does not carry parasympathetic fibers?**

A. Vagus nerve

B. Glossopharyngeal nerve

C. Hypoglossal nerve

D. Facial nerve

**50. Following are the parts of the uveal tract** *except*:

A. Ciliary body

B. Iris

C. Sclera

D. Choroid

**51. The normal intraocular pressure is about:**

A.  5–10 mm of Hg

B. 15–20 mm of Hg

C. 30–50 mm of Hg

D. 50–70 mm of Hg

**52. Aqueous humour is drained by:**

A. Capillaries of the ciliary body

B. Sinus venosus sclerae

C. Cornea

D. Ciliary body

**53. Hypermetropia is:**

A. Increase in the transverse diameter of eyeball

B. Increase in the anteroposterior diameter of eyeball

C. Decrease in the anteroposterior diameter of eyeball

D. Decrease in the transverse diameter of eyeball

**54. Follwing are the cell types present in the retina** *except*:

A. Amacrine cells

B. Bipolar cells

C. Purkinje cells

D. Rods and cones

**55. Cornea is supplied by:**

A. Maxillary nerve

B. Facial nerve

C. Ophthalmic nerve

D. None of the above

**56. Maculae are the receptors present in:**

A. Membranous semicircular duct

B. Bony semicircular canals

C. Saccule and utricle

D. Bony vestibule

**57. Scala tympani opens at the:**

A. Fenestra vestibuli

B. Fenestra cochleae

C. Saccule

D. Utricle

**58. The auditory tube opens at:**

A. The posterior wall of middle ear

B. The anterior wall of middle ear

C. The lateral wall of middle ear

D. The medial wall of middle ear

**59. The suprarenal medulla secretes:**

A. Aldosterone

B. Cortisol

C. Estrogen

D. Noradrenaline and adrenalin

**60. The parafollicular cells of the thyroid gland secrete:**

A. Calcitonin

B. Thyroxin

C. Parathormone

D. Thyroglobulin

**61. The vasopressin hormone is secreted by:**

A. Preoptic nucleus of hypothalamus

B. Paraventricular nucleus of hypothalamus

C. Supraoptic of hypothalmus

D. Posterior lobe of the pituitary

**62. Following are the parts of adenohypophysis** *except*:

A. Pars anterior

B. Pars tuberalis

C. Pars nervosa

D. Pars intermedia

**63. Pituitary gland is located in the body of:**

A. Frontal bone

B. Parietal bone

C. Temporal bone

D. Sphenoid bone

**64. The superior cerebral veins drains into:**

A. Cavernous sinus

B. Superior sagittal sinus

C. Inferior sagittal sinus

D. Sigmoid sinus

IV

**65. The right and left internal cerebral veins join to form:**
A. Thalamostriate vein
B. Basal vein
C. Great cerebral vein
D. Straight sinus

**66. Which of these cranial nerves carry parasympathetic fibers to heart?**
A. Facial
B. Glossopharyngeal
C. Cranial part of the accessory
D. Vagus

**67. The preganglionic sympathetic fibers are mainly located in:**
A. Cervical segment of the spinal cord
B. Thoracic segment of the spinal cord
C. Lower lumbar segment of the spinal cord
D. Sacral segment of the spinal cord

**68. The neurons of the sympathetic ganglia are:**
A. Unipolar
B. Bipolar
C. Multipolar
D. Pseudo unipolar

**69. On each side the cervical part of the sympathetic chain presents:**
A. 7 ganglia
B. 6 ganglia
C. 3 ganglia
D. 8 ganglia

**70. The stimulation of sympathetic system is manifested by following conditions *except*:**
A. Increased heart rate
B. Increased blood pressure
C. Suppressed peristalsis
D. Constriction of pupil

**71. Following are the parasympathetic ganglia *except*:**
A. Ciliary ganglion
B. Submandibular ganglion
C. Pterygopalatine ganglion
D. Dorsal root ganglion

**72. The pyramids of medulla oblongata are produced by underlying:**
A. Corticopontine fibers
B. Corticospinal fibers
C. Fasciculus gracilis
D. Fasciculus cuneatus

**73. Which of these cranial nerves emerge between pyramid and olive of the medulla oblongata?**
A. Abducent nerve
B. Facial nerve
C. Cranial part of the accessory nerve
D. Hypoglossal nerve

**74. Motor fibers to the muscles of palate, pharynx and larynx is derived from:**
A. Nucleus ambiguus
B. Inferior olivary nucleus
C. Solitarius nucleus
D. Hypoglossal nucleus

**75. The ventral part of the pons is traversed by:**
A. Basilar artery
B. Vertebral artery
C. Posterior cerebral artery
D. Middle cerebral artery

**76. The middle cerebellar peduncle consists of:**
A. Olivocerebellar fibers
B. Vestibulocerebellar fibers
C. Pontocerebellar fibers
D. Posterior spinocerebellar fibers

**77. The upward continuation of lateral spinothalamic tract is called:**
A. Medial lemniscus
B. Lateral lemniscus
C. Trigeminal lemniscus
D. Spinal lemniscus

**78. The pontine nuclei receive fibers from:**
A. Cerebellum
B. Spinal cord
C. Cerebral cortex
D. Basal nuclei

## Short Note Questions (3 *marks*)

1. Lumbar puncture
2. Motor decussation
3. Sensory decussation
4. Basilar part of the pons
5. Facial colliculus
6. Crus cerebri
7. Substantia nigra
8. Cerebellar nuclei
9. Middle cerebellar peduncle
10. Superior cerebellar peduncle
11. Arterial supply to cerebellum
12. Lateral sulcus

13. Central sulcus
14. Calcarine sulcus
15. Interpeduncular fossa
16. Red nucleus
17. Primary motor cortex
18. Primary sensory area
19. Primary visual area
20. Speech area
21. Auditory area
22. Corpus callosum
23. Association fibers of cerebrum
24. Caudate nucleus
25. Lentiform nucleus
26. Hypothalamohypophyseal tract
27. Hippocampus
28. Choroid plexus
29. Iris
30. Epidermis of the skin

## Brief Essays (5 or 6 marks)

1. Falx cerebri
2. Tentorium cerebelli
3. Subarachnoid cisternae
4. Spinal piamater
5. External features of spinal cord
6. Anatomy of the pyramidal tract
7. Origin, termination and functions of posterior column tract
8. Extrapyramidal tracts
9. Spinothalamic tracts
10. Spinocerebellar tracts
11. External features of medulla oblongata
12. Lateral medullary syndrome
13. Medial medullary syndrome
14. Cochlear nuclei
15. Colliculi of midbrain
16. External features of cerebellum
17. Morphological subdivision of cerebellum
18. Inferior cerebellar peduncle
19. Arterial supply to the cerebral cortex
20. External features of thalamus
21. Name the parts of limbic system. Mention their functions
22. Third ventricle
23. Formation, circulation and absorption of CSF
24. Circle of Willis
25. Sympathetic chain
26. Visual pathway

27. Oculomotor nerve
28. Glossopharyngeal nerve
29. Hypoglossal nerve
30. Accomodation reflex
31. Light reflex
32. Blood supply to pituitary gland
33. Blood supply to thyroid gland
34. Parathyroid glands
35. Tympanic membrane
36. Medial wall of the middle ear
37. Cornea
38. Ciliary body
39. Retina

## Major Questions (10 marks)

1. Discuss the external features of the spinal cord. Draw a neat labeled diagram of cross-section of spinal cord showing ascending and descending tracts.
2. Discuss the ascending and descending tracts of the spinal cord.
3. List the main nuclei present inside the medulla oblongata. Add a note on their functions.
4. Name the different lemnisci present in the brainstem. Give a brief account of each of them.
5. Describe the external features of cerebellum. Add a note on its microscopic structure.
6. Discuss the connections of cerebellum. Add a note on its function.
7. With the help of a diagram discuss the major functional areas of cerebrum.
8. Draw a neat labeled diagram showing gyri and sulci on superolateral surface of cerebrum. Name the functional areas present in this surface.
9. Draw a neat labeled diagram of the medial surface of the cerebrum. Name the functional areas present in this surface.
10. Classify the white matter of the cerebrum, giving examples to each variety. Give a detailed account of internal capsule.
11. Name the parts of basal nuclei. Discuss their connections and functions.
12. Discuss the main nuclei of thalamus. Give their connections and functions.
13. Discuss the position, main nuclei and connections of hypothalamus.
14. Discuss the wall (boundaries) of different parts of the lateral ventricle.
15. Discuss the boundaries of fourth ventricle. With the help of a diagram discuss the features of its floor.

16. Discuss the main branches of vertebral (cranial part) and internal carotid artery supplying the brain.
17. Name the peripheral parasympathetic ganglia. Give their location and distribution.
18. Name the cranial nerve. Give an account of their functions in brief.
19. Discuss the facial nerve/trigeminal nerve/vagus nerve under:
    A. Nuclei of origin
    B. Course and branches
    C. Distribution and applied aspects
20. Discuss the pituitary gland under:
    A. Position and parts
    B. Microscopic structure and hormones
    C. Blood supply
21. Discuss the thyroid gland under:
    A. Position and parts
    B. Blood supply
    C. Microscopic structure and hormones
22. Discuss the suprarenal gland under:
    A. Position and parts
    B. Blood supply
    C. Microscopic structure and hormones

23. Discuss the microscopic structure of the skin. Add a note on its appendages
24. Discuss the walls of the middle ear. Give its communication and contents
25. Draw a neat labeled diagram showing the sagittal section of eyeball. Discuss the structure of the uveal tract in brief.

## Answers to Single Best Response Questions

| | | | | | |
|---|---|---|---|---|---|
| 1. C | 2. D | 3. A | 4. B | 5. A | 6. D |
| 7. C | 8. C | 9. B | 10. D | 11. B | 12. D |
| 13. B | 14. A | 15. B | 16. B | 17. A | 18. C |
| 19. A | 20. A | 21. A | 22. A | 23. A | 24. B |
| 25. C | 26. B | 27. D | 28. B | 29. C | 30. C |
| 31. C | 32. A | 33. B | 34. D | 35. B | 36. B |
| 37. D | 38. C | 39. C | 40. B | 41. A | 42. D |
| 43. B | 44. D | 45. A | 46. C | 47. A | 48. B |
| 49. C | 50. C | 51. B | 52. B | 53. C | 54. C |
| 55. C | 56. C | 57. B | 58. B | 59. D | 60. A |
| 61. C | 62. C | 63. D | 64. B | 65. C | 66. D |
| 67. B | 68. C | 69. C | 70. D | 71. D | 72. B |
| 73. D | 74. A | 75. A | 76. C | 77. D | 78. C |

IV

# Anatomy of Certain Clinical Procedures

The understanding of human anatomy is very essential for undergraduate students of nursing and medical laboratory technology to perform various clinical procedures. This chapter is uniquely designed to cater to these students.

## ARTERIAL PULSATION

The arterial pulse is the abrupt expansion of an artery resulting from the ejection of blood from the left ventricle into the aorta and its transmission throughout the arterial tree in the body. The pulse may be palpated in any place that allows an artery to be compressed against hard rigid structures like bone, tendon or ligaments. Feeling the pulse of an artery provide information about the arterial blood flow through that particular vessel.

*Brachial artery:* The pulsation of the brachial artery is felt in front of the elbow in the cubital fossa against (medial to) tendon of the biceps brachii muscle

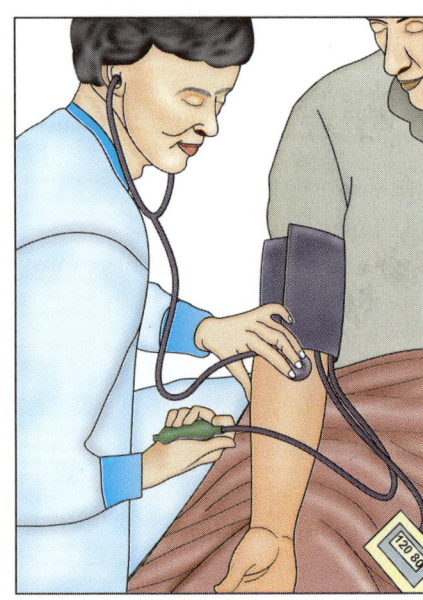

**Fig. 38.1b:** Measuring blood pressure by using branchial artery

(Fig. 38.1a). The brachial artery is also compressed for measuring blood pressure (Fig. 38.1b).

*Radial artery:* It is felt at the distal end of the forearm, anterior to the lower end of the radius lateral to the tendon of flexor carpi radialis (Fig. 38.2).

*Femoral artery:* Pulsation of the femoral artery is felt in front of the upper thigh, just below the mid-inguinal point (mid-point between the anterior superior iliac spine and pubic symphysis) against the tendon of psoas major muscle (Fig. 38.3).

*Popliteal artery:* Popliteal artery is the deepest structure in the popliteal fossa at the back of the knee, hence, it is difficult to feel its pulse. However pulsation can be felt in semiflexed knee. The fingertips of both hands are

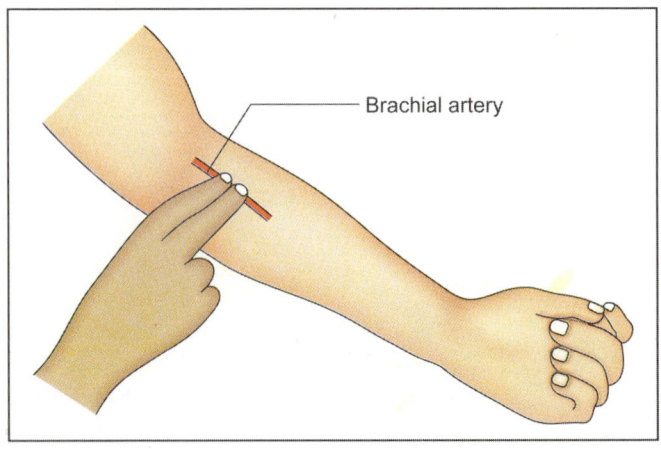

Brachial artery

**Fig. 38.1a:** Pulsation of brachial artery

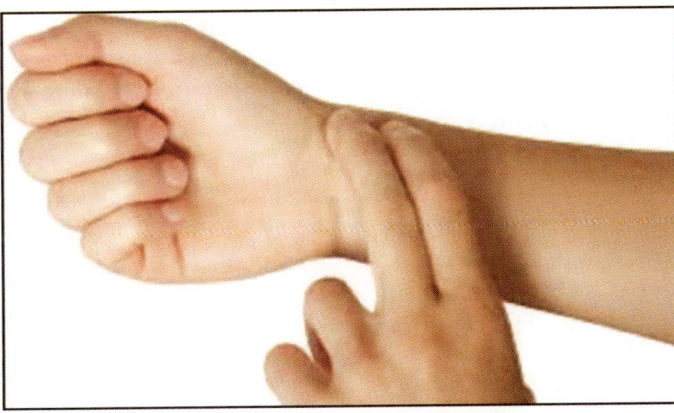

Fig. 38.2: Pulsation of radial artery

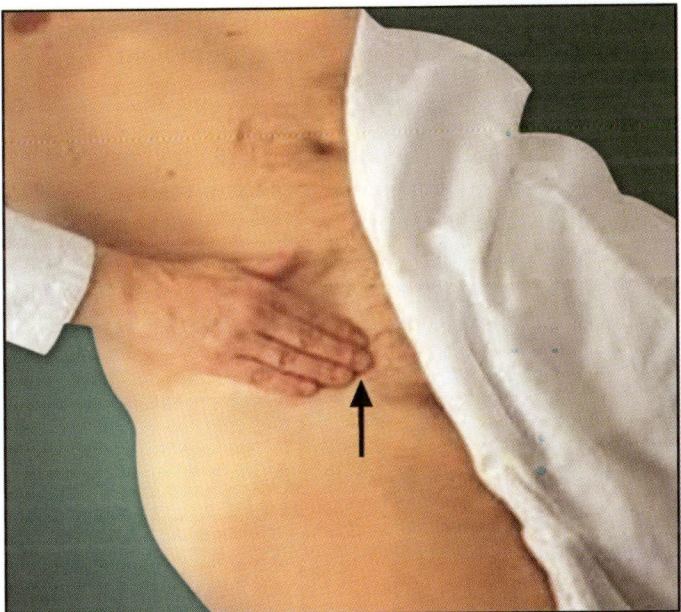

Fig. 38.3: Pulsation of the femoral artery

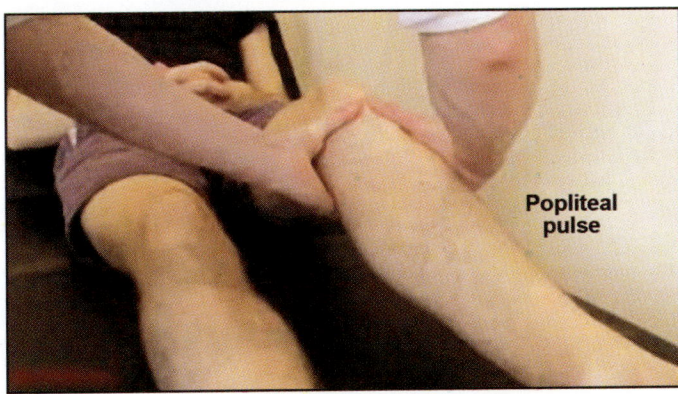

Fig. 38.4: Pulsation of the popliteal artery

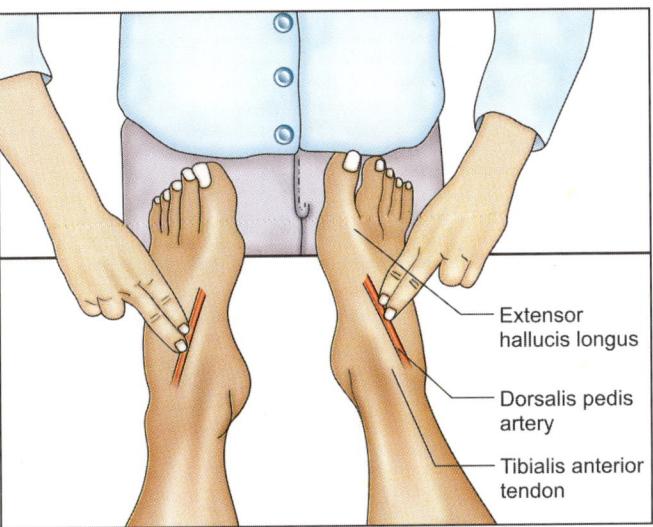

Extensor hallucis longus

Dorsalis pedis artery

Tibialis anterior tendon

Fig. 38.5: Pulsation of the dorsalis pedis artery

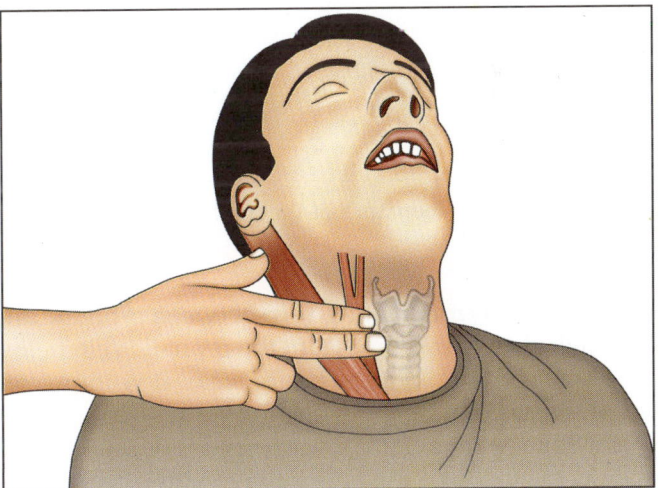

Fig. 38.6: Pulsation of the carotid artery

*Dorsalis pedis artery:* It is felt at the midpoint between the two malleoli in front of the ankle just lateral to the tendon of extensor halluces longus against tarsal bone (Fig. 38.5).

*Carotid pulse:* The common carotid artery is felt at the side of the neck, where it lies in a groove between trachea and infrahyoid muscle. It is usually palpated just deep to the anterior border of the sternocleidomastoid muscle at the level of upper border of thyroid cartilage (Fig. 38.6).

## INTRAVENOUS INFUSION

The intravenous route is chosen when rapid action of the drug is required. Apart from infusion of drugs it is also utilized for venipuncture (taking a blood sample) and blood transfusion because the veins are superficial compare to artery.

placed in the popliteal fossa with the thumbs resting on patient's patella (Fig. 38.4).

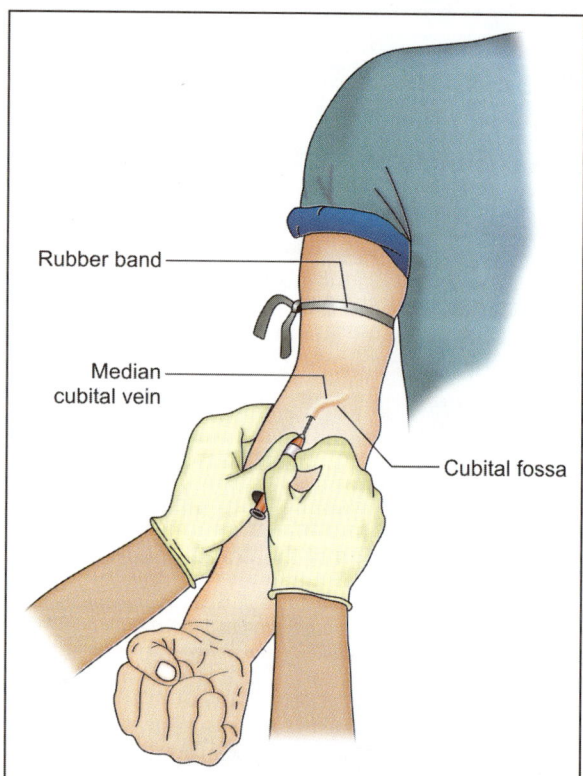

Fig. 38.7: Venipuncture of the median cubital vein

### Median Cubital Vein

It is a large communicating vein between cephalic and the basilic veins. It begins from the cephalic vein below the elbow and ends in the basilic vein. It is connected to the deep veins by perforating and veins, which perforates the bicipital aponeurosis. Since it is fixed to deep veins through the perforating veins, it is the vein of choice for intravenous injections and for cardiac catheterization. There is a possibility of injuring brachial artery and median nerve during intravenous injection or procedures through median cubital vein. Variations in the median cubital vein are also possible. Injury to the brachial artery results in spurting of blood from the injured vessel (Fig. 38.7). The following procedures are customarily employed while doing venipuncture.

a. Keeping the arm in dependent position for sometime which slows the venous return
b. Compressing the veins by a tourniquet 1.5 to 2 inches proximal to the site of puncture
c. Applying heat by means of hot water bag, moist towels or by immersing the hand and forearm into a basin of warm water
d. Alternating opening and closing of the hand

Muscular activity will increase the amount of arterial blood flow to the distal portion of the upper limb. It is also possible that the opening and closing of the hand

will enhance the blood flow from the deep to superficial veins by means of perforating veins. On the other hand, applying tight tourniquets may obstruct the arterial flow to the forearm.

### Great Saphenous Vein

In case of an emergency, when all the superficial veins are collapsed, venous cut down is performed through great saphenous vein just in front of the medial malleolus. The position of the vein is constant at this site, but care has to be taken to avoid damage to the saphenous nerve (Fig. 38.8).

### Femoral Vein

In infants and children femoral vein is selected for intravenous injections. It is also used to reach the right side of the heart (right atrium and right ventricle).

### Internal Jugular Vein

Internal jugular vein or sometimes subclavian veins are used for central venous access for measuring the pressure in the pulmonary artery and intracardiac pressure. Internal jugular vein can be approached through supraclavicular triangle between the two heads of the sternocleidomastoid muscle (Fig. 38.9).

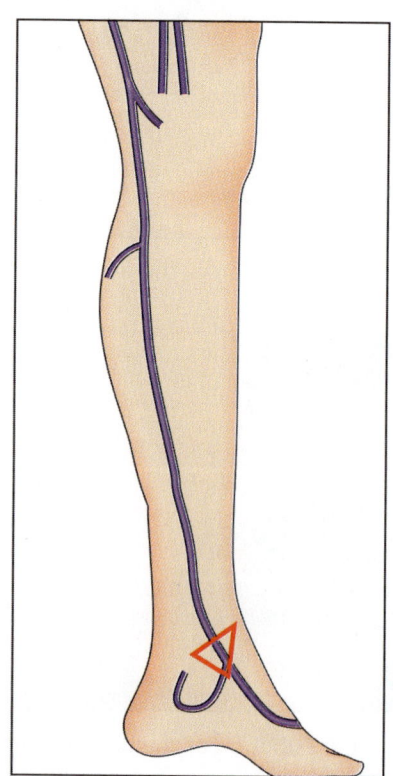

Fig. 38.8: Great saphenous vein and marked area is the preferred site for venesection

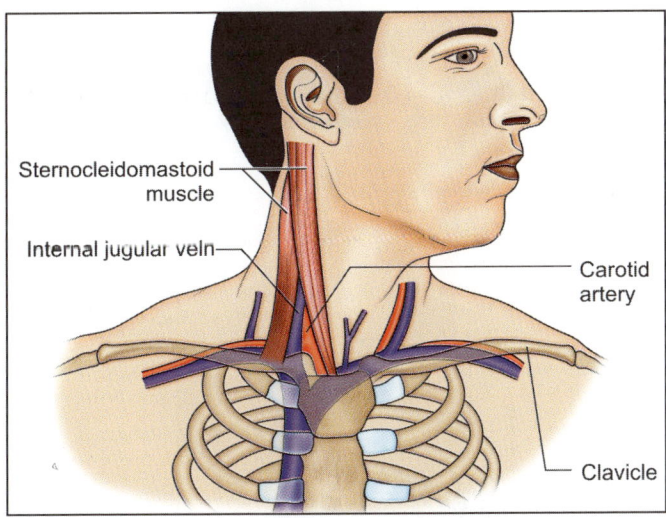

Fig. 38.9: Site of venesection of internal jugular vein

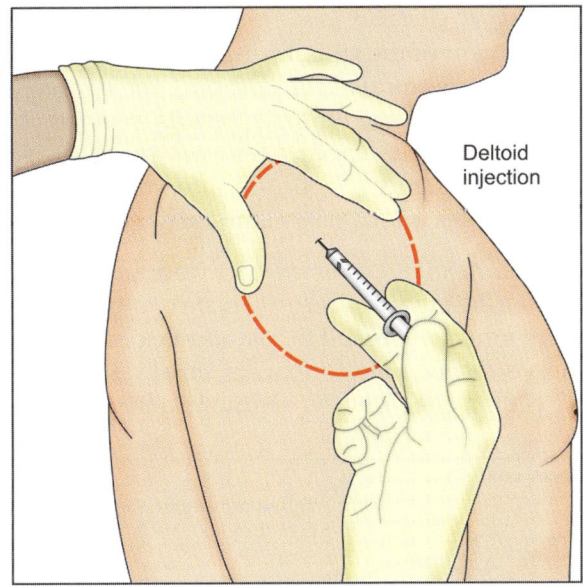

Fig. 38.10: Intramuscular injection over the deltoid

## ARTERIAL CATHETERIZATION

### Femoral Artery

Femoral artery is superficial in position in the upper part of the thigh and often selected for various procedures like angiographic studies (by injecting radiopaque dye through a catheter inserted to femoral artery) of abdominal, lower limb arteries and even coronary arteries.

### Radial Artery

The arterial blood for blood gas analysis is often obtained from radial artery as it is superficial in the distal part of the forearm. It is also used for procedures like coronary angiographic studies

### INTRAMUSCULAR INJECTIONS

*Deltoid muscle:* It is often a site for intramuscular injection. The needle is inserted at 90° angle on the multipennate portion of the deltoid, 1–2 inches below the acromion process (about the level of the armpit). This site should not be used if the person is very thin or the muscle is very small (Fig. 38.10).

*Vastus lateralis muscle:* The site of injection is on the lateral side of the thigh. This part of the thigh can be arbitrarily divided into upper, middle and lower one-thirds. The injection is given in the middle third. The thigh is a good place to give an injection for children younger than 3 years old.

*Gluteus maximus muscle:* Intramuscular injections are often preferred in the gluteal region. The gluteal muscle provides a large surface area for absorption of drugs. The superolateral quadrant is safe site for intramuscular injection. An injection, little below and behind the anterior superior iliac spine involves following structures successively—skin, superficial fascia, deep fascia and gluteus medius. Injecting superomedial quadrant, endanger the superior gluteal nerve and inferomedial quadrant, endanger the sciatic nerve and also inferior gluteal nerves and vessels (Fig. 38.11).

## TENDON REFLEXES

A reflex is defined as automatic/involuntary, stereotyped/repetitive, purpose serving response for stimulation. The components of the reflex arc include, receptor, afferent limb, center, efferent limb and effector organ. Clinically the reflexes are classified into superficial (plantar, corneal), deep (knee jerk, ankle jerk) and visceral (micturition, defecation). Knowledge of reflexes are important in differentiating upper motor versus lower motor neuron lesions and also assess the level of lesions.

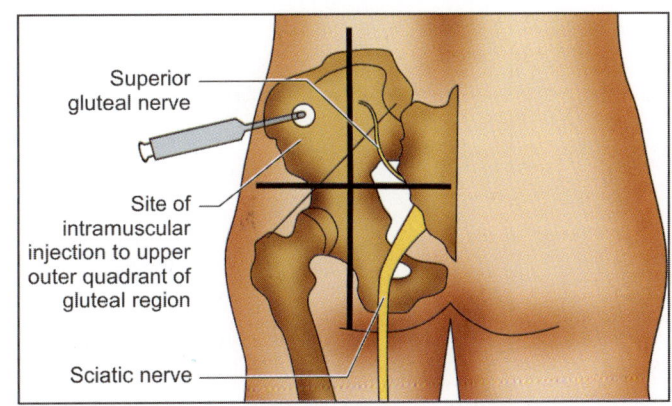

Fig. 38.11: Intramuscular injection in the gluteal region

38

*Knee jerk reflex (Patellar tendon reflex):* It tests the $L_2$, $L_3$ and $L_4$ segment of the spinal cord or these spinal nerve roots forming femoral nerve. Tapping the ligamentum patellae with the knee hammer results in extension of the knee joint (quadriceps femoris muscle) under normal circumstances. Both the afferent and efferent limb of the reflex is formed by femoral nerve (Fig. 38.12).

*Ankle jerk or Achillis tendon reflex:* On tapping the tendon with knee hammer, there is reflex contraction of gastrocnemius with resultant plantar flexion of the foot. The nerve responsible for this is tibial nerve and the spinal center is $S_1$ and $S_2$ segments. In paralysis of

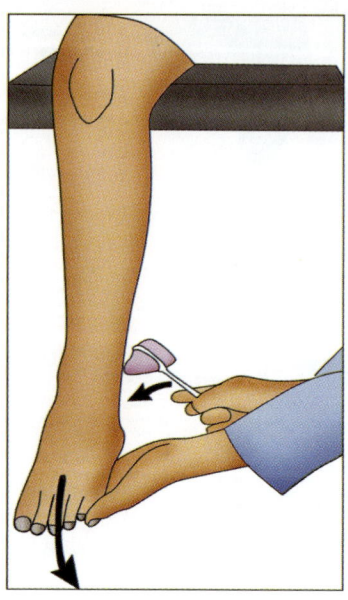

**Fig. 38.13:** Ankle jerk reflex

gastrocnemius or involvement of $S_1$ segment the patient will not be able to stand on the toes and there will be loss of ankle jerk/Achilis tendon reflex (Fig. 38.13)

*Plantar reflex:* The lateral aspect of the sole ($S_1$ dermatome) of the foot is stroked with a blunt object. Flexion of the toes is a normal response. Slight fanning of the lateral 4 toes and dorsiflexion of the great toe is an abnormal response (Babinski sign). It indicates brain injury (upper motor neuron) or cerebral disease, but considered normal in infants (Fig. 38.14).

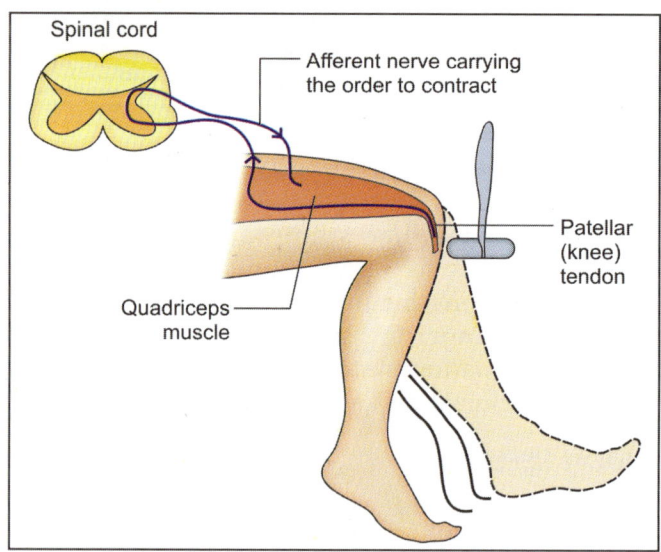

**Fig. 38.12:** Knee jerk reflex

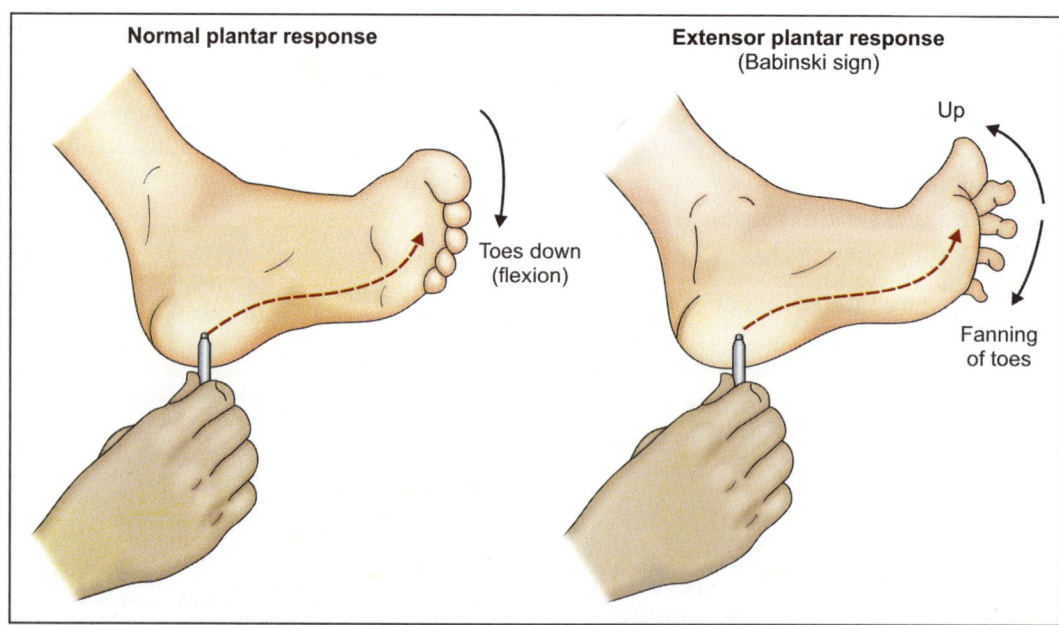

**Fig. 38.14:** Plantar reflex

## AUSCULTATION OF CARDIAC VALVES (Fig. 38.15)

*Pulmonary valve:* 2nd intercostal space to the left of the sternum (pulmonary valve murmurs, ventricular septal defect murmurs, continuous murmurs of patent ductus arteriosus).

*Aortic valve:* 2nd intercostal space to the right of the sternum.

*Tricuspid valve:* Left 4th intercostal space (tricuspid and aortic regurgitation).

*Mitral valve:* Left 5th intercostal space 9 cm away from midline (apex of the heart).

### Anatomy of Certain Other Procedures

*Tracheostomy:* Tracheostomy is a lifesaving surgical procedure, when there is upper respiratory obstruction (in case of impaction of foreign body in the larynx or in laryngeal edema). In low tracheostomy, the head of the patient is kept in the extended position by keeping a pillow under the shoulders. The vertical incision is placed in 2nd to 4th tracheal rings (at 3rd tracheal ring) and endotracheal tube is inserted through the opening in the trachea. The incision passes successively through skin, superficial fascia, deep fascia (investing layer). The interval between right and left sternohyoid muscle is opened up and sternothyroid muscles are retracted. The pretracheal fascia is incised and isthmus of the thyroid is retracted upwards.

### Urinary Catherization

Sometimes a catheter is introduced through urethra (in case of retention of urine in the bladder). It is also performed to obtain an uncontaminated sample of urine. In such procedures one should know about the curves of male urethra and presence of lacunae (small pit like recesses in spongy part) which may intercept the tip of the catheter. The membranous part of the urethra is the least dilatable part of male urethra and is vulnerable to rupture during catheterization. Urethral stricture results from infection of the urethra. The external urethral orifice is the narrowest and least distensible part of the urethra; hence an instrument that passes through this opening normally passes through remaining parts of the urethra. Just beyond the terminal fossa of the penile urethra, a fold of mucous membrane projects downward from the roof of the urethra. This fold will sometimes completely obstruct the passage of a catheter if the point is directed toward the roof. With the patient lying in a supine position, hold the penis vertically. Introduce the catheter into the external meatus in such a way that the point is directed first toward the floor of the urethra until this fold is passed (Fig. 38.16).

*Thoracocentesis or pleural tap:* It is a procedure to remove excess fluid or blood or pus from the pleural cavity. This is performed with the patient in sitting posture. Usually the needle is inserted in the posterior axillary line or the midaxillary line through the lower part of 8th or 9th intercostal space. The excess fluid accumulates in costodiaphragmatic recess. Performing thoracocentesis in either of these spaces during expiration will avoid the injury to the lung. The needle passes in succession the skin, fasciae, serratus anterior, intercostal muscles, endothoracic fascia and the costal pleura. To avoid damage to the intercostal nerve and vessels, the needle is inserted to superior to the rib, high enough to avoid the collateral branch (which runs along the upper border of the rib).

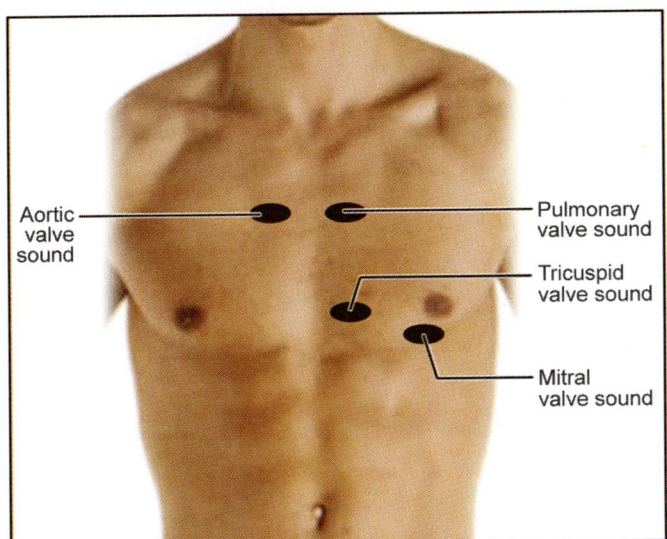

**Fig. 38.15:** Auscultation areas of cardiac valves

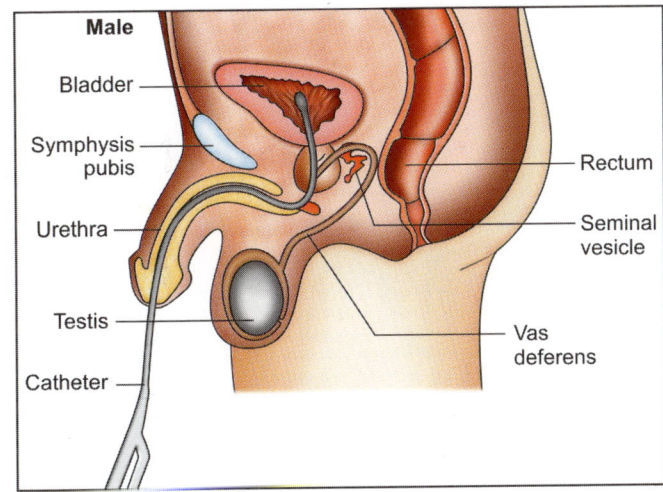

**Fig. 38.16:** Urinary catheterization in males

38

*Insertion of a chest tube:* This is a procedure to remove major amount of air, blood, fluid, pus or any combination of these substances from the pleural cavity. A short incision is made in the 5th or 6th intercostal space in the midaxillary line. The tube inserted is directed upwards towards cervical pleura for removal of air or the tube can be directed downwards for fluid drainage. The outer end of the tube is connected to a controlled suction, to prevent air from being sucked back into the pleural cavity. Failure of removal of fluid may cause the lung to develop a resistant fibrous covering that inhibits expansion unless it is peeled.

## Lumbar Puncture

It is a procedure in which the spinal cistern is approached for aspiration of CSF. It is usually performed between $L_3$ and $L_4$ spines (line passing through the highest point of the iliac crest-corresponds to $L_4$ spine will be a guideline), since this part of the vertebral canal is not occupied by the spinal cord (Fig. 38.16). The patient lies in curled position to flex the lumbar spine to open up the interval between the laminae. The needle successively passes through skin,

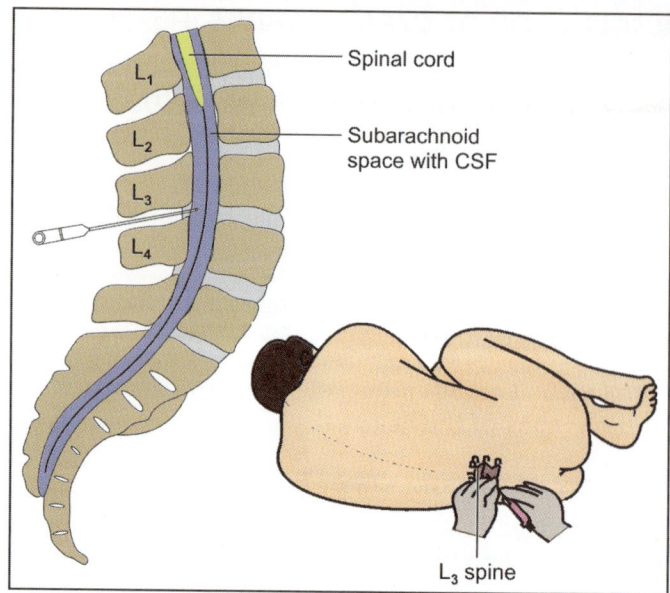

Fig. 38.17: Lumbar puncture

fasciae, supraspinous ligament, infraspinous ligament, ligamentum flavum, dura and arachnoid mater. Certain drug which cannot cross the blood–brain barrier is also administered through this route (Fig. 38.17).

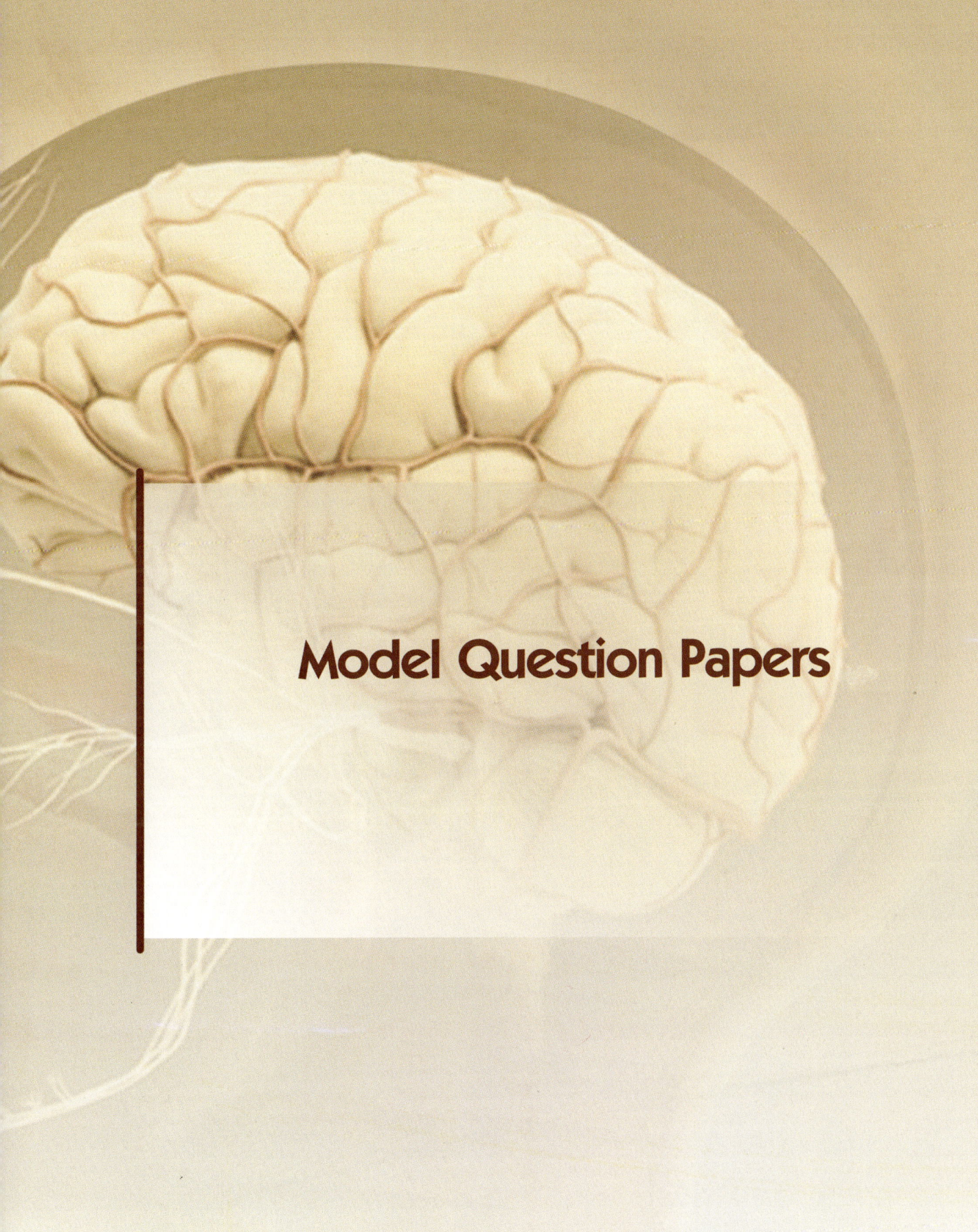

# Model Question Papers

# BPT QUESTION PAPERS

## RGUHS, Karnataka

Time: Three Hours        **First Year BPT Exam**        Maximum Marks: 100

**Anatomy (RS-3 & RS-4)—Q.P. Code: 2701**

### Long Essays

Answer any two questions   (10 × 2 = 20 marks)
Questions 1 to 3

### Short Essays

Answer any twelve questions   (5 × 12 = 60 marks)
Questions 4 to 17

### Short Answers

Answer all 10 questions   (2 × 10 = 20 marks)
Questions 18 to 27

### Sample question paper-1 (September 2015)

*Long essays (answer any two) 2 × 10 = 20 marks*

1. Describe the femoral triangle in detail
2. Classify the white matter of the cerebrum. Describe the internal capsule in detail
3. Describe the attachments of the deltoid. Name the structures undercovering deltoid

*Short essays (answer any twelve) 12 × 5 = 60 marks*

4. Bronchopulmonary segments
5. Axillary nerve
6. Third ventricle
7. Cubital fossa
8. Dorsalis pedis artery
9. Fetal circulation
10. Femoral nerve
11. Trachea
12. Arterial supply to heart
13. Ovarian follicles
14. Abdominal aorta
15. Extraocular muscles and their nerve supply
16. External carotid artery
17. Supports of the bladder

*Short answers (answer all questions) 10 × 2 = 20 marks*

18. Name the carpal bones
19. Name the sinuses of the pericardium
20. Name the attachments of the coracoid process
21. Name the branches of the medial cord of the brachial plexus
22. Parts of the pancreas
23. Name the hamstring muscles
24. Parts of the corpus callosum
25. Name the paranasal air sinuses
26. Skeletal muscle histology (only diagram)
27. Ligaments of wrist joint

### Sample-2 (September 2012)

*Long essays (answer any two)  2 × 10 = 20 marks*

1. Describe the origin, course, relations, branches of the radial nerve till it reaches the elbow
2. Discuss the lymphatic drainage of the lower limb
3. Write about the adductor pollicis and 1st carpometacarpal joint

*Short essays (answer any twelve) 12 × 5 = 60 marks*

4. Describe the superficial palmar arch, its formation and branches
5. Lower end of the femur
6. Classify muscles with examples
7. Floor of the IV ventricle
8. Splenic artery and its branches
9. Muscles of tongue
10. Deltoid muscle
11. Write briefly about median nerve in the forearm
12. Discuss about the blood supply to the cecum
13. Discuss the origin, course and relations of axillary artery with its branches
14. Bronchopulmonary segments of right lung
15. Great saphenous vein
16. Femoral triangle
17. Describe the right atrium of the heart

*Short answers (answer all questions) 10 × 2 = 20 marks*

18. Name six structures passing through foramen magnum
19. Mention the joint where inversion and eversion takes place
20. Name the ear ossicles
21. Attachments of sternocleidomastoid muscle
22. Name the parts of the hip bone
23. Function of gallbladder
24. Femoral artery and its branches
25. Boundaries of cubital fossa
26. Mention the structures passing through foramen ovale
27. Name the nuclei present in the cerebellum

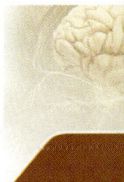

## MGR Health University, Tamil Nadu
### First Year BPT Exam (Common to BPT and BOT Exam)
### Paper II – Anatomy (Code: 6252)

Time: Three Hours      **Q.P. Code: 746252**      Maximum Marks: 100

### Elaborate on (major question)

1. Major question–20 marks
2. Major questions–20 marks

### Write notes on

5-mark questions × 8 = 40 marks

### Short answers

2-mark questions × 10 = 20 marks

### Sample question paper-1 (August 2014)

I. *Elaborate on*   *(2 × 20 = 40 marks)*

1. Describe in detail about the facial nerve.
2. Describe in detail about the shoulder joint.

II. *Write notes on*   *(8 × 5 = 40 marks)*

1. Wrist drop
2. Popliteal fossa
3. Spleen
4. Levator ani
5. Inversion and eversion
6. Movements of thoracic cage
7. Right atrium
8. Bronchopulmonary segments of left lung

III. *Short answers*   *(10 × 2 = 20 marks)*

1. Name the branches of axillary artery
2. Give formation of great saphenous vein
3. Name the structures opening into second part of duodenum
4. Name the contents of middle mediastinum
5. Name the structures opening into the middle meatus of nose
6. Name the structures forming the medial longitudinal arch
7. Name the types of sulci in cerebrum
8. Name the major openings and the structures passing through the diaphragm
9. Erb's point
10. Name the branches of coeliac trunk

### Sample question paper-2 (August 2013)

I. *Elaborate on*   *(2 × 20 = 40 marks)*

1. Explain in detail about hip joint under the following headings: (a) type of joint, (b) articulating bones, (c) ligaments, (d) movements, (e) relations, (f) blood supply and nerve supply. Add a note on its applied anatomy.
2. Describe in detail about ulnar nerve under the following headings: (a) root value, (b) course, (c) branches, (d) muscles supplied by it, and (e) applied anatomy

II. *Write notes on*   *(8 × 5 = 40 marks)*

1. Lower end of humerus
2. Screw home movement
3. Radial nerve
4. Femoral artery
5. Muscles of respiration
6. Styloid process
7. Blood supply of brain
8. Extraocular muscles

III. *Short answers*   *(10 × 2 = 20 marks)*

1. Contents of cubital fossa
2. Winging of scapula
3. Name the branches arising from arch of aorta
4. Name the contents in rectus sheath
5. Name the invertors and evertors of foot
6. Hilar structures of lung
7. Name the muscles of mastication
8. Contents of carotid triangle
9. Name the ventricles of brain
10. Name the flexors of arm

### Sample question paper-3 (February 2013)

I. *Elaborate on*   *(2 × 20 = 40 marks)*

1. Explain the anatomy of ear.
2. Explain in detail about right lung (coverings, external features, impressions. Blood supply and bronchopulmonary segments).

## II. Write Notes on  (8 × 5 = 40 marks)

1. Sternum
2. Rotator cuff of shoulder joint
3. Cruciate ligaments of knee
4. Radial nerve
5. Great saphenous vein
6. Spinal cord
7. Intercostal muscles
8. Male urethra

## III. Short answers  (10 × 2 = 20 marks)

1. Nerve supply of urinary bladder
2. Name the muscles of pelvic floor
3. Organ of Corti
4. Branches of posterior cord of brachial plexus
5. Brainstem
6. Foramen magnum
7. Coronary sinus
8. Conducting system of heart
9. Nerves of lumbar plexus
10. Carpal bones

## Sampe question paper-4 (February 2014)

### I. Elaborate on  (2 × 20 = 40 marks)

1. Write in detail about shoulder joint—type, articulating surfaces, relations, rotator cuff, ligaments, movements, muscles producing those movements and its applied anatomy.

2. Explain diaphragm under the following subdivisions: (i) origin, (ii) insertion, (iii) blood supply, (iv) nerve supply, (v) action, (vi) orifices present, (vii) structures passing through it, and (viii) applied anatomy.

### II. Write notes on  (8 × 5 = 40 marks)

1. Define supination and pronation, its mechanism of action and muscles producing it.
2. Cubital fossa
3. Lateral compartment of leg
4. Sciatic nerve
5. Sternocleidomastoid
6. Internal jugular vein
7. Rectus sheath
8. Circle of Willis

### III. Short answers  (10 × 2 = 20 marks)

1. Define sesamoid bone with two examples
2. Constrictions of ureter
3. Openings in right atrium
4. Branches of brachial artery
5. Saturday night palsy
6. Trendelenburg's sign
7. Any two features of atypical intercostal nerve
8. Structures passing through stylomastoid foramen
9. Frowining muscles
10. Achilles tendon

---

## Kerala Health University
## First Year BPT Degree Examinations (2012-scheme)

Time: Three Hours                **Anatomy**                Maximum Marks: 100

### Essays (major questions)

1. Essay question – 14 marks
2. Essay question – 14 marks

### Short notes

Question 3 to 6   (8 × 4 = 32 marks)

### Answer briefly

Question 7 to 16   (4 × 10 = 40 marks)

## Sample question paper-1 (March 2014)

### Essays  (2 × 14 = 28 marks)

1. Describe the sciatic nerve under the following headings:
   • Root value

   • Course and relations
   • Branches
   • Applied anatomy            (2+6+3+3)
2. Describe the superolateral surface of left cerebral hemisphere under the following headings:
   • Lobes
   • Sulci and gyri
   • Functional areas
   • Blood supply            (2+5+5+2)

### Short notes  (4 × 8 = 32 marks)

3. Thyroid gland
4. Femoral triangle
5. Muscles of mastication
6. Pericardium

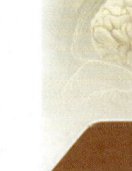

*Answer briefly (10 × 4 = 40 marks)*

7. Microscopic structure of thick skin
8. Ossification
9. Arches of foot
10. Rotator cuff
11. Digastric triangle
12. Formation of germ layers
13. Soft palate
14. Maxillary artery and its branches
15. Lobes of prostate gland
16. Interossei of hand

## Sample question paper-2 (September 2013)

*Essays (2 × 14 = 28 marks)*

1. Describe the brachial plexus under the following headings:
   - Roots
   - Trunks
   - Cords
   - Branches.
   - Add a note on Erb's paralysis    (3+3+3+3+2)
2. Give classification of synovial joints. Describe shoulder joint in detail      (7+7)

*Short notes (4 × 8 = 32 marks)*

3. Adductors of the thigh
4. Midbrain at the level of superior colliculus
5. Diaphragm
6. Posterior triangle of neck

*Answer briefly (10 × 4 = 40 marks)*

7. Wrist drop
8. Sesamoid bone
9. Microscopic structure of elastic cartilage

10. Spermatogenesis
11. Bronchopulmonary segments
12. Dorsalis pedis artery
13. Nucleus of animal cell
14. Epiphysis
15. Lumbricals of hand
16. Name the muscles of soft palate

## Sample question paper-3 (September 2014)

*Essays (2 × 14 = 28 marks)*

1. Draw a neat diagram of the formation of brachial plexus. Explain the root value, course, relations, branches of distribution and applied anatomy of radial nerve.      (4+10)
2. Explain the type, articulating bones, ligaments, relations and movements of knee joint. Describe locking and unlocking of the joint.      (10+4)

*Short notes (4 × 8 = 32 marks)*

3. Joints involved in pronation and supination
4. Right lung and its bronchopulmonary segments
5. External features and cross-section of spinal cord
6. Gluteal muscles

*Answer briefly (10 × 4 = 40 marks)*

7. Blood supply of a long bone
8. Plantar aponeurosis
9. Urinary bladder
10. Pivot joint
11. Boundaries and contents of femoral triangle
12. Rectus abdominis muscle
13. Arch of aorta
14. Curvatures of spinal column
15. Deltoid muscle
16. Differences between male pelvis and female pelvis

---

## Manipal University, Manipal
### I Year BPT/BOT Examination
### Anatomy

Time: Three Hours                                  Maximum Marks: 100

1. Major question–20 marks
2. Major questions–20 marks
3. Write briefly on (5 × 5 = 25 marks)
4. Write short notes on (3 × 5 = 15 marks)

## Sample question paper-1 (August 2013)

1. Describe the radial nerve under the following headings:

1A. Origin
1B. Course
1C. Branches and distribution
1D. Clinical anatomy      (1+5+ 10+4 = 20)

2. Describe the ankle joint under the following headings:

2A. Articulating parts

2B. Type and subtype
2C. Capsule and ligaments
2D. Movements and muscles producing them
2E. Applied anatomy          (2+2+7+7+2 = 20)

3. Write briefly on:          (5 × 5 = 25 marks)
3A. Circle of Willis
3B. Facial nerve
3C. Classification and functions of cerebellum
3D. Corticospinal tract
3E. Parts and functions of basal nuclei

4. Write short notes on:          (3 × 5 = 15 marks)
4A. Fibrous joints
4B. Parts and position of uterus
4C. Arch of aorta
4D. Pleura
4E. Esophagus

## Sample-2 (May/June 2013)
1. Describe the hip joint under the following headings:
1A. Type and subtype
1B. Bones taking part

1C. Ligaments
1D. Movements and muscles producing each of those
movements          (2+2+8+8 = 20)

2. Describe the radial nerve under the following headings:
2A. Origin and course
2B. Branches and distribution
2C. Applied anatomy          (8+ 10+2 = 20)

3. Write short notes on    (5 × 5 = 25 marks)
3A. Spinothalamic tracts
3B. Cerebellum
3C. Internal capsule
3D. Anterior cerebral artery
3E. Internal structure of medulla oblongata

4. Write short notes on    (3 × 5 = 15 marks)
4A. Thyroid gland
4B. Ovary
4C. Spermatic cord
4D. Stomach
4E. Nasal septum

# BSc NURSING QUESTION PAPERS

Time: Three Hours

**RGUHS, Karnataka**
**1st Year BSc Nursing**

Maximum Marks: 100

## Section A—ANATOMY (37 marks)
*Long essays (answer any one)*
1. One question (10 marks)
   OR
2. One question (10 marks)

*Short essays (answer any three)* 5 × 3 = 15 marks
3 to 6

*Short answers*   2 × 6 = 12 marks
7 to 12

## Sample question paper-1 (Aug/Sept 2011)
*Long essays (answer any one)   (10 marks)*
1. Enumerate the different parts of the excretory system with neat diagram. Describe the kidney in detail.
2. Enumerate the different parts of the respiratory system. Describe the lungs in detail.

*Short esays (answer any three)*      (5 × 3 = 15 marks)
3. Testis
4. Duodenum
5. Gluteus maximus muscle
6. Structure and functions of heart

*Short answers*          (2 × 6 = 12 marks)
7. Great saphenous vein
8. Parts of thyroid gland
9. Name the carpal bones
10. Name the arteries supplying the stomach
11. Name the meninges of the brain
12. Various positions of vermiform appendix

## Sample question paper-2 (Feb/March 2012)
*Long essays (answer any one)          (10 marks)*
1. a). Describe the gross anatomy of the stomach, (b). add a note on its lymphatic drainage and nerve supply.
2. Describe the female reproductive system.

*Short esays (answer any three) (5 × 3 = 15 marks)*

3. Upper end of the femur
4. Urinary bladder
5. Tongue
6. Thoracic duct

*Short answers*      *(2 × 6 = 12 marks)*

7. Microscopic structure of pancreas

8. Name the parts of the brainstem
9. Name four muscles of larynx
10. Give the attachment of the biceps brachii muscle
11. Name the air sinuses opening into the middle meatus of the nose
12. Name four branches of femoral nerve

---

## MGR Health University, Tamil Nadu

### First Year BSc Nursing
### (New Regulations for the candidates admitted from 2006-07 onwards)
### Paper I – Anatomy (Part A), Physiology (Part B)

Time: Three Hours (For Anatomy and Pysiology together)

Anatomy 37, Physiology 38, Total 75

### Answer all questions

  I. Essay (12 marks)
  II. Write notes on (5 × 3 = 15 marks)
  III. Short answer questions (2 × 5 = 10 marks)

### Sample question paper-1 (February 2014)

*I. Essay*      *(1 × 12 = 12 marks)*

1. Name the endocrine glands and describe about the thyroid gland in detail.

*II. Write notes on*      *(3 × 5 = 15 marks)*

1. Classification of bones
2. Cerebellum
3. Vermiform appendix

*III. Short answer questions*      *(5 × 2 = 10 marks)*

1. Costodiaphragmatic recess
2. Parts of pituitary gland
3. Transitional epithelium

4. Median cubital vein
5. Coverings of eyeball

### Sample question paper-2 (August 2014)

*I. Essay*      *(1 × 12 = 12 marks)*

1. Name the sensory organs and write in detail about the tongue.

*II. Write notes on*      *(3 × 5 = 15 marks)*

1. Testis
2. Differences between small and large intestines
3. Great saphenous vein

*III. Short answer questions*      *(5 × 2 = 10 marks)*

1. Pleuritis
2. Parts of a young bone
3. Openings of diaphragm
4. Name the lymphoid organs
5. Ear ossicles

## Dr. NTR Health University
## 1st Year BSc Nursing
## Section A- ANATOMY (37 marks)

Write an essay on any one of the following:

1. One question (10 marks)    Or
2. One question (10 marks)

*Write short notes on any three:* 3 to 7   (5 × 3 = 15 marks)
*Write brief answer:* 7 to 12            (2 × 6 = 12 marks)

### Sample question paper-1

*Write an essay on any one of the following (10 marks)*

1. Name the parts of the female reproductive system. Describe the uterus in detail.
2. Name the parts of the central nervous system. Describe the brainstem in detail.

*Write short notes on any three of the following:*

(5 × 3 = 15 marks)

3. Hyaline cartilage
4. Tongue
5. Lateral wall of the nasal cavity
6. Duodenum
7. Gluteus maximus

*Write brief answers to the following:*

(2 × 6 = 12 marks)

8. Define epiphysis
9. Name 4 lower limb muscles
10. Name 2 features of large intestine
11. Name 3 body cavities
12. Name 4 lymphatic tissues in the body

### Sample question Paper-2

*Write an essay on any one of the following (10 marks)*

1. Name the endocrine glands in the body. Explain the pituitary gland in detail.
2. Name the parts of the urinary system. Explain kidney in detail.

*Write short notes on any three of the following*

(5 × 3 = 15 marks)

3. Fibrocartilage
4. Pharynx
5. Synovial joint
6. Right atrium
7. Spinal cord

*Write brief answers to the following (2 × 6 = 12 marks)*

8. Name four tarsal bones
9. Name parts of the inner ear
10. Name the layers of the epidermis of the skin
11. Name the nuclei of the cerebellum
12. Draw and label a neuron

### Sample question paper-3

*Write an essay on any one of the following (10 marks)*

1. Describe the coronary circulation.
2. Name the parts of the gastrointestinal system and describe stomach in detail.

*Write short notes on any three of the following*

(5 × 3 =15 marks)

3. Bronchopulmonary segments of lung
4. Uterus
5. Paransal air sinuses
6. Deltoid muscle
7. Classification of glands with examples

*Write brief answers to the following (2 × 6 = 12 marks)*

8. Name four muscles of lower limb
9. Microscopic differences in skeletal and cardiac muscles
10. Name four branches of abdominal aorta
11. Name four parts of the eye
12. Name the parts of the uterine tube

### Sample question paper-4

*Write an essay on any one of the following (10 marks)*

1. Name the parts of the gastrointestinal tract. Describe the liver in detail.
2. Name the organs of female reproductive system and explain the uterus.

*Write short notes on any three of the following*

(5 × 3 = 15 marks)

3. Medial wall of the nasal cavity
4. Diaphragm
5. Biceps brachii muscle
6. Great saphenous vein
7. Transitional epithelium

*Write brief answers to the following (2 × 6 = 12 marks)*

8. Name four upper limb muscles
9. Name ossicles of middle ear
10. Name four organells of cell
11. Name the parts of nephron
12. Mention the parts of the central nervous system

**Kerala Health University**

Time: Three Hours

**I Year BSc Nursing – Anatomy**

Maximum Marks: 100

## Essays

1. 10 marks
2. 10 marks

## Short notes                  (5 × 7 = 35 marks)

Questions 3 to 9

## Answer briefly              (3 × 5 =15 marks)

Questions 10 to 14

## Match the following      (1 × 5 = 5 mark)

Questions 15 to 18

## Sample question paper -1 (May 2013)

*Essays*                            (2 × 10 = 20 marks)

1. Describe the uterus under the following headings:
   - Parts
   - Supports
   - Layers of uterine wall          (3+4+3=10)
2. Enumerate the parts of the respiratory system. Describe the right lung under the following headings:
   - Lobes and fissures
   - Relations of mediastinal surface
   - Bronchopulmonary segments          (2+2+3+3=10)

*Short notes*                        (7 × 5 = 35 marks)

3. Skin
4. Clavicle
5. Right atrium
6. Mammary gland
7. Pancreas
8. Diaphragm
9. Anal canal

*Answer briefly*                    (5 × 3 =15 marks)

10. Median cubital vein
11. Ureter
12. Coronary sinus
13. Sciatic nerve
14. Ear ossicles

*Match the items in column A with items in column B:*                        (5 × 1= 5 marks)

| A | B |
|---|---|
| 15. Pulmonary veins | a. Medium sized artery |
| 16. Smooth muscle | b. Axillary nerve |

| 17. Deltoid | c. Tongue |
|---|---|
| 18. Spleen | d. Kidney |
| 19. Filiform papilla | e. Lymphatic organ |
| | f. Left atrium |

## Sample question paper-2 (August 2011)

1. Draw labelled diagram of parts of female reproductive system and describe uterus in detail          (5+5= 10 marks)
2. Classify epithelium with example and draw a neat labelled diagram of human cell    (6+4 = 10 marks)

*Write short notes on the following (7 × 5 =35marks)*

3. Right atrium
4. Types of bone
5. Tongue
6. Histology of muscles
7. Pituitary gland
8. Blood supply of spinal cord
9. Spleen

*Write briefly on the following*    (5 × 3 = 15 marks)

10. Caecum
11. Meninges
12. Relations of right kidney
13. Structure of thick skin
14. Diaphragm

*Match the items in column A with items in column B*                        (5 × 1= 5 marks)

| A | B |
|---|---|
| 15. Shoulder joint | a. Right lung |
| 16. Cardiac notch | b. Hinge type |
| 17. Three lobes | c. Left lung |
| 18. Chorda tympani | d. Smell |
| 19. Olfactory cells | e. Taste |

## Sample question paper-3 (April 2012)

1. Describe shoulder joint under the following headings:
   - Type and articular surfaces of bones
   - Relations
   - Ligaments          (3+3+4 = 10)
2. Draw a neat labelled diagram of chambers of heart and describe coronary artery under the following headings:
   - Origin

- Branches of right and left coronary arteries
- Applied anatomy                                   (3+2+3+2 = 10)

### Short notes                                   (7 × 5 = 35 marks)

3. Fallopian tube
4. Large intestine
5. Urinary bladder
6. Multipolar neuron labelled diagram
7. Thyroid gland
8. Histology of tonsil
9. Deltoid muscle

### Answer briefly                                   (5 × 3 = 15 marks)

10. Male urethra
11. Ligaments of liver
12. Cross section of spinal cord
13. Structure of hairy skin
14. Classify glands with example

### Match the items in column A with items in column B
(5 × 1 = 5 marks)

| A | B |
|---|---|
| 15. Pons | a. Middle ear |
| 16. Trasitional epithelium | b. Nose lateral wall |
| 17. Portahepatis | c. Lung |
| 18. Stapes | d. Brainstem |
| 19. Concha and meatus | e. Urinary bladder |

### Sample question paper-4

1. Describe the cerebrum under the following headings:
   - Lobes and surfaces

- Sulci, gyri and functional areas
- Blood supply                                   (3+5+2 = 10)

2. Describe the kidney under the following headings:
   - Parts and relations
   - Structure
   - Applied anatomy                                   (4+4+2=10)

### Write short notes on the following (5×7=35 marks)

3. Ligaments of uterus
4. Middle ear
5. Pituitary gland
6. Compound epithelium
7. Liver
8. Coronary arteries
9. Bronchopulmonary segments

### Write briefly on the following:   (3 × 5 = 15 marks)

10. Neuron
11. Deltoid muscle
12. Pleural recesses
13. Haversian system
14. Papillae of tongue

### Match the items in column A with items in column B
(5 × 1 mark = 5)

| A | B |
|---|---|
| 15. Foramen magnum | a. Spleen |
| 16. Myelin sheath | b. Islets of Langerhans |
| 17. Hassall's corpuscles | c. Schwann cell |
| 18. Red pulp | d. Suprarenal gland |
| 19. Pancreas | e. Thymus |
| | f. Occipital bone |

---

### Manipal University
### I Year BSc Nursing
### Section A – Anatomy
### Max marks: 22

### Sample question paper-1 (September 2014)

#### 1. Write briefly on                                   (3 × 4 = 12 marks)

1A. Liver
1B. Urinary bladder
1C. Prostate
1D. Right lung

#### 2. Write short notes on each of the following
(2 × 5 = 10 marks)

2A. Lymph node

2B. Uterine tube
2C. Pancreas
2D. Middle ear
2E. Enumerate the parts of respiratory system

### Sample Question paper-2 (June 2014)

#### 1. Write briefly on                                   (3 × 4 = 12 marks)

1A. Uterine tube
1B. Duodenum
1C. Posterior relations of right kidney
1D. Interior of larynx

2. *Write short notes on each of the following*

*(2 × 5 = 10 marks)*

2A. Urothelium
2B. Coronary arteries
2C. Extrinsic muscles of tongue
2D. Neurohypophysis
2E. Microscopic structure of lung

## Sample question paper-3 (September 2013)

1. *Write briefly on*  *(3 × 4 = 12 marks)*

1A. Right lung
1B. Pharynx
1C. Duodenum
1D. Pituitary gland

2. *Write short notes on*  *(2 × 5 = 10 marks)*

2A. Right atrium
2B. Superior vena cava
2C. Nasal septum
2D. Middle ear
2E. Uterine tube

# Index